American Cancer Society
Atlas of
Clinical Oncology

American Cancer Society

Atlas of

Clinical Oncology

Editors

GLENN D. STEELE JR, MD
Geisinger Health System

THEODORE L. PHILLIPS, MD
University of California

BRUCE A. CHABNER, MD
Harvard Medical School

Managing Editor

TED S. GANSLER, MD, MBA
Director of Health Content, American Cancer Society

Every Decker book is accompanied by a CD-ROM.

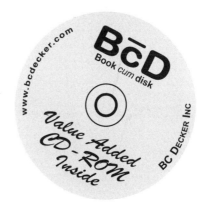

The disk appears in the front of each copy, in its own sealed jacket. Affixed to the front of the book will be a distinctive BcD sticker **"Book *cum* disk"**.

The disk contains the complete text and illustrations of the book, in fully searchable PDF files. The book and disk will be sold *only* as a package; neither will be available independently, and no prices will be available for the items individually.

BC Decker Inc is committed to p   electronic
publications that will compliment   1 and
learning methods.

find the Book/CD
valuable and invite your
comments and suggestions.

Brian C. Decker
CEO and Publisher

American Cancer Society

Atlas of
Clinical Oncology

Cancer of the Head and Neck

Editor

**Jatin P. Shah, MD, MS (Surg.), FACS,
Hon. FRCS (Edin), Hon. FDSRCS (Lond)**

Chief, Head and Neck Service
E.W. Strong Chair in Head and Neck Oncology
Memorial Sloan-Kettering Cancer Center
Professor of Surgery, Weill Medical College, Cornell University
New York, New York

Assistant Editor

Snehal G. Patel, MD, MS (Surg.), FRCS

Clinical Research Associate
Head and Neck Service
Memorial Sloan-Kettering Cancer Center
New York, New York

Illustrator

Alice Y. Chen

2001
BC Decker Inc
Hamilton • London

BC Decker Inc
20 Hughson Street South
P.O. Box 620, L.C.D. 1
Hamilton, Ontario L8N 3K7
Tel: 905-522-7017; 1-800-568-7281
Fax: 905-522-7839
E-mail: info@bcdecker.com
Website: www.bcdecker.com

ISBN 1–55009–084-4
Printed in Canada

Sales and Distribution

United States
BC Decker Inc
P.O. Box 785
Lewiston, NY 14092-0785
Tel: 905-522-7017; 1-800-568-7281
Fax: 905-522-7839
E-mail: info@bcdecker.com
Website: www.bcdecker.com

Canada
BC Decker Inc
20 Hughson Street South
P.O. Box 620, L.C.D. 1
Hamilton, Ontario L8N 3K7
Tel: 905-522-7017; 1-800-568-7281
Fax: 905-522-7839
E-mail: info@bcdecker.com
Website: www.bcdecker.com

Foreign Rights
John Scott & Company
International Publishers' Agency
P.O. Box 878
Kimberton, PA 19442
Tel: 610-827-1640
Fax: 610-827-1671

U.K., Europe, Scandinavia,
Middle East
Harcourt Publishers Limited
Customer Service Department
Foots Cray High Street
Sidcup, Kent
DA14 5HP, UK
Tel: 44 (0) 208 308 5760
Fax: 44 (0) 181 308 5702
E-mail: cservice@harcourt_brace.com

Australia, New Zealand
Harcourt Australia Pty. Limited
Customer Service Department
STM Division
Locked Bag 16
St. Peters, New South Wales, 2044
Australia
Tel: (02) 9517-8999
Fax: (02) 9517-2249
E-mail: stmp@harcourt.com.au
Website: www.harcourt.com.au

Japan
Igaku-Shoin Ltd.
Foreign Publications Department
3-24-17 Hongo
Bunkyo-ku,Tokyo, Japan 113-8719
Tel: 3 3817 5680
Fax: 3 3815 6776
E-mail: fd@igaku.shoin.co.jp

Singapore, Malaysia, Thailand,
Philippines, Indonesia, Vietnam,
Pacific Rim, Korea
Harcourt Asia Pte Limited
583 Orchard Road
#09/01, Forum
Singapore 238884
Tel: 65-737-3593
Fax: 65-753-2145

Contributors

PETER E. ANDERSEN, MD, FACS
Associate Professor
Department of Otolaryngology, Head and
  Neck Surgery
Oregon Health Sciences University
Portland, Oregon
Management of Cervical Metastasis

JAY O. BOYLE, MD
Assistant Attending Surgeon
Head and Neck Service
Memorial Sloan-Kettering Cancer Center;
  Assistant Professor
Department of Otorhinolaryngology
  —Head and Neck Surgery
Weill Medical College of Cornell University
New York, New York
Oral Cavity Cancer

JOHN F. CAREW, MD
Assistant Attending Surgeon
Department of Otorhinolaryngology
  —Head and Neck Surgery
New York Presbyterian Hospital;
  Assistant Professor
Department of Otorhinolaryngology
  —Head and Neck Surgery
The Weill Medical College of Cornell University
New York, New York
The Larynx: Advanced Stage Disease

LANCEFORD M. CHONG, M.D.
Associate Attending Radiation Oncologist
Department of Radiation Oncology
Memorial Sloan-Kettering Cancer Center
New York, New York
Head and Neck Radiation Oncology

PETER G. CORDEIRO, MD, FACS
Associate Attending Surgeon
Plastic and Reconstructive Surgery Service
Memorial Sloan-Kettering Cancer Center;
  Associate Professor of Surgery
Department of Surgery
Weill Medical College of Cornell University
New York, New York
*General Principles of Reconstructive Surgery
  for Head and Neck Cancer*
Mandible Reconstruction

BRUCE J. DAVIDSON, MD, FACS
Assistant Professor
Deartment of Otolaryngology
  —Head and Neck Surgery
Georgetown University Medical Center
Washington, District of Columbia
Epidemiology and Etiology

JOSEPH J. DISA, MD
Assistant Attending Surgeon
Plastic and Reconstructive Surgery Service
Memorial Sloan-Kettering Cancer Center;
  Assistant Professor
Department of Surgery
Weill Medical College of Cornell University
New York, New York
*General Principles of Reconstructive Surgery
  for Head and Neck Cancer*
Mandible Reconstruction

ANDREW G. HUVOS, MD
Attending Pathologist
Memorial Sloan-Kettering Cancer Center;
  Professor of Pathology
Weill Medical College of Cornell University
New York, New York
Pathology of Head and Neck Tumors

PAUL A. KEDESHIAN, MD
Visiting Assistant Professor
Division of Head and Neck Surgery
University of California Medical Center
Los Angeles, California
Skull Base: Anterior and Middle Cranial Fossa
Neurogenic and Vascular Tumors of the Head
  and Neck

DANIEL J. KELLEY, MD
Director, Head and Neck Oncology
  and Skull Base Surgery
Department of Otolaryngology—
  Bronchoesophagology
Assistant Professor
Temple University School of Medicine
Philadelphia, Pennsylvania
Cancer of the Hypopharynx and Cervical
  Esophagus

DENNIS H. KRAUS, MD, FACS
Associate Attending Surgeon
Head and Neck Service
Memorial Sloan-Kettering Cancer Center;
  Associate Professor
Department of Otorhinolaryngology
  —Head and Neck Surgery
Weill Medical College of Cornell University
New York, New York
Cancer of the Nasal Cavity and Paranasal Sinuses
Skull Base: Anterior and Middle Cranial Fossa

DANIEL D. LYDIATT, DDS, MD, FACS
Associate Professor
Department of Otolaryngology/Head and Neck
  Surgery
University of Nebraska Medical Center
Omaha, Nebraska
The Larynx: Early Stage Disease

WILLIAM M. LYDIATT, MD, FACS
Associate Professor
Department of Otolaryngology/Head and Neck
  Surgery
University of Nebraska Medical Center
Omaha, Nebraska
The Larynx: Early Stage Disease

FERNANDO C. MALUF, MD
Associate Professor
Division of Solid Tumor, Department of Medicine
Sirio Libanes Hospital
Sao Paolo, Brazil
Chemotherapy and Chemoprevention in
  Head and Neck Cancer

BERNARD B. O'MALLEY, MD
Attending Radiologist
The Princeton Medical Center
Princeton, New Jersey
Head and Neck Imaging

SNEHAL G. PATEL, MD, MS, FRCS
Clinical Research Associate
Head and Neck Service
Memorial Sloan-Kettering Cancer Center
New York, New York
Tumors of the Oropharynx
Soft Tissue and Bone Tumors
Thyroid and Parathyroid Tumors

DAVID G. PFISTER, MD
Associate Attending Physician
Division of Solid Tumor
Memorial Sloan-Kettering Cancer Center;
  Associate Professor, Department of Medicine
Weill Medical College of Cornell University
New York, New York
Chemotherapy and Chemoprevention in
  Head and Neck Cancer

MANJU L. PRASAD, MD
Assistant Professor
Department of Pathology
Ohio State University Hospital
Columbus, Ohio
Pathology of Head and Neck Tumors

SCOTT SAFFOLD, MD
Resident, Department of Otolaryngology
  —Head and Neck Surgery
Oregon Health Sciences University
Portland, Oregon
Management of Cervical Metastasis

ERIC SANTAMARIA, MD
Associate Professor
Department of Surgery
Hospital General Dr. Manuel Gea Gonzalez
Mexico City, Mexico
*General Principles of Reconstructive Surgery
   for Head and Neck Cancer*
Mandible Reconstruction

JATIN P. SHAH, MD, FACS
Chief and Attending Surgeon
Elliot W. Strong Chair in Head and Neck Oncology
Head and Neck Service
Memorial Sloan-Kettering Cancer Center;
   Professor, Department of Surgery
Weill Medical College of Cornell University
New York, New York
Skin Cancers of the Head and Neck
Tumors of the Oropharynx
Skull Base: Anterior and Middle Cranial Fossa
*Neurogenic and Vascular Tumors of the
   Head and Neck*
Soft Tissue and Bone Tumors

ASHOK R. SHAHA, MD, FACS
Attending Surgeon
Head and Neck Service
Memorial Sloan-Kettering Cancer Center;
   Professor, Department of Surgery
Weill Medical College of Cornell University
New York, New York
Thyroid and Parathyroid Tumors

ERIC J. SHERMAN, MD
Assistant Member
Division of Population Science
Department of Medical Oncology
Fox Chase Cancer Center
Philadelphia, Pennsylvania
*Chemotherapy and Chemoprevention in
   Head and Neck Cancer*

BHUVANESH SINGH, MD
Assistant Attending Surgeon
Head and Neck Service
Memorial Sloan-Kettering Cancer Center;
   Assistant Professor

Department of Otorhinolaryngology
   —Head and Neck Surgery
Weill Medical College of Cornell University
New York, New York
Skin Cancers of the Head and Neck
*Rehabilitation and Quality of Life Assessment in
   Head and Neck Cancer*

JEFFREY D. SPIRO, MD, FACS
Professor of Surgery
University of Connecticut Health Science Center
Farmington, Connecticut
Salivary Tumors

RONALD H. SPIRO, MD, FACS
Professor of Surgery
Head and Neck Service
Memorial Sloan-Kettering Cancer Center
New York, New York
Salivary Tumors

ELLIOT W. STRONG, MD, FACS
Professor Emeritus
Head and Neck Service
Memorial Sloan-Kettering Cancer Center
New York, New York
Oral Cavity Cancer

SUZANNE L. WOLDEN, MD
Assistant Attending Radiation Oncologist
Memorial Sloan-Kettering Cancer Center;
   Assistant Professor of Radiation Oncology
Weill Medical College of Cornell University
New York, New York
Cancer of the Nasopharynx

RICHARD J. WONG, MD
Fellow, Head and Neck Service
Memorial Sloan-Kettering Cancer Center
New York, New York
Cancer of the Nasal Cavity and Paranasal Sinuses

IAN M. ZLOTOLOW, DMD
Chief and Attending Dental Surgeon
Dental Service
Memorial Sloan-Kettering Cancer Center
New York, New York
Dental Oncology and Maxillofacial Prosthetics

Contents

Preface

Although oral cancer is the sixth most common cancer worldwide, cancer of the head and neck is a rare disease in the western world. A higher incidence is reported in Southeast Asia as well as certain parts of Europe and Latin America. Tobacco and alcohol remain the most important etiologic factors; however, the primary site incidence of head and neck cancer varies throughout the world depending on the type of substance abuse and the extent of consumption.

Management of these patients requires a team effort with expertise in various disciplines. As our understanding of the biology and natural history of cancers of the head and neck increases, efforts at preservation or restoration of form and function become increasingly important. These efforts are not only important in the surgical treatment of these tumors but are also important in the multidisciplinary, integrated treatment programs delivered by comprehensive treatment teams. Most major cancer centers, not only in the United States but also worldwide, now deliver optimal care for patients with cancers of the head and neck through the integrated efforts of multidisciplinary "disease-management" teams. Such disease-management teams work to develop treatment algorithms and establish guidelines for a unified treatment approach in order to maintain internal consistency, initiate investigative protocols, and push the frontiers in the battle against cancer. Such guidelines are also developed by the American Head and Neck Society (AHNS) and the National Cancer Center Network (NCCN). The focus has clearly been on outcome analysis and (whenever feasible), implementation of evidence-based medicine. These have provided excellent practice guidelines for the practitioner in the community and are rapidly becoming standards of care.

The contributing authors in this book are or have been members of the head and neck disease-management team at Memorial Sloan-Kettering Cancer Center in New York. As a result, the treatment programs practiced at Memorial Sloan-Kettering Cancer Center tend to be reflected in the philosophies expressed in this book, though every attempt has been made to be comprehensive and to give a balanced view of other treatment approaches and report results. Thus, in spite of being a multi-authored book, the strength of this work is its internal consistency of diagnostic approaches, therapeutic decisions, multidisciplinary treatment programs, and surgical techniques. It is obviously impossible for a work of this nature to be either complete or permanently up-to-date; new technology will offer newer diagnostic approaches that will impact on the development of newer treatment strategies and therapeutic protocols. However, this book represents the art and science of head and neck surgery and oncology as well as the current approach to the multidisciplinary management of tumors of the head and neck. Accurate clinical staging of head and neck tumors is crucial to treatment planning and for comparison of outcomes. However, we have deliberately not included the AJCC/UICC staging system in the book due to the anticipated revision of the AJCC/UICC staging system this year. It is expected that the sixth edition of the AJCC/UICC staging manual will be published in the year 2002 and we recommend that the reader refer to this manual for information on details of staging criteria. This book will not only be a valuable resource to aspiring head and neck surgeons and oncologists but also to surgeons, medical oncologists, radiation oncologists, and physicians in other specialties as it will act as a reference volume for current concepts in the management of cancer of the head and neck.

Jatin P. Shah, MD
August 2001

Dedication

This work is dedicated to our patients who have endured the ravages of head and neck cancer and who have demonstrated extraordinary strength in their struggle to preserve life. These exceptional human beings, who join hands with us in the dogged pursuit of a cure for their cancer and a better quality of life, have a special place in our hearts. We salute their courage, understanding, and perseverance. We are thankful to them for putting their trust and lives in our hands, for giving us the opportunity to understand the disease, and for inspiring us to put this work together.

Acknowledgments

I would like to express my sincere appreciation to the American Cancer Society for asking me to edit this volume in their series of clinical atlases. I am equally grateful for the contributions of each of the authors who so willingly and promptly provided up-to-date, generously illustrated, comprehensive but concise chapters on their assigned topics. But for their diligence and promptness, it would not have been possible to compile this work on schedule.

My special thanks are owed to Ms. Alice Chen for the artwork in this book, Ms. Nancy Bennett for the graphics and editorial responsibilities, and Ms. Arlene Cooper for transcription of the text.

Jatin P. Shah, MD

Epidemiology and Etiology

BRUCE J. DAVIDSON, MD, FACS

INCIDENCE

Current Incidence Data

The global incidence of cancers of the oral cavity, pharynx and larynx is about 500,000 cases per year with mortality of 270,000 cases per year.[1] Excluding skin cancers, this represents about 6 percent of the incidence and 5 percent of the mortality of all cancers.[1] About three-fourths of these are cancers of the oral cavity and pharynx and the remainder are laryngeal cancers. Figure 1–1 describes the incidence of oral and pharyngeal cancers by world region. As demonstrated here, the areas of the world with the greatest incidence are Melanesia (Papua, New Guinea and adjacent islands), Western Europe and South Central Asia (India and the Central Asian republics of the former Soviet Union).[1]

Figure 1–2 details the oral and pharyngeal cancer mortality rates for selected countries. In 2001, oral, pharyngeal and laryngeal cancers are expected to occur in approximately 40,100 individuals in the United States and result in death in 11,860.[2] In United States males, oral and pharyngeal cancer comprise the seventh most common cancer and larynx cancer ranks fifteenth.[2] In females, the incidence of oral and pharyngeal cancers ranks fourteenth and laryngeal cancer and anal cancer (2,000 each) share the twenty-seventh and twenty-eighth positions.[2]

Trends Over Time

United States

Head and neck cancer incidence in the United States has shown declines in the past 2 decades after pre-vious increases. From 1940 to 1985, there was an increase in laryngeal cancer incidence in men and women reflecting the increase in cigarette use in this century.[3] Oral and pharyngeal cancer incidence was stable in men and increased in women over this time period.[3] Between 1973 and 1997, a decrease in oral and pharyngeal cancer and in laryngeal cancer appeared.[4] This decrease was primarily determined by large rate decreases in men. During this same period, females showed an increase in laryngeal cancer rates and no change in oral cancer.[4] Most recently, 1990s United States cancer registry data shows a significant drop in the incidence rates of oral cavity and pharyngeal cancers for both sexes.[5] A steady drop in oral and pharyngeal cancer mortality has also been noted.[6] Mortality trends differ by race, which will be explored later in this chapter.

Europe

While United States' rates (incidence and mortality) for oral and pharyngeal cancer have recently been falling, European mortality rates for these cancers among males rose between 1983 and 1993.[7] Laryngeal cancer mortality increased in Eastern Europe.[7] Studies from individual European countries tend to reflect a rising mortality from oral,[8,9] pharyngeal,[9,10] and laryngeal[9,10] cancers from the early 1950s through about 1980. One exception to this is a Swiss study showing a decrease in laryngeal cancer mortality in males, but an increase in females.[11] More recent studies, spanning the mid 1970s into the 1990s, show decreases in oral cancer mortality in France[12] and laryngeal cancer mortality in France,[12] Italy,[13] Switzerland,[11] and Sweden.[14] These reductions may be secondary to decreased cigarette con-

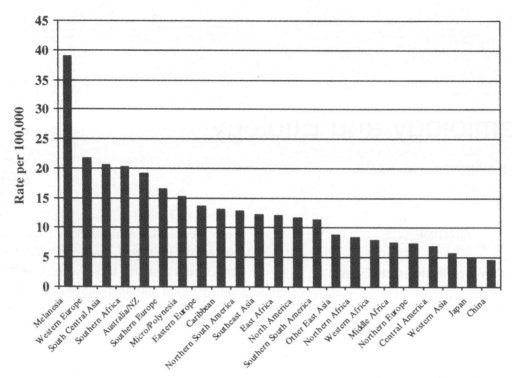

Figure 1–1. Incidence (cases/100,000) of cancer of the lip, oral cavity and pharynx in males by geographic area. (Data from: Parkin DM, Pisani P, Ferlay J. Global cancer statistics. CA Cancer J Clin 1999;49:33–64.)

sumption or a change to less carcinogenic tobacco products (eg, filtered cigarettes or less carcinogenic blond tobacco products).

Variations in alcohol use may also explain some cancer incidence changes over time. A Scottish study showed an increased incidence of oropharyngeal and

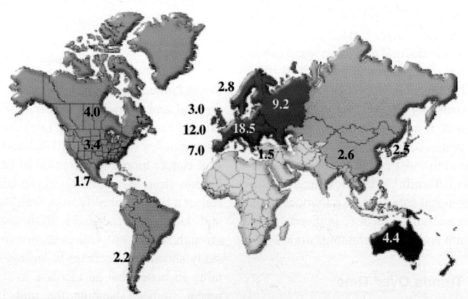

Figure 1–2. World map with death rates for oral and pharyngeal cancer in males indicated for selected countries. Units are age-adjusted death rates per 100,000 population. Countries shown are: Canada (4.0), United States (3.4), Chile (2.2), Norway (2.8), United Kingdom (3.0), France (12.0), Spain (7.0), Hungary (18.5), Russian Federation (9.2), Israel (1.5), China (2.6), Japan (2.5), and Australia (4.4). Source document does not include data from several high-incidence areas such as Melanesia, India and Brazil. (Data from: Landis SH, Murray T, Bolden S, Wingo PA. Cancer statistics, 1998. CA Cancer J Clin 1998;48:6–29.)

hypopharyngeal cancers with stable incidence of nasopharyngeal cancer between 1960 and 1989.[15] As a possible predictor of future trends, young adult males (ages 20 to 44) have shown an increase in oral and pharyngeal cancer mortality between the 1950s and the late 1980s in a Swiss study[16] as well as in studies across Europe.[17] Increased incidence and mortality rates from hypopharyngeal cancers in individuals under 60 years of age have also been shown since 1960 in an Austrian study.[18] These data are thought to be a reflection of increased alcohol consumption over time.[15]

Former Soviet Union

A long-term study of cancer mortality in the former Soviet Union showed an increase in oral, pharyngeal and laryngeal cancer mortalities between 1965 and 1990.[19] Estonia (former Eastern European Soviet Union member) showed increased mortality rates for cancers of the oral cavity, pharynx and larynx in men and oral cavity and pharynx in women, between 1965 and 1989.[20] Trends in the former Soviet Union and in Eastern Europe appear to reflect continued high rates of tobacco consumption. Figure 1–3 shows oral and pharyngeal mortality rates for several countries in Western Europe, Eastern Europe and the former Soviet Union. From the figure, wide variations in mortality are indicated.

Asia

Japanese males showed an increase in oral and pharyngeal cancers mortality between 1950 and 1994, although no change was seen in females. Analysis specified by tumor site showed a decrease in oral tongue and tongue-base cancer mortality, with increases in mortality from other oral and oropharyngeal sites. It was suggested that these changes were reflective of increased tobacco consumption for pharyngeal cancers, increased alcohol consumption for oral cancers and were unrelated to tobacco or alcohol for tongue cancers.[21]

The incidence of head and neck cancer in India is variable, with some areas showing rates of cancer among the highest in the world and other areas with rates comparable to the United States. Oral and pharyngeal cancers are highest in the area of Ahmedabad in West India. Between the 1960s and 1980s, a drop in head and neck cancer incidence was seen across India. This decrease has been attributed to decreased consumption of oral tobacco and an increase in cigarette and bidi (tobacco rolled in a tendu leaf) smoking.[22]

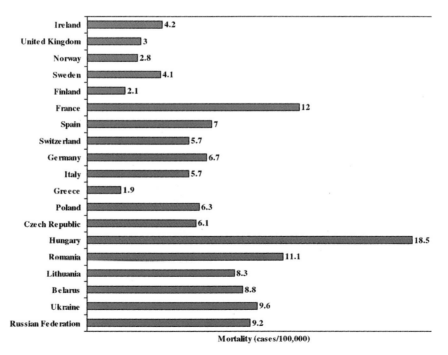

Figure 1–3.   Death rates for oral and pharyngeal cancer in males indicated for Europe and Russia. Units are age-adjusted death rates per 100,000 population. (Data from: Landis SH, Murray T, Bolden S, Wingo PA. Cancer statistics, 1998. CA Cancer J Clin 1998;48:6–29.)

EPIDEMIOLOGY

Geographic Variation

Incidence and Tumor Site Differences

As indicated in Figure 1–1, the incidence of head and neck cancer varies throughout the world. For instance, mouth cancers are 45 times more common in certain areas of France than in The Gambia.[4] The Basque region of Spain has an incidence of laryngeal carcinoma (20/100,000) that is about 200 times greater than the incidence of laryngeal cancer in Qidong, China (0.1/100,000).[4]

Mortality also differs throughout the world. Mortality differences are influenced by incidence of disease as well as survival rates after diagnosis. The 5-year survival rate for cancers of the oral cavity and pharynx is 46 percent worldwide, but differs between developed (59%) and developing (39%) countries. The larynx cancer 5-year survival rate is 46 percent with similar differences between developed (51%) and developing (41%) countries.[1]

Table 1–1 lists the countries with the highest rates of oral and pharyngeal cancer mortality over two periods in the past 20 years. Unfortunately, the source documents fail to report mortality data on several high-incidence areas such as India, Melanesia and Brazil. In the mid 1980s, the highest rates of oral and pharyngeal cancer mortality for males were seen in Hong Kong, France, Singapore and Hungary

(all 10–15/100,000).[4] The rates for females were highest in Singapore, Hong Kong, and Kuwait (2–5/100,000).[4] In the more recent period, four of the five countries with the highest mortality in males are in Eastern Europe.[117] Hungary has shown a rise in mortality rates from 12.5 to 18.5 in less than a decade. In females, two of the top five are in Eastern Europe and the other three are in the Central Asian republics of the former Soviet Union.[117] The comparison between 1986 to 1988 and 1992 to 1995 shows the effect of geopolitical changes on cancer statistics with several newly independent countries reporting high mortality rates from these cancers.

Race

Significant racial differences are seen in cancer demographics in the United States. According to SEER statistics from 1973 to 1997, the incidence of oral and pharyngeal cancer was shown to be higher in blacks than in whites from 1975 onward. Similarly, the incidence of laryngeal cancer has been higher in blacks since 1973.[118] While oral/pharyngeal cancer is the sixth most common cancer in the United States, this represents the fourth most common cancer in blacks.[119] An exploration of this observation has found that most of the increased incidence in blacks can be attributed to higher tobacco and alcohol consumption among this group. Controlling for these exposures results in almost equivalent risk of oral and pharyngeal cancers by race.[120]

Table 1–1. COUNTRIES WITH THE HIGHEST MORTALITY RATES FOR ORAL AND PHARYNGEAL CANCER
(AGE-ADJUSTED DEATH RATES / 100,000)

1986–1988				1992–1995			
Male		Female		Male		Female	
Country	Rate	Country	Rate	Country	Rate	Country	Rate
Hong Kong	14.8	Singapore	4.8	Hungary	18.5	Hungary	2.4
France	14.3	Hong Kong	4.8	France	12	Kazakhstan	1.9
Singapore	12.8	Kuwait	2.4	Croatia	11.7	Turkmenistan	1.7
Hungary	12.5	Cuba	1.8	Slovenia	11.2	Albania	1.6
Puerto Rico	9	Malta	1.7	Romania	11.1	Uzbekistan	1.5
Czechoslovakia	8.2	Panama	1.7	Ukraine	9.6	Denmark	1.4
Luxembourg	7.6	Hungary	1.6	Russian Federation	9.2	France	1.3
Uruguay	6.9	Australia	1.4	Estonia	9	Australia	1.3
Soviet Union	6.6	Denmark	1.4	Belarus	8.8	United States	1.2
Switzerland	6.5	Venezuela	1.4	Lithuania	8.3	Canada	1.2

Adapted from Ries LAG. Rates. In: Harras A, editor. Cancer: Rates and risks. Washington, DC, National Institutes of Health; 1996. p.9–55. and from Li FP, Correa P, Fraumeni JF. Testing for germ line p53 mutations in cancer families. Cancer Epidemiol Biomarkers Prev 1991;1:91–4.

Trends in oral and pharyngeal cancer and laryngeal cancer incidence are favorable when evaluated by race. For oral and pharyngeal cancers, the trend in cancer incidence is downward since about 1984 in whites and since 1980 in blacks. For laryngeal cancer the negative trend began in 1988 in whites and 1990 in blacks.[118]

Mortality rates are also significantly higher for blacks than for whites for both oral/pharyngeal and laryngeal cancers. For both types of cancer, between 1973 and 1997, mortality was higher in blacks every year, and from 1993 to 1997, mortality rates in blacks were approximately double that seen in whites. Oral and pharyngeal cancer mortality has been trending downward since 1973 for whites, but for blacks, mortality rates rose from 1973 to 1980 and since then have been falling. For laryngeal cancer, mortality has also fallen since 1973 in whites, but rose in blacks from 1973 to 1992. Mortality rates in blacks have more recently been trending downward (trend not statistically significant).[118]

The differences in oral and pharyngeal cancer mortality between African Americans and Caucasians have been attributed in part to differences in survival rates. Five-year survival rates for these cancers from 1989 to 1996 were 56 percent for Caucasians and 35 percent for African Americans.[118] Data shows that African Americans are more likely to be diagnosed at a higher tumor stage, but that even after adjustment for stage, the mortality is greater in African Americans (see Figure 1–8).[2] Access to health care may play a role as 21 percent of African American adults lack a health care plan while only 13 percent of Caucasians are without coverage.[119] Racial differences in prevention appear to exist, in that a higher proportion of African Americans over Caucasians continue to smoke—34 percent versus 28 percent respectively.[119]

Gender

Gender differences in head and neck cancer incidence and mortality appear to reflect differences in risk factor exposure. The rise in tobacco consumption by women since the 1950s has resulted in an increased proportion of female cancer incidence and mortality for these cancers. A study from Houston compared the male-to-female ratio of laryngeal cancer over two periods in the past four decades. The proportion of male-to-female cases dropped from 5.6:1 to 4.5:1 between the periods 1959 to 1973 and 1974 to 1988.[121] Other studies have reflected similar trends.[122,123] Significant differences in the site of laryngeal cancer development has been suggested, with a ratio of glottic to supra-glottic sites of 22.1:1 in men and 0.6:1 in women.[124]

Among nonsmokers who develop oral and pharyngeal cancer, a higher proportion of women than men is seen in patients over the age of 50.[29] Analyzing oral cancers by site relative to gender reveals that the ratio of males to females is highest for floor-of-mouth cancers (ratio=3.4:1), and lowest for gingival cancers (ratio=0.5:1).[125]

SEER data suggests a downward trend for oral and pharyngeal cancer incidence for both males and females since the early 1980s. Mortality has also been declining for both males and females since 1979. For laryngeal cancer, incidence has declined since the mid to late 1980s for both males and females. Mortality has been falling since 1973 for males, but rose until 1992 in females. Recently a downward trend in laryngeal cancer mortality rate (not statistically significant) has been seen in females.[118]

ETIOLOGY

It has been estimated that in the United States, well over three-fourths of all head and neck cancers can be attributed to tobacco and alcohol use.[23] This section will explore these risk factors for head and neck squamous cell carcinoma and will describe other factors that may play a role in the etiology of these cancers. As with most cancers, age itself may be a risk factor for the development of head and neck cancer. In nonsmokers and nondrinkers, the average age of onset of laryngeal cancer is about 10 years later than in patients with a history of tobacco or alcohol use.[24]

Tobacco

Cigarettes

Cigarette smoking is the single most important risk factor in head and neck cancer. For oral cancers in men, 90 percent of cancer risk can be attributed to tobacco. The attributable risk of tobacco for oral cancer development is lower in females at 59 percent.[4] The smoking attributable risk for laryngeal cancer in males and females is more similar at 79 and 87 percent respectively.[4] The relative risk of laryngeal cancer between smokers and nonsmokers is 15.5 in men and 12.4 in women.[14] In support of the association between tobacco and head and neck cancer is information associating cigarette consumption with oral dysplasia (Odds Ratio [OR] = 4.1), a premalignant oral lesion.[25]

Discontinuation of smoking reduces the risk of head and neck premalignant and malignant lesions. Smoking cessation results in a decreased risk of oral dysplasia that reaches that of "never-smokers" after 15 years.[25] The risk of oral cancer has been suggested to be reduced by 30 percent for those who have discontinued tobacco for 1 to 9 years and by 50 percent for those who have abstained for over 9 years.[26] No excess risk of oral and pharyngeal cancer has been shown among individuals who have abstained for over 10 years.[23,27] These results emphasize the importance of smoking cessation efforts.

Tobacco contains over thirty known carcinogens. The majority of these are polycyclic aromatic hydrocarbons and nitrosamines.[28] Increasing tar consumption has been associated with oral and pharyngeal cancer in a dose-dependent manner. Interestingly, when this is evaluated by gender, the risks of cancer associated with tar exposure increase more sharply for women than men.[29] Specific tobacco use habits appear to alter the risk of head and neck cancer. Exclusive use of filtered cigarettes is protective when compared to unfiltered cigarette use.[27,30] Inhalation increases the risk of cancer of the endolarynx, although it does not alter the risk of hypopharyngeal or epilaryngeal (suprahyoid epiglottis and aryepiglottic folds) cancer.[31]

Cigars, Pipe Smoking

An increased risk of incidence for cancers of the oral cavity, pharynx and larynx has been shown for pipe and cigar smokers.[28] Risk of cancer from pipe smoking tends to be higher for oral cavity sites than pharyngeal or laryngeal sites.[32] Mashberg found

that cigar or pipe smoking without a history of cigarette smoking was associated with a relative risk of oral and pharyngeal cancer of 3.3. When mixed exposures (ie, pipe and cigarette or cigar and cigarette) were analyzed, the relative risk of oral and pharyngeal cancer was 2.6 for cigar smokers and 3.2 for pipe smokers.[27]

Smokeless Tobacco

Smokeless tobacco use has gained popularity in the United States over the past 25 years. The habit was traditionally practiced by women in the rural south as an alternative to cigarette smoking. In this population, a four- to six-fold increase in risk of oral cancer has been shown.[23,33] Cancers are typically well-differentiated and occur on the alveolar ridge or buccal mucosa.[34] Snuff-related oral cancer appears to require prolonged exposure. Patients developing oral cancers who have a history of snuff use without other risk factors typically are in their 60s and have been using oral tobacco for 40 years.[34]

Recent attempts to define the risk of oral cancer related to this increasingly popular practice has been difficult. The state with the highest per capita consumption of smokeless tobacco, West Virginia, has not shown an increased incidence of or mortality from oral or pharyngeal cancer when compared with national averages.[35] These results are possibly reflective of the low prevalence of alcohol abuse in West Virginia. In addition, a Swedish case-control study showed no increased risk for oral cancer in current or former snuff users.[36] These results may be a reflection of the prolonged exposure to oral tobacco required for the development of oral cancer.

Types of Tobacco

Two major types of tobacco exist. Black or dark (air-cured) tobacco is used in the manufacture of cigars, pipe-blends and certain cigarettes. Blond (flue-cured) tobacco is used more commonly for cigarettes. A major difference in these two tobacco types is that the alkalinity of black tobacco causes it to be irritating to the respiratory mucosa. Deep inhalation is less well-tolerated than with blond tobacco products. For this reason, it is theorized that black tobacco products might exert a greater effect on the upper aerodigestive mucosa while blond products have a greater effect on the lower respiratory mucosa. This is supported by data showing a greater risk of larynx cancer than lung cancer in persons using black tobacco products.[32]

Experimental studies have shown the extract of black tobacco cigarettes to be more carcinogenic than blond tobacco cigarettes.[37] As a reflection of this, epidemiologic studies have shown that the type of tobacco consumed is associated with the risk of aerodigestive tract cancer. Dark (air-cured) tobacco use was associated with a 59-fold increased risk of laryngeal cancer while blond (flue-cured) tobacco was associated with a 25-fold risk.[38] After control for socioeconomic factors, alcohol consumption, length of smoking exposure, and filter use, the user of black tobacco cigarettes has a threefold relative risk of oral cavity and pharyngeal cancer when compared with the user of blond tobacco cigarettes.[39]

When studies compare the use of blond tobacco only, with black tobacco only, with mixed exposures, a dose-response effect is demonstrated. A multi-institutional case-control study from Europe showed such an effect with an increased relative risk of cancer of the endolarynx, epilarynx and hypopharynx associated with increasing use of black tobacco relative to blond tobacco.[31] Analogous data from Thailand has shown that certain Thai tobacco preparations, specifically the more alkaline and less easily inhaled varieties, are associated with an increased risk of laryngeal cancer over other Thai preparations.[40]

The difference in popularity of black and blond tobacco cigarettes is likely to influence the geographic variations in laryngeal cancer incidence and subsite distribution throughout the world (Figure 1–4, A and B). Countries with the highest death rates from laryngeal cancer are France, Uruguay, Spain and Italy. Each of these countries, along with Cuba, Argentina, Brazil, Columbia and Greece has a relatively high prevalence of black tobacco cigarette consumption. Several of these countries also show a greater prevalence of supraglottic cancers than glottic cancers.[38] This is in contrast to the United States where blond tobacco cigarettes are typical and laryngeal glottic cancer is more common.

Alcohol

Head and neck squamous cell carcinoma is a disease occurring most often in individuals with heavy tobacco and alcohol use. Tobacco has gained the majority of attention in terms of public health education and many lay persons are unaware of the association of alcohol with upper aerodigestive squamous cell carcinoma. The cancer risk associated with alcohol consumption varies among upper aerodigestive tract sites.

The association between alcohol and head and neck cancer is stronger for pharyngeal cancer than for other head and neck sites. A dose-response effect has been shown between alcohol and pharyngeal cancer in a German study. After adjustment for tobacco consumption, the relative risk of pharyngeal cancer is seen to rise progressively from 1.0 for those consuming < 25 g/day (> 2 drinks) to 125 for those consuming > 100 g/day (> 7 drinks).[41] High alcohol consumption (> 100 g/day) represents less of a risk for oral cancers (RR=11)[42] and laryngeal cancers (RR=15) (unpublished data described in[41]). Figure 1–5 describes the difference in relative risk of cancer for several head and neck sites when compared to various levels of alcohol consumption.[43] These data support a strong association between alcohol use and pharyngeal cancer.

This variation in the risk of alcohol on the development of head and neck cancer has also been shown to differ for subsites of the larynx. Patients with glottic cancer are more likely than those with supraglottic cancer to be nondrinkers.[43] When comparison is made between drinkers and nondrinkers, the nondrinkers more often develop glottic cancer than supraglottic cancer. By comparison, the distribution is about equal for drinkers. Similarly, the association between alcohol and cancer varies between oral cavity sites, with a higher risk of buccal cancer than floor-of-mouth cancer in the nondrinkers and a higher risk of lateral tongue cancer than other tongue cancers in the nondrinkers. In drinkers, lateral tongue cancer is less common than other tongue cancers (includes base of tongue), and floor-of-mouth cancer is twice as common as buccal mucosa cancer.[43]

Multiplicative Effect of Alcohol and Tobacco

The synergistic effects of tobacco and alcohol have been shown in head and neck cancer in multiple studies.[38,44–46] Figure 1–6 shows data from a multicenter case-control study for oral and pharyngeal cancers in the United States. The combined use of tobacco and alcohol increases the risk of laryngeal cancer by about 50 percent over the estimated risk if these factors are

considered using an additive risk model.[47] Other studies have also supported a synergistic effect of tobacco and alcohol on head and neck cancer risk.[38,44]

Types of Alcohol and Risk

There are significant differences of content between various alcoholic beverages. Beer contains the carcinogen nitrosodimethylamine, while distilled wines have a high content of tannin, another carcinogen. When comparing various hard liquors, dark liquors (eg, whiskey, dark rum, cognac) contain greater

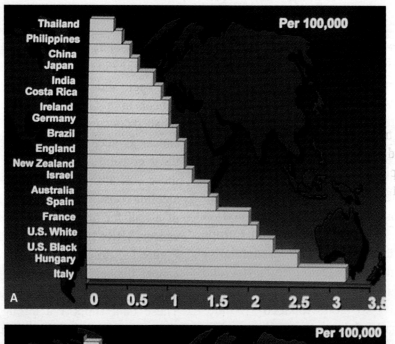

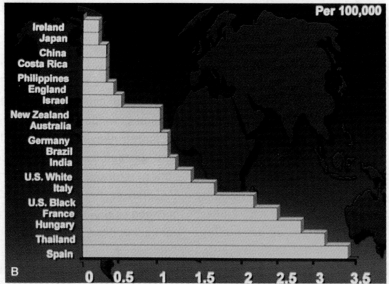

Figure 1–4.   *A,* Worldwide incidence of supraglottic cancer. *B,* Worldwide incidence of glottic cancer.

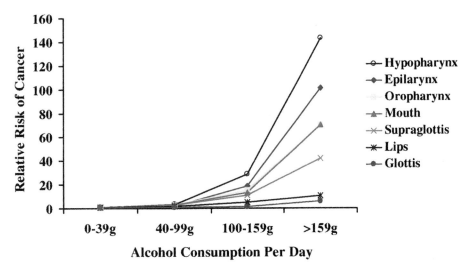

Figure 1–5. Relative risk of cancer for various head and neck sites relative to history of daily alcohol consumption adjusted for tobacco use. (Data from: Brugere J, Guenel P, Leclerc A, Rodriguez J. Differential effects of tobacco and alcohol in cancer of the larynx, pharynx and mouth. Cancer 1986;57:391–5.)

amounts of organic compounds than light liquors (eg, vodka, gin, light rum). These include higher alcohols, esters and acetaldehyde.[48] The risk of laryngeal and hypopharyngeal cancers is increased with dark liquor intake when compared with light liquor intake. The risk is greater for hypopharyngeal cancer than for laryngeal cancers.[48]

The relationship between type of liquor consumed and cancer risk has not been consistent. Mashberg reported on a series of oral cavity cancers and found

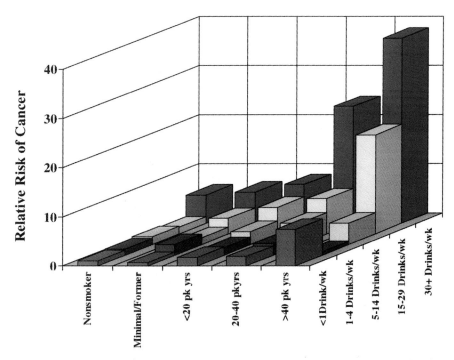

Figure 1–6. Relative risk of oral and pharyngeal cancer relative to tobacco and alcohol intake. The synergistic effect of tobacco and alcohol exposure is shown. One pack-year is equivalent to smoking 20 cigarettes perday per one year. (Data from: Blot WJ, McLaughlin JK, Winn DM, et al. Smoking and drinking in relation to oral and pharyngeal cancer. Cancer Res 1988;48:3282–7.).

that after controlling for total alcohol consumption, beer and wine intake were more strongly associated with oral cancer risk than was whiskey consumption.[49] On the other hand, Blot showed increased risk of oral and pharyngeal cancer for beer and whiskey intake, but no excess risk for wine consumption.[23]

The type of alcohol consumed may influence the site of aerodigestive cancer development. A study from the Institut Curie in France attempted to evaluate these differences, but was limited by the fact that > 90 percent of patients were wine drinkers, and the majority drank other liquors as well.[43] However, tongue cancer was associated with wine drinking while supraglottic cancer was associated with aniseed liquor consumption.

The synergistic effect of tobacco and alcohol consumption has been shown to vary with the type of tobacco used as well as the type of alcohol. Upon comparing the level of consumption of blond and black tobacco as well as the level of wine intake versus spirits, heavy use of black tobacco and heavy wine consumption showed the greatest synergistic effect. Blond tobacco and spirit consumption showed a lesser, but still considerable synergistic effect (Figure 1–7).[50]

Alcohol and Carcinogenesis

The mechanisms by which alcohol use contributes to the risk of head and neck cancer is not clearly defined, while systemic and local effects have been proposed. While alcohol itself is not a known carcinogen, it may act as a solvent, allowing increased cellular permeability of other carcinogens through mucosa of the upper aerodigestive tract. As noted above, the non-alcohol constituents of various alcoholic beverages may have carcinogenic activities.[48]

As summarized in Maier,[41] chronic alcohol use may upregulate enzymes of the cytochrome P-450 system. This enzyme system can contribute to activation of procarcinogens to carcinogens. This upregulation may be critical to activation of many carcinogens, as the vast majority of environmental carcinogens exist in their procarcinogenic form. Alcohol has also been shown to decrease the activity of DNA-repair enzymes, and increased chromosomal damage has been documented in chronic alcohol users. Other possible effects of alcohol include impaired immunity resulting from a reduction in T cell number, decreased mitogenic activity and/or reduced macrophage activity.

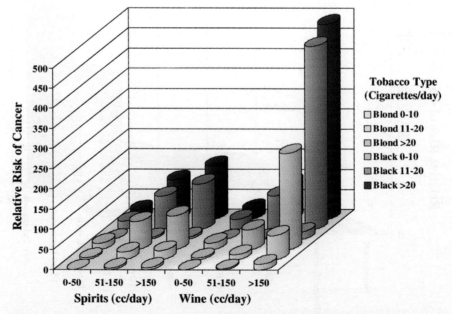

Figure 1–7. Graph demonstrating the odds ratio for exposure to alcohol and tobacco exposure in pharyngeal and laryngeal cancer patients. Odds ratio highest with heavy wine and black tobacco consumption. (Data from: Sancho-Garnier H, Theobald S. Black (air-cured) tobacco and blond (flue-cured) tobacco and cancer risk II: Pharynx and larynx cancer. Eur J Cancer 1993; 29A:273–6.).

The greater significance of the solvent activity of alcohol, as opposed to its systemic effect, is supported by data comparing dark and light liquor intake and the risk of hypopharyngeal cancer. Only dark liquor consumption was related to the risk of hypopharyngeal cancer. After controlling for total alcohol use and tobacco use, heavy dark liquor consumption was associated with an increased risk of cancer while no such risk was seen with light liquor intake.[48] These data argue against a systemic effect of alcohol on hypopharyngeal cancer risk and instead argue for the solvent effect of alcohol along with the carcinogenicity of the nonalcoholic components of dark liquors.

Injury to mucosa of the upper aerodigestive tract may relate to a toxic metabolite of alcohol, acetaldehyde. The enzyme aldehyde dehydrogenase-2 (ALDH-2) is a strong determinant of blood acetaldehyde concentration following alcohol ingestion. A small group of Japanese patients was studied, and those with an inactive ALDH-2 phenotype more often had multiple primary esophageal cancers (77%) versus those with an active ALDH-2 phenotype (31%).[51]

Other Carcinogens

Betel Quid

In India and parts of Asia, oral tobacco is commonly consumed in a preparation known as "pan," which combines tobacco with betel leaf, slaked lime and areca nut. These betel quid are associated with the risk of oral cancer. Oral cancer risk increases in a dose-dependent manner when classified by years of betel quid use and by numbers of betel quid per day.[52] Like the relationship between tobacco and alcohol exposure, the use of betel quid has been shown to act synergistically with tobacco and alcohol to promote oral cancer.[53]

Maté

Maté is a hot drink made from the herb *Ilex paraguariensis* and is commonly consumed in South America. It has been associated with an increased risk of cancer of the esophagus and larynx. It has been estimated that up to 20 percent of head and neck squamous cell carcinoma in southern South America may be linked to maté ingestion.[54] The odds ratio for maté ingestion has been reported as 3.0 for glottic cancer and 3.3 for cancer of the supraglottis.[38] Others have demonstrated a significant association with oral cancers.[54] Maté consumption is more strongly associated with the risk of laryngeal cancer in patients with a history of heavy tobacco or alcohol use. Maté itself has not been shown to be carcinogenic but, similar to alcohol, may act as a solvent for other carcinogens or as a promoter.[38]

Dental Considerations

Hygiene

Poor oral hygiene is associated with oral cancer, but no causal relationship has been established. A case-control study of patients with upper aerodigestive tract squamous cell carcinoma matched 100 patients with 214 age- and sex-matched controls and found significantly worse oral hygiene and dental status in the tumor patients. Chronic inflammation of the gingiva was more often seen in the cancer patients.[55] Similarly, oral cancers have been significantly associated with a history of chronic oral infections (OR = 3.8).[56]

Other studies have also supported the relationship between poor oral hygiene and increased risk of oral cancer.[57] Less-than-daily brushing has been associated with an approximate twofold increased risk of tongue and other oral cancers in a Brazilian population,[58] but no association was seen in a United States study.[59] The absence of multiple teeth may represent a surrogate marker of dental hygiene and has been associated with oral cancer in multiple studies.[60,61] However, a history of multiple broken teeth has not been associated with oral cancer risk.[59,62]

The frequent use of mouthwash has been discouraged due to the fact that several preparations contain ethanol. The association between mouthwash use and risk of oral or pharyngeal cancer has been the subject of previous studies with mixed results.[59,63,64] When controlled for total tobacco and alcohol intake, users of alcohol-containing mouthwashes appear to be at increased risk.[64] Women, especially those who are not tobacco users, appear to be most consistently associated with this risk factor.[65] However, it is possible that the cancer risk of mouthwash use may be confounded by other unmeasured factors. In one study of oral cancer in women, the reasons for mouthwash use were explored. While mouthwash use per se was not associated with a risk of cancer in this particular study, the use to "disguise the smell of tobacco" or "disguise the smell of alcohol" was seen more commonly in cancer cases.[60]

Dentures

A large Brazilian case-control study has demonstrated an association between oral sores from loose-fitting dentures and risk of oral cancer.[58] Painful or ill-fitting dentures have also been associated with oral or oropharyngeal cancer in a study from Wisconsin.[59] However, in these and other studies, long-term use of dentures has not been shown to increase the risk of oral cancers.[62,66,67] These results and those relating hygiene to oral cancer may describe the role of chronic inflammation as a risk for oral cancer.

Occupational Exposure

Occupational risks for head and neck squamous cell cancer development have been suggested in epidemiologic data. Wood dust exposure is associated with the risk of oral cancer[68] as well as pharyngeal and laryngeal cancer.[69] Other occupations associated with increased risk of head and neck squamous cell carcinoma include machinists[70–72] and automobile mechanics.[70] Occupations which involve exposure to organic chemicals, coal products, cement, and paint, laquer or varnish are also associated with increased risk of head and neck cancer.[69] A risk of cancer of the upper aerodigestive tract has also been shown in cases of long-term exposure to high concentrations of sulfuric or hydrochloric acid as found in battery plant workers.[73] While it has been suggested that an increased risk of oral and pharyngeal cancer is seen in bartenders,[27] no excess risk has been found when analysis includes adjustment for alcohol and tobacco consumption.[74]

Premalignant laryngeal lesions have also been associated with occupational exposures, with a relative risk of 10 for laryngeal dysplasia for blue-collar compared with white-collar workers even after con-

trolling for tobacco use.[75] Laryngeal cancers have been associated with nickel and mustard gas exposure.[4] An association between asbestos exposure and laryngeal cancer has been suggested, but contradictory results have been reported.[4,71,76,77]

Social and Economic Factors

Associations between oral, pharyngeal and laryngeal cancers and marital status (cancer patients more often unmarried or divorced) and educational status (cancer patient less often with college education) have been described.[78] However, a study in the United States failed to show any relationship between oropharyngeal cancer and education or occupational status. This United States study did show an inverse relationship between the percentage of potential working life spent in employment and the risk of cancer.[79] While this study attempted to adjust for tobacco and alcohol consumption, alcohol consumption may confound the employment measure used. Regularity and consistency of employment may be reduced by excessive alcohol use which, in turn, contributes to cancer risk.

Infections

Human Papillomavirus

Evidence of human papillomavirus (HPV) genetic material has been identified in a proportion of head and neck squamous cell cancers.[80] Verrucous carcinomas have the squamous histology with the strongest association with HPV, as HPV genomic material is found in 30 to 100 percent of these tumors.[80] For squamous cell cancers in general, the proportion of cancers with evidence of HPV genomic material appears to vary, depending upon the upper aerodigestive tract site analyzed. As reviewed and compiled by Steinberg,[80] the tumor site most often revealing HPV infection is tonsil (74%), with lesser evidence of HPV in larynx (30%), tongue (22%), nasopharynx (21%) and floor-of-mouth (5%) carcinomas. The role of HPV in these cancers is confounded by the fact that HPV genomic material may also be found in normal head and neck mucosa in up to 64 percent of samples.[80,81]

Cofactors for HPV induction of oral cancers have been investigated in a handful of studies. Tobacco

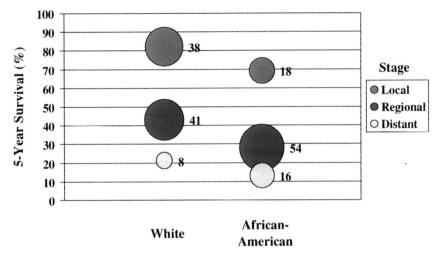

Figure 1–8. Incidence and survival of oral and pharyngeal cancer for Caucasian and African American males, 1986 to 1993. Circle position indicates percent 5-year survival for each stage. Circle size indicates stage distribution for each race. Numbers correspond to circle size and indicate percent of tumors presenting at each stage. Figure indicates a higher stage at diagnosis for African Americans and poorer survival at each stage. (Data from: Landis SH, Murray T, Bolden S, Wingo PA. Cancer statistics, 1998. CA Cancer J Clin 1998;48:6–29.)

and alcohol habits have not been associated with the likelihood of detecting HPV in tumor tissue.[82] However, use of betel quid has been associated with HPV detection in 9 of 11 (82%) cases of tongue cancer.[83]

Human Immunodeficiency Virus

Human immunodeficiency virus (HIV) has shown an emerging association with head and neck squamous cell carcinoma. In a recent study from New York, HIV infection was present in almost 5 percent of patients with head and neck cancer.[84] Patients with HIV were younger than non-HIV patients and HIV infection was present in over 20 percent of head and neck cancer patients who were under 45 year of age. The site of tumor presentation did not vary with respect to HIV status, but tumors were larger and more advanced in the HIV group. As in most cases of head and neck squamous cell carcinoma, a history of tobacco and alcohol use is prevalent in the HIV population.[85]

Herpes Simplex Virus

Herpes simplex virus (HSV) has been associated with cancer of the oral cavity. In a study utilizing patient questionnaires for data collection, a history of *proven* HSV-1 infections was associated with oral cancer (OR=1.9). A stronger association was seen with a history of a *suspected* HSV-1 infection (OR=3.3).[56] While this study raises concerns about reporting bias, support for this association is provided by a finding of HSV type 1 protein in 42 percent of patients with oral cancer and no positive results in control patients.[86]

Epstein-Barr Virus

Epstein-Barr virus (EBV) has been associated with nasopharyngeal carcinoma. The association appears strongest with World Health Organization (WHO) types II and III while a minority of WHO type I carcinomas have revealed EBV.[87] Type I tumors make up one-third of cancers in non-endemic populations. The presence of EBV DNA in upper aerodigestive mucosa samples seems to vary geographically. An 81 percent prevalence has been found in Greenland Eskimos, a population with a high incidence of undifferentiated nasopharyngeal cancer. Among the Danish population, the prevalence is only 35 percent.[88] Despite the fact that over 90 percent of the world's population shows serologic evidence of prior EBV infection, evidence of persistent EBV DNA was seen in less than 1 percent of normal upper aerodigestive mucosa samples in a large North American series.[89] These results suggest that an EBV

chronic
Howeve
sample:
require

Chronic
ynx and
tor for
reflux h
study in
and pha
lence is
lence in
nonmal
been dif
describe
geal ca
patients

Several
and vege
neck squ
between
reduced
such mi
carotene
serum m
upper ae
after ser
alpha an
opment c
dietary c
and esop
tein intak
and flavc
shown th
ated with
cancers.
ryngeal a
with high
vitamin C

22. Sanghvi LD, Rao DN, Joshi S. Epidemiology of head and neck cancers. Semin Surg Oncol 1989;5:305–9.

23. Blot WJ, McLaughlin JK, Winn DM, et al. Smoking and drinking in relation to oral and pharyngeal cancer. Cancer Res 1988;48:3282–7.

24. Agudelo D, Quer M, Leon X, et al. Laryngeal carcinoma in patients without a history of tobacco and alcohol use. Head Neck 1997;19:200–4.

25. Morse DE, Katz RV, Pendrys DG, et al. Smoking and drinking in relation to oral epithelial dysplasia. Cancer Epidemiol Biomarkers Prev 1996;5:769–77.

26. MacFarlane GJ, Zheng T, Marshall JR, et al. Alcohol, tobacco, diet and the risk of oral cancer: a pooled analysis of three case-control studies. Eur J Cancer B Oral Oncol 1995;31B:181–7.

27. Mashberg A, Boffetta P, Winkelman R, Garfinkel L. Tobacco smoking, alcohol drinking, and cancer of the oral cavity and oropharynx among U.S. veterans. Cancer 1993;72:1369–75.

28. International Agency for Research on Cancer. Tobacco Smoking: IARC Monograph on the Evaluation of the Carcinogenic Risk of Chemicals to Humans. Washington (DC): IARC; 1986.

29. Muscat JE, Richie JP Jr, Thompson S, Wynder EL. Gender differences in smoking and risk for oral cancer. Cancer Res 1996;56:5192–7.

30. Moulin JJ, Mur JM, Cavelier C. [Comparative epidemiology, in Europe, of cancers related to tobacco (lung, larynx, pharynx, oral cavity)]. Bull Cancer 1985;72:155–8.

31. Tuyns AJ, Esteve J, Raymond L, et al. Cancer of the larynx/hypopharynx, tobacco and alcohol: IARC international case-control study in Turin and Varese (Italy), Zaragoza and Navarra (Spain), Geneva (Switzerland) and Calvados (France). Int J Cancer 1988;41:483–91.

32. Kahn HA. The Dorn study of smoking and mortality among U.S. veterans: report on eight and one-half years of observation. Natl Cancer Inst Monogr 1966;19:1–25.

33. Winn DM, Blot WJ, Shy CM, et al. Snuff dipping and oral cancer among women in the southern United States. N Engl J Med 1981;304:745–8.

34. Wray A, McGuirt WF. Smokeless tobacco usage associated with oral carcinoma. Arch Otolaryngol Head Neck Surg 1993;119:929–33.

35. Bouquot JE, Meckstroth RL. Oral cancer in a tobacco-chewing U.S. population—no apparent increased incidence or mortality. Oral Surg Oral Med Oral Pathol Oral Radiol Endod 1998;86:697–706.

36. Schildt EB, Eriksson M, Hardell L, Magnuson A. Oral snuff, smoking habits and alcohol consumption in relation to oral cancer in a Swedish case-control study. Int J Cancer 1998;77:341–6.

37. Munoz N, Correa P, Bock FG. Comparative carcinogenic effect of two types of tobacco. Cancer 1968;21:376–89.

38. De Stefani E, Correa P, Oreggia F, et al. Risk factors for laryngeal cancer. Cancer 1987;60:3087–91.

39. De Stefani E, Boffetta P, Oreggia F, et al. Smoking patterns and cancer of the oral cavity and pharynx: a case-control study in Uruguay. Oral Oncol 1998;34:340–6.

40. Simarak S, de Jong UW, Breslow W, et al. Cancer of the oral cavity, pharynx/larynx and lung in Northern Thailand: Case-control study and analysis of cigar smoke. Br J Cancer 1977;36:130–40.

41. Maier H, Sennewald E, Heller GF, Weidauer H. Chronic alcohol consumption—the key risk factor for pharyngeal cancer. Otolaryngol Head Neck Surg 1994;110:168–73.

42. Chu KC, Baker SG, Tarone RE. A method for identifying abrupt changes in U.S. cancer mortality trends. Cancer 1999;86:157–69.

43. Brugere J, Guenel P, Leclerc A, Rodriguez J. Differential effects of tobacco and alcohol in cancer of the larynx, pharynx, and mouth. Cancer 1986;57:391–5.

44. Maier H, Dietz A, Gewelke U, et al. [Tobacco- and alcohol-associated cancer risk of the upper respiratory and digestive tract]. Laryngorhinootologie 1990;69:505–11.

45. Olsen J, Sabreo S, Fasting U. Interaction of alcohol and tobacco as risk factors in cancer of the laryngeal region. J Epidemiol Community Health 1985;39:165–8.

46. Guenel P, Chastang JF, Luce D, et al. A study of the interaction of alcohol drinking and tobacco smoking among French cases of laryngeal cancer. J Epidemiol Community Health 1988;42:350–4.

47. Flanders WD, Rothman KJ. Interaction of alcohol and tobacco in laryngeal cancer. Am J Epidemiol 1982;115:371–9.

48. Rothman KJ, Cann CI, Fried MP. Carcinogenicity of dark liquor. Am J Public Health 1989;79:1516–20.

49. Mashberg A, Garfinkel L, Harris S. Alcohol as a primary risk factor in oral squamous carcinoma. CA Cancer J Clin 1981;31:146–55.

50. Sancho-Garnier H, Theobald S. Black (air-cured) and blond (flue-cured) tobacco and cancer risk II: Pharynx and larynx cancer. Eur J Cancer 1993;29A:273–6.

51. Yokoyama A, Muramatsu T, Ohmori T, et al. Multiple primary esophageal and concurrent upper aerodigestive tract cancer and the aldehyde dehydrogenase-2 genotype of Japanese alcoholics [published erratum appears in Cancer 1996; 78(3):578]. Cancer 1996;77:1986–90.

52. Lu CT, Yen YY, Ho CS, et al. A case-control study of oral cancer in Changhua County, Taiwan. J Oral Pathol Med 1996;25:245–8.

53. Ko YC, Huang YL, Lee CH, et al. Betel quid chewing, cigarette smoking and alcohol consumption related to oral cancer in Taiwan. J Oral Pathol Med 1995;24:450–3.

54. Pintos J, Franco EL, Oliveira BV, et al. Maté, coffee, and tea consumption and risk of cancers of the upper aerodigestive tract in southern Brazil. Epidemiology 1994;5:583–90.

55. Maier H, Zoller J, Herrmann A, et al. Dental status and oral hygiene in patients with head and neck cancer. Otolaryngol Head Neck Surg 1993;108:655–61.

56. Schildt EB, Eriksson M, Hardell L, Magnuson A. Oral infections and dental factors in relation to oral cancer: a Swedish case-control study. Eur J Cancer Prev 1998;7:201–6.

57. Marshall JR, Graham S, Haughey BP, et al. Smoking, alcohol, dentition and diet in the epidemiology of oral cancer. Eur J Cancer B Oral Oncol 1992;28B:9–15.

58. Velly AM, Franco EL, Schlecht N, et al. Relationship between dental factors and risk of upper aerodigestive tract cancer. Oral Oncol 1998;34:284–91.

59. Young TB, Ford CN, Brandenburg JH. An epidemiologic study of oral cancer in a statewide network. Am J Otolaryngol 1986;7:200–8.

60. Kabat GC, Hebert JR, Wynder EL. Risk factors for oral cancer in women. Cancer Res 1989;49:2803–6.

61. Bundgaard T, Wildt J, Frydenberg M, et al. Case-control study of squamous cell cancer of the oral cavity in Denmark. Cancer Causes Control 1995;6:57–67.

62. Levi F, Pasche C, La Vecchia C, et al. Food groups and risk of oral and pharyngeal cancer. Int J Cancer 1998;77:705–9.

63. Mashberg A, Barsa P, Grossman ML. A study of the relationship between mouthwash use and oral and pharyngeal cancer. J Am Dent Assoc 1985;110:731–4.

64. Winn DM, Blot WJ, McLaughlin JK, et al. Mouthwash use and oral conditions in the risk of oral and pharyngeal cancer. Cancer Res 1991;51:3044–7.

65. Jaber MA, Porter SR, Scully C, et al. The role of alcohol in non-smokers and tobacco in non-drinkers in the aetiology of oral epithelial dysplasia. Int J Cancer 1998;77:333–6.

66. Campbell BH, Mark DH, Soneson EA, et al. The role of dental prostheses in alveolar ridge squamous carcinomas. Arch Otolaryngol Head Neck Surg 1997;123:1112–5.

67. Zheng TZ, Boyle P, Hu HF, et al. Dentition, oral hygiene, and risk of oral cancer: a case-control study in Beijing, People's Republic of China. Cancer Causes Control 1990;1:235–41.

68. Schildt EB, Eriksson M, Hardell L, Magnuson A. Occupational exposures as risk factors for oral cancer evaluated in a Swedish case-control study. Oncol Rep 1999;6:317–20.

69. Maier H, Dietz A, Gewelke U, Heller WD. [Occupational exposure to hazardous substances and risk of cancer in the area of the mouth cavity, oropharynx, hypopharynx and larynx. A case-control study]. Laryngorhinootologie 1991;70:93–8.

70. Flanders WD, Rothman KJ. Occupational risk for laryngeal cancer. Am J Public Health 1982;72:369–72.

71. Zagraniski RT, Kelsey JL, Walter SD. Occupational risk factors for laryngeal carcinoma: Connecticut, 1975–1980. Am J Epidemiol 1986;124:67–76.

72. Tisch M, Enderle G, Zoller J, Maier H. [Cancer of the oral cavity in machine workers]. Laryngorhinootologie 1996;75:759–63.

73. Coggon D, Pannett B, Wield G. Upper aerodigestive cancer in battery manufacturers and steel workers exposed to mineral acid mists [see comments]. Occup Environ Med 1996;53:445–9.

74. Huebner WW, Schoenberg JB, Kelsey JL, et al. Oral and pharyngeal cancer and occupation: a case-control study. Epidemiology 1992;3:300–9.

75. Grasl MC, Neuwirth-Riedl K, Vutuc C, et al. Risk of vocal chord dysplasia in relation to smoking, alcohol intake and occupation. Eur J Epidemiol 1990;6:45–8.

76. Hinds MW, Thomas DB, O'Reilly HP. Asbestos, dental X-rays, tobacco, and alcohol in the epidemiology of laryngeal cancer. Cancer 1979;44:1114–20.

77. Burch JD, Howe GR, Miller AB, et al. Tobacco, alcohol, asbestos and nickel in the etiology of cancer of the larynx: a case-control study. J Natl Cancer Inst 1981;67:1219–21.

78. Maier H, Dietz A, Zielinski D, et al. [Risk factors for squamous epithelial carcinoma of the mouth, the oropharynx, the hypopharynx and the larynx]. Dtsch Med Wochenschr 1990;115:843–50.

79. Greenberg RS, Haber MJ, Clark WS, et al. The relation of socioeconomic status to oral and pharyngeal cancer. Epidemiology 1991;2:194–200.

80. Steinberg BM. Viral etiology of head and neck cancer. In: Harrison LB, Sessions RB, Hong WK, editors. Head and neck cancer: a multidisciplinary approach. Philadelphia (PA): Lippincott-Raven; 1999. p. 35–47.

81. McKaig RG, Baric RS, Olshan AF. Human papillomavirus and head and neck cancer: epidemiology and molecular biology. Head Neck 1998;20:250–65.

82. Brandwein M, Zeitlin J, Nuovo GJ, et al. HPV detection using "hot start" polymerase chain reaction in patients with oral cancer: a clinicopathological study of 64 patients. Mod Pathol 1994;7:720–4.

83. Balaram P, Nalinakumari KR, Abraham E, et al. Human papillomaviruses in 91 oral cancers from Indian betel quid chewers—high prevalence and multiplicity of infections. Int J Cancer 1995;61:450–5.

84. Singh B, Balwally AN, Shaha AR, et al. Upper aerodigestive tract squamous cell carcinoma. The human immunodeficiency virus connection [published erratum appears in Arch Otolaryngol Head Neck Surg 1996; 122(9):944]. Arch Otolaryngol Head Neck Surg 1996;122:639–43.

85. Spitz MR, McPherson RS, Jiang H, et al. Correlates of mutagen sensitivity in patients with upper aerodigestive tract cancer. Cancer Epidemiol Biomarkers Prev 1997;6:687–92.

86. Kassim KH, Daley TD. Herpes simplex virus type proteins in human oral squamous cell carcinoma. Oral Surg Oral Med Oral Pathol Oral Radiol Endod 1988;65:445–8.

87. Hording U, Nielson HW, Albeck H, Daugaard S. Nasopharyngeal carcinoma: histopathologic types and association with Epstein-Barr virus. Eur J Cancer B Oral Oncol 1993;29B:137–9.

88. Hording U, Albeck H, Katholm M, Kristensen HS. Epstein-Barr virus in exfoliated cells from the postnasal space. Viral detection by polymerase chain reaction is not a useful means of screening for nasopharyngeal carcinoma in high-risk populations. APMIS 1994;102:367–70.

89. Liavaag PG, Cheung RK, Kerrebijn JD, et al. The physiologic reservoir of Epstein-Barr virus does not map to upper aerodigestive tissues. Laryngoscope 1998;108:42–6.

90. Freije JE, Beatty TW, Campbell BH, et al. Carcinoma of the larynx in patients with gastroesophageal reflux. Am J Otolaryngol 1996;17:386–90.

91. Ward PH, Hanson DG. Reflux as an etiological factor of carcinoma of the laryngopharynx. Laryngoscope 1988;98:1195–9.

92. Biacabe B, Gleich LL, Laccourreye O, et al. Silent gastroesophageal reflux disease in patients with pharyngolaryngeal cancer: further results. Head Neck 1998;20:510–4.

93. Chen MY, Ott DJ, Casolo BJ, et al. Correlation of laryngeal and pharyngeal carcinomas and 24-hour pH monitoring of the esophagus and pharynx. Otolaryngol Head Neck Surg 1998;119:460–2.

94. Baron AE, Franceschi S, Barra S, et al. A comparison of the

joint effects of alcohol and smoking on the risk of cancer across sites in the upper aerodigestive tract. Cancer Epidemiol Biomarkers Prev 1993;2:519–23.

95. Winn DM, Ziegler RG, Pickle LW, et al. Diet in the etiology of oral and pharyngeal cancer among women from the southern United States. Cancer Res 1984;44:1216–22.

96. Esteve J, Riboli E, Pequignot G, et al. Diet and cancers of the larynx and hypopharynx: the IARC multi-center study in southwestern Europe. Cancer Causes Control 1996;7: 240–52.

97. La Vecchia C, Negri E, D'Avanzo B, et al. Dietary indicators of laryngeal cancer risk. Cancer Res 1990;50:4497–500.

98. McLaughlin JK, Gridley G, Block G, et al. Dietary factors in oral and pharyngeal cancer. J Natl Cancer Inst 1988; 80:1237–43.

99. Nomura AM, Ziegler RG, Stemmermann GN, et al. Serum micronutrients and upper aerodigestive tract cancer. Cancer Epidemiol Biomarkers Prev 1997;6:407–12.

100. De Stefani E, Ronco A, Mendilaharsu M, Deneo-Pellegrini H. Diet and risk of cancer of the upper aerodigestive tract—II. Nutrients. Oral Oncol 1999;35:22–6.

101. Rogers MA, Thomas DB, Davis S, et al. A case-control study of element levels and cancer of the upper aerodigestive tract. Cancer Epidemiol Biomarkers Prev 1993;2:305–12.

102. La Vecchia C. Mediterranean epidemiological evidence on tomatoes and the prevention of digestive-tract cancers. Proc Soc Exp Biol Med 1998;218:125–8.

103. Franceschi S, Bidoli E, La Vecchia C, et al. Tomatoes and risk of digestive-tract cancers. Int J Cancer 1994;59: 181–4.

104. De Stefani E, Ronco A, Mendilaharsu M, Deneo-Pellegrini H. Case-control study on the role of heterocyclic amines in the etiology of upper aerodigestive cancers in Uruguay. Nutr Cancer 1998;32:43–8.

105. De Stefani E, Oreggia F, Ronco A, et al. Salted meat consumption as a risk factor for cancer of the oral cavity and pharynx: a case-control study from Uruguay. Cancer Epidemiol Biomarkers Prev 1994;3:381–5.

106. Notani PN, Jayant K. Role of diet in upper aerodigestive tract cancers. Nutr Cancer 1987;10:103–13.

107. Riboli E, Kaaks R, Esteve J. Nutrition and laryngeal cancer. Cancer Causes Control 1996;7:147–56.

108. Li FP, Correa P, Fraumeni JF. Testing for germ line p53 mutations in cancer families. Cancer Epidemiol Biomarkers Prev 1991;1:91–4.

109. Berkower AS, Biller HF. Head and neck cancer associated with Bloom syndrome. Laryngoscope 1988; 98:746–8.

110. Hecht F, Hecht BK. Cancer in ataxia-telangiectasia patients. Cancer Genet Cytogenet 1990;46:9–19.

111. Snow DG, Campbell JB, Smallman LA. Fanconi's anemia and post-cricoid carcinoma. J Laryngol Otol 1991;105:125–7.

112. Lisner M, Patterson B, Kandel R, et al. Cutaneous and mucosal neoplasms in bone marrow transplant recipients. Cancer 1990;65:473–6.

113. Socie G, Scieux C, Gluckman E, et al. Squamous cell carcinomas after allogenic bone marrow transplantation for aplastic anemia: further evidence of a multistep process. Transplantation 1998;66:667–70.

114. Benner SE, Pajak TF, Lippman SM, et al. Prevention of second primary tumors with isotretinoin in patients with squamous cell carcinoma of the head and neck: long-term follow-up. J Natl Cancer Inst 1994;86:140–1.

115. Schwartz LH, Ozahin M, Zhang GN, et al. Synchronous and metachronous head and neck carcinomas. Cancer 1994;74:1933–8.

116. Nees M, Homann N, Discher H, et al. Expression of mutated p53 occurs in tumor-distant epithelia of head and neck cancer patients: a possible molecular basis for the development of multiple tumors. Cancer Res 1993;53:4189–96.

117. Landis SH, Murray T, Bolden S, Wingo PA. Cancer statistics, 1998. CA Cancer J Clin 1998;48:6–29.

118. Ries LAG, Eisner MP, Kosary CL, editors. SEER Cancer Statistics Review, 1973–1997. Bethesda (MD): National Cancer Institute; 2000.

119. Parker SL, Davis KJ, Wingo PA, et al. Cancer statistics by race and ethnicity. CA Cancer J Clin 1998;48:31–48.

120. Day GL, Blot WJ, Austin DF, et al. Racial differences in risk of oral and pharyngeal cancer: alcohol, tobacco, and other determinants. J Natl Cancer Inst 1993;85:465–73.

121. DeRienzo DP, Greenberg SD, Fraire AE. Carcinoma of the larynx. Changing incidence in women. Arch Otolaryngol Head Neck Surg 1991;117:681–4.

122. Harris JA, Meyers AD, Smith C. Laryngeal cancer in Colorado. Head Neck 1993;15:398–404.

123. Wynder EL, Covey LS, Mabuchi K, Mushinski M. Environmental factors in cancer of the larynx: a second look. Cancer 1976;38:1591–601.

124. Stephenson WT, Barnes DE, Holmes FF, Norris CW. Gender influences subsite of origin of laryngeal carcinoma. Arch Otolaryngol Head Neck Surg 1991;774–8.

125. Barasch A, Morse DE, Krutchkoff DJ, Eisenberg E. Smoking, gender, and age as risk factors for site-specific intraoral squamous cell carcinoma. A case-series analysis. Cancer 1994;73:509–13.

2

Pathology of Head and Neck Tumors

MANJU L. PRASAD, MD
ANDREW G. HUVOS, MD

TUMORS OF THE UPPER AERODIGESTIVE TRACT MUCOSA

Neoplasias of the upper aerodigestive tract histologically tend to mimic the normal constituent cells in this region. The most common neoplasias show differentiation toward lining epithelium.

Benign Papillary Lesions

Squamous papilloma is a solitary papillary lesion of the squamous epithelium which has a white, frond-like gross appearance. Microscopically, it consists of multiple papillae of benign, stratified squamous cells arranged around central fibrovascular cores. They usually occur in adults. Although a viral etiology is suspected, human papillomavirus (HPV) types 6 and/or 11 have been detected in only some of the cases. Juvenile laryngeal papillomatosis are histologically similar to squamous papilloma but occur in children and are characteristically multiple. They tend to recur and sometimes can be florid enough to cause asphyxiation. Sometimes the recurrences cease at puberty. Squamous cell carcinoma may follow radiation therapy for treatment of juvenile papillomatosis (Figure 2–1).

Schneiderian papillomas arise in the sinonasal region and may be fungiform (exophytic), inverted (endophytic) or oncocytic (Figure 2–2). The role of HPV in their development is controversial. The patients are middle-aged. Although benign, the recurrence rate with local excision is almost 70 percent. The inverted papilloma may erode bone by

pressure. Synchronous or metachronous association with squamous cell carcinoma as well as progression to it may occur in some patients with inverted

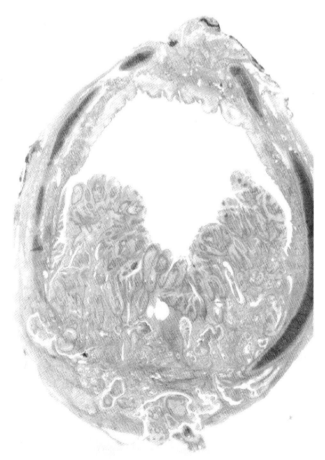

Figure 2–1. Infiltrating squamous cell carcinoma developing in a solitary tracheal papilloma in a 31-year-old male. The papillary lesion occupied the anterior half of the tracheal lumen. The carcinoma infiltrated the anterior wall of the trachea. The patient had a benign solitary tracheal papilloma since the age of 2 and had suffered many recurrences.

and oncocytic papillomas. The histologic appearance does not help in predicting the occurrence of recurrence or carcinomatous change.[1]

Verruca vulgaris and condyloma can be seen in the oral mucosa and their appearance is similar to that occurring elsewhere in the body.

Malignant and Premalignant Squamous Cell Lesions

Squamous cell carcinoma (SCC) is the most common malignant tumor of the upper aerodigestive mucosa, and shows a distinct male predilection. Tobacco and alcohol consumption are significant risk factors. Several HPV DNA subtypes have been found in association with SCC; however, their role in carcinogenesis remains conjectural.

Precancerous Lesions

Leukoplakia is a whiter patch on the oral mucosa which cannot be scraped off; nor can it be attributed to any other disease entity. Histologically, it is represented by hyperkeratosis with acanthosis with or without dysplasia. Erythroplakia is a red, velvety mucosal patch that represents epithelial atrophy, inflammation and subepithelial telangiectasia. Erythroplakia or erythroleukoplakia (speckled white and red patches) confer a greater risk of being associated with dysplasia with 91 percent being in situ or invasive SCC.[2,3] Proliferative verrucous leukoplakia (PVL) is an idiopathic condition occurring typically in the oral mucosa of elderly women which pursues a recurrent and progressive clinical course. Histologically, it appears with innocuous hyperkeratosis of the squamous epithelium and progresses to verrucous hyperplasia and dysplasia with the ultimate development of verrucous or conventional SCC over a protracted period of time.[4] This has led some to advocate that verrucous hyperplasia, the earliest histologically definable event in PVL, should be treated like verrucous carcinoma.[5]

Dysplasia is architecturally disordered proliferation of epithelial cells displaying abnormal cytologic appearance and maturation. Graded along a 3-tier system, mild dysplasia manifests as an increase in mitotic activity in the basal layer. It is difficult to distinguish it from reactive/repair activity of the squamous epithelium. Suprabasal mitosis heralds moderate dysplasia, the diagnosis of which may be aided by immunohistochemical staining for cell proliferation markers, eg, Ki-67 (MIB1) and proliferating cell nuclear antigen (PCNA). Overexpression of p53, although uncommon, signifies malignant transformation of moderate dysplasia to carcinoma in situ.[6]

Carcinoma in Situ

Carcinoma in situ (CIS)/severe dysplasia of the oral mucosa is usually of the keratinizing type, in which the abundant eosinophilic cytoplasm continues to show some degree of differentiation as the atypical epithelial cells migrate from basal to more superficial layers while still retaining their mitotic activity. The basaloid type, in which atypical, undifferentiated, basaloid cells with high nuclear cytoplasmic ratio

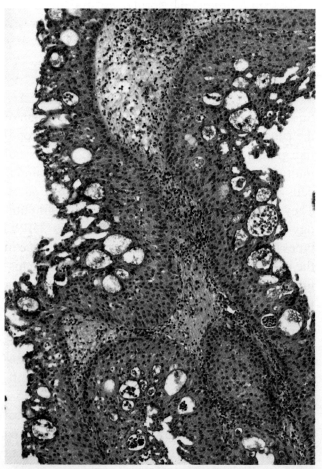

Figure 2–2. Fungiform schneiderian papilloma. The lesion is exophytic, lined with multiple layers of cells with a morphology transitional between squamous and columnar cells. Mucous cells containing blue mucin are scattered throughout. Acute and chronic inflammation is characteristically present.

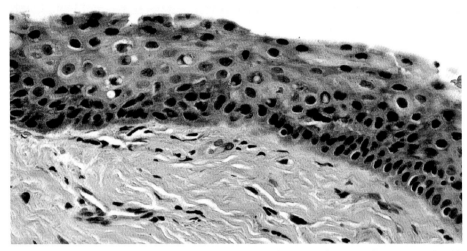

Figure 2–3. Carcinoma in situ/severe dysplasia in atrophic laryngeal mucosa. Dysplastic cells with hyperchromatic nuclei and increased nuclear cytoplasmic ratio are present even in the superficial layer of the squamous mucosa. The basement membrane is intact.

occupy all layers of the epithelium, is usually seen in the oropharynx and the larynx (Figure 2–3).

Field cancerization is the appearance of multiple synchronous or metachronous primary carcinomas in a mucosal field exposed to the same local carcinogen. The synchronous lesions are separated by so-called skip areas of histologically normal mucosa. Metachronous second primary lesions are accompanied by CIS.

Invasive Squamous Cell Carcinoma

Squamous cell carcinoma (SCC) consists of malignant cells with squamous differentiation as evinced by the presence of intercellular bridges and keratin formation. The conventional SCC is histologically graded on a scale of 3: well-, moderately- and poorly-differentiated SCC, depending upon the presence of intra- and extracellular keratin. However, this scheme has little bearing on prognosis. Better prognostic indicators and predictors of lymph node metastasis are enumerated in Table 2–1. Excellent prognosis is expected for so-called thin tumors versus thick ones, ie, less than 1.5 mm in the floor of the mouth,[7] 2 mm in the tongue,[8] and 3 mm in the buccal mucosa.[9] Tumor thickness is an independent predictor of recurrence, lymph node metastasis and survival. It has been shown that when the invasive front is well demarcated, blunt and of pushing type (grade 1) (Figure 2–4), the tumors have a better

prognosis and lower rate of lymph node metastasis than when it is jagged, irregularly infiltrative in the form of short cords and even single cells (grade 3 to 4) (Figure 2–5).[10,11] Assessment of surgical margins by intraoperative pathology consultation helps ensure complete removal of tumor. In situ or invasive carcinoma at or close (less than 5 mm) to the inked margin of resection increases the risk of recurrence and may require postsurgical radiotherapy. Tumors of the lower alveolar ridge infiltrate the mandible by direct extension and either spread between the medullary bony trabeculae or perineurally around the inferior alveolar nerve. The latter is significantly more common in edentulous patients than in the dentate ones. The mandibular extension

Table 2–1. PATHOLOGIC PROGNOSTIC FACTORS IN UPPER AERODIGESTIVE SQUAMOUS CELL CARCINOMA	
Factors Related to Primary Tumor	**Factors Related to Regional Lymph Nodes**
Size	Positive/negative
Thickness	Number of positive nodes
Invasive front	Size of largest positive node
Vascular and perineural invasion	Laterality of positive nodes
Margins of resection	Presence/absence of
Morphology	extracapsular extension
Well/poorly differentiated	
Exophytic/endophytic	
Mitotic index	
Presence of carcinoma in situ and multifocality	

is, however, limited and corresponds to the extent of the tumor in the overlying mucosa.[12]

In node-positive carcinomas, the number of positive nodes, their location and the size of the largest positive lymph node are important predictors of survival. The presence of extracapsular extension of tumor is a poor prognostic feature requiring postsurgical radiotherapy (see Table 2–1). Some conventional SCC may show cystic degeneration, pseudoglands and extracellular mucinous substance, but intracytoplasmic mucin is not seen in SCC. Several variants of SCC are recognized.

Verrucous carcinoma is an exophytic, warty, low-grade, well-differentiated SCC predominantly occurring in men in their seventh decade of life. It has a well-defined, broad, pushing invasive front. The cytomorphology of tumor cells is bland (Figure 2–6). Therefore, a superficial biopsy may not establish the

diagnosis, as it may not include the invasive base of the tumor which is essential for a histologic diagnosis. The prognosis is excellent, marred only by local recurrences. Pure verrucous carcinoma does not have metastatic potential. However, approximately 20 percent of verrucous carcinomas are hybrid, having an additional component of conventional SCC that confers metastatic potential to it.[13]

Papillary SCC is also exophytic but has a frond-like appearance with a central fibrovascular core usually lined by layers of poorly-differentiated tumor cells. Infiltration of the stroma and/or the base of the neoplasm is necessary to establish invasion (Figure 2–7).

Basaloid SCC usually arises in the posterior oral cavity and is highly aggressive. These patients fare much worse as compared to even the poorly-differentiated SCC in terms of metastasis and survival. Nodal

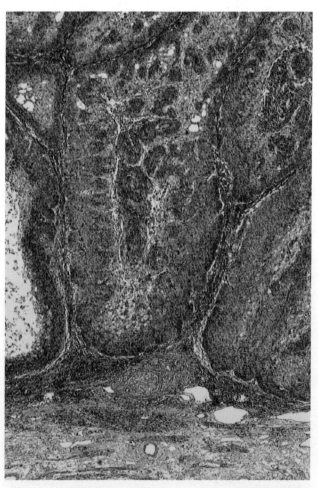

Figure 2–4. Moderately-differentiated squamous cell carcinoma of the tongue with a pushing type (grade 1) of infiltrating pattern at the tumor's growing edge.

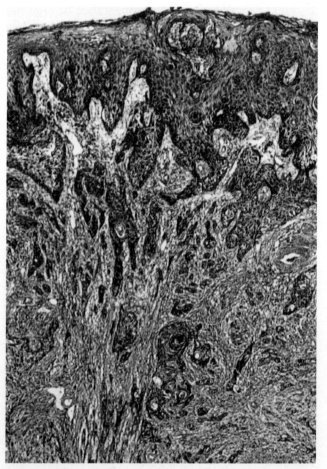

Figure 2–5. Moderately-differentiated squamous cell carcinoma of the tongue infiltrating the lamina propria. The invasive front shows a grade 3 infiltrating pattern by small clusters and cords of malignant cells.

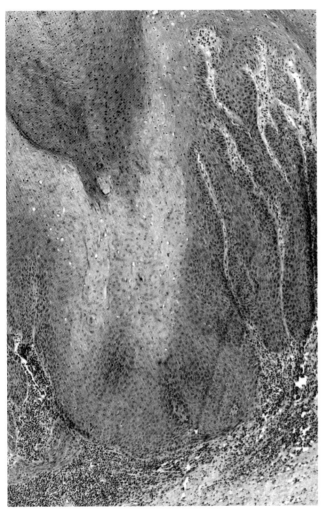

Figure 2–6. Verrucous carcinoma of the vocal cord. The malignant squamous cells are extremely well-differentiated with maturation and abundant keratinization toward the surface. The deep edge of the tumor is broad and of the pushing type. Grossly, the carcinoma was exophytic and warty.

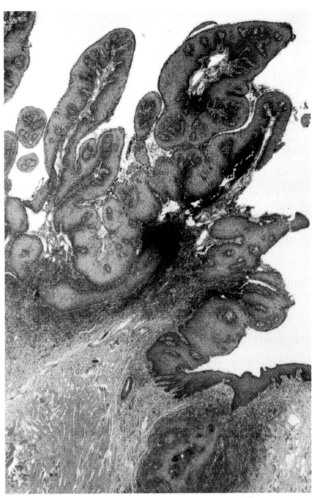

Figure 2–7. Papillary squamous cell carcinoma of the tongue. The tumor is exophytic with a focus of infiltration in the lamina propria. The papillae have fibrovascular cores and are lined by non-keratinizing moderately-differentiated squamous carcinoma cells in contrast with verrucous carcinoma. The prognosis is worse than the verrucous carcinoma as this tumor has metastatic capabilities.

metastasis is detected at initial presentation in almost two-thirds of the patients, and one-half of them develop distant metastasis with the lung being the most common site. This mandates a metastatic survey at initial diagnosis.[14] Median survival is 18 months.[15]

Sarcomatoid (spindle cell) SCC is usually exophytic and polypoid with the same clinical profile as conventional SCC. Histologically, the tumor has remarkable resemblance to malignant fibrous histiocytoma. Lymph node metastasis can show either or both epithelial and sarcomatous components. Immunohistochemically, cytokeratin can be demonstrated in the epithelial as well as spindle cell components. Ultrastructurally, tonofilaments and desmosomes, two of the hallmarks of squamous cells, have been demonstrated in the spindle cells. Expression of smooth muscle actin and occasionally desmin points to myofibroblastic differentiation of the spindle cells.[16]

Adenocarcinoma and adenosquamous carcinoma of the upper aerodigestive tract are believed to arise in the submucosal glands. They may resemble salivary gland tumors and are discussed in that section.

Undifferentiated Carcinoma

Lymphoepithelial carcinoma occurs most commonly in the nasopharynx where it is also designated as World Health Organization (WHO) type 3 nasopharyngeal carcinoma (Table 2–2). Cervical lymph

Table 2–2. CLASSIFICATION OF NASOPHARYNGEAL CARCINOMA WORLD HEALTH ORGANIZATION, 1991

1. Squamous cell carcinoma, keratinizing
2. Non-keratinizing carcinoma
   A. Differentiated non-keratinizing carcinoma
   B. Undifferentiated carcinoma

node metastasis from an occult primary is a frequent presentation. There is a bimodal age distribution with peaks in the second and sixth decades. There is a predilection for people of southern China and a well-established association with Epstein-Barr virus (EBV) infection.[17] The tumor is heavily infiltrated by lymphocytes and sometimes eosinophils and may mimic Hodgkin's or non-Hodgkin's lymphoma (Figure 2–8). The sinonasal undifferentiated carcinoma (SNUC) usually occurs in middle-aged patients and has a slight female preponderance. The tumor is characterized by numerous mitoses, necroses and extensive vascular invasion—features supportive of its high-grade nature (Figure 2–9).

Lymphoma

The sinonasal region is the most frequent site for lymphomas of the upper aerodigestive tract, most of which are diffuse large B-cell lymphomas with clin-

icopathologic characteristics similar to anywhere else in the body. The nasal NK/T-cell lymphomas (synonyms: polymorphic reticulosis, angiocentric lymphoma, lethal midline granuloma) is a distinct clinicopathologic entity affecting Asians and Native Americans. It is a destructive sinonasal disease presenting usually in the midline. It is a tumor of the natural killer cells and T cells, and is frequently associated with EBV infection. The prognosis is extremely poor in Asians and Native Americans in contrast to Caucasians.

Plasmacytoma, either solitary or in association with multiple myeloma, may occur in relation to the upper aerodigestive tract. It may be associated with amyloid.

Neuroendocrine carcinoma and malignant melanoma are discussed in a separate section on tumors of neurogenic origin.

TUMORS OF THE SALIVARY GLANDS

The distribution of tumors among different salivary glands studied at the Memorial Sloan-Kettering Cancer Center is given in Figure 2–10.[18] Benign tumors occur more frequently in the parotid glands of women in their fourth to fifth decades of life (Figure 2–11). Tumors in the minor salivary glands are

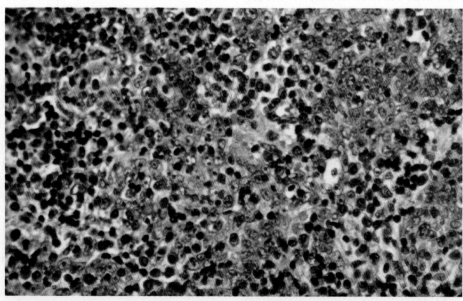

Figure 2–8. Lymphoepithelial carcinoma of the nasopharynx. The tumor cells have large, vesicular nuclei with prominent nucleoli and indistinct cytoplasm. They appear to be in a syncytium with an intimate admixture of lymphocytes (Schmincke pattern). Another pattern (not seen here) consists of cells arranged in loosely cohesive groups (Régaud pattern).

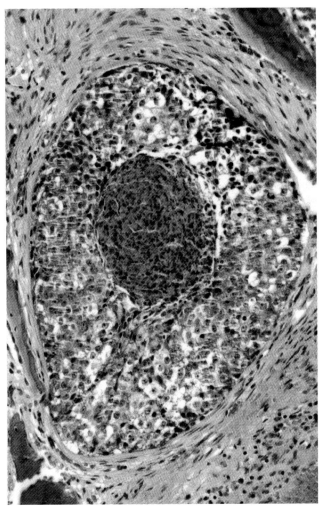

Figure 2–9. Sinonasal undifferentiated carcinoma (SNUC). Poorly-differentiated tumor cells with central comedo-type necrosis infiltrating bone.

more likely to be malignant than parotid tumors (see Figure 2–11). Salivary gland tumors tend to recapitulate the normal histology of the salivary glands (Figure 2–12).

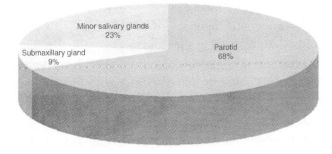

Figure 2–10. Relative distribution of 2,743 salivary gland tumors at the Memorial Sloan-Kettering Cancer Center, New York.

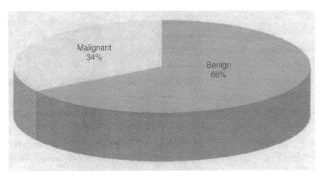

Figure 2–11. Relative distribution of benign versus malignant tumors among 1,875 parotid tumors at the Memorial Sloan-Kettering Cancer Center, New York.

Pleomorphic Adenoma

Pleomorphic adenoma or benign mixed tumor is the most frequent of parotid tumors. It occurs usually in the third to fifth decades with a female preponderance. The usual history is that of a slow growing tumor present for a long time. Grossly, the tumor is usually located in the superficial lobe of the parotid gland, and is well circumscribed with a gray-white, lobulated cut surface (Figure 2–13A). Histologically, it is composed of a varied mixture of epithelial and stromal components giving rise to its name "pleomorphic" or "mixed" tumor (Figure 2–13B). The tumor is believed to arise in the myoepithelial cells

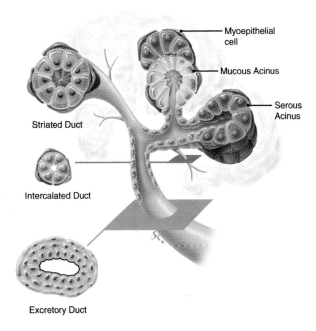

Figure 2–12. Schematic diagram of the histology of the normal salivary gland. A uniform layer of myoepithelial cells invests the terminal secretory unit—the acinus and the intercalated duct.

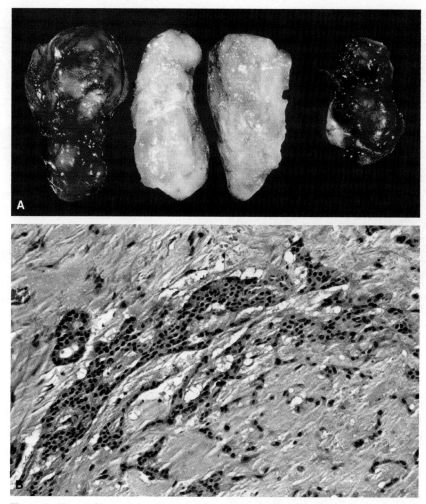

Figure 2–13. *A*, Pleomorphic adenoma. The tumor has a nodular external surface and a gray-white cut surface which may display focal chondroid differentiation. *B*, Histology shows prominent blue mucinous/myxoid component with small cuboidal bland cells forming cords and duct-like structures.

which retain their capacity for dual differentiation. Although these tumors are well-circumscribed, multiple microscopic pseudopods of the tumor can be left behind if resected by "shelling out" which can lead to multifocal recurrences. A cellular mixed tumor has an excess of epithelial and myoepithelial cells with sparse chondromucinous stroma.

Malignant transformation occurs in 5 to 10 percent of cases and is much more common than the de novo malignant mixed tumor. Clinically, recent rapid growth and nerve palsy, while microscopically, cellular atypia, mitosis, invasion of the surrounding tissue, nerves and vessels constitute features of malignancy. Although both the epithelial and the mesenchymal components of the mixed tumor can undergo malignant transformation, the former is much more frequent, giving rise to the designation "carcinoma ex mixed tumor" and "carcinoma ex pleomorphic adenoma." They represent about 11 percent of all malignant salivary gland neoplasms.[19] The patients are usually in their fifth decade with a slight female predilection. Most tumors are more than 3 cm in size. Important histologic prognostic factors are morphology of carcinoma (low vs. high grade) and degree of infiltration (in situ or minimally vs. extensively invasive).[20] Almost all patients have local treatment failure. Distant metastasis can occur in 33 percent of cases, with lungs and bones being common sites. The less commonly occurring biphasic carcinosarcoma or "true" malignant mixed tumor has a very aggressive and lethal behavior.[21]

Monomorphic Adenoma

Monomorphic adenomas are relatively uncommon benign epithelial tumors predominantly occurring in the parotid glands. They lack the myxoid stroma of the pleomorphic adenoma. Various morphologic types are described. The canalicular adenoma occurs most frequently in the upper lip. The basal cell adenoma is composed of basal cells surrounded by a thick, hyaline basement membrane material containing stroma. The malignant counterpart, basal cell adenocarcinoma, is characterized by an infiltrative growth pattern.

Oncocytic Tumors

The parotid gland is the most common site for oncocytic tumors which tend to occur in the fifth to sixth decades and which have shown a relationship to previous radiation exposure. Oncocytomas are solid tumors composed of cells with abundant mitochondria-rich cytoplasm which is intensely eosinophilic and granular in texture (Figure 2–14). The much more common papillary and cystic Warthin's tumor has a male predilection and a strong association with smoking. A characteristic non-neoplastic lymphocytic component with activated follicles containing germinal centers is present, justifying the synonym papillary cystadenoma lymphomatosum (Figure 2–15). It may be bilateral in a small but significant number of cases. The extremely rare oncocytic carcinoma has an infiltrative growth pattern and an aggressive clinical behavior.

Malignant salivary gland tumors account for approximately 7 percent of all carcinomas arising in the upper aerodigestive tract.[22] Risk factors include exposure to radiation, tobacco, chemicals, and viruses, and genetic predisposition. About 15 percent of all parotid, 35 percent of submandibular, 45 percent of minor salivary and 80 percent of sublingual gland tumors are malignant.[23] Men and women are almost equally affected. In most instances, the clinical stage of the disease has greater influence on prognosis than the histologic grade, except in mucoepidermoid and adenocarcinoma, not otherwise specified.

Mucoepidermoid Carcinoma

The most frequent site for a mucoepidermoid carcinoma is the parotid, followed by intraoral minor salivary glands. Most patients are in their early fifties. Grossly, the tumor is poorly circumscribed and measures from 3 to 5 cm. The cut surface is solid but may be cystic. The tumor is composed of glandular and epidermoid cells, the latter characteristically of intermediate basaloid type (Figure 2–16). The histologic grading scheme is prognostically significant. Low-grade tumors form cysts lined by a single layer of glandular mucinous cells with an admixture of

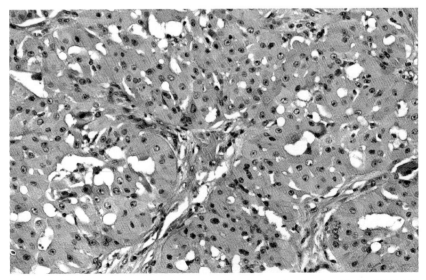

Figure 2–14. Oncocytoma. The tumor is solid with sheets of cells with abundant acidophilic cytoplasm. The nuclei have characteristic prominent nucleoli.

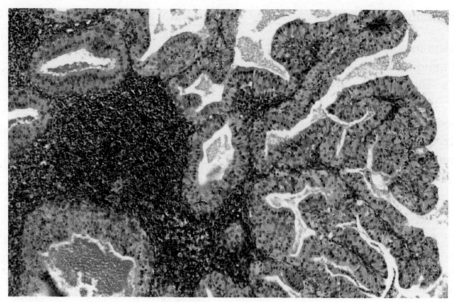

Figure 2–15.   Warthin's tumor. The lesion is predominantly cystic with an exuberant lymphoid follicular reaction. The cyst is lined by oncocytic cells which are arranged in papillary structures.

epidermoid cells. The epidermoid and intermediate basaloid-type cells tend to form solid areas in intermediate grade, and predominate in high-grade lesions along with scant evidence of glandular differentiation, increased cytologic atypia, mitosis, necrosis and perineural invasion. Using these grading criteria, 90 percent of the low-grade as compared to 42 percent of the high-grade mucoepidermoid carcinoma patients were found to be alive at 10 years after treatment.[24] An important differential diagnosis is primary or metastatic squamous cell carcinoma, which is rare in the parotid and lacks intracellular mucin. Sebaceous and clear cell neoplasms are additional differential diagnostic concerns.

Adenoid Cystic Carcinoma

The most frequent site of origin of adenoid cystic carcinoma is in the minor salivary glands, especially in the palate, followed by the sinuses and nasal cavity and the parotid glands. The patients are usually in their fifties and may be of either sex. On microscopic examination, the tumor has a characteristic cribriform appearance formed by the interruption of sheets of tumor cells by cylindrical pseudo-spaces or pseudo-lumina, giving rise to the designation cylindroma (Figure 2–17). Although clinically indolent, these tumors are relentlessly infiltrative with a local

recurrence rate of 47 percent. Perineural invasion is frequent and extensive, requiring intraoperative assessment of the neural margin of resection. Distant metastasis has been reported in 38 percent of cases with lung and bones being common sites. The microscopic grading system does not appear to be useful. Clinical stage is the most important factor in determining prognosis.[25]

Polymorphous Low-Grade Adenocarcinoma

This tumor is increasingly being recognized as one of the more frequent salivary gland adenocarcinomas ever since it was described under synonyms such as lobular, terminal duct or trabecular carcinoma.[26,27] The patients usually are in their fifth decade. The tumors involve the minor salivary glands almost exclusively, and rarely, the nasal cavity or nasopharynx. The lesion may be relatively well-circumscribed but can extensively invade the adjacent bone. Microscopically, there is great architectural diversity (Figure 2–18). A single file arrangement may be seen as in the infiltrating lobular carcinoma of breast. In spite of their low-grade, usually indolent biologic behavior, 76 percent show perineural invasion and up to 29 percent may metastasize to the cervical lymph nodes.[28] Differential diagnosis includes adenoid cystic carcinoma and pleomorphic adenoma.

Acinic Cell Carcinoma

Acinic cell carcinoma (ACC) comprises 17 percent of primary malignant salivary gland tumors.[25] Almost 90 percent of them arise in the parotid gland, making it the second most common malignant tumor at this site. The age varies widely with a small peak in the fourth decade. Grossly, the tumor usually measures less than 3 cm, and is well-defined with a friable, tan cut surface. The most characteristic tumor cells are the acinic cells which contain periodic acid Schiff's reagent (PAS)-positive cytoplasmic glycogen granules resembling the serous cells of salivary glands (Figure 2–19A). Histologic features used for grading are increased mitosis, necrosis, neural invasion, infiltration, pleomorphism and stromal hyalinization. Although the histologic grading system is not always useful, the conventional ACC should be separated from the papillocystic variant (Figure 2–19B) believed to have a particularly bad prognosis, and a highly aggressive dedifferentiated variant.[29,30] The conventional ACC is a low-grade malignant tumor characterized by prolonged disease-free survival, late recurrences and late distant metastasis to bone, lung and brain.[31]

Adenocarcinoma, Not Otherwise Specified

These are adenocarcinomas lacking any characteristic feature that helps in classifying them as other specific types of epithelial tumors of salivary origin. Thus, it is a diagnosis by exclusion. There is a slight

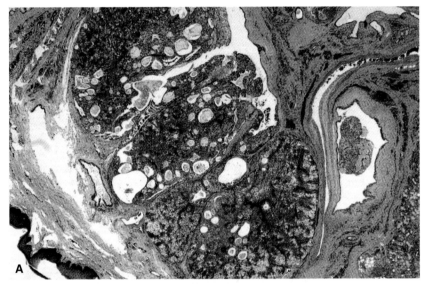
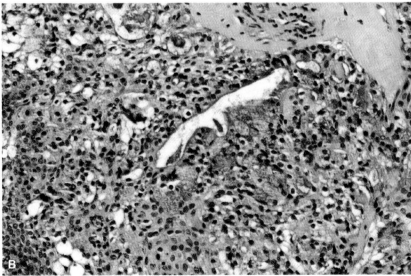

Figure 2–16. *A*, A partly cystic mucoepidermoid carcinoma involving a dilated minor salivary gland duct. Although the tumor forms numerous cysts, the solid areas indicate its intermediate grade. *B*, The intracytoplasmic, as well as extracytoplasmic, neutral mucin stains bright pink with mucicarmine stain. The former is diagnostic of mucoepidermoid carcinoma.

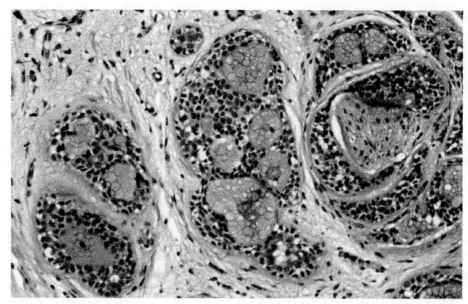

Figure 2–17.   Adenoid cystic carcinoma showing tumor cell nests with a cribriform/cylindromatous pattern. The pseudolumina may contain acidic mucin (as in this figure) or basement membrane-like material which may also surround tumor nests. The pseudolumina shows two layers of tumor cells with small, cuboidal cells towards the center and clear myoepithelial cells at the periphery.

male preponderance with a median age of 58 years. The minor salivary glands are more frequently involved followed by the parotid glands. Microscopically, the cells may display a glandular, papillary or mucinous growth pattern, and sometimes even resemble colonic adenocarcinoma. The histologic grading which takes into account cytologic atypia, pleomorphism, mitosis and necrosis, identifies low, intermediate and high grades. Prognosis depends on site (better in oral cavity tumors), histologic grade and clinical stage.[32]

Rare Tumors

Myoepithelioma and myoepithelial carcinoma are rare neoplasms composed almost entirely of myoepithelial cells. The parotid is the most common site. Multiple recurrences, distant metastasis and death due to disease occur in one-third of the patients suffering from myoepithelial carcinoma, suggesting an intermediate- to high-grade malignant potential.[31] Epithelial-myoepithelial carcinoma is an uncommon, low-grade, multilobular, malignant neoplasm that shows both epithelial and myoepithelial differentiation and occurs most commonly in the parotid glands of elderly women. Clear cell adenocarcinoma occurs in the fifth to seventh decade and is comprised of

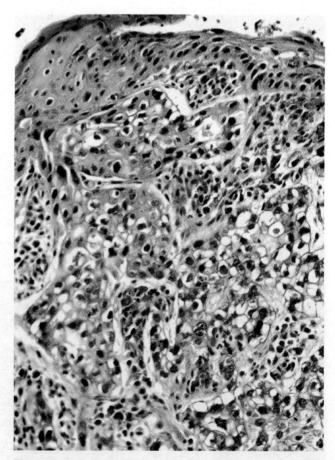

Figure 2–18.   Polymorphous low-grade adenocarcinoma. The squamous mucosa of the oral cavity is visible above. The tumor cells are squamoid near the surface and become clear and form glandular structures below.

glycogen-rich cells. It affects both sexes equally. Lymphoepithelial carcinoma may arise in the salivary glands, usually de novo but sometimes in association with Sjögren's syndrome. A female predilection and a higher incidence among the Inuit is noted.[33] The parotid is the most frequently involved salivary gland. The morphology is similar to the nasopharyngeal variant—metastasis from which should be ruled out before considering a primary parotid tumor. Salivary duct carcinoma is a very aggressive neoplasm that resembles intraductal carcinoma of the breast replete with comedo-necrosis, "Roman bridges" and cribriform pattern. Most tumors occur in the parotid glands of elderly men.[31] Perineural and vascular invasion and dense fibrosis are commonly present. Primary squamous cell carcinoma of the salivary gland is a rarity. It probably arises in the part of the excretory salivary duct which is closer to the oral cavity. A prerequisite for diagno-

sis is ruling out mucoepidermoid carcinoma and metastatic squamous cell carcinoma. Cystadenoma and cystadenocarcinoma are rare tumors characterized by cysts lined by columnar cells and resemble their counterparts in the pancreas and ovary.[31]

TUMORS OF THYROID AND PARATHYROID GLANDS

Thyroid tumors affect females more often than men. Radiation is an important predisposing factor, especially for papillary thyroid carcinoma. A close association of Hashimoto's thyroiditis to many thyroid malignancies, eg, lymphoma, papillary and Hürthle cell carcinoma, sclerosing mucoepidermoid thyroid carcinoma and squamous cell carcinoma has been noted. Malignant cells arising in the follicular epithelium express thyroglobulin, a feature that may be used to support their thyroid origin at metastatic sites.

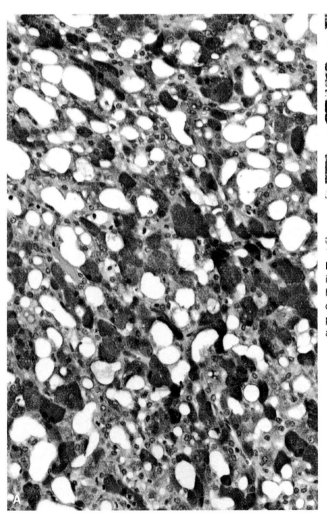

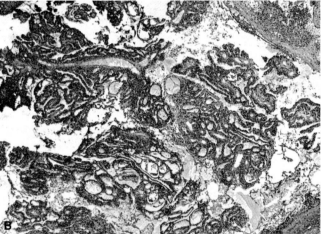

Figure 2–19. *A*, Acinic cell carcinoma—conventional type. The tumor is predominently solid with microcyst formation. Several tumor cells have the typical granular cytoplasm of serous acinic cells. *B*, Acinic cell carcinoma—papillocystic variant. The tumor is predominantly cystic with papillary proliferation in the cyst lumen. This variant is believed to have a poorer prognosis than the conventional type.

Papillary Carcinoma

This is the most common thyroid carcinoma affecting patients at a young age. The size of the tumor varies widely from microscopic to massive tumors that may completely replace the thyroid and extend outside of it. Incidental or occult presentation and multifocality is well known. The characteristic nuclear features (Figure 2–20A), when present, are sufficient for the diagnosis of papillary carcinoma, even in the presence of a capsule and in the absence of invasion. Psammoma bodies may be present in nearly half of the cases. The nuclear morphology, papillary tissue fragments and psammoma bodies can also be appreciated in fine-needle aspiration cytology facilitating correct diagnosis. Several histologic variants have been described. The conventional papillary carcinoma with true papillae, and the follicular variant recapitulating the follicular architecture of the thyroid gland, have similar biologic behavior and a good prognosis (see Figure 2–20). The size of the papillary microcarcinoma is by definition less than 1 cm. It is usually incidentally discovered in association with a fibrous scar and has an excellent prognosis as has the encapsulated variant. The diffuse sclerosing variant is characterized by the patient's younger age, extensive involvement of the thyroid gland with a predominantly fibrosing, psammomatous papillary carcinoma with frequent squamous metaplasia, lymphocytic infiltration and vascular invasion. More than half of the patients develop regional lymph node involvement, and metastasis to lungs are frequent. In spite of the higher incidence of distant metastasis, death rate due to tumor is extremely low.[34] The tall cell (Figure 2–21) and columnar cell variants have extremely poor prognosis.[35,36] The former occurs in older patients and presents with large tumor size while the

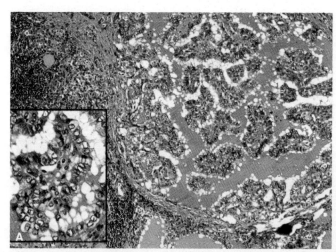

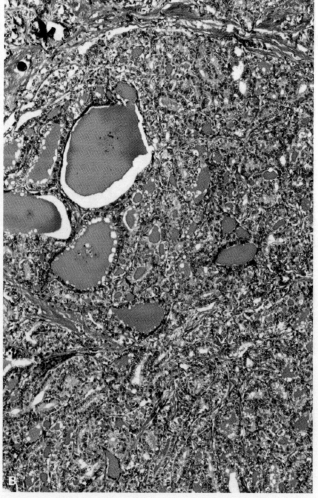

Figure 2–20. *A*, Papillary thyroid carcinoma—conventional type with well-formed papillae with fibrovascular cores. A psammoma body is seen in the upper right corner. The surrounding non-neoplastic tissue shows lymphocytic thyroiditis with which it is commonly associated. Inset shows the characteristic nuclear clearing, overlapping nuclei ("eggs in a basket") and nuclear grooves. *B*, Papillary carcinoma—follicular variant. The diagnosis is based on the similarity of nuclear features to conventional papillary carcinoma. A psammoma body is seen in the upper left corner.

latter is reported in young men who die of disease within 2 years of presentation. Other morphologic indicators of poor prognosis are extra-thyroidal extension and vascular invasion. A cribriform-morular variant has been described in young women in association with familial adenomatous polyposis.[37]

Follicular Neoplasm

Follicular adenoma is a benign, solitary, encapsulated tumor of the thyroid follicular epithelium. Follicular carcinoma is a malignant neoplasm which is distinguished from its benign counterpart by the presence of vascular and full-thickness capsular invasion into the surrounding non-neoplastic thyroid parenchyma (Figure 2–22). Thus, all follicular

lesions should be completely excised with their capsule and the adjacent thyroid, so as to permit histologic evaluation of the entire capsule for infiltration. For this reason, distinction between follicular adenoma and carcinoma cannot be made on fine-needle aspiration cytology. Mitosis and nuclear atypia may be present in adenomas which are then designated atypical follicular neoplasms, the overwhelming majority of which behave in a benign fashion. Most patients with follicular carcinoma are in their fifth decade of life and present with a solitary neck mass. Blood-borne metastasis to lungs and bones is more common than lymphatic spread to regional nodes. A minimally invasive (encapsulated) follicular carcinoma needs to be distinguished from an extensively invasive one, as fewer than 5 percent of the former

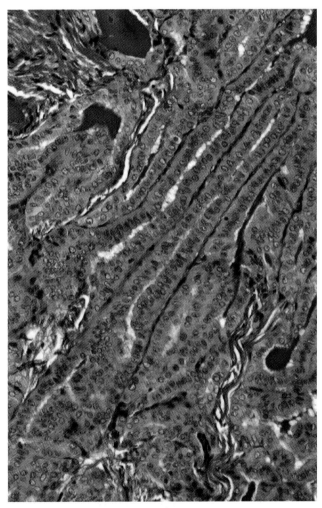

Figure 2–21. Papillary carcinoma—tall cell variant. The cells are twice as tall as broad while the nuclear features remain the same as in papillary carcinoma. This morphologic variant is believed to have a worse prognosis than the conventional papillary thyroid carcinoma.

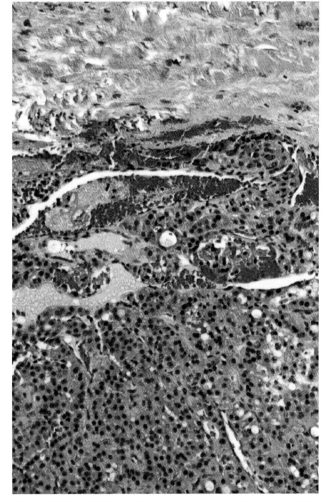

Figure 2–22. Hürthle cell carcinoma—minimally invasive. The tumor cell cytoplasm is deeply acidophilic. Although the fibrous capsule is present all around the tumor, at this focus the tumor shows vascular invasion.

metastasize.[38,39] In the encapsulated variant, capsular invasion in the absence of vascular invasion has little value in predicting outcome. Figure 2–23 schematically enumerates all follicular neoplasms in order of their malignant potential.

Hürthle Cell Neoplasms

Hürthle cell or oncocytic neoplasms are composed of cells with abundant pink (oxyphilic) cytoplasm containing ample abnormal mitochondria on ultrastructural examination. The majority of these tumors are benign. The lesion is often divided into lobules by thick fibrous septa. As in follicular carcinoma, presence of capsular or vascular invasion is a prerequisite for the diagnosis of malignancy (see Figure 2–22). As a result, fine-needle aspiration cytology can at best suggest a Hürthle cell neoplasm, but cannot distinguish between a benign or malignant lesion. These tumors tend to occur in an older age group with only a slight female preponderance. They are more aggressive than the conventional papillary or follicular carcinomas, suggesting an intermediate-grade malignant behavior.[40]

Poorly-Differentiated (Insular) Carcinoma

This tumor is viewed as a poorly-differentiated variant of the well-differentiated papillary or follicular thyroid carcinoma and occurs in a relatively older age group. The tumor cells are uniformly small with mild atypia and variable mitosis. Focal necrosis may be present. The cells are arranged in a solid or micro-follicular, nested or insular pattern. They express thyroglobulin which is useful in distinguishing them from medullary carcinoma. The biologic behavior is aggressive, resulting in recurrences and distant metastases (Figure 2–24).

Undifferentiated/Anaplastic Carcinoma

This is a high-grade malignant neoplasm which usually affects older patients and has a female preponderance. Patients present with a recent-onset rapidly-enlarging mass frequently associated with dyspnea, dysphagia and/or hoarseness, indicating extra-thyroidal extension at presentation. Histologically, the tumor may be composed of three types of

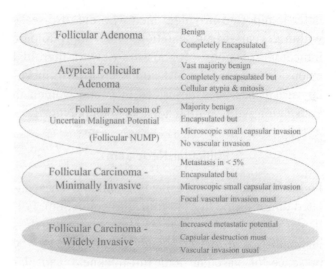

Figure 2–23. Follicular neoplasms arranged in order of worsening prognosis from above down.

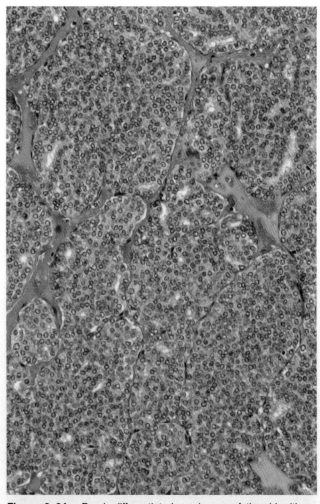

Figure 2–24. Poorly-differentiated carcinoma of thyroid with an insular and barely discernible micro-follicular growth pattern. This tumor showed nuclear features of papillary carcinoma at higher magnification, suggesting that it may have progressed from a well-differentiated papillary carcinoma.

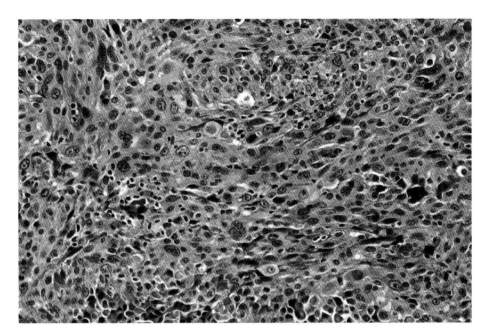

Figure 2–25. Anaplastic carcinoma of the thyroid. The tumor cells are spindle-shaped with markedly anaplastic nuclei resembling a high-grade sarcoma. Due to their extreme degree of dedifferentiation, the tumor cells do not (or only focally) express thyroglobulin, requiring a combined clinicopathologic effort to make a definite diagnosis of primary thyroid carcinoma.

cells: anaplastic spindle cells resembling a sarcoma, bizarre pleomorphic multinucleate giant cells and squamoid cells (Figure 2–25). Severe nuclear atypia, cellular pleomorphism, brisk mitosis, large foci of necrosis and extensive invasion are characteristic features. Rarely, metaplastic bone or cartilage may be present. Immunohistochemically, thyroglobulin expression is variable—usually weak or even negative. The undifferentiated carcinomas may arise from dedifferentiation in a well-differentiated papillary or follicular carcinoma (Figure 2–26). The tumor metastasizes widely using both blood and lymphatic vessels. All patients die, mostly due to respiratory compromise caused by the tumor.

Medullary Thyroid Carcinoma

Medullary thyroid carcinoma (MTC) is a malignant tumor of the calcitonin-secreting parafollicular C cells of the thyroid. It accounts for less than 10 percent of all thyroid malignancies. Characteristically, MTCs secrete calcitonin, produce amyloid and, in about 20 percent of cases, are familial. In the latter situation, it may be inherited in an autosomal dominant manner either in association with multiple endocrine neoplasia (MENIIa and MENIIb) syndromes or as familial MTC, and affects children and adolescents with an equal gender distribution. Mutations in the RET proto-oncogene on chromosome 10

have been found to be associated with all familial and some sporadic cases.[41] The tumor usually involves the upper two-thirds of the thyroid, the area of maximum concentration of C cells in the normal gland. The sporadic cases are unifocal and discrete while the familial cases are more likely to be multifocal and involve both lobes. Less than 50 percent of tumors contain the characteristic stromal amyloid which may be focally calcified (Figure 2–27). Immunohistochemistry shows that the tumor cells and sometimes the stromal amyloid are positive for calcitonin (Figure 2–28). The tumor cells also

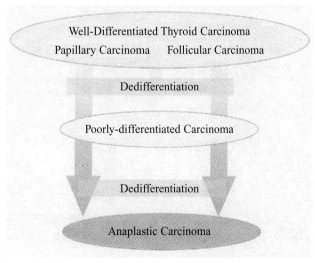

Figure 2–26. Schematic diagram showing possible progression of well-differentiated thyroid carcinoma to anaplastic carcinoma.

express calcitonin gene-related peptide and carcinoembryonic antigen, and are negative for thyroglobulin. However, immuno-stain for chromogranin, a marker for neuroendocrine differentiation, is more sensitive than calcitonin for MTC. Ultrastructurally, multiple intracytoplasmic membrane-bound secretory granules are demonstrated. It is possible to diagnose MTC by fine-needle aspiration because of the typical plasmacytic tumor cell morphology and demonstration of amyloid and calcitonin. The tumor tends to be indolent in familial MTC, and aggressive in sporadic MTC and MENIIb, leading to metastasis due to lymphatic and vascular invasion of cervical nodes, lung, liver and bone. Death is usually due to uncontrolled local disease. It is important to recognize a small cell (anaplastic) variant of MTC which resembles small (oat) cell neuroendocrine carcinoma

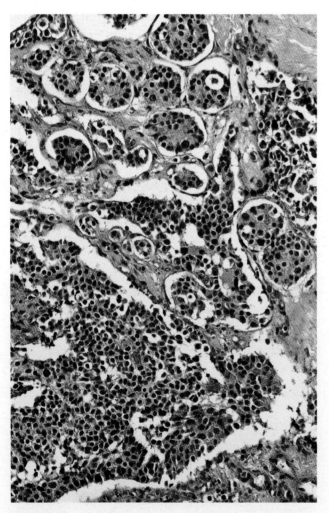

Figure 2–27. Medullary carcinoma of the thyroid showing an insular pattern of growth interrupted by hyalinized fibrous septa which may contain amyloid.

of the lung. It is mitotically more active, less likely to produce calcitonin and amyloid, and is believed to have a slightly worse prognosis than the conventional MTC. Mixed medullary-follicular and medullary-papillary carcinomas have also been described.

Uncommon Tumors of the Thyroid

Primary squamous cell carcinoma is extremely rare in the thyroid. Direct extension from the larynx, metastasis, or a nonsquamous thyroid carcinoma, eg, papillary or undifferentiated carcinoma with extensive squamous metaplasia should be ruled out. Mucoepidermoid carcinoma in the thyroid is a rare, low-grade neoplasm postulated to arise as a metaplastic change in the thyroid follicular epithelium. A sclerosing variant with eosinophilia has been described.[42] Carcinoma showing thymus-like differentiation is a rare, low-grade tumor believed to arise in branchial pouch remnants capable of thymic differentiation with resemblance to a thymic carcinoma.[43] Lymphomas of the thyroid are usually non-Hodgkin's lymphomas of B-cell type spanning the spectrum of low-grade to high-grade diffuse large cell type. The low-grade lymphomas are similar to the mucosa-associated lymphoid tissue lymphomas elsewhere in the body. Frequent association with Hashimoto's thyroiditis is noted. Transformation of low- to high-grade lymphoma is well documented.

Parathyroid Adenoma and Carcinoma

Parathyroid adenoma is a solitary, well-defined, hyperfunctional benign neoplasm which accounts for the majority of cases of primary hyperparathyroidism. Its distinction with hyperplasia is important for correct surgical management, as the former is treated by removal of only the adenomatous gland while the latter requires resection of all four glands. The distinction between normal and hyperplastic glands is made by weight as the histologic appearance may be similar. Most adenomas are composed of chief cells which completely replace the intraglandular fat that is present in normal and hyperplastic glands. Ectopic adenomas may be found in association with the thymus in the mediastinum and in intrathyroidal locations. Extremely high serum calcium levels are generally indicative of

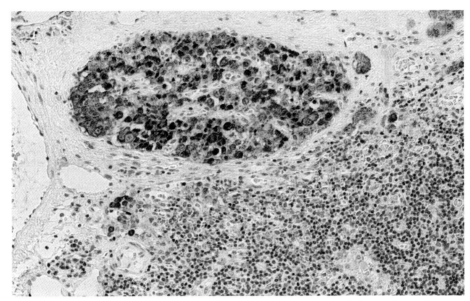

Figure 2–28. Immunohistochemistry for calcitonin highlights a metastatic focus of medullary carcinoma in a lymph node.

parathyroid carcinoma. This is an infiltrative tumor characterized by vascular and capsular invasion, dense fibrosis, nuclear atypia, increased mitosis and regional and distant metastasis (Figure 2–29).

NEURONAL, NEUROENDOCRINE AND NEUROECTODERMAL TUMORS

Paraganglioma

Extra-adrenal paragangliomas can occur in the head and neck. They secrete norepinephrine and are functional. Patients (most of whom are adults) present with hypertensive headaches, tachycardia and sweating. The carotid body tumors occur at the bifurcation of the carotid artery. The jugulotympanic paraganglioma (glomus jugulare tumor) may present as mass in temporal bone extending to the middle ear or external auditory canal or involve the jugular bulb in the jugular foramen. There is a female predilection. Angiographic findings are characteristic as the tumor is very vascular. Because of poor accessibility in the jugulotympanic region, the tumors are removed in a piece-meal fashion destroying the typical "zellballen" arrangement of the tumor cells, making histologic diagnosis difficult (Figure 2–30A). The cells express several neuroendocrine markers by immunohistochemistry and contain

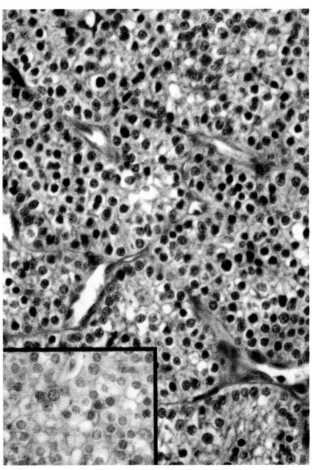

Figure 2–29. Parathyroid carcinoma in a 51-year-old man with hyperparathyroidism. The cells have uniform morphology and frequent cytoplasmic clearing. The tumor invaded blood vessels, adjacent soft tissue, and thyroid gland in other sections. Immunostaining with anti-parathyroid hormone antibody is characteristically positive (inset).

dense core neurosecretory granules on ultrastructural examination (Figure 2–30B). Ten percent of these tumors metastasize. Histologic criteria such as nuclear atypia, pleomorphism and mitosis are not reliable in predicting malignant behavior. The vagal paraganglioma may be seen in association with the vagus nerve in the anterolateral portion of the neck.

Olfactory Neuroblastoma

Olfactory neuroblastoma or esthesioneuroblastoma is a rare malignancy with a bimodal age distribution in adolescents and adults and without any gender predilection. It is believed to arise in the specialized neurosecretory cells of the olfactory mucosa in the

superior one-third of the nasal septum, superior turbinate and the cribriform plate, which may be broken with intracranial extradural extension of the tumor. The usual presentation is as a polypoid nasal mass with epistaxis and nasal obstruction, usually of long duration. Microscopically, the tumor is submucosal and is composed of nests of monomorphous cells in a fibrillary background of neuropil (Figure 2–31A). Immunohistochemically, the tumor cells are positive for neural and neuroendocrine markers, eg, synaptophysin, neurofilament protein, and chromogranin among others (Figure 2–31B). Ultrastructural examination can help in the differential diagnosis by demonstrating neurosecretory granules, microtubules and neuritic processes. We believe that

Figure 2–30. *A*, Paraganglioma—carotid body tumor. The cells have moderate-to-abundant cytoplasm, and are arranged in well-defined nests ("zellballen"). There is occasional binucleation and nuclear atypia. Cytologic criteria are of no help in predicting biologic behavior. *B*, Intense and diffuse cytoplasmic staining of tumor cells with anti-chromogranin antibody by immunohistochemistry supporting their neuroendocrine nature.

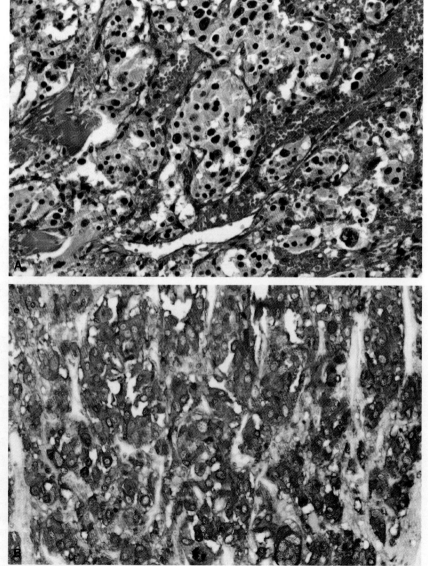

the olfactory neuroblastoma is different from Ewing's sarcoma/primitive neuroectodermal tumors at both the molecular and immunohistochemical level.[44] Higher incidence of S100 protein expression and low expression of Ki 67, a cell proliferation marker, have been linked to better survival.[45] Most tumors are slow growing, locally destructive and have a favorable prognosis although regional and distant metastasis can occur at prolonged follow-up.

Ewing's Sarcoma/Primitive Neuroectodermal Tumor

Skeletal or extraskeletal Ewing's sarcoma/primitive neuroectodermal tumor (ES/PNET) is extremely rare in the head and neck. It is characterized by the chromosomal translocation t(11:22)(q24;q12) leading to the EWS/FLI1 fusion protein MIC2 which can be detected immunohistochemically by O13 (CD99) antibody.[44] Metastasis should be ruled out before considering the lesion as a primary tumor in the head and neck.

Neuroendocrine Carcinoma

Small cell neuroendocrine carcinoma is extremely rare in the head and neck and may be seen in the nasal cavity, paranasal sinuses, salivary or thyroid glands. It resembles the small (oat) cell carcinoma of the respiratory tract. The tumor cells are positive for markers

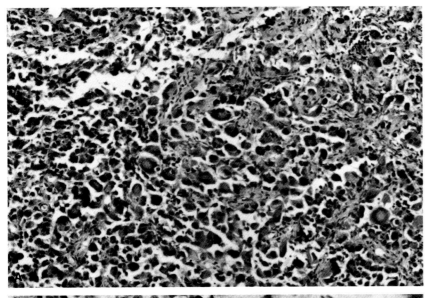
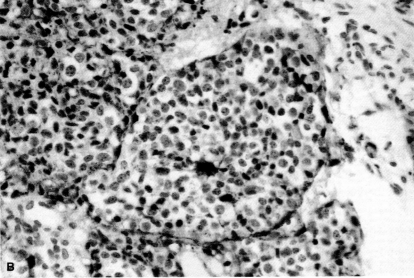

Figure 2–31. *A*, Olfactory neuroblastoma showing a cellular small blue cell neoplasm in a fibrillary background of neuropil. Homer-Wright rosettes formed by the arrangement of tumor cells around central neurofibrillary collections are seen. *B*, Immunohistochemistry with S100 protein shows staining of sustentacular cells around the periphery of tumor cell nests, an important feature in the differential diagnosis with other relatively high-grade neuroendocrine/ neuroectodermal neoplasms in this area.

of neuroendocrine differentiation and cytokeratin. In the nose, it needs to be distinguished from an olfactory neuroblastoma because of different prognosis and management. In the thyroid, lack of calcitonin expression and amyloid production are helpful hints to distinguish it from medullary carcinoma.

Merkel cell carcinoma (MCC) is a variant of neuroendocrine carcinoma of the dermis and subcutaneous tissue. There is a male predilection with a median age of 70 years. Most MCCs arise in the skin of the head and neck. They differ from the small cell neuroendocrine carcinoma in having a distinct pale nucleus with fine speckled chromatin, a characteristic perinuclear dot-like reaction with cytokeratin 20 and neurofilament protein[46] on immunohistochemistry (Figures 2–32 and 2–33.). This is a high-grade tumor and has rarely been reported in the salivary gland and oral mucosa.

Malignant Melanoma

Head and neck melanomas can be categorized into cutaneous and mucosal types. Cutaneous melanomas occur most commonly in the face, followed by scalp, neck and external ear in decreasing order of frequency. They have a slightly worse prognosis than similar lesions outside of the head and neck. The tumor may be in the radial growth phase which is completely excisable and therefore curable, and/or in the vertical growth phase. In the latter, the malignant cells invade and grow within the dermis and acquire metastatic potential The two phases are clinically definable. The superficial spreading melanoma is an in situ, and usually microinvasive, radial growth phase malignant melanoma etiologically associated with recreational sun exposure (Figure 2–34A). Lentigo maligna is usually in situ and occurs in the background of epidermal atrophy and severe sun damage as a result of chronic exposure in an elderly person. If invasion is also present, the diagnosis is lentigo maligna melanoma (Figure 2–34B). In contrast, the nodular melanoma is completely within the dermis without any associated radial growth phase and needs to be differentiated from metastatic melanoma. The cells may be epithelioid or spindle-shaped giving the tumor a biphasic appearance. Immunohistochemically, malignant melanoma stains

diffusely for S100 protein, and markers for melanocytic differentiation gp-100 (HMB 45) and Melan-A/ MART-1.[47] The clinical outcome depends upon several clinical criteria, eg, age, sex (younger and female patients have a better outcome than older and males), location (neck and ear better than scalp and face) and several histopathologic criteria enumerated in Table 2–3. Of these, the thickness of the lesion and Clark's level are the most powerful predictors of outcome (Figure 2–35).[49] In the radial growth phase, regressive changes have a negative effect on survival. The desmoplastic melanoma is a spindle cell, collagen producing, usually amelanotic melanoma which is usually a vertical growth phase tumor but may be associated with a radial growth phase (Figure 2–36). The prognosis is good despite a tendency to neurotropism (nerve invasion).

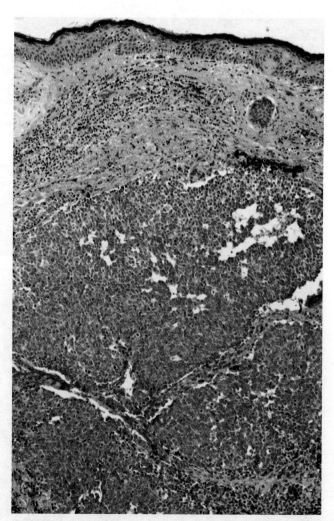

Figure 2–32. Merkel cell carcinoma in the skin showing nests of small blue cells.

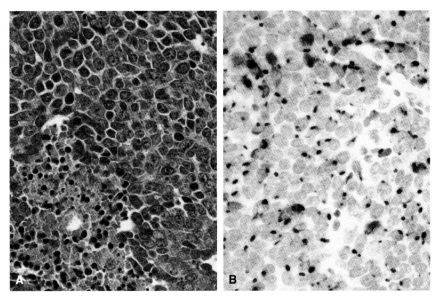

Figure 2–33. *A*, Merkel cell carcinoma—higher magnification shows the typical hyperchromatic endocrine type of nucleus, necrosis and brisk mitosis. *B*, Immunostain with neurofilament shows characteristic dot-like positivity in the paranuclear golgi area. Similar positivity is also seen with cytokeratin (CK20).

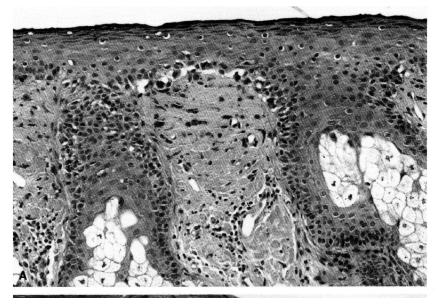

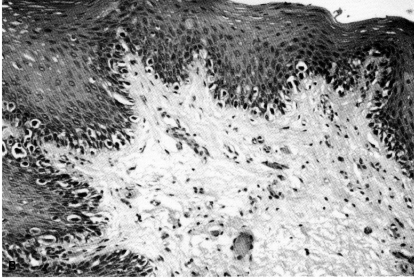

Figure 2–34. *A*, Cutaneous superficially-spreading malignant melanoma in situ (Clark level 1). Single cell proliferation of malignant melanocytes is seen in contact with the basal layer of the epidermis while single atypical melanocytes are identified migrating into upper dermis-like "buckshots." The tumor does not acquire metastatic potential even when microinvasion is present. *B*, Malignant melanoma in situ—lentiginous type involving the buccal mucosa. The malignant melanocytes spread along the basal layer of the squamous epithelium.

Table 2–3. HISTOPATHOLOGIC CRITERIA AFFECTING THE PROGNOSIS OF CUTANEOUS MALIGNANT MELANOMA

Radial versus vertical growth pattern
Breslow's thickness
Clark's level
Nodular morphology
Regressive changes
Mitosis
Ulceration
Lymphocytic response
Microsatellitosis

Primary mucosal melanoma of the upper aerodigestive mucosa is a rarity. It may arise from pre-existing melanocytes in the squamous or respiratory mucosa and usually presents as polypoid growths. In a series of 259 patients from the United Kingdom, 69 percent of mucosal melanoma occurred in the nasal cavities and sinuses (Figure 2–37), 22 percent in the oral cavity and 9 percent in the pharynx, larynx and upper esophagus.[50] In contrast to skin melanomas, no race distribution or relationship to exposure to sunlight has been noted. The mucosal-lentiginous melanoma is an in situ radial phase lesion where the tumor cells are arranged basally in the mucosa (see Figure 2–34B). Nodular and desmoplastic melanomas can also present in the mucosa. Presence of an in situ component or junctional activity helps to differentiate primary from metastatic mucosal melanoma. A significant number of mucosal melanomas are amelanotic. The typical immunohistochemical profile helps in the differential diagnosis of amelanotic melanoma from other undifferentiated tumors of the head and neck. The prognosis is generally poor although patients with melanomas less than 1 mm thick appear to do better.[51]

TUMORS OF THE SOFT TISSUES AND BONES

Almost any soft-tissue tumor (Table 2–4) occurring elsewhere in the body may be seen in the head and neck region. Only the more frequent ones will be described here.

The most frequent benign mesenchymal tumors of the head and neck are vascular in nature and

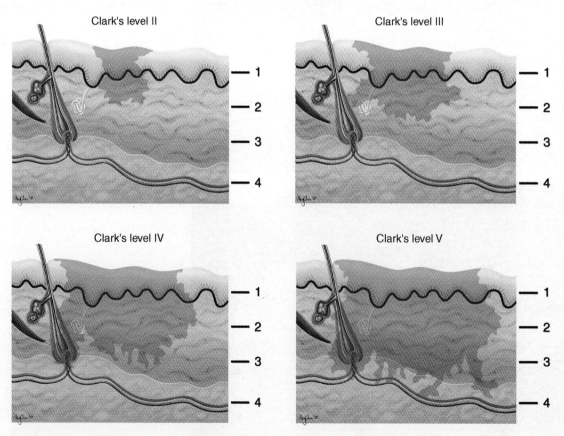

Figure 2–35. Microstaging vertical growth phase of malignant melanoma—Clark levels II to IV. The tumor has acquired metastatic potential.

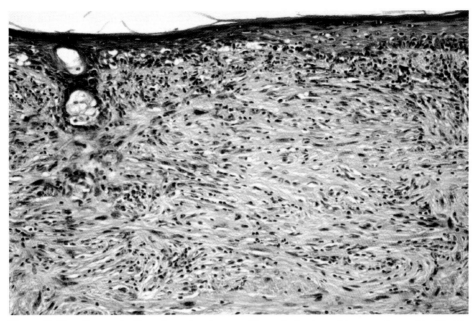

Figure 2–36. Desmoplastic malignant melanoma. The spindle-shaped tumor cells are identified in a very collagenous stroma.

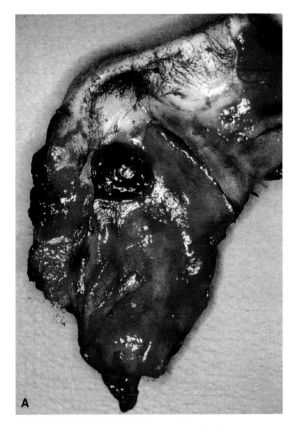

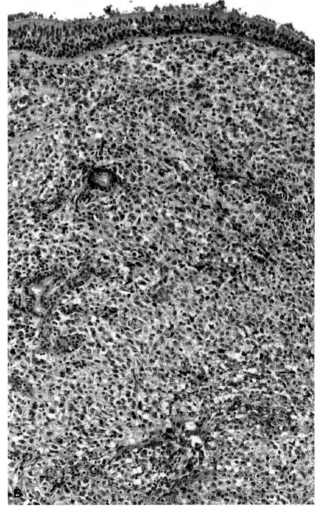

Figure 2–37. *A*, Mucosal malignant melanoma in the nasal septum. The tumor forms a raised, darkly pigmented nodule. *B*, Another sinonasal melanoma. This tumor is composed of amelanotic epithelioid cells which form a polypoid nodule underneath columnar ciliated respiratory mucosa.

include hemangioma and lymphangioma. Their frequent presence in childhood suggests a hamartomatous nature with congenital origin. The distinction between capillary and cavernous hemangiomas lies in the size of the vascular lumina and the thickness of the vessel wall (larger lumina and thicker walls in cavernous angiomas) (Figure 2–38). Lymphangiomas or cystic hygromas usually are congenital and occur in the neck. Angiosarcoma may be seen in the skin of the scalp and face in elderly individuals (Figure 2–39). The tumor may be indolent with a better prognosis than post-radiation and deep soft tissue angiosarcomas.

Lipoma are common, superficial, benign tumors of mature adipose tissue derivation (Figure 2–40). A special variant, the spindle cell lipoma has a propensity to occur in the back of the neck.

Granular cell tumor is a benign solitary subepithelial tumor characterized by large pink cells with abundant granular cytoplasm, bland nuclear morphology and diffuse positive reaction to S100 proteins on immunohistochemistry. Although a myogenous origin was once favored, hence the older term

Table 2–4. MESENCHYMAL TUMORS

Fatty Tumors
Benign: Lipoma
  Variants:
    Spindle cell
    Intra- and intermuscular
    Pleomorphic
    Myolipoma
    Angiolipoma
Malignant: Liposarcoma
  Variants:
    Atypical lipomatous tumor (well-differentiated liposarcoma)
    Myxoid
    Pleomorphic

Fibrous Tumors
Benign: Fibromatosis
Malignant: Fibrosarcoma
  Sclerosing epithelioid fibrosarcoma
  Fibromyxoid sarcoma
  (nodular and cranial fascitis—pseudotumor)

Fibrohistiocytic Tumors
Benign: Xanthoma
  Benign fibrous histiocytoma/ dermatofibroma
Borderline: Dermatofibrosarcoma protuberans
Malignant: Atypical fibroxanthoma (superficial MFH)
  Malignant fibrous histiocytoma (MFH)
  Variants:
    Pleomorphic
    Myxofibrosarcoma

Vascular Tumors
Benign: Hemangioma
  Variants:
    Capillary
    Cavernous
    Intramuscular
  Glomus tumor
  Lymphangioma
  Lymphangiomyoma
Borderline: Atypical vascular proliferation
  Hemangioendothelioma
  Hemangiopericytoma
Malignant: Angiosarcoma
  Kaposi's sarcoma

Neural Tumors
Benign: Schwannoma
    Cellular
    Ancient
  Neurofibroma
    Traumatic neuroma
    Plexiform neurofibroma
    Neurofibromatosis
Malignant: Malignant peripheral nerve sheath tumor

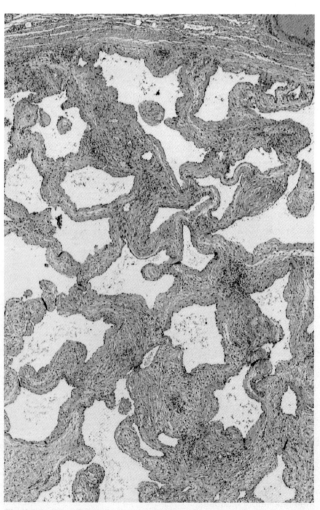

Figure 2–38. Cavernous hemangioma. The tumor is encapsulated and contains cavernous vascular spaces.

granular cell "myoblastoma," it is now believed to be of nerve sheath origin. The tongue and skin are frequent sites.

The desmoid tumor or fibromatosis usually presents in the neck of a young woman as a slow-growing mass. Grossly, the tumor is related to skeletal muscle and fascia, and is firm and white on cut surface. Microscopically, the tumor cells are bland, uniform, spindle-shaped with myofibroblastic differentiation (Figure 2–41). The tumor is locally infiltrative with frequent involvement of several resection margins and has a great tendency for multiple recurrences. It should be distinguished from a fibrosarcoma, as the latter has metastatic capabilities even when it is low grade.

Dermatofibrosarcoma protuberans is an uncommon, locally aggressive fibrohistiocytic neoplasm of trunk and lower extremity which may rarely occur in the head and neck in middle-aged patients. There is a slight male preponderance. Microscopically, the tumor is composed of uniform, benign-appearing spindle cells arranged in a "storiform" pattern infiltrating into the dermis and subcutaneous tissue. A pigmented variant, the so-called Bednar tumor is also known. A dermatofibroma (benign fibrous histiocytoma), on the other hand, is a non-infiltrative benign dermal tumor, usually less than 3 cm in size which can be cured by local excision alone.

Atypical fibroxanthoma (superficial malignant fibrous histiocytoma) is a dermal tumor characterized by markedly atypical mitotically-active spindle cells with paradoxically low-grade behavior. The typical patient is elderly and the lesion may affect the face or scalp. The tumor has low metastatic potential which may be heralded by multiple recurrences, deep soft tissue and vascular invasion and necrosis.

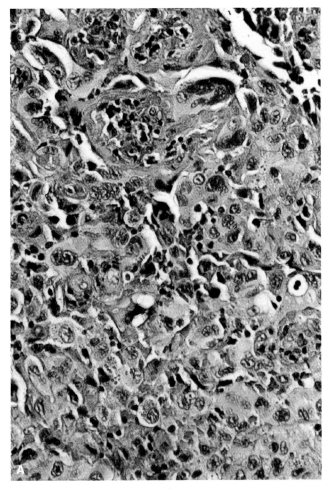 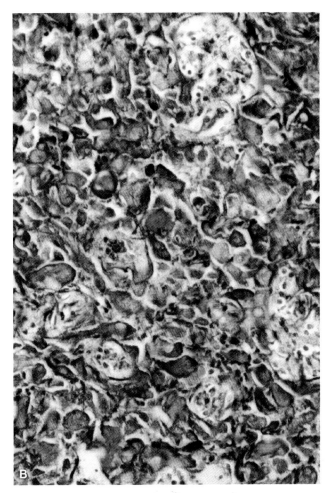

Figure 2–39. *A*, Epithelioid angiosarcoma in the skin of the forehead of an 85-year-old man. The bizarre, pleomorphic tumor cells are lining clefts and spaces, recapitulating the tendency of the endothelial cells to line blood vessels. *B*, Immunohistochemistry for CD31, an endothelial cell marker, shows strong, diffuse positive cytoplasmic reaction.

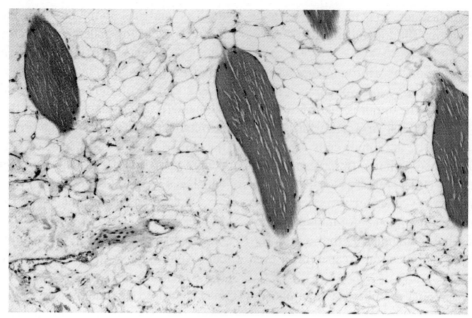

Figure 2–40. Intramuscular infiltrating lipoma of the retropharynx. Mature adipose tissue is seen dissecting skeletal muscle fibers. Although benign, this tumor is difficult to excise completely and may recur.

Malignant fibrous histiocytoma (MFH), a usually high-grade spindle cell sarcoma of fibrohistiocytic origin rarely presents in the deep soft tissue of the head and neck. Most patients are elderly males. This is the most common post-radiation sarcoma. The most frequent variant, pleomorphic MFH, is composed of highly atypical cells arranged in a storiform pattern and shows brisk mitosis, tumor necrosis and giant cells (Figure 2–42). The myxoid variant, myxofibrosarcoma is relatively low grade.

Rhabdomyosarcoma

Rhabdomyosarcoma (RMS) is the most frequent soft-tissue sarcoma in the head and neck. It occurs most commonly in the pediatric age group and rarely in older people. The common sites are orbit, nose and paranasal sinuses, the middle ear and the mastoid. In the nose, they may present as polypoid, grape-like masses giving rise to the name sarcoma botryoides. Microscopically , the majority of tumors are alveolar RMS (Figure 2–43). Immunohistochemical demonstration of myoid differentiation such as positive staining for desmin, actin, and myosin among many others helps distinguish them from other small "blue" cell tumors, eg, non-Hodgkin's lymphoma, olfactory neuroblastoma, Ewing's sarcoma/primitive

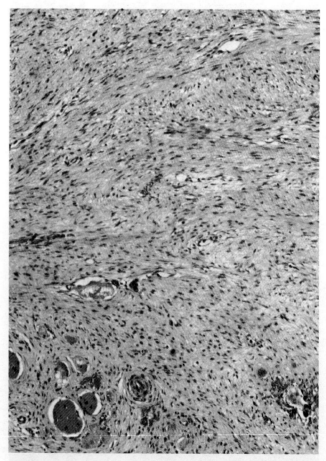

Figure 2–41. Fibromatosis of the neck in a young woman. The tumor is highly collagenous (desmoid) and composed of spindle cells with bland uniform nuclei which have infiltrated the adjacent skeletal muscle.

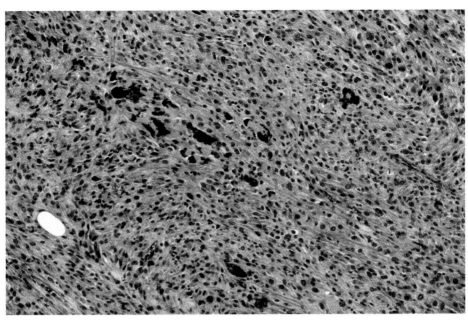

Figure 2–42. Malignant fibrous histiocytoma—pleomorphic variant. This is a high-grade spindle cell neoplasm demonstrating marked pleomorphism and multinucleated tumor giant cells.

neuroectodermal tumor, other neuroectodermal, neuroendocrine and in adults amelanotic melanoma. The embryonal RMS is hypocellular and myxoid with no fibrosis and has a better prognosis than the alveolar RMS. The sarcoma botryoides, a variant of embryonal RMS, is characterized by a thin, submucosal "cambium" layer of hypercellularity overlying areas of loose, edematous, hypocellular tumor. This variant has an excellent prognosis. A characteristic finding of all RMSs is the presence of at least a few tumor cells with abundant pink cytoplasm. Although the older literature shows a distinct survival disadvantage in RMS, with the new multimodal therapy, survival appears to depend on the clinical stage.[52]

Osteoma is a common benign bone tumor of the head and neck microscopically composed of lamellar bone which may be arranged into outer cortical and inner cancellous bone with marrow elements (ivory osteomas). They are common in the paranasal sinuses, frontal being most frequently affected. Multiple osteomas are associated with Gardner's syndrome.

Benign fibro-osseous lesions run the gamut from fibrous dysplasia to ossifying fibroma to cemento-ossifying fibroma. Fibrous dysplasia is an ill-defined solid lesion consisting of thin trabeculae of irregular, curvilinear woven bone directly formed by fibrous tissue. Ossifying fibroma (OF) is rare and is composed of fibrous tissue and woven bone trabeculae which have osteoblastic rimming. Radiologically, OF is well defined whereas fibrous dysplasia has merging outlines. Cemento-ossifying fibroma has, in addition to bone, cementum formation (Figure 2–44). A juvenile aggressive form of ossifying fibroma occurs in patients in their early teens.

Eosinophilic granuloma of the bone has been noted in the skull or skull base where it can involve the sella turcica and present with symptoms attributable to pituitary dysfunction. The tumor is composed of Langerhans' cells which demonstrate S100 protein and CD1 immunoreactivity and contain an admixture of other inflammatory cells including eosinophils. Birbeck granules are ultrastructural hallmarks of the Langerhans' cells.

Osteosarcoma

This is the most frequent malignant bone tumor of the head and neck. About 6 percent of all osteosarcoma occur in the jaw.[53] They are usually spontaneous, but risk factors include radiation, Paget's disease and retinoblastoma, among others.[54] There is an almost equal distribution in the maxilla and mandible. A male preponderance with a peak incidence in the early fourth decade is noted. Histologically, most

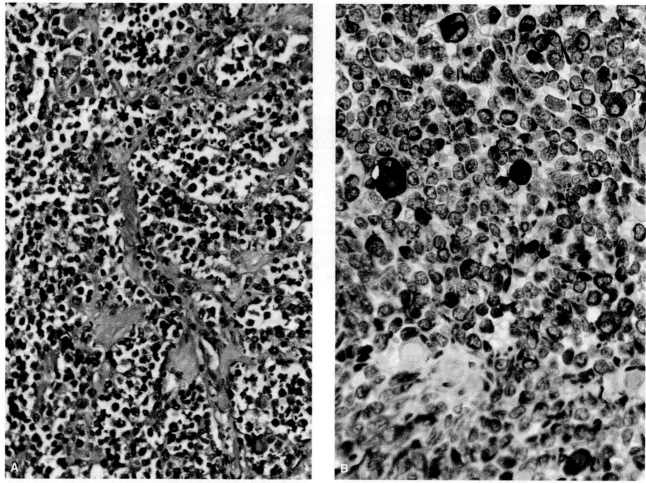

Figure 2–43. *A,* Solid alveolar rhabdomyosarcoma of left periparotid soft tissue in a 47-year-old male consisting of predominantly round tumor cells with hyperchromatic nuclei and scant cytoplasm. Presence of occasional cells with abundant deep pink, glassy cytoplasm is a clue to rhabdoid differentiation. The alveolar pattern is produced by thin fibrous septa intersecting the tumor. *B,* Immunohistochemistry with anti-desmin antibody shows several cells expressing this cytoplasmic protein and further supporting the skeletal muscle differentiation.

Figure 2–44. Cementifying fibroma. The tumor occurred in the maxilla of a 15-year-old boy and shows cementicles within fibrous tumor tissue.

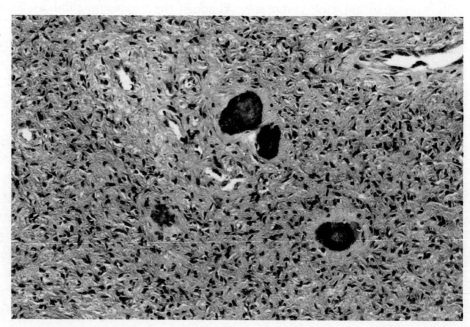

gnathic osteosarcomas are well-differentiated low-grade tumors and may show osteoblastic, fibroblastic and chondroblastic differentiation (Figure 2–45). The direction of differentiation does not have prognostic significance. The prognosis is better than extra-gnathic osteosarcoma and distant metastasis is infrequent. Radical surgical resection with negative margins as initial therapy is more effective than combined modality treatment. There is no well-documented relationship between response to chemotherapy and degree of tumor necrosis in gnathic osteosarcomas in contrast to the extra-gnathic osteosarcomas.

Chondrosarcoma may occur in the base of the skull, in the craniofacial bones, larynx, trachea or the cervical vertebrae. Most are low-grade conventional chondrosarcomas (Figure 2–46), although mesenchymal, skeletal and extra-skeletal myxoid and dedifferentiated chondrosarcomas are also described.[55–57]

Chordomas arising in the spheno-occipital area and the upper cervical vertebrae can present as nasopharyngeal tumors. These are low-grade, locally aggressive tumors believed to derive from embryonal notochordal remnants and are comprised of lobules of cells with abundant foamy cytoplasm and the characteristic physaliphorous cells. Immunohistochemically, the cells are positive for cytokeratin and S100 protein.

TUMORS OF THE SKIN

Several benign tumors of the skin appendages frequently affect the head and neck. The classic cylindroma (turban tumor) is a tumor of eccrine origin which is usually solitary but can be multiple. It produces abundant basement membrane material and shows myoepithelial differentiation. Syringomas are eccrine tumors usually occurring in the lower eyelid

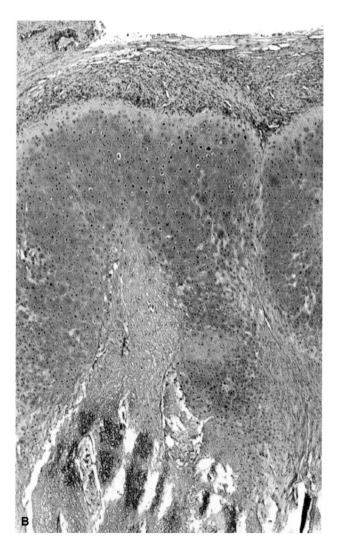

Figure 2–45. *A,* Osteosarcoma of the right maxilla in a 37-year-old woman. The tumor is gray-white and bone-hard, and replaces the maxillary sinus entirely. *B,* At low magnification, the tumor is lobulated and shows a zonation from extremely cellular to chondroblastic to osteogenic areas, which is characteristic of osteosarcomas in the maxilla.

in women and which may be multiple. Chondroid syringoma (mixed tumor) is the cutaneous counterpart of the pleomorphic adenoma of the salivary glands and shows myoepithelial differentiation. It is believed to be eccrine in origin. Pilomatrixoma (synonym: pilomatricoma, calcifying epithelioma of Malherbe) is a benign tumor of the pilar apparatus and occurs in children and young adults. Another benign tumor of the hair follicle cells is the pilar tumor which usually affects women; it occurs in the scalp and at the base of neck and can grow quite large.

Squamous Cell Carcinoma

The squamous cell carcinoma is the most common malignant tumor of the skin, particularly in the head and neck. A relationship with cumulative sun exposure, actinic keratosis and SCC has been noted; p53 mutation by ultraviolet light is a postulated mechanism. Actinic keratosis is characterized by atrophy of the epidermis with dysplasia of the basal layer in a background of solar elastosis. All morphologic variants of SCC have been identified in the skin of the head and neck. In addition, an excessively keratinized variant, SCC with horn formation, may also be seen. Verrucous SCC needs to be differentiated from keratoacanthoma which is a rapidly-growing benign lesion affecting males more frequently than females. The diagnosis is made on the characteristic architecture which shows a keratin-filled epidermal crater with overhanging edges. Most lesions regress spontaneously after a few weeks, suggesting a viral etiology. Because of the cytologic overlap with SCC and the reports of metastasizing keratoacanthomas, it has been suggested that all keratoacanthomas should be considered variant SCC.

Basal Cell Carcinoma

Basal cell carcinoma (BCC) is a malignant tumor of the basal layer of the epidermis arising in a background of prolonged cumulative exposure to sun and therefore is seen in older people. Although many morphologic forms are described, the superficial and sclerosing BCCs require special mention because of a high propensity for local recurrence. The superficial BCC is a clinically subtle in situ change in the basal layer of epidermis characterized

by multifocality and skip lesions. The sclerosing or morpheaform BCC is accompanied by a pseudosarcomatous stroma with very few infiltrating carcinoma cells. In a surgical excision, it is difficult to assess the margins without the help of immunohistochemistry. This usually indolent tumor can be locally destructive and may metastasize if neglected. Basal cell nevus syndrome is discussed in tumors of the dentoalveolar structures (Figure 2–47).

Sebaceous carcinoma is a rare high-grade tumor showing sebaceous differentiation (Figure 2–48). The majority of these carcinomas arise in the eyelid in association with meibomian glands.[58] It may be associated with multiple visceral malignancies (Muir-Torre syndrome). Rarely, it has been reported in the parotid glands.

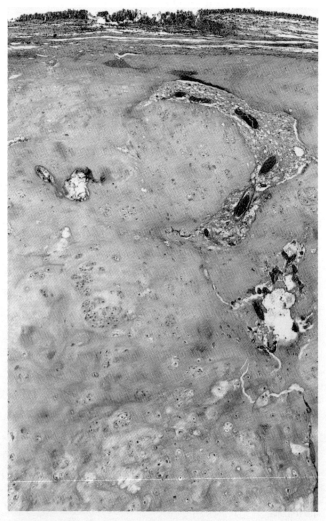

Figure 2–46. Chondrosarcoma of the larynx in an 84-year-old man. Lobules of tumor cartilage push the respiratory epithelium of the larynx.

Sweat gland carcinoma is another rare skin-appendage carcinoma that can occur in the face and the scalp. The adenoid cystic carcinoma, sclerosing sweat duct carcinoma and mucinous carcinoma are some of the variants.

Merkel cell carcinoma and malignant melanoma are discussed in the section on neuroendocrine and neuroectodermal tumors.

TUMORS AND CYSTS OF THE DENTOALVEOLAR STRUCTURES

About 9 percent of all tumors in the oral cavity are odontogenic and may differentiate toward epithelial or the odontogenic ectomesenchymal line and are classified accordingly (Table 2–5). They are predominantly benign with rare exceptions.

Ameloblastoma is a locally aggressive, usually intraosseous tumor of odontogenic epithelium most commonly involving the posterior part of mandible and sometimes the posterior maxilla. The tumor affects both sexes at all ages, with a higher incidence in the third to fifth decades. The tumors are usually multicystic with solid areas (Figure 2–49). Various histologic types are described, the most common being follicular and plexiform. The uncommon unicystic variant may be radiologically misinterpreted as an odontogenic cyst. The peripheral ameloblas-

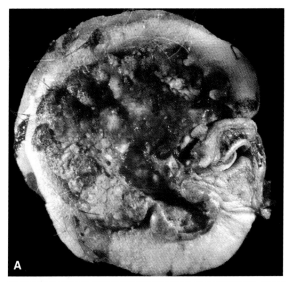

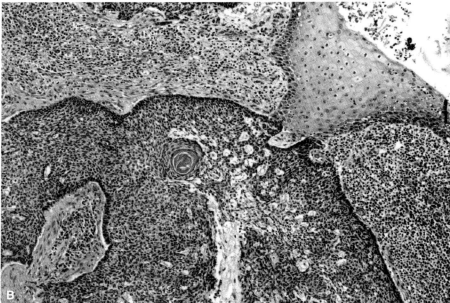

Figure 2–47. *A*, A neglected basal cell carcinoma of the skin of face. The patient was a 73-year-old woman who had the lesion for many years. The eye is identified in the right side of the photograph. *B*, Microphotograph shows nests of cellular blue basaloid cells with peripheral pallisading, central small cyst formation and a single keratin pearl. The tumor is connected to the overlying epidermis.

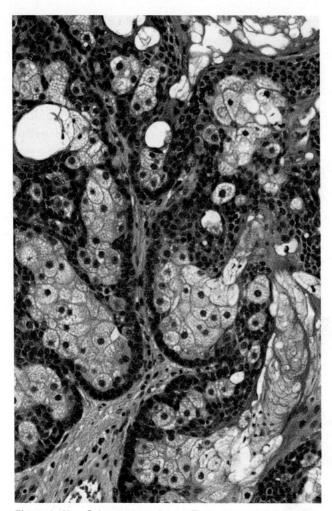

Figure 2–48. Sebaceous carcinoma. The tumor shows sebaceous differentiation with large cells with multiple small vacuoles. The smaller cells with hyperchromatic nuclei can show brisk mitosis. Keratinization is identified.

Table 2–5. BENIGN TUMORS OF THE ODONTOGENIC TISSUE
Tumors related to Odontogenic Epithelium
Ameloblastoma: central and peripheral
Squamous odontogenic tumor
Clear cell odontogenic tumor
Calcifying epithelial odontogenic tumor
Tumors related to Odontogenic Mesenchyme
Odontogenic fibroma: central and peripheral
Odontogenic myxoma/fibromyxoma
Cementifying tumors
Cementoblastoma (cementoma)
Cementifying and cemento-ossifying fibroma
Mixed Tumors related to Odontogenic Epithelium
and Mesenchyme
Ameloblastic fibroma
Ameloblastic fibrodentinoma
Ameloblastic fibro-odontoma
Odontoameloblastoma
Odontoma: complex and compound
Adenomatoid odontogenic tumor
Calcifying odontogenic cyst

demonstrates additional formation of dentine, and the latter both dentine and enamel. The tumors show variable radio-opacity depending upon the amount of dentine and enamel formation.

Squamous odontogenic tumor is an intraosseous infiltrative tumor composed of islands of well-differentiated squamous cells, sometimes with central cystic change. Most behave in a benign fashion requiring curettage only. The clear cell odontogenic tumor consists of islands of clear epithelial cells. Most tumors are benign though locally aggressive, and clinical behavior appears to be slightly worse than ameloblastoma. Rarely, primary intraosseous squamous cell carcinoma

toma is extraosseous, located in the gingiva or buccal mucosa. The unicystic peripheral and desmoplastic ameloblastoma have lower recurrence rates than the conventional multicystic ameloblastoma. Rare metastasis after prolonged illness punctuated by multiple surgeries and/or radiotherapy is known (malignant ameloblastoma). Odontoameloblastoma is an extremely rare, composite, true neoplasm consisting of an ameloblastoma and hard dental tissue eg, dentine, cementum or enamel. The clinical behavior is similar to ameloblastoma.

The ameloblastic fibroma is essentially a solid intraosseous fibrous lesion with scattered foci of attenuated ameloblastic epithelium. Ameloblastic fibrodentinoma (dentinoma) and fibro-odontoma are similar to ameloblastic fibroma, but the former

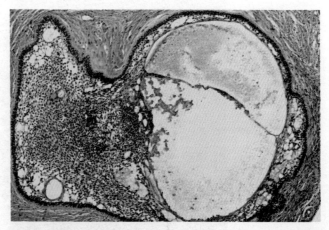

Figure 2–49. Ameloblastoma. The central cystic portion of the tumor contains a loose reticulum of stellate cells. There is a peripheral layer of tall columnar cells with dark nuclei resembling the inner dental epithelium.

and clear cell adenocarcinoma (odontogenic carcinoma) occur and are believed to arise in intraosseous remnants of the odontogenic epithelium. They may be seen in association with an odontogenic cyst (type 1), ameloblastoma (type 2) or may arise de novo (type 3), and may be keratinizing or non-keratinizing.

The calcifying epithelial odontogenic tumor (Pindborg tumor) presents as a painless slow-growing mass of variable radiolucency, most commonly in the posterior lower jaw, in adults between the ages of 20 to 60 years. It may be associated with an unerupted tooth. One-third of cases may present in the maxilla. Microscopically, the tumor shows sheets of polyhedral, sometimes pleomorphic epithelial and clear cells in a fibrous stroma. Characteristically, large globular masses of acidophilic amyloid-like material and variable degrees of calcification may be seen. The clinical behavior is similar to ameloblastoma. The adenomatoid odontogenic tumor occurs commonly in the anterior maxilla in the second decade of life. The presence of a capsule, duct-like structures and dentine are characteristic. Enucleation may be adequate treatment. Calcifying odontogenic cyst has a cystic component lined by odontogenic epithelium containing characteristic "ghost" epithelial cells, and a mesenchymal component which may contain dental hard tissue. It usually presents as an intraosseous lesion in the second decade of life and may not be a true neoplasm.

Odontoma is a developmental anomaly occurring in association with the crown of a developing tooth in young individuals. The complex odontoma consists of a disordered mixture of dentine, enamel, cementum and odontogenic epithelium whereas the same components are more orderly with tooth-like formations in the compound odontoma.

Mesenchymal odontogenic tumors are usually tumors of young people affecting the mandible. The odontogenic fibroma may be intraosseous (central) or in the gingiva (peripheral) and contains odontogenic epithelium. Myxoma is locally destructive and extends through the bone into the soft tissue, making complete surgical resection difficult. Cementoblastoma (cementoma) consists of large fusing globules and masses of cementum associated with the root of a tooth. A special variant, the gigantiform cementoma is a bilateral deposition of cementum in both jaws of young black women with an autosomal dominant inheritance pattern.

Most cysts of the jaw are not true neoplasms. They may arise in the odontogenic epithelium or in developmental fissures. A diagrammatic representation of the different odontogenic cysts is depicted in Figure 2–50.

The most common cyst is the periapical or radicular cyst, an incidental radiologic discovery. The cyst is usually less than 1 cm in size with stratified squamous lining associated with inflammation.

The dentigerous cyst is a destructive cyst associated with the crown of an unerupted and displaced permanent tooth (Figure 2–51). Rarely, neoplastic transformation to ameloblastoma can occur.

Odontogenic keratocyst is another destructive uni- or multiloculated cystic lesion in the posterior mandible and maxilla (Figure 2–52). These cysts

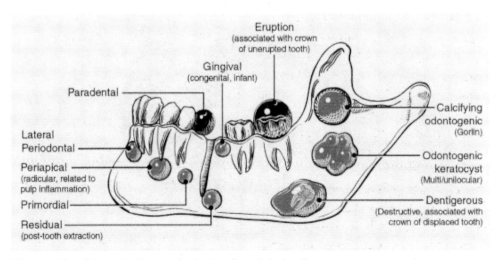

Figure 2–50. Schematic diagram of odontogenic cysts by location.

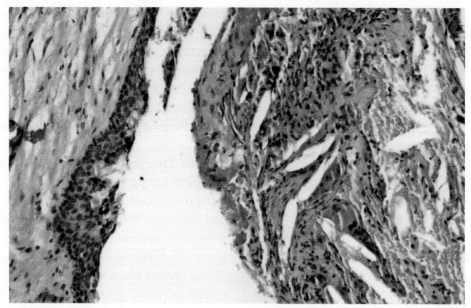

Figure 2–51. Dentigerous cyst. The cyst is lined by stratified squamous epithelium with an admixture of mucus-secreting cells. The lumen contains hemorrhagic debris showing cholesterol clefts.

have a high propensity for destructive growth and recurrence. They may be associated with the nevoid basal cell carcinoma syndrome, an autosomal dominant condition with high penetrance described by Gorlin and Goltz.[59] Other components of the syndrome include skeletal abnormalities, ectopic calcification and dyskeratotic pitting of the hands and feet.

Fissural or developmental cysts are believed to arise in the epithelium entrapped between the bony parts of the jaw bones during embryologic development. The different types are depicted in the diagram (Figure 2–53). The most common is the midline nasopalatine cyst which may be within the bone or in the soft tissue. The lateral nasolabial cyst is also a soft-tissue cyst. The other types of cysts are intraosseous.

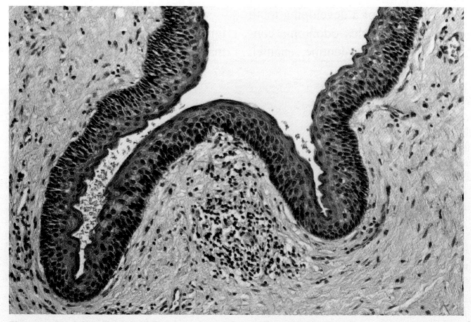

Figure 2–52. Odontogenic keratocyst. The cyst is lined by stratified squamous cells showing keratinization toward the surface.

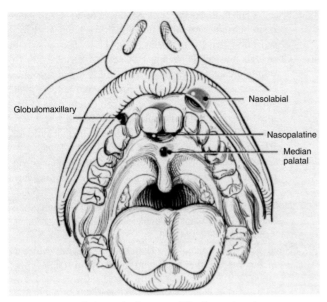

Globulomaxillary

Nasolabial

Nasopalatine

Median
palatal

Figure 2–53.   Schematic diagram of the fissural cysts.

REFERENCES

1. Ridolfi RL, Lieberman PH, Erlandson RA, Moore OS. Schneiderian papillomas: a clinicopathologic study of 30 cases. Am J Surg Pathol 1977;1:43–53.

2. Mashberg A. Erythroplasia: the earliest sign of asymptomatic oral cancer. J Am Dent Assoc 1978;96:615–20.

3. Shafer WG, Waldron CA. Erythroplakia of the oral cavity. Cancer 1975;36:1021–8.

4. Silverman S Jr, Gorsky M. Proliferative verrucous leukoplakias: a follow-up of 54 cases. Oral Surg Oral Med Oral Pathol Oral Radiol Endod 1997;84:154–7.

5. Batsakis JG, Suarez P, El-Naggar AK. Proliferative verrucous leukoplakia and its related lesions. Oral Oncol 1999; 35:354–9.

6. Coltrera MD, Zarbo RJ, Sakr WA, Gown AM. Markers of dysplasia of the upper aerodigestive tract. Suprabasal expression of PCNA, p53 and CK19 in alcohol fixed paraffin embedded tissue. Am J Pathol 1992;141:817–25.

7. Mohit-Tabatai MA, et al. Relation of thickness of floor of mouth stage I and II cancers to regional metastasis. Am J Surg 1986;152:351.

8. Spiro RH, Huvos AG, Wong GY, et al. Predictive value of tumor thickness in squamous carcinoma confined to the tongue and floor of mouth. Am J Surg 1986;152:345–50.

9. Urist M, O'Brien CJ, Soong SJ, et al. Squamous cell carcinoma of the buccal mucosa: analysis of prognostic factors. Am J Surg 1987;154:411.

10. Yamamoto E, Miyakawa A, Kohama G. Mode of invasion and lymph node metastasis in squamous cell carcinoma of the oral cavity. Head Neck Surg 1984;6:938–47.

11. Spiro RH, Guillamondegui O Jr, Paulino AF, Huvos AG. Pattern of invasion and margin assessment in patients with oral tongue cancer. Head Neck 1999;21:408–13.

12. McGregor AD, MacDonald DG. Patterns of spread of squamous cell carcinoma within the mandible. Head Neck 1989;11:457–61.

13. Medina JE, Dichtel W, Luna MA. Verrucous squamous carcinomas of the oral cavity. A clinicopathologic study of 104 cases. Arch Otolaryngol 1984;110:437–40.

14. Winzenburg SM, Nichans GA, George E, et al. Basaloid squamous cell carcinoma: a clinical comparison of two histologic types with poorly differentiated squamous cell carcinoma. 1998;119:471–5.

15. Banks ER, Frierson HF Jr, Mills SE, et al. Basaloid squamous cell carcinoma of the head and neck: a clinicopathologic and immunohistochemical study of 40 cases. Am J Surg Pathol 1992;16:939–46.

16. Nakhleh RE, et al. Myogenic differentiation in spindle cell (sarcomatoid) carcinomas of the upper aerodigestive tract. Appl Immunohistochem 1993;1:58–68.

17. Gaffey MJ, Weiss LM. Association of Epstein-Barr virus with human neoplasia. Pathol Annu 1992;27(Pt 1):55–74.

18. Spiro RH. Salivary neoplasms, overview of a 35 year experience with 2,807 patients. Head Neck Surg 1986;8: 177–84.

19. Spiro RH, Huvos AG, Strong EW. Malignant mixed tumor of salivary origin, a clinicopathologic study of 146 cases. Cancer 1977;39:388–96.

20. Tortoledo ME, Luna MA, Batsakis JG. Carcinoma ex pleomorphic adenoma and malignant mixed tumor. Histomorphologic indexes. Arch Otolaryngol 1984;110:172–6.

21. Bleiweiss IJ, Huvos AG, Lara J, Strong EW. Carcinosarcoma of the submandibular salivary gland. Immunohistochemical findings. Cancer 1992;69:2031–35.

22. Spiro RH. Management of malignant tumors of the salivary glands. Oncology 1998;12:671–80.

23. Eveson JW, Cawson RA. Salivary gland tumors. A review of 2,410 cases with particular reference to histological types, site, age and sex distribution. J Pathol 1985;146:51–8.

24. Spiro RH, Huvos AG, Berk R, Strong EW. Mucoepidermoid carcinoma of salivary gland origin. A clinicopathologic study of 367 cases. Am J Surg 1978;136:461–8.

25. Spiro RH. Distant metastasis in adenoid cystic carcinoma of salivary origin. Am J Surg 1997;174:495–8.

26. Freedman PD, Lumerman H. Lobular carcinoma of intraoral minor salivary gland origin. Report of twelve cases. Oral Surg 1983;56:157–65.

27. Batsakis JG, Pinkston GR, Luna MA, et al. Adenocarcinoma of the oral cavity: A clinicopathologic study of terminal duct carcinoma. J Laryngol Otol 1983;97:825–35.

28. Perez-Ordonez B, Linkov I, Huvos AG. Polymorphous low-grade adenocarcinoma of minor salivary glands: a study of 17 cases with emphasis on cell differentiation. Histopathology 1998;32:521–9.

29. Spiro RH, Huvos AG, Strong EW. Acinic cell carcinoma of salivary origin: a clinicopathologic study of 67 cases. Cancer 1978;41:924–35.

30. Stanley RJ, Weiland LH, Olsen KD, et al. Dedifferentiated acinic (acinus) cell carcinoma of the parotid gland. Otolaryngol Head Neck Surg 1988;98:155–61.

31. Ellis GL, Auclair PL. Tumors of the salivary gland. 3rd series. Washington (DC): Armed Forces Institute of Pathology; 1996. p.183–203.

32. Spiro RH, Huvos AG, Strong EW. Adenocarcinoma of salivary origin. Clinicopathologic study of 204 patients. Am J Surg 1982;144:423–31.

33. Arthaud JB. Anaplastic parotid carcinoma (malignant lymphoepithelial lesion) in seven Alaskan natives. Am J Clin Pathol 1972;57:275–86.

34. Fujimoto Y, Obara T, Ito Y, et al. Diffuse sclerosing variant of papillary carcinoma of thyroid. Clinical importance, surgical treatment and follow-up study. Cancer 1990;66:2306–12.

35. Johnson TL, Lloyd RV, Thompson NW, et al. Prognostic implication of the tall cell variant of papillary thyroid carcinoma. Am J Surg Pathol 1988;12:22–7.

36. Evans HL. Columnar-cell carcinoma of the thyroid. A report of two cases of an aggressive variant of thyroid carcinoma. Am J Clin Pathol 1986;85:77–80.

37. Harach HR, Williams GT, Williams ED. Familial adenomatous polyposis-associated thyroid carcinoma: a distinct type of follicular cell neoplasm. Histopathology 1994;25:549–61.

38. Lang W, Choritz H, Hundeshagen H. Risk factors in follicular thyroid carcinomas. A retrospective follow-up study covering a 14-year period with emphasis on morphological findings. Am J Surg Pathol 1986;10:246–55.

39. Mueller-Gaertner HW, Brzac HT, Rehpenning W. Prognostic indices for tumor relapse and tumor mortality in follicular thyroid carcinoma. Cancer 1991;67:1903–11.

40. Har-El G, Hadar T, Segal K, et al. Hürthle cell carcinoma of the thyroid gland. A tumor of moderate malignancy. Cancer 1986;57:1613-7.

41. Hofstra RM, Landsvater RM, Ceccherini I, et al. A mutation of RET proto-oncogene associated with MEN2B and sporadic medullary thyroid carcinoma. Nature 1994;367:375–6.

42. Chan JK, Albores-Saavedra J, Battifora H, et al. Sclerosing mucoepidermoid thyroid carcinoma with eosinophilia. A distinctive low grade malignancy arising from the metaplastic follicles of Hashimoto's thyroiditis. Am J Surg Pathol 1991;15:438–48.

43. Chan JK, Rosai J. Tumors of the neck showing thymic or related branchial pouch differentiation. A unifying concept. Hum Pathol 1991;22:349–67.

44. Argani P, Perez-Ordonez B, Xiao H, et al. Olfactory neuroblastoma is not related to the Ewing family of tumors. Absence of EWS/FLI1 gene fusion and MIC2 expression. Am J Surg Pathol 1998;22:391–8.

45. Frierson HF Jr, Ross GW, Mills SE, Frankfurter A. Olfactory neuroblastoma. Additional immunohistochemical characterization. Am J Clin Pathol 1990;94:547–53.

46. Chan JK, Suster S, Wenig BM, et al. Cytokeratin 20 immunoreactivity distinguishes Merkel cell (primary cutaneous neuroendocrine) carcinomas and salivary gland small cell carcinomas from small cell carcinomas of various sites. Am J Surg Pathol 1997;21:226–34.

47. Busam KJ, Jungbluth AA. Melan A. A new melanocytic differentiation marker. Adv Anat Pathol 1999;6:12–8.

48. Huvos AG, Shah JP, Mike V. Prognostic factors in cutaneous malignant melanoma. A comparative study of long term and short term survivors. Hum Pathol 1974;5:347–57.

49. Donnellan MJ, Seemayer T, Huvos AG, et al. Clinicopathologic study of cutaneous melanoma of the head and neck. Am J Surg 1972;124:450–5.

50. Nandapalan V, Roland NJ, Helliwell TR, et al. Mucosal melanoma of the head and neck. Clin Otolaryngol 1998;23:107–16.

51. McKinnon JG, Kokal WA, Neifeld JP, Kay S. Natural history and treatment of mucosal melanoma. J Surg Oncol 1989;41:222–5.

52. Kraus DH, Saenz NC, Gollamudi S, et al. Pediatric rhabdomyosarcoma of the head and neck. Am J Surg 1997;174:556–60.

53. Clark JL, Unni KK, Dahlin DC, Devine KD. Osteosarcoma of the jaw. Cancer 1983;51:2311–6.

54. Kassir RR, Rassekh CH, Kinsella JB, et al. Osteosarcoma of the head and neck: meta-analysis of nonrandomized studies. Laryngoscope 1997;107:56–61.

55. Arlen M, Follefsen HR, Huvos AG, Marcove RE. Chondrosarcoma of the head and neck. Am J Surg 1970;120:456–60.

56. Ruark DS, Schlehaider UK, Shah JP. Chondrosarcoma of the head and neck. World J Surg 1992;16:1010–6.

57. Huvos AG, Rosen G, Dabska M, Marcove RC. Mesenchymal chondrosarcoma: a clinicopathologic analysis of 35 patients with emphasis on treatment. Cancer 1983;51:1230–7.

58. Zurcher M, Hintschich C, Garner A, et al. Sebaceous carcinoma of the eyelid: a clinicopathological study. Br J Ophthalmol 1989;82:1049–55.

59. Gorlin RJ, Goltz RW. Multiple nevoid basal cell epithelioma, jaw cysts and syndrome. N Engl J Med 1962;262:908–14.

3

Head and Neck Imaging

BERNARD B. O'MALLEY, MD

Imaging the neck is unlike imaging any region of the torso or brain since maximal contrast resolution is necessary to differentiate lesions in cross-sectional exams of those solid organs. Because of the various organ systems, the neck has very good native contrast resolution between lesions and adjacent normal structures and at the interface with the skull base and thoracic inlet. Intravenous contrast is necessary, however, to differentiate veins (and arteries) from adenopathy and masses (Figure 3–1). Once a baseline scan has been obtained, contrast is less important for this particular consideration. Intravenous contrast also helps characterize internal lymph node architecture for necrosis. Bolus timing parameters are dependent on the equipment used[1] and the medical condition of the patient. Oral contrast in the form of barium paste is helpful for lesions of the hypopharyngo-esophageal complex. The throat, being a semi-collapsed tube, is difficult to evaluate on cross-sectional images. The importance of cross-sectional imaging is in evaluating the submucosal component of lesions (Figure 3–2), complementing the clinical and endoscopic exam. Imaging is therefore not valuable for detection of mucosal disease and cannot be a substitute for clinical inspection. Evaluating a palpable neck mass[2] and staging a known mucosal or sinonasal lesion is the primary role for imaging of the neck and head. Lesions of the nasopharynx, parapharyngeal space, sinonasal tract and subglottic space are better staged by the cross-sectional exam, however. Familiarity with the imaging of lymphomas and benign[3] or inflammatory lesions of the neck can prevent unnecessary surgical explorations in this functionally and cosmetically sensitive region.[4] Imaging exams have been docu-

mented to improve upon the accuracy of clinical lymph node staging. This is true of either computed tomography (CT), magnetic resonance imaging (MRI) or sonography and nuclear imaging including fluorodeoxyglucose-positron emission tomography (FDG-PET). Intravenous contrast is necessary to characterize internal lymph node architecture on CT, but less important on MRI. Careful attention to lymph node sub-sites is needed at the lateral retropharyngeal (Figure 3–3) and tracheo-esophageal groove (Figure 3–4) when appropriate. The added value of sonography is the capacity to perform fine-needle aspiration (FNA) of suspicious lymph nodes,[5] which might otherwise look unremarkable on other imaging modalities or feel unimportant to the examiner. With proper attention to technique,

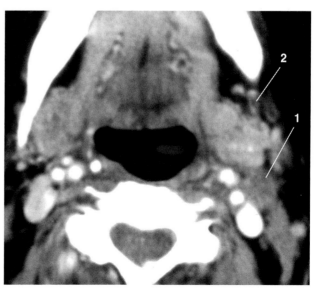

Figure 3–1. Enhanced axial CT image through the oropharynx. (1) Partially necrotic pathologic lymph node (level II). (2) Normal submandibular node (level I-b) with fatty hilum.

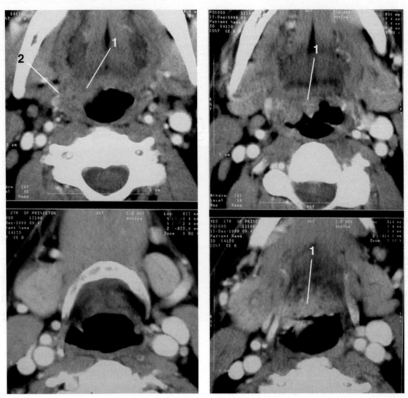

Figure 3–2.   Enhanced axial CT images through the oropharynx. (1) Base of tongue squamous cancer extending to lateral pharyngeal wall. (2) Early extra-pharyngeal extension into parapharyngeal space.

both the neck and the primary lesion can be adequately scanned at one imaging visit. Whether or not there is a known primary tumor, the contrast bolus should be peak for the axial survey of the neck. The primary site, if it is known, can be scanned in whatever plane necessary in the post-bolus phase of the scan. These issues are less important in MRI. As many as one-third of all N0 neck dissections show histologically positive metastatic adenopathy.[6] Imaging may demonstrate some of these occult metastases and thus improves upon the clinical exam.[7] In the N0 neck, FDG-PET (Figure 3–5) has been reported to be more sensitive than CT or MRI[8] and to have a sensitivity and specificity of approximately 90 percent.[9] However, true micro-metastases will remain below the resolution of cross-sectional exams and current FDG-PET technology, but enlarged lymph nodes should not be overlooked. One half of all missed lymph nodes are less than or equal to one centimeter in size. Careful analysis of high quality scans is necessary to maintain a respectable accuracy rate for staging the neck. Both

CT and MRI improve upon the clinical accuracy of 71 percent.[7] Conventional MR is not adequate[10] and has no benefit over CT.[11] The neck can be adequately staged if MR is chosen for staging of the primary site. FDG-PET is very accurate in the post-treatment setting compared to either CT or MRI.[12,13]

As in other body regions, a diagnosis has often been established and the imaging is performed to round out the TNM staging. While radiology is complementary to the clinical staging, it is responsible for so-called stage creep,[14,15] increasing the T, N, or M component of the diagnosis. The radiologist and clinical oncologist need to establish a rapport and select the modality most appropriate for their collective expertise and imaging armamentarium. Scan protocols must be established for consistency within a practice and at the very least among sequential follow-up surveillance-type scans on a given patient. Consistent imaging parameters from contrast injection rates through scan technique[16] to photography facilitate detection of subtle changes lending confidence to the diagnosis of often clinically occult

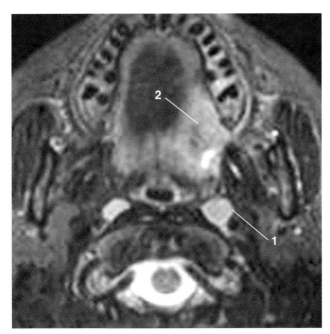

Figure 3–3. Axial T2-weighted MR image through the maxilla. (1) Metastatic left lateral retropharyngeal lymph node. (2) Palate tumor (hard and soft palate).

changes. Consistency also allows the other members of the clinical oncology team to work with reliable images for treatment planning.

Staging the index lesion involves evaluating for the possibility of clinical underestimation of the submucosal extent of disease[17] (Figure 3–6), invasion of adjacent vital structures[18] (Figure 3–7), and non-palpable adenopathy. Imaging for determination of the M stage of disease begins (and usually ends) with the chest radiograph. Cross-sectional imaging of the chest should be productive given the prevalence of smoking exposure in the head and neck cancer population. This would also serve as a baseline against which any developing apical pulmonary radiation changes or aspiration infiltrates could be compared. A well-designed scan of the neck that covers the superior mediastinum should provide adequate evaluation of the apical pulmonary region.

Detection and staging of neck lesions are very important for accurate assignment of initial treatment pathways for individual patients. High quality CT is usually adequate for most upper aerodigestive subsites. MRI is useful for skull base, larynx[19] and equivocal CT findings.[20] Follow-up imaging is very challenging, especially for the uninitiated. Distortion of tissue planes by biopsy, resection, neck dissection,

flap reconstruction (Figure 3–8) and/or radiation therapy can be very distracting and misleading.[21] Inflammatory changes related to chemotherapy-induced mucositis and superimposed radiation changes[22] limit our ability to diagnose mucosal recurrences. Lymph node metastases take unconventional pathways after neck dissection.[23] Different phases of contrast are beneficial for different modalities. Early phases are better for MRI[1] and later phases are better for CT.[24] Metabolic imaging in the form of FDG-PET will find a more important role for this stage of patient evaluation.[13,25,26] This tool, while not perfect,[27] will help triage previously operated patients into categories such as intervention or continued surveillance. In the "unresectable" or organ preservation groups, determining the relative degree of metabolic activity of a tumor prior to being treated will help determine the effects of radiation treatment[28] or combined therapies.[29] These images are best interpreted with some form of co-registration with a cross-sectional scan.[30] Less expensive methods of imaging FDG-PET without a dedicated PET scanner (Figure 3–9) can be competitive.[31] If the PET radionuclides are not available, SPECT imaging with Tl-201 can be used as an adjunct to the clinical exam.[32,33]

The Paranasal Sinuses

Tumors of the nasal cavity and paranasal sinuses are the most challenging lesions to stage. The cosmetic

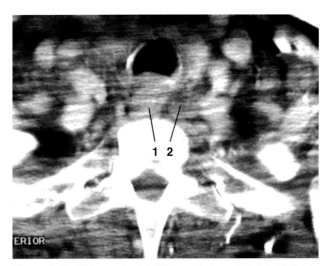

Figure 3–4. Enhanced axial CT through thoracic inlet. (1) Thickened esophagus related to squamous cancer. (2) Necrotic lymph node in the left tracheo-esophageal groove.

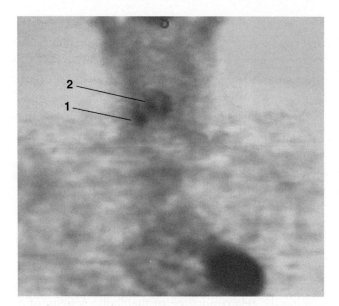

Figure 3–5. Corongal FDG-PET image of torso. (1) Activity related to unsuspected lymph node metastasis. (2) Activity related to glottic squamous cancer.

and functional impact of these tumors is immediately apparent. They rarely present at an early stage. There are few, if any, discriminating imaging features among the various subtypes of tumors in this region. The challenge is to accurately predict the tissue compartments that have been violated without overestimating the boundaries of the tumor. Unlike the neck, this region requires multiplanar imaging. Radiographs and tomographic radiographs no longer have a role in this work-up. The coronal view is the single most important imaging plane (Figure 3–10) for the orbital margin and for the cribriform plate for high naso-ethmoidal lesions.[34] Prior to MRI, high resolution CT was used to evaluate these thin osseous barriers. Any distortion of the bone texture raised the suspicion of involvement of the adjacent soft-tissue space. With the advent of MRI, not only is the coronal plane easier to acquire but also the soft tissue within any compartment is directly evaluated,[35] not inferred from bony change. MRI is probably the single best baseline-imaging exam for paranasal neoplasms.[36] Certain vagaries of physics disturb tissue signal at these bone tissue air interfaces, but this is less problematic when tumor or fluid replaces the air of the sinus cavity. The critical determination of whether or not an orbit should be exenterated demands the application of *both* modalities (CT and MRI). These complementary modali-

ties each provide vital but incomplete information. Nowhere else than the skull-base margin is perineural extension more problematic.[37] Some very small and very peripheral lesions track deep into the skull base foramina (Figure 3–11) while other larger, more centrally located masses grow in a simple centrifugal manner. The interpretation must be made with a high index of suspicion while the oncologist must have a great deal of confidence in the interpretation. A brain imaging protocol is often applied but is inadequate in its standard form. A standard neck imaging protocol will not provide adequate spatial resolution at the skull base. A well-designed CT or MR imaging protocol with appropriate plane, range and section thickness is necessary for accurate diagnosis. Coronal, axial and sometimes sagittal views track the deep margin to best advantage. The cavernous sinus is the most difficult compartment to confidently pronounce clear of disease with imaging. The vascular channels intermixed with fat are alternately bright and dark on MR imaging and inhomogeneously bright on CT. Tumor extension within the cavernous sinus can actually be identified on non-contrast images (Figure 3–12). Contrast images are necessary, however, to exclude disease

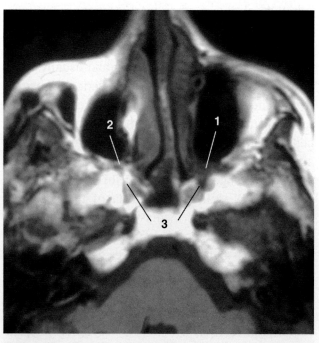

Figure 3–6. Axial T1-weighted MR image through maxilla in a patient with squamous cancer of the soft palate. (1) Neurotropic extension to the left pterygopalatine fossa (PPF). (2) Normal appearance of right PPF. (3) Vidian canals, diseased on the left.

beyond the cavernous sinus, within the basal cisterns (Figure 3–13). Axial views are familiar to most observers and easily outline the deep posterolateral extracranial extension to the masticator and para-

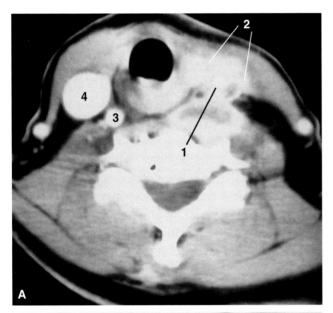

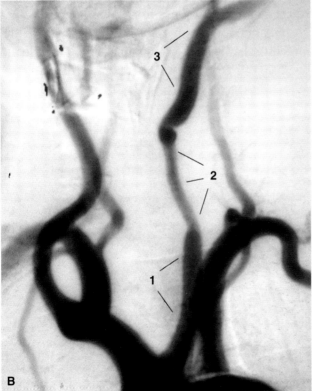

Figure 3–7. *A,* Enhanced axial CT through lower neck. (1) Left common carotid artery (CCA). (2) Recurrent squamous cancer surrounding the CCA. (3) Normal right CCA. (4) Normal right internal jugular vein. *B,* Nonselective cervical catheter angiogram. (1) Proximal left CCA. (2) Extrinsic compromise of distal left CCA. (3) Normal caliber proximal left internal carotid artery.

pharyngeal spaces. The lateral retropharyngeal lymph node station can also be cleared in this view. Extra-paranasal extension into the clinically suspected buccal and pre-maxillary spaces is confirmed in this plane as well. Involvement of the palate must be determined to allow appropriate preoperative consultation with the maxillofacial prosthodontist.

Epithelial tumors of the hard palate are best staged by cross-sectional imaging protocols that evaluate deep extension such as a paranasal sinus protocol. The larger lesions are staged for the deep margin that is neither visible nor palpable. Both advanced and apparently early/small lesions are at risk for central neurotropic extension to and through the foramina at the skull base (Figure 3–14). Distant perineural extension is more typical of the minor salivary histologies but can be seen in squamous neoplasms, particularly those with desmoplastic features. MRI has the distinct advantage over CT by revealing abnormal perineural enhancement before evidence of widening of the corresponding fissure or foramen. These images help determine the extent and appropriateness of skull base resection and portal planning for radiation therapy in anticipation of a positive margin.

Oral Cavity

Oral cavity lesions rarely require imaging without clinical suspicion of deep infiltration. Patients with floor of mouth, retromolar gum and endophytic lesions of the tongue are imaged to rule out deeper involvement. Key landmarks are the midline lingual septum, mylohyoid sling, extrinsic muscles and cortical margin of mandible. Although axial images are most familiar, the coronal view is crucial for the above determination. The sagittal view is important to exclude extension of anterior tongue lesions into the root of the tongue base (Figure 3–15). As with surgical margins, the confidence in diagnosing involvement of the intrinsic tongue is limited by the heterogeneous signal of the interlacing muscle and fat. Pre-contrast and fat-suppressed post-contrast views must be carefully matched to improve confidence. Involvement of the extrinsic muscles must also be carefully excluded. Determining T stage by measuring size

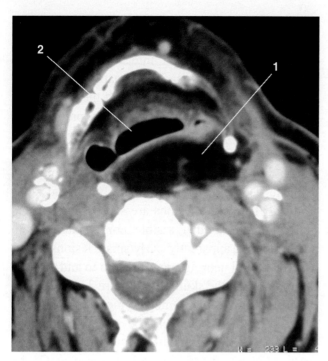

Figure 3–8. Enhanced axial CT image through reconstructed hypopharynx. (1) Composite free tissue graft at hypopharynx produces a pseudo-mass. (2) Partial airway compromise at supraglottic airway.

may be difficult to determine by any means and any radiographic description must be considered an estimated margin.

Retromolar lesions sit within one of the most asymmetrically shaped structures, the trigone. Furthermore, imaging artifacts most often degrade this area, especially CT. Upward posterior extension along the lateral pterygoid fascia and neurotropic extension along the mandibular segment of the Vth nerve can be clinically silent but should be excluded in all cases.

Buccal mucosal lesions are not usually imaged until they become problematic due to multiple recurrences and limitations to clinical evaluation due to trismus. Submucosal, periosteal and perineural extension is difficult to evaluate and close correlation with the clinical findings is necessary to avoid over- or underestimating disease which becomes difficult to stage given the loss of tissue planes after multiple treatments.

Nasopharynx

Imaging of nasopharyngeal tumor requires the greatest expenditure of techniques to confirm the status of bone as well as perineural involvement.[38] Confirming that disease is limited to the mucosal compartment allows treatment of nasopharyngeal lesions with a standard radiation portal while sparing the cranial nerves (particularly cranial nerve II) and the temporal lobes is the main goal of imaging. While one modality may be adequate and efficient for follow-up surveillance, it is the combination of CT and MRI that is crucial at the baseline for this disease. MRI is more sensitive than CT for invasion of the cancellous bone of the central skull base. CT is more sensitive to early involvement of the overlying cortical bone of the sphenoid and basi occiput. The minor change in the bone cortex that is not well shown with MRI may have prognostic implications, but will not likely change the treatment portal. MRI may be the single best staging exam (Figure 3–16) given the greater sensitivity to perineural extension,[39] cavernous sinus extension[4] and the more accurate estimation of cancellous bone involvement. MRI is adequate for nodal staging. Treatment planning is widely performed with CT although MRI-based planning continues to develop.

Imaging follow-up is best performed with the modality that is most compatible with the patients' condition. CT remains an efficient method for fol-

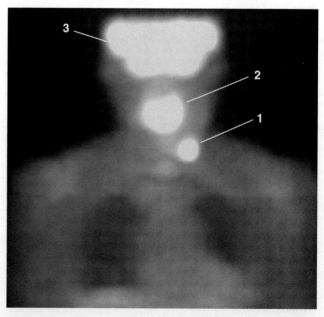

Figure 3–9. Coronal coincidence FDG image of the upper body. (1) Clinically symptomatic metastatic lower left cervical lymph node. (2) Primary base of tongue lesion, occult on cross-sectional imaging. (3) Normal intensity brain activity.

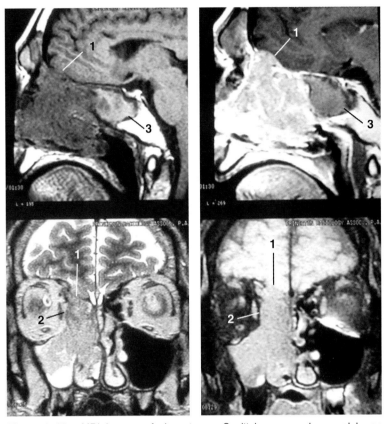

Figure 3–10. MRI images of sinus tumor. Sagittal upper and coronal lower images with T1 and T2 weighting. (1) Penetration through fovea ethmoidalis into extradural space. No brain invasion. (2) Displaced lamina papyracea without invasion of orbital fat or muscle cone. (3) Obstructed sphenoid sinus secretions, not tumor extension.

low-up surveillance imaging of the primary site and the neck. It is very reproducible between patients' visits and among different institutions. CT does require intravenous contrast for detailed restaging, however. Patients receiving nephrotoxic chemotherapeutic agents should be followed with

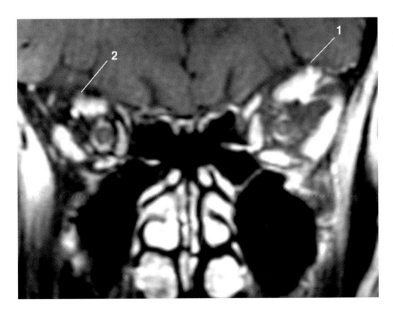

Figure 3–11. Enhanced coronal T1-weighted MR image through mid-orbits. (1) Thickened first division of left trigeminal nerve due to neurotropic skin tumor at forehead. (2) Normal appearing first division of left trigeminal nerve.

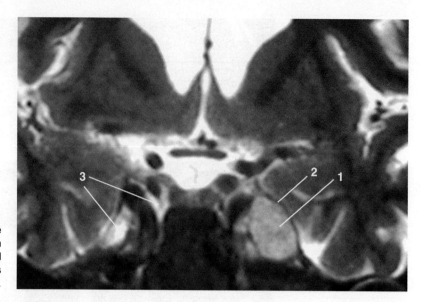

Figure 3–12. Coronal T2-weighted MR image through cavernous sinuses. (1) Tumor extension into left cavernous sinus. (2) Intact dura stretched by expanding tumor. (3) Normal heterogeneous appearance of non-contrast MR of cavernous sinus.

MRI if their mucositis doesn't produce too much swallowing motion artifact. Scanning of both the primary site and comprehensive evaluation of the neck does result in a lengthy exam, however. A bonus for the MRI cohort is evaluation of the CNS white matter injury of the spinal cord, brainstem and optic nerves.

Oropharynx

Most of the oropharyngeal sub-sites are easily evaluated in the axial plane with cross-sectional imaging. Pharyngeal wall lesions rarely penetrate the tough pharyngo-basilar fascia in their early stages. Retropharyngeal extension and adenopathy are clinically occult and must be excluded radiographically. Invasion of the masticator space by tonsillar lesions (Figure 3–17) can be detected with a good contrast-enhanced scan. The index of suspicion must be high particularly when trismus is present. Axial views also outline base of tongue lesions across the glosso-tonsillar sulcus, which may be difficult to appreciate clinically. Base of tongue lesions are best supplemented by sagittal views to outline the status of the preepiglottic space. This also determines the extent of involvement anteriorly into the intrinsic muscles of the tongue for accurate T staging.

Follow-up images need careful correlation with pretreatment scans because of the variability of native lymphoid tissue during treatment. Often regrowth of lymphoid tissue produces pseudotumor contralateral to the original primary tumor. Misinterpretation of this phenomenon could falsely suggest locoregional failure. Imaging artifact can be avoided in the oropharynx with direct coronal views behind the dental work that would otherwise obscure the lesion in the axial plane.

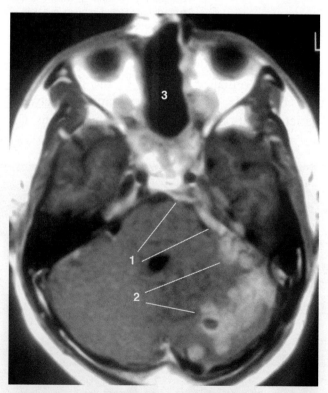

Figure 3–13. Axial contrast T1-weighted MR image through skull base. (1) Neurotropic intracranial extension along cisternal segment of Vth nerve. (2) Leptomeningeal growth along cerebellar folia. (3) Operative bed of original ethmoid sinus tumor remains free of disease.

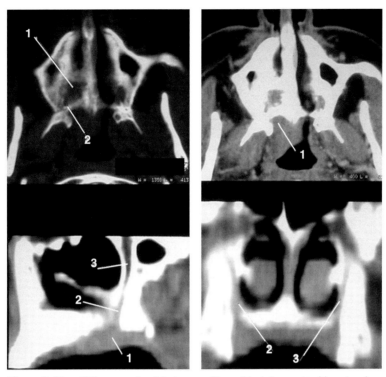

Figure 3–14. CT images of palate tumor with centripetal neurotrophic extension. Upper panel: axial bone (L) and tissue (R) windows through palate. Lower panel: coronal (L) and para-sagittal (R) tissue windows. (1) Palate tumor involving hard and soft segments. (2) Extension upward through widened left greater palatine foramen. (3) Normal bilateral palatine canals.

Soft palate lesions are difficult to discriminate with conventional imaging because of the curved contour of the structure, the poor conspicuity of these lesions and motion artifact from the soft palate resting on the tongue. This organ is best imaged in the semi-coronal plane (Figure 3–18) with special attention to the tonsillar margin.

Larynx and Hypopharynx

Imaging findings in the larynx have, in the past, helped confirm the limited extent of *early* larynx cancer allowing patients to decide between radiation and surgery for primary management. Imaging for advanced larynx and hypopharynx lesions helps confirm the need for surgery and single out the patients appropriate for organ preservation. Post-biopsy changes distort the narrow tissue planes within the larynx and patients should not be scanned prior to any endoscopic manipulation or biopsy. MRI provides exquisite soft tissue resolution[40] even

without intravenous contrast. That benefit is not necessary in early larynx cancer but has a bearing on prognosis for local recurrence for more locally advanced lesions.[41] A negative CT is adequate for

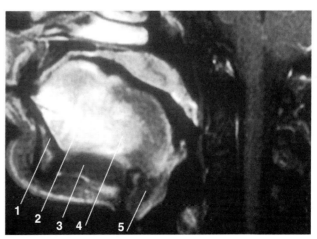

Figure 3–15. Midline sagittal MR tongue with undifferentiated carcinoma. (1) Intact bone cortex of buccal plate at symphysis. (2) Tumor originating at oral tongue. (3) Intact geniohyoid muscle. (4) Tumor extension toward base of tongue. (5) Preserved pre-epiglottic space.

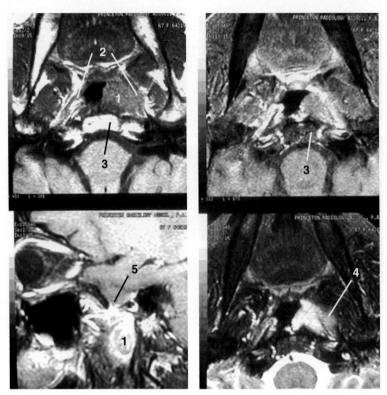

Figure 3–16. Nasopharynx cancer. Clockwise from upper left: semi-coronal T1-weighted, contrast T1-weighted, and fat-suppressed T2-weighted MR images and para-sagittal contrast T1-weighted MR images. (1) Mucosal mass. (2) Levator veli palatini muscles (invaded on the left). (3) Intact skull base (clivus) with normal marrow signal. (4) Early invasion of parapharyngeal space. (5) Benign reactive enhancement at foramen ovale, intracranial extension.

clearance of the paraglottic space and preepiglottic space[42] (Figure 3–19). MRI better evaluates the subglottic extent and is more sensitive to early cartilage involvement.[43] Neither of these features is common with early glottic cancer. Either modality can confirm a locally advanced lesion being restricted to the supraglottis or hemilarynx permitting a primary surgical approach.[44,45] Advanced cancers of the larynx cause pain and difficulty managing secretions—limiting the success of MRI for staging. Tracheostomy alleviates some of these problems. Rapid CT scanners coupled with "slip ring" (helical/spiral) technology help produce images with less patient motion artifact.[46] Reformatted images can be produced in the sagittal and coronal planes from the original axial scan plane (Figure 3–20). Either modality provides adequate surgical planning or baseline information prior to treatment. MRI is more sensitive but less specific than CT for cartilage invasion.[47] Imaging of primary tumors of the hypopharynx is per-

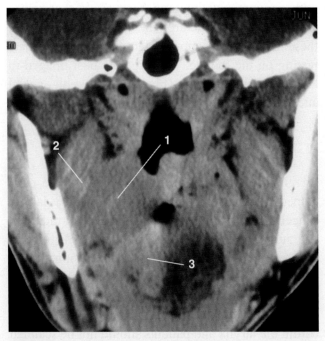

Figure 3–17. Squamous cancer tonsillar pillar. (1) Large mass arising in right palatine tonsil. (2) Right medial pterygoid invaded. (3) Right base of tongue extension.

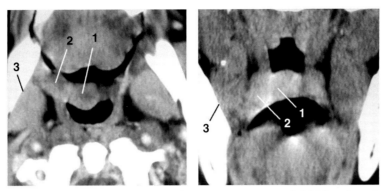

Figure 3–18. CT images of soft palate squamous cancer. Axial (L) and semi-coronal (R) tissue windows. (1) Soft palate component. (2) Tonsillar pillar extension. (3) Medial pterygoid muscle (normal).

formed with larynx style protocols. Local extension to the laryngeal framework is the most important component of extra-pharyngeal extension. Imaging detects cartilage invasion that can be clinically occult.[48] CT can detect inferior extension of pyriform sinus tumor (Figure 3–21) that cannot be assessed clinically.[49] Surveillance follow-up imaging should take into account the risk for patient motion with MRI and the ability of the patient to tolerate intravenous contrast for CT.

One method to reduce the need for re-biopsy and avoid the difficulties of follow-up cross-sectional imaging is PET imaging.[13,26] Non-surgical or organ preservation patients treated by chemo/radiotherapy frequently have persistent morphologic abnormalities on follow-up clinical evaluation and imaging despite maximal therapy. Often this represents sterilized tumor and fibrosis. Pain or dysfunction influence the decision to re-biopsy the primary site. In an effort to avoid the post-biopsy injury, a baseline

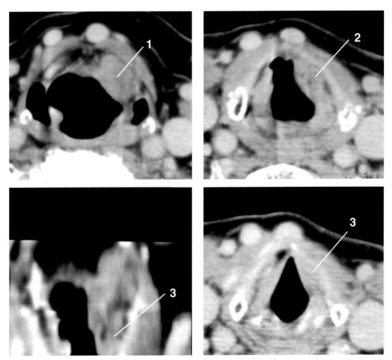

Figure 3–19. CT images of left transglottic squamous cancer. Clockwise from upper left panel: axial images through epiglottic, false cord and true cord levels of larynx and coronal reformatted image of same. (1) Supraglottic lesion. (2) Paraglottic component at false cord level. (3) Paraglottic extension to true cord level.

FDG-PET scan should be obtained and repeated after treatment.[50] If the degree of metabolic activity has improved, biopsy could be deferred unless cross-sectional imaging shows a distinct progression and resection deferred unless the correlation of modalities indicates severe tissue necrosis. Another secondary benefit of the FDG-PET scan would be surveillance for second primaries. Nuclear scans with thallium-201 on more conventional equipment with single photon emission computed tomography (SPECT) capacity has been shown to be competitive with CT in the post-treatment larynx population.[51] This method had an accuracy of 90 percent and does not require investment in PET technology.

Follow-up imaging of the reconstructed and irradiated laryngopharyngectomy is very important given the difficulty of examining the irradiated/operated neck. Familiarity with the type of resections, flap reconstructions and patterns of recurrence is essential for accurate interpretation.[52,53] Careful attention should be directed to the anastomotic level and peristomal region.

Esophagus

The cervical segment of the esophagus is difficult to evaluate clinically. It remains one of the sites in the head and neck best evaluated with fluoroscopy (Figure 3–22). Mural and exophytic lesions can be detected prior to advanced dysphagia, which is usually the accompanying chief complaint. Like other segments of the esophagus, complete staging is best performed with a combination of endo-sonography,[54] and cross-sectional imaging. These techniques are complementary, with the endoscopic exam providing information about the depth of invasion relative to the muscularis, the linear extent of the lesion and characterization of internal architecture of posterior mediastinal lymph nodes. Synchronous lesions can be excluded at other levels of the esophagus at baseline. Cross-sectional exams provide a more complete locoregional N staging and can be extended for regional M staging. Neither CT nor MRI has sufficient negative predictive value for adenopathy, however.

Salivary Glands

Imaging of cancer of the *minor* salivary glands is covered in the corresponding sub-sites. Imaging of the major salivary gland masses is usually performed when the clinical exam does not provide accurate assessment of the anatomic extent of the tumor or when surgical excision is likely to have a positive margin on a vital structure. Imaging

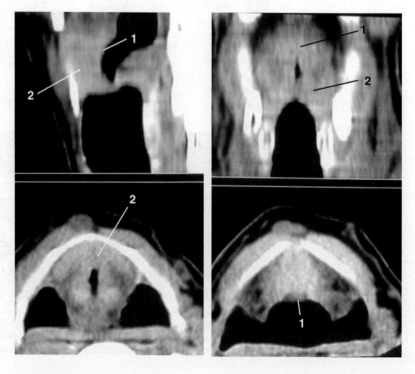

Figure 3–20. Large supraglottic cancer. Upper panel: sagittal (L) and coronal (R) reformatted CT images. Lower panel: glottic (L) and epiglottic (R) axial CT source images. (1) Mucosal lesion at laryngeal surface of epiglottis. (2) Inferior preepiglottic extension.

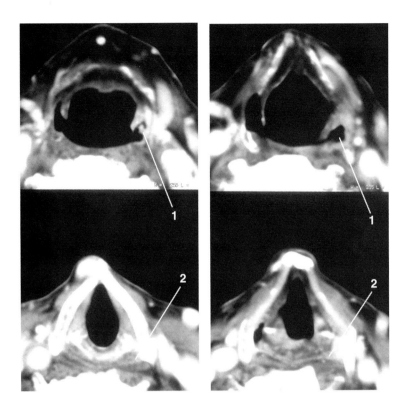

Figure 3–21. Contrast CT images of left pyriform squamous cell carcinoma. Clockwise from upper left: serial images through the laryngo-pharynx. (1) Diseased left pyriform aperture. (2) Preserved left pyriform apex.

should also be considered in the setting of cranial nerve palsy.[55]

Parotid lesions are easily outlined with CT when high quality multiplanar images can be acquired and intravenous contrast used. Contrast helps outline the lesion relative to the gland and provides better characterization of the vascular margin at the carotid sheath. The benefits of MRI over CT are better discrimination of the lesion relative to background parotid tissue (Figure 3–23) and slightly better discrimination of proximal neurotropic extension of disease along the VIIth nerve.

Image-guided biopsy is helpful when there is a need to establish the diagnosis prior to treatment. Follow-up imaging is best performed with the modality that revealed the lesion prior to treatment. Radiation changes produce extensive regional hyperintensity[22] of the parotid bed and mastoid, limiting the value of T2-weighted images. Contrast-enhanced fat-suppressed T1-weighted images are important at this stage.[1]

Submandibular lesions are often managed without imaging prior to resection. Imaging of the neck can be performed to confirm the completeness of the resection and determine whether a limited neck dissection

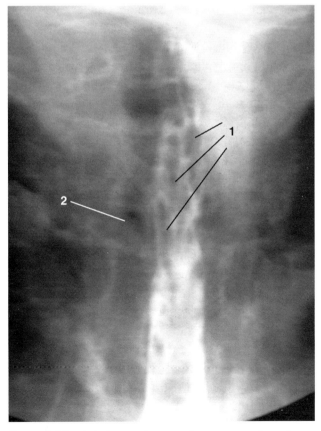

Figure 3–22. Anterior esophagram of squamous cell carcinoma upper esophagus. (1) Varicoid appearance of squamous cancer cervicothoracic esophagus. (2) Trachea.

is appropriate. Both sublingual and submandibular salivary gland lesions are imaged with an oral cavity-type imaging protocol with careful attention to the floor of mouth and the status of Wharton's duct.

Thyroid

Imaging of the thyroid gland and neck for thyroid cancer varies because of the variety of disciplines that manage this disorder. Imaging of the gland is only part of a comprehensive clinical and laboratory evaluation. Whether the imaging is cross-sectional, functional (radioiodine), or metabolic (FDG-PET) should be determined by the evaluation and the chief complaint. Persons with metabolic complaints should be imaged with radioiodine to supplement their work-up, if necessary. Persons with palpable abnormalities don't necessarily need radioiodine scanning initially. Sonography is often used to confirm multiplicity and consistency of lesions, favoring a benign condition. Neither CT, MRI, sonography nor radioiodine scans can confirm or exclude cancer, however. FNA is essential for lesions considered at risk for cancer by clinical or imaging grounds. Sonography preceding or as an adjunct to the FNA may reveal a cyst, which could be aspirated or followed, as clinically indicated. When cancer has been confirmed, sonography (Figure 3–24) can establish the size of the lesion(s), the status of any pseudo-capsule, and the condition of the capsule of the gland.[56] Sonographic staging of the lymph nodes is limited[5] and CT or MRI is better at covering the high level II nodes and the lower tracheo-esophageal nodes. Cross-sectional imaging of the neck is not necessary prior to thyroid surgery in the absence of clinical features suspicious for extra-thyroidal or mediastinal extension. Since iodinated intravenous contrast alters the accuracy of radioiodine scans, CT is a less useful modality for baseline staging. Imaging artifacts at the thoracic inlet and upper mediastinum are difficult to sort out in the absence of contrast with CT. MRI is not prone to these artifacts (Figure 3–25) and can be performed with contrast without interference with radioiodine scans. Neck scans by either modality should be extended to the level of the tracheal carina to cover the lower

tracheoesophageal lymph nodes at risk. Correlation of the cross-sectional views with the radioiodine scans is more productive than either scan alone. Lesions that accumulate iodine less well can be imaged with thallium[57] or FDG-PET.[58,59] This agent accumulates in metabolically active tissue, and to a greater degree in tumor. Although costly and less specific, FDG-PET can be used without interruption of thyroid replacement. Another definite advantage of PET is the ability to co-register the images in any plane with cross-sectional exams in a way that cannot be done with I-131.

Unknown Primary

No discussion of head and neck imaging would be complete without a discussion of the occult primary presumed to be within the upper aerodigestive tract. If one looks at the larger picture of patients with metastatic adenopathy above the clavicles, the role of imaging has increasing value. CT of the neck, chest, abdomen and pelvis usually follows the traditional method of panendoscopy and exam under anesthesia after an unproductive office exam. The advent of FDG-PET can obviate the need for such comprehensive searching[60] and might even be sequenced between the office exam and any subse-

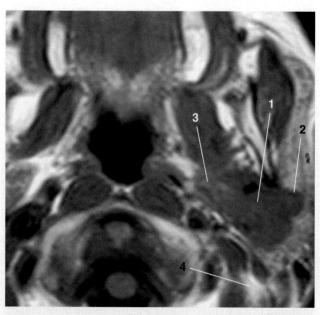

Figure 3–23. Parotid tumor. (1) Parotid tumor along expected course of facial nerve. (2) Superficial lobe involvement. (3) Deep lobe extension to paraphayngeal space. (4) Preserved stylomastoid foramen.

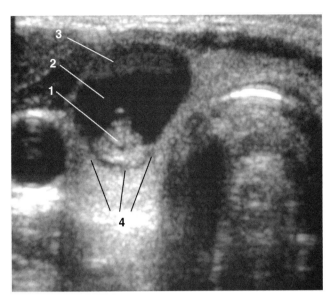

Figure 3–24. Throid cancer sonogram. Transverse sonogram through right thyroid bed. (1) Solid component of complex mass. (2) Cystic component of complex mass. (3) Artifact. (4) Intact pseudocapsule of lesion.

quent procedure requiring anesthesia. The results of the PET scan can show other sites of adenopathy and locate the primary tumor[25] (see Figure 3–9). PET images are best reviewed in correlation with a cross-

sectional exam of the neck. The majority of patients with positive FDG-PET scans are found to have a corresponding tumor and most of those with negative scans never manifest a head or neck primary on follow-up (after treatment).[61,62] At the very least, patients with no identifiable primary or one localized to the head and neck have a better prognosis than those discovered to have a visceral primary below the clavicles.[63]

Sarcomas

Soft tissue sarcomas and other tumors usually present within the lateral neck or paraspinal compartments. These are imaged equally well with MRI[64] or contrast enhanced CT. CT tends to overestimate the overall size of neck masses[65] compared with MRI—probably because of its multiplanar capacity. Vascular integrity and margins can also be surveyed at the initial MRI visit with the help of magnetic resonance angiography (MRA). Many patients can be spared catheter angiography. Sarcomas developing within sub-sites of the aerodigestive tract are imaged according to those protocols. Combining informa-

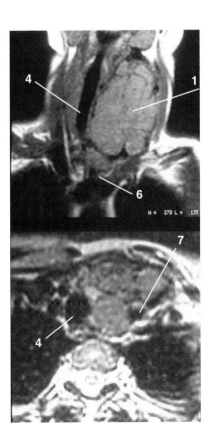
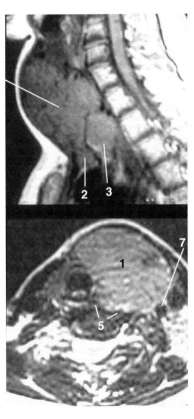

Figure 3–25. Throid cancer MRI. Clockwise from upper left: Coronal and sagittal T1-weighted non-contrast images and axial T2-weighted images through base of neck and thoracic inlet. Note the lack of imaging artifacts. (1) Left lobe thyroid mass. (2) Extracapsular extension. (3) Tracheoesophageal lymph node metastasis. (4) Trachea. (5) Invasion of prevertebral muscles. (6) Plane of brachiocephalic vein. (7) Left common carotid artery.

tion from pretreatment MRI with CT based treatment planning lends confidence to those plans.

FUTURE DIRECTIONS

Cross-sectional imaging will continue to develop computer assisted interactive methods for operative guidance[66] and treatment based on pre-procedure scans. These procedures are best performed by practitioners with prior experience without the aid of imaging support. Further development of interactive types of software should allow trainees to develop skills on so-called virtual patients, providing that experience base. Performing procedures under imaging guidance is advancing from simple biopsies and ablations to realtime guidance on "fluoroscopic-CT" and "open architecture" MRI equipment.

Developments in sonography with color flow imaging of lymph nodes and power Doppler imaging of masses and lymph nodes is being explored to better characterize for neoplastic features.

Continued improvement in CT scanner technology allows for performance of CT angiography in selected cases for patients that may not be able to undergo MRA.

Continued development of iron-coated dextran may provide more accurate evaluation of borderline sized lymph nodes.[11]

Nuclear imaging will come to play a greater role in triage of patients along treatment pathways, pre- and post-treatment. New ligands, combined with conventional radionuclides, are being explored for the detection of squamous cell carcinoma with cross-sectional nuclear imaging (SPECT).[67,68] More specific isotopes for head and neck neoplasms will replace FDG for PET imaging.[69] The continued exploration of monoclonal antibodies[70] holds promise for detection of more specific tissue antigens.[71,72] Novel combinations of established nuclear agents are being explored to reduce the need for obtaining both a nuclear and a cross-sectional exam, simply for correlation.[73]

The thrust of much of the past decade of research has been to find an efficient pathway of patient management where selection of an imaging modality provides pertinent and accurate informa-

tion. Ideally the technique would provide anatomic staging of the primary site, comprehensive lymph node staging and functional information regarding nerves and blood vessels. One of the original goals of MRI was to provide in vivo tissue characterization on human subjects. Twenty years after its introduction, MR shows promise for "one-stop shopping" for all vital information: MR imaging, MR angiography, and now MR spectroscopy.[74] Improvements in software have followed necessary improvements in hardware and magnetic field strength. Sampling a small volume of tissue from a cross-sectional image and analyzing for relative amounts of known metabolites can predict the likelihood of neoplasm.[75] As with other modalities, a physician is responsible for determining the presence of a target on the image for sampling. Like FDG-PET, this noninvasive technique allows one to follow a trend during treatment in order to confirm treatment response.

REFERENCES

1. Baba Y, Furusawa M, Murakami R, et al. Role of dynamic MRI in the evaluation of head and neck cancers treated with radiation therapy. Int J Radiat Oncol Biol Phys 1997;37(4):783–7.
2. Fife DG. The management of lumps in the neck. Br J Hosp Med 1997;57(10):522–6.
3. Morley SE, Ramesar KC, Macleod DA. Cystic hygroma in an adult: a case report. J R Coll Surg Edinb 1999;44(1):57–8.
4. Chong J, Som PM, Silvers AR, Dalton JF. Extranodal non-Hodgkin's lymphoma involving the muscles of mastication [see comments]. AJNR Am J Neuroradiol 1998; 19(10):1849–51.
5. Ahuja A, Ying M, King W, Metreweli C. A practical approach to ultrasound of cervical lymph nodes. J Laryngol Otol 1997;111(3):245–56.
6. Shah JP. Patterns of cervical lymph node metastasis from squamous carcinomas of the upper aerodigestive tract. Am J Surg 1990;160(4):405–9.
7. Friedman M, Mafee MF, Pacella BL Jr, et al. Rationale for elective neck dissection in 1990. Laryngoscope 1990; 100(1):54–9.
8. Myers LL, Wax MK, Nabi H, et al. Positron emission tomography in the evaluation of the N0 neck. Laryngoscope 1998;108(2):232–6.
9. Braams JW, Pruim J, Freling NJ, et al. Detection of lymph node metastases of squamous-cell cancer of the head and neck with FDG-PET and MRI. J Nucl Med 1995;36(2): 211–6.
10. Yucel T, Saatci I, Sennaroglu L, et al. MR imaging in squamous cell carcinoma of the head and neck with no palpable lymph nodes. Acta Radiol 1997;38(5):810–4.

11. Anzai Y, Brunberg JA, Lufkin RB. Imaging of nodal metastases in the head and neck. J Magn Reson Imaging 1997;7(5):774–83.

12. Adams S, Baum RP, Stuckensen T, et al. Prospective comparison of 18F-FDG PET with conventional imaging modalities (CT, MRI, US) in lymph node staging of head and neck cancer. Eur J Nucl Med 1998;25(9):1255–60.

13. Fischbein NJ, AAssar OS, Caputo GR, et al. Clinical utility of positron emission tomography with 18F-fluorodeoxyglucose in detecting residual/recurrent squamous cell carcinoma of the head and neck [see comments]. AJNR Am J Neuroradiol 1998;19(7):1189–96.

14. Stevens MH, Harnsberger HR, Mancuso AA, et al. Computed tomography of cervical lymph nodes. Staging and management of head and neck cancer. Arch Otolaryngol 1985;111(11):735–9.

15. Prehn RB, Pasic TR, Harari PM, et al. Influence of computed tomography on pretherapeutic tumor staging in head and neck cancer patients. Otolaryngol Head Neck Surg 1998; 119(6):628–33.

16. Escott EJ, Rao VM, Ko WD, Guitierrez JE. Comparison of dynamic contrast-enhanced gradient-echo and spin-echo sequences in MR of head and neck neoplasms. AJNR Am J Neuroradiol 1997;18(8):1411–9.

17. Loevner LA, Ott IL, Yousem DM, et al. Neoplastic fixation to the prevertebral compartment by squamous cell carcinoma of the head and neck. AJR Am J Roentgenol 1998;170(5):1389–94.

18. Yousem DM, Hatabu H, Hurst RW, et al. Carotid artery invasion by head and neck masses: prediction with MR imaging. Radiology 1995;195(3):715–20.

19. Curtin HD. Importance of imaging demonstration of neoplastic invasion of laryngeal cartilage [editorial; comment]. Radiology 1995;194(3):643–4.

20. Lemort M. Computed tomography (CT) in head and neck tumors: technique and indications. [review] [14 refs]. Journal Belge de Radiologie 1994;77(2):60–6.

21. Som PM, Urken ML, Biller H, Lidov M. Imaging the postoperative neck. [review] [30 refs]. Radiology 1993; 187(3):593–603.

22. Becker M, Schroth G, Zbaren P, et al. Long-term changes induced by high-dose irradiation of the head and neck region: imaging findings. Radiographics 1997;17(1):5–26.

23. Koch WM. Axillary nodal metastases in head and neck cancer. Head Neck 1999;21(3):269–72.

24. Harris EW, LaMarca AJ, Kondroski EM, et al. Enhanced CT of the neck: improved visualization of lesions with delayed imaging. AJR Am J Roentgenol 1996;167(4):1057–8.

25. Bailet JW, Abemayor E, Jabour BA, et al. Positron emission tomography: a new, precise imaging modality for detection of primary head and neck tumors and assessment of cervical adenopathy. Laryngoscope 1992;102(3):281–8.

26. Wong WL, Chevretton EB, McGurk M, et al. A prospective study of PET-FDG imaging for the assessment of head and neck squamous cell carcinoma. Clin Otolaryngol 1997;22(3):209–14.

27. Paulus P, Sambon A, Vivegnis D, et al. 18FDG-PET for the assessment of primary head and neck tumors: clinical, computed tomography, and histopathological correlation in 38 patients. Laryngoscope 1998;108(10):1578–83.

28. Greven KM, Williams DW III, Keyes JW Jr, et al. Positron emission tomography of patients with head and neck carcinoma before and after high dose irradiation [see comments]. Cancer 1994;74(4):1355–9.

29. Haberkorn U, Strauss LG, Dimitrakopoulou A, et al. Fluorodeoxyglucose imaging of advanced head and neck cancer after chemotherapy. J Nucl Med 1993;34(1):12–7.

30. Sercarz JA, Bailet JW, Abemayor E, et al. Computer coregistration of positron emission tomography and magnetic resonance images in head and neck cancer. Am J Otolaryngol 1998;19(2):130–5.

31. Zimny M, Kaiser HJ, Cremerius U, et al. F-18-FDG positron imaging in oncological patients: gamma camera coincidence detection versus dedicated PET. Nuklearmedizin 1999;38(4):108–14.

32. Valdes Olmos RA, Balm AJ, Hilgers FJ, et al. Thallium-201 SPECT in the diagnosis of head and neck cancer. J Nucl Med 1997;38(6):873–9.

33. Yigitbasi OG, Tutus A, Bozdemir K, et al. 201Tl imaging for differentiating between malignant and benign neck masses. Nucl Med Commun 1998;19(6):555–60.

34. Derdeyn CP, Moran CJ, Wippold FJ II, et al. MRI of esthesioneuroblastoma. J Comput Assist Tomogr 1994;18(1): 16–21.

35. Allbery SM, Chaljub G, Cho NL, et al. MR imaging of nasal masses. [review] [17 refs]. Radiographics 1995;15(6): 1311–27.

36. Held P, Breit A. [Comparison of CT and MRI in diagnosis of tumors of the nasopharynx, the inner nose and the paranasal sinuses]. [German] Vergleich von CT und MRT in der Diagnostik von Tumoren des Nasopharynx, der inneren Nase und der Nebenhohlen. Bildgebung 1994; 61(3):187–96.

37. Nemzek WR, Hecht S, Gandour-Edwards R, et al. Perineural spread of head and neck tumors: how accurate is MR imaging? AJNR Am J Neuroradiol 1998;19(4):701–6.

38. Su CY, Lui CC. Perineural invasion of the trigeminal nerve in patients with nasopharyngeal carcinoma. Imaging and clinical correlations. Cancer 1996;78(10):2063–9.

39. Majoie CB, Hulsmans FJ, Verbeeten B Jr, et al. Perineural tumor extension along the trigeminal nerve: magnetic resonance imaging findings. Eur J Radiol 1997;24(3): 191–205.

40. Zbaren P, Becker M, Lang H. Pretherapeutic staging of hypopharyngeal carcinoma. Clinical findings, computed tomography, and magnetic resonance imaging compared with histopathologic evaluation [published erratum appears in Arch Otolaryngol Head Neck Surg 1998 Feb;124(2):231]. Arch Otolaryngol Head Neck Surg 1997;123(9):908–13.

41. Castelijns JA, van den Brekel MW, Smit EM, et al. Predictive value of MR imaging-dependent and non-MR imaging-dependent parameters for recurrence of laryngeal cancer after radiation therapy. Radiology 1995;196(3):735–9.

42. Thabet HM, Sessions DG, Gado MH, et al. Comparison of clinical evaluation and computed tomographic diagnostic accuracy for tumors of the larynx and hypopharynx. Laryngoscope 1996;106(5 Pt 1):589–94.

43. Zbaren P, Becker M, Lang H. Pretherapeutic staging of laryngeal carcinoma. Clinical findings, computed tomography,

and magnetic resonance imaging compared with histopathology. Cancer 1996;77(7):1263–73.

44. Williams DW III. Imaging of laryngeal cancer [review] [51 refs]. Otolaryngol Clin N Am 1997;30(1):35–58.

45. Weinstein GS, Laccourreye O, Brasnu D, Yousem DM. The role of computed tomography and magnetic resonance imaging in planning for conservation laryngeal surgery [review] [25 refs]. Neuroimaging Clin N Am 1996;6(2):497–504.

46. Korkmaz H, Cerezci NG, Akmansu H, Dursun E. A comparison of spiral and conventional computerized tomography methods in diagnosing various laryngeal lesions. Eur Arch Otorhinolaryngol 1998;255(3):149–54.

47. Becker M, Zbaren P, Laeng H, et al. Neoplastic invasion of the laryngeal cartilage: comparison of MR imaging and CT with histopathologic correlation [see comments]. Radiology 1995;194(3):661–9.

48. Zbaren P, Becker M, Lang H. Staging of laryngeal cancer: endoscopy, computed tomography and magnetic resonance versus histopathology. Eur Arch Otorhinolaryngol Suppl. 1997;1:S117–S22.

49. Saleh EM, Mancuso AA, Stringer SP. Relative roles of computed tomography and endoscopy for determining the inferior extent of pyriform sinus carcinoma: correlative histopathologic study. Head Neck 1993;15(1):44–52.

50. Kitagawa Y, Sadato N, Azuma H, et al. FDG-PET to evaluate combined intra-arterial chemotherapy and radiotherapy of head and neck neoplasms. J Nucl Med 1999;40(7):1132–7.

51. Mukherji SK, Gapany M, Phillips D, et al. Thallium-201 single-photon emission CT versus CT for the detection of recurrent squamous cell carcinoma of the head and neck [see comments]. AJNR Am J Neuroradiol 1999;20(7):1215–20.

52. Misiti A, Macori F, Caimi M, et al. Computerized tomography in the evaluation of the larynx after surgical treatment and irradiation. Radiol Med (Torino) 1997;94(6):600–6.

53. Hudgins PA, Burson JG, Gussack GS, Grist WJ. CT and MR appearance of recurrent malignant head and neck neoplasms after resection and flap reconstruction. AJNR Am J Neuroradiol 1994;15(9):1689–94.

54. Doldi SB, Lattuada E, Zappa MA, et al. Ultrasonographic imaging of neoplasms of the cervical esophagus. Hepatogastroenterology 1997;44(15):724–6.

55. Ariyoshi Y, Shimahara M. Determining whether a parotid tumor is in the superficial or deep lobe using magnetic resonance imaging. J Oral Maxillofac Surg 1998;56(1):23–6.

56. Shimamoto K, Satake H, Sawaki A, et al. Preoperative staging of thyroid papillary carcinoma with ultrasonography. Eur J Radiol 1998;29(1):4–10.

57. Lin JD, Kao PF, Weng HF, et al. Relative value of thallium-201 and iodine-131 scans in the detection of recurrence or distant metastasis of well differentiated thyroid carcinoma. Eur J Nucl Med 1998;25(7):695–700.

58. Wang W, Macapinlac H, Larson SM, et al. [18F]-2-fluoro-2-deoxy-D-glucose positron emission tomography localizes residual thyroid cancer in patients with negative diagnostic (131)I whole body scans and elevated serum thyroglobulin levels. J Clin Endocrinol Metab 1999;84(7):2291–302.

59. Jadvar H, McDougall IR, Segall GM. Evaluation of suspected recurrent papillary thyroid carcinoma with [18F]fluorodeoxyglucose positron emission tomography. Nucl Med Commun 1998;19(6):547–54.

60. Mendenhall WM, Mancuso AA, Parsons JT, et al. Diagnostic evaluation of squamous cell carcinoma metastatic to cervical lymph nodes from an unknown head and neck primary site. Head Neck 1998;20(8):739–44.

61. AAssar OS, Fischbein NJ, Caputo GR, et al. Metastatic head and neck cancer: role and usefulness of FDG PET in locating occult primary tumors. Radiology 1999;210(1):177–81.

62. Schipper JH, Schrader M, Arweiler D, et al. [Positron emission tomography for primary tumor detection in lymph node metastases with unknown primary tumor]. HNO 1996;44(5):254–7.

63. Jones AS, Roland NJ, Hamilton J, et al. Non-squamous malignancy in lymph nodes: the occult primary. Clin Otolaryngol 1996;21(1):49–53.

64. Hirsch RJ, Yousem DM, Loevner LA, et al. Synovial sarcomas of the head and neck: MR findings. AJR Am J Roentgenol 1997;169(4):1185–8.

65. Rasch C, Keus R, Pameijer FA, et al. The potential impact of CT-MRI matching on tumor volume delineation in advanced head and neck cancer. Int J Radiol 1997;39(4):841–8.

66. Davis SP, Anand VK, Dhillon G. Magnetic resonance navigation for head and neck lesions. Laryngoscope 1999;109(6):862–7.

67. Shen YY, Kao CH, Changlai SP, et al. Detection of nasopharyngeal carcinoma with head and neck Tc-99m tetrofosmin SPECT imaging. Clin Nucl Med 1998;23(5):305–8.

68. Flamen P, Bernheim N, Deron P, et al. Iodine-123 alpha-methyl-l-tyrosine single-photon emission tomography for the visualization of head and neck squamous cell carcinomas. Eur J Nucl Med 1998;25(2):177–81.

69. Lindholm P, Leskinen S, Lapela M. Carbon-11-methionine uptake in squamous cell head and neck cancer. J Nucl Med 1998;39(8):1393–7.

70. De Rossi G, Maurizi M, Almadori G, et al. The contribution of immunoscintigraphy to the diagnosis of head and neck tumours. Nucl Med Commun 1997;18(1):10–6.

71. de Bree R, Roos JC, Quak JJ, et al. Radioimmuno-scintigraphy and biodistribution of technetium-99m-labeled monoclonal antibody U36 in patients with head and neck cancer. Clin Cancer Res 1995;1(6):591–8.

72. Ramos-Suzarte M, Rodriguez N, Oliva JP, et al. 99mTc-labeled antihuman epidermal growth factor receptor antibody in patients with tumors of epithelial origin: Part III. Clinical trials safety and diagnostic efficacy. J Nucl Med 1999;40(5):768–75.

73. Leitha T, Glaser C, Pruckmayer M, et al. Technetium-99m-MIBI in primary and recurrent head and neck tumors: contribution of bone SPECT image fusion. J Nucl Med 1998;39(7):1166–71.

74. Adalsteinsson E, Spielman DM, Pauly JM, et al. Feasibility study of lactate imaging of head and neck tumors. NMR Biomed 1998;11(7):360–9.

75. Star-Lack J, Spielman D, Adalsteinsson E, et al. In vivo lactate editing with simultaneous detection of choline, creatine, NAA, and lipid singlets at 1.5 T using PRESS excitation with applications to the study of brain and head and neck tumors. J Magn Reson 1998;133(2):243–54.

4

Skin Cancers of the Head and Neck

BHUVANESH SINGH, MD

JATIN P. SHAH, MD, FACS

SKIN PATHOLOGY

Benign epidermal tumors
Fibroepithelial polyp
Keratoacanthoma
Actinic keratosis

Adnexal tumors
Benign tumors
Malignancies

Dermal tumors
Malignant fibrous histiocytoma
Dermatofibrosarcoma protuberans
Kaposi's sarcoma
Hemangioma
Xanthoma

Malignant epidermal tumors
Basal cell carcinoma
Squamous cell carcinoma

Other cancers
Merkel cell carcinoma
Dermatofibrosarcoma protuberans
Malignant fibrous histiocytoma

Melanocytic lesions
Malignant melanoma

The skin is by far the largest organ in humans. It has several functions, but mainly acts as a barrier against the outside environment. Given its chronic exposure to environmental carcinogens, it is not surprising that cancers of cutaneous origin are the most common human malignancies. Embryologically, the skin is derived from ectoderm, neuroectoderm and meso-derm, and correspondingly supports the development of a myriad of benign and malignant processes. Approximately 1 million new cases of basal or squamous cell carcinoma, 51,400 melanomas, and 5,000 non-epithelial skin cancers occur yearly in the United States, with the head and neck region as the site of origin in over 80 percent of these cases.[1]

Benign Epidermal Tumors

Fibroepithelial Polyp

Also known as skin tags, fibroepithelial polyps typically develop in middle-aged persons and are of limited consequence. These lesions are usually removed for cosmetic reasons, although they may become quite large and symptomatic due to irritation or trauma. The pedunculated lesions are usually fleshy and are composed of an epithelial covering and a fibrovascular core. Occasional case reports have demonstrated the presence of coexistent carcinoma; but this is rare, with one series showing only 5 of 1,335 fibroepithelial polyps containing malignancy.[2,3] The neck is the most common site of involvement. Local excision is sufficient for management of symptomatic lesions or for cosmetic concerns.

Keratoacanthoma

These are lesions of middle-aged people that typically begin as a keratosis, firm papule, or wart-like lesion. Keratoacanthomas often display rapid enlargement into a dome-shaped lesion with a central crater filled with keratin. These lesions typically grow over a period of 2 to 4 weeks, to a size of 1 to

2 cm, although giant, >5 cm lesions rarely do develop. The natural course of these lesions after the rapid growth phase is involution, leaving a scar or hypopigmented region on the skin. Clinically and histologically, these lesions can resemble squamous cell carcinoma, with cytologic atypia often present.[4] An evaluation of the overall architecture of the lesion, with accompanying hyperkeratosis, parakeratosis, acanthosis, and hypergranulosis, is diagnostic. The lesions typically occur on the central portion of the face, usually involving the cheek and nose. Solitary lesions are present in the majority of cases, but multiple lesions may occur infrequently. Observation and local care usually suffice for management, although vigilance for the presence of squamous cell carcinoma must remain.[5]

Actinic Keratosis

Actinic keratoses are common premalignant lesions of the skin that are associated with chronic sun exposure. Although lesions are reported to progress into squamous cell carcinoma in up to 25 percent of cases, most studies suggest that the true progression rate is closer to 0.01 to 0.24 percent.[6–11] Clinically these lesions have an erythematous papular or plaque-like appearance, a rough texture, and can form conical projections called cutaneous horns. Histologically, these tumors contain anaplastic keratinocytes in the basal layers of aplastic or hyperplastic epidermis. The lesions are typically multiple and most often involve the sun-exposed regions of the head, neck and arms. Some authors advocate intervention in all cases, given the high rates of transformation to carcinoma and an inability to identify high-risk lesions.[12] Treatment typically consists of cryosurgery and curettage, topical chemotherapy with 5-fluorouracil (5-FU), or surgical excision.[13,14] Topical 5-FU is usually applied as a 5 percent cream twice daily for 2 weeks. An intense local reaction results, followed by resolution of the lesion, with no effects to the remaining skin. More recently, novel therapies have shown promise in treating these lesions. A double-blind controlled study demonstrated an enhanced efficacy of 5-FU with the addition of tretinoin cream.[15] Another randomized paired comparison showed a single treatment with photodynamic therapy with topical δ-aminolevulinic acid to be as effective as 5-fluorouracil treatment.[16, 17]

Adnexal Tumors

Benign Tumors

These tumors arise from the skin appendages and can show pilosebaceous, eccrine, or apocrine differentiation. Common benign adnexal tumors include nevus sebaceous, trichoepithelioma, pilomatricoma, cylindroma, syringocystadenoma papilliferum, syringoma, and eccrine spiradenoma.

Nevus sebaceous tumors are congenital hamartomas of the skin that probably arise from basal cells. These lesions typically involve the face and scalp regions of children, ranging in appearance from slightly raised flesh-colored plaques to verrucous nodular lesions. Although it is controversial, excision is usually recommended due to the risk of transformation to basal cell carcinoma. A study by Cribier and colleagues showed that of 596 excised cases of nevus sebaceous tumor, 0.8 percent contained coexistent basal cell carcinoma, while 13.6 percent of cases contained benign pathology, mainly syringocystadenoma papilliferum (37%) and trichoblastoma (35%).[18] Similarly, a study by Chun and colleagues also observed low transformation rates, suggesting that excision of sebaceous nevi should be performed only in cases where transformation of benign to malignant pathology is suspected.[19]

Trichoepithelioma is a tumor displaying hair follicle differentiation that occurs in two forms: a sporadic form that typically presents as a solitary lesion, and a familial form with multifocal lesions. Multiple familial trichoepithelioma (MFT) has an autosomal dominant inheritance pattern with the gene located on chromosome 9p21.[29] MFT may degenerate into basal cell carcinoma in a small number of cases. The lesions appear as flesh-colored papules and nodules of the facial or scalp skin, and less commonly that of the neck and trunk.

Pilomatricomas or Malherbe's calcifying epitheliomas are tumors of hair follicle origin, derived from the adnexal keratinocytes. Although these tumors can occur at any age, they typically occur in the first and sixth decades of life.[20] The lesions involve the face or arms and can range from subcutaneous nodules to superficial lesions with rare ulceration. A familial association to myotonic dystrophy has been suggested.[21,22] Fifty-five cases of degeneration into malignant pilomatricomas have been reported in the literature.[23] Surgical excision is usually sufficient for management.[24] A malignant variant of this lesion has been reported, which has locally aggressive features and rare metastasis. Recurrence of malignant pilomatricoma is common after simple excision, requiring aggressive local surgical treatment and adjuvant radiation as required.[25–27]

Cylindroma, also known as turban tumor, can either be apocrine or eccrine in origin. These lesions arise in the scalp and facial region in early adulthood. The lesions can be single, but are more often multiple. A familial syndrome of multiple cylindromas is inherited via an autosomal dominant pattern of inheritance with a linkage to chromosome 16q12-13.[28] Briggs and colleagues, using loss of heterozygosity (LOH) analysis, suggested that CYLD1, a tumor suppressor gene, is involved in both familial and sporadic types.[28] Malignant transformation may occur in both the sporadic and familial varieties, but is rare. Typically, the presence of rapid growth and frequent recurrence after excision should raise suspicion for malignant transformation. These tumors are locally aggressive with frequent regional and distant metastasis.[25, 29, 30]

Syringocystadenoma papilliferum is a lesion occurring in the scalp and facial region of patients entering puberty. It can have either eccrine or apocrine differentiation and clinically presents as a plaque or nodule of the scalp or face.[31] It is usually associated with a pre-existing nevus sebaceous.[32]

Syringomas are derived from the eccrine duct and typically occur in adulthood. The majority of patients present with generalized syringomas, although solitary lesions can occur. These lesions typically occur on the face (especially the lower eyelid), abdomen and vulva.[33] The lesions are multiple flesh top yellowish-colored, 1 to 2 mm subcutaneous nodules. Reports have suggested a higher rate of palpebral syringomas in patients with Down's syndrome.[34] A malignant variant of this lesion has been reported, but is more common in the trunk and extremity.[35] These lesions show locally aggressive

behavior with a tendency toward regional and distant metastasis.[36,37] Multimodality treatment with aggressive surgical resection, adjuvant radiation therapy, and consideration for chemotherapy has been recommended for malignant syringomas.[36,37]

Eccrine spiradenoma are derived from eccrine glandular structures. These tumors typically present as painful subcutaneous nodules in young adults.[38] No anatomical predilection has been reported. Degeneration of eccrine spiradenoma to a malignant variant has been reported, which usually presents as an expanding solitary painful nodule. Malignant tumors are rare, have no site predilection, and display locally aggressive behavior with a propensity for regional and distant metastasis.[39,40] These tumors occur in older patients and manifest as rapidly enlarging lesions which incite a local inflammatory response and an accompanying change in the color of the overlying skin.[41]

Malignant Tumors

Malignant sweat gland tumors can be divided into those of apocrine or eccrine origin and typically occur in older patients in their fifth to sixth decades of life. Unlike most other skin cancers, these lesions do not have a racial predilection, although apocrine tumors may be more common in African Americans.[25,42] Surgical excision is recommended for all types of sweat gland carcinomas, with regional node dissection advocated for patients with clinically palpable lymphadenopathy and electively in selected high risk cases.[43] Taken as a whole, recurrence in sweat gland cancers occurs in the majority of cases, with up to 56 percent having more than one recurrence.[25] Although these tumors tend to be radiation-resistant, adjuvant radiation treatment should be considered in selected cases.[43, 44] *Apocrine gland carcinomas* are less common, occurring most often in the axilla of elderly individuals.[42] In the head and neck, the eyelid region is the one most often involved. In the eyelid, the origin of these tumors are Moll's glands, which are modified apocrine glands.[25] The mortality associated with these tumors is approximately 39 percent.[42] *Eccrine gland carcinomas*, the most common type of sweat gland carcinoma, can arise either de novo or from pre-existing benign lesions. Primary eccrine gland cancers typically present as asymptomatic subcutaneous nodules in elderly individuals. Histologic variants include syringoid, mucinous, microcystic eccrine carcinomas, and adenocarcinomas. Lesions most often involve the extremity and head and neck, with the eyelid as the most common site.[45] Secondary eccrine gland carcinomas are more common, arising from pre-existing benign lesions. Overall, malignant transformation should be suspected when rapid change in size, color, or appearance manifest in a long-standing benign lesion. Details of the most common secondary eccrine gland carcinomas are discussed above as part of the precursor benign lesions.

Sebaceous gland carcinomas typically arise in older females, from the ocular adnexa, including the meibomian glands, Zeis' glands, and the pilosebaceous glands. The facial region is the most common site for extraocular involvement, with rare cases of tumor arising from upper aerodigestive tract mucosa and salivary glands. Prior irradiation may increase the risk for the development of sebaceous carcinoma.[46–48] Local invasion and regional lymphatic metastasis followed by distant metastasis often occurs.

Basal Cell Carcinoma

Basal cell carcinomas (BCC) account for the vast majority of non-melanoma skin cancers (75%) and well over 25 percent of all cancers diagnosed in the United States each year.[49–51] Five clinical histopathologic subtypes of basal cell carcinoma have been described of which nodular ulcerative is most common, followed by pigmented, superficial, morphea-like, and fibroepithelioma.[51] BCC has a predilection for fair-skinned individuals but can occur in Latin American and African American patients.[52] A causative association with chronic ultraviolet radiation exposure has been established.[53] Other factors linked with the development of BCC include immunosuppression and several genetic syndromes. The genetic syndromes include basal cell nevus syndrome, Basex's syndrome and Rambo's syndrome, all of which are associated with the development of multiple basal cell carcinomas.[54]

BCC typically occurs in older individuals in their fourth to eighth decades of life, with a slight male predominance, reflecting the effects of chronic sun exposure. The majority of lesions present with an ulceration, surrounded by a pearly rolled border, thereby earning the appellation of "rodent ulcer." The head and neck region is involved in over 85 percent of cases.[49–51] Within the head and neck region, the nasal tip is the most common site followed by other areas of the face, scalp and neck. These lesions generally display a locally infiltrative behavior pattern but can occasionally metastasize to regional lymph nodes and distant sites. The location of the lesion has been purported to have some influence on behavior, with those occurring in the center of the face having a greater risk for recurrence than other sites.[55] This probably reflects the difficulty of excision to obtain satisfactory margins in central facial lesions. One study showed that the relative risk of recurrence was highest for lesions of the nose, followed by ears, periorbital areas, remainder of the face, neck and scalp and finally, the lowest risk at the trunk and upper extremity. Size greater than 2 cm increased the recurrence rate from 13 percent to 46 percent in one series of 1,620 cases of basal cell carcinoma.[49–51,56]

Metastasis occurs in less than 1 percent of cases and is associated with a dismal outcome.[56] The average survival after the development of a lymph node metastasis is 3.6 years but the metastasis can present as late as 15 years after initial treatment of the primary lesion.[57] Accordingly, long-term follow-up of a patient with this histopathology is required. The rate of metastasis to cervical nodes from basal cell carcinoma is reported to range from 0.0028 to 0.4 percent.[58] Other sites of metastasis include the bones and lungs. The 1-year and 5-year survival rates for metastatic basal carcinoma are reported to be approximately 10 percent and 20 percent respectively.[58]

Treatment of this tumor revolves around surgical excision or radiation therapy.[59] Surgical excision can be accomplished using a variety of techniques including curettage and electrodesiccation, Mohs' surgery, and wide surgical excision. The recurrence rates are purported to be lower for the Mohs' surgery approach, however this likely represents a significant selection bias in the studies reporting these results.[60] The rate of recurrence increases with the margin status, with a recurrence rate of 1.2 percent in absence of tumor at the margin, 12 percent when the tumor is within one high power field, and 33 percent when gross tumor is present at the margin. Surgical margins of 2 to 3 mm are adequate with 85 percent of cases adequately treated in this manner based on results from Mohs' surgical excision.[61,62] Larger lesions and morphea-like lesions require larger margins up to 1 cm.

Squamous Cell Carcinoma

After basal cell carcinoma, squamous cell carcinoma (SCC) is the next most common type of skin cancer accounting for 20 percent of all cutaneous malignancies and occurring in approximately 40 people per 100,000 population annually.[49,63,64] Well over 90 percent of cutaneous squamous cell carcinomas arise in the head and neck and most commonly involve the ears and upper face.[49,64] Like basal cell carcinoma, these lesions have been associated with chronic exposure to UVB radiation.[53] There is a significant increase in the rate of development of squamous cell carcinomas in immunosuppressed patients including patients undergoing medical immunosuppression for organ transplantation, as well as patients with lymphoma and acquired immunodeficiency syndrome.[65–68] Although an increasing proportion of squamous cell carcinoma is seen with age, age is felt to be a coexistent rather than independent variable with respect to causation.

SCC can be effectively treated with either surgery or radiation therapy with equal efficacy.[59,63] Factors associated with poor outcome include size greater than 3 cm, prior treatment, immunosuppression, tumor thickness, perineural invasion, and possibly anatomic site of the lesion—with lesions of the external ear, lip and temple having the worst outcome within the head and neck region.[49,63,64,69] The development of locoregional or distant metastasis has a grave implication for patients with head and neck squamous cell carcinoma and occurs in approximately 0.3 to 13.7 percent of all cases.[70] These metastases can develop in a delayed fashion as seen for basal cell carcinomas. Once local or regional metastasis develops, the 5-year disease free rate drops from approximately 90 percent down to

34 percent.[70] The overall 2- and 5-year survival rates drop to 33 percent and 22 percent respectively. Clinical staging of the neck is the most important prognostic factor once metastasis develops.[49,63,64,69]

Melanocytic Lesions

Malignant Melanoma

The incidence of malignant melanoma in the United States increased by approximately 69 cases per year during the 1970s and by approximately 39 cases per year during the 1980s and 1990s.[70] The death rate from melanoma, however, has not changed during that period, suggesting the impact of more aggressive efforts at early detection. Approximately 20 percent of these tumors involve the head and neck region and occur in patients in their fifth and sixth decades of life.[71–73]

Like non-melanomatous skin cancers, melanoma is more common in fair-skinned individuals but also occurs in darker-skinned populations, albeit at a lower rate. An association with chronic, intense sun exposure has been implicated in the development of melanomas.[71-73] Clinical syndromes such as xeroderma pigmentosum and basal cell nevus syndrome have also been associated with a high rate of melanoma development.[54] A family history of melanoma is associated with a two to eight times increased risk for developing melanoma.[54] Patients undergoing immunosuppression for renal transplantation and those with hematologic malignancies also appear to have a higher risk for melanoma development.

The treatment and prognosis of melanoma is most consistently associated with depth of invasion. Patients with thin lesions less than 0.75 mm tend to have an excellent prognosis and require only local excision. Patients with intermediate thickness melanoma ranging in size from 0.76 to 3.99 mm have a significantly increased risk for development of lymphatic metastasis and therefore require not only adequate surgical resection but also consideration for treatment of regional metastasis.[71–73] Patients with lesions greater than 4 mm in thickness have a dismal prognosis with distant metastasis being the most common source for failure.

Adjuvant therapy should be considered in patients with locally advanced melanoma as well as those with regional or distant metastasis. Adjuvant radiation therapy has been supported by studies from Harwood and colleagues, reporting a 75 percent 4-year locoregional control rate in 89 patients with stage III melanoma who were treated with 3 doses of 800 cGy over a 3-week period.[74–76] Ang and colleagues from M.D. Anderson reported similar control rates for patients with high-risk melanoma using a treatment regimen of 600 cGy fraction × 4 over 2 weeks or × 5 over 2.5 weeks postoperatively.[77–79] Systemic adjuvant therapy is not as well established as yet. Interferon has been approved by the FDA for adjuvant treatment of high-risk patients with melanoma. However, more recent randomized trials have shown disappointing results for interferon use with respect to overall survival.[80–91] Studies looking at gene therapy, immunotherapy, chemotherapy and combinations thereof have been similarly disappointing.[80–91]

Other Cancers

Merkel Cell Carcinoma

Merkel cell carcinomas (MCC) are rare tumors originating from neuro-tactile cells in the epidermis.[92] These lesions present as 0.5 to 5 cm smooth, dome-shaped lesions, with telangiectasias and red to violaceous color. MCCs tend to be indolent, slow-growing tumors, which often display sudden rapid enlargement.[93–97] These tumors typically occur in elderly Caucasian individuals, involving the head and neck region in 49 percent of cases. The distribution of MCC leads to speculation of a relationship to sun exposure, but no definitive association has been established. A study by Goepfert and colleagues reported a 19 percent incidence of excessive sun exposure in patients with head and neck MCC.[93]

MCC occurs in decreasing order of frequency on the skin of the cheek, upper neck, and nose. Treatment requires excision with wide surgical margins and regional nodal dissection in patients with metastasis.[93–97] Elective nodal dissection should be considered in tumors occurring in close proximity to draining lymphatics, having >10 mitotic figures per high power field, displaying histologic evidence of lymphatic involvement, or containing predominantly small cells.

The failure rate is reported to be as high as 75 percent in cases where regional lymphatics are not electively treated. In addition, MCC is a radiosensitive tumor. Therefore, the use of adjuvant radiation may improve local and regional control. Morrison and colleagues recommend the addition of adjuvant radiation in cases with primary lesions over 1.5 cm, narrow resection margins (< 2 cm), or those showing evidence of lymphatic penetration. Dose recommendations for adjuvant treatment are 46 to 50 Gy in 2 Gy fractions and 56 to 60 Gy for unresectable disease.[98]

Even with radical treatment, MCC has an aggressive course. Local recurrence occurs in 40 percent of cases, regional nodal involvement in 46 percent, and distant metastasis in upward of 36 percent of cases. For head and neck primaries, disease control above the clavicles is associated with a lower rate of distant metastasis (69% in patients who fall locoregionally versus 17% in thoses who are free of locoregional disease).[25,92–97] Although a wide variety of locations can be involved, distant metastasis usually occurs to the liver, bone, brain, lung, or skin. Survival is reported to be 88 percent at one year, 72 percent at 2 years, 55 percent at 3 years, and 30 percent at 5 years.[25, 92–97]

Dermatofibrosarcoma Protuberans

Dermatofibrosarcoma protuberans (DFSP) is a low-to intermediate-grade sarcoma that involves the head and neck region in 14 percent of cases, accounting for 1.4 percent of all head and neck sarcomas.[99–102] In the head and neck region, the scalp and supraclavicular fossae are most often involved.[102,103] There is a 3:2 male to female ratio and a predominance in the fourth to fifth decade of life. These tumors typically display a locally aggressive course, with local recurrence rates as high as 60 percent.[99,100,102,103] This reflects the propensity of tumor cells to invade the local tissue with tentacle-like projections within clinically normal-appearing skin. Recurrence rates appear to be higher for head and neck lesions (up to 75% of cases) than those at other sites, probably due to limitations[99,100,102,103] in the extent of surgical resection. Regional and distant metastasis is uncommon, occurring in 1 percent and 4 percent of cases respectively.[99, 100]

The treatment of these neoplasms is wide surgical resection, with resection margins of ≥ 3 cm. The rates of recurrence are directly associated with extent of resection. In a review of series of DFSP treated with conservative margins the rate of recurrence was 44 percent in contrast to 18 percent for series treated with greater than 2 cm margins. Many authors, suggesting a better local control rate with this modality, have advocated the use of Mohs' surgery in the management of DFSP. The use of adjuvant radiation has been suggested to be of benefit in selected cases, but this has not been clearly substantiated.[99,100,102,103] Factors influencing outcome are the size of the primary tumor, extent of resection margins, mitotic index, and the presence of fibrosarcomatous change.

Malignant Fibrous Histiocytoma

Malignant fibrous histiocytoma (MFH) is the most common soft tissue sarcoma in adults, but involves the head and neck region in only 1 to 3 percent of cases.[104–106] There is a 3:2 male to female predominance, and the majority of cases occur in patients 50 to 70 years of age. Subcutaneous lesions form only a small proportion of head and neck MFH, with the majority arising from the upper aerodigestive tract and deep tissues of the neck. Overall, MFH accounts for only 0.01 percent of cutaneous malignancies.[104,106] Studies suggest that MFH in the subcutis has a more infiltrative growth pattern and higher rate of recurrence after surgical treatment. A study by Fanburg-Smith and colleagues showed that 83 percent of subcutaneous MFH displayed an infiltrative growth pattern in contrast to only 24 percent of intramuscular cases.[107,108] Higher rates of involved margins occurred in cases displaying infiltrative growth, advocating a need for wide surgical margins. Local recurrences occurred exclusively in cases displaying infiltrative growth. Wide resection, with margins over 2 cm, is advocated for cutaneous MFH. Adjuvant radiation therapy should be considered in locally advanced cases.

SURGICAL MANAGEMENT OF SKIN CANCER

Anatomic Considerations

The scalp is a unique adaptation of the epithelial covering of the body. Anatomical variations present in the scalp modify both tumor behavior and the treatment of tumors in this area. The hair-bearing area of the scalp consists of a thick padding of hair follicles, sweat glands, fat fibrous tissue and lymphatics that are interspersed with numerous arteries and veins (Figure 4–1). This thick padding is supported by a tough aponeurotic layer that is fused in the anterior region with the frontalis muscle, and in the posterior region with the occipital muscle. This inelastic layer rests loosely on the periosteum of the

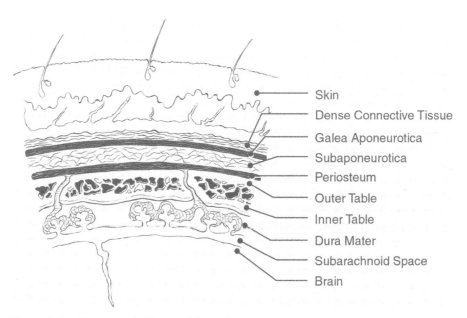

Skin
Dense Connective Tissue
Galea Aponeurotica
Subaponeurotica
Periosteum
Outer Table
Inner Table
Dura Mater
Subarachnoid Space
Brain

Figure 4–1. The anatomical layers of the scalp.

skull creating a potential subaponeurotic space. Laterally, the temporalis muscle provides an additional barrier between the galea and the periosteum.

Three principal arteries provide a rich blood supply to each side of the scalp. Two of these, the superficial temporal and occipital, are branches of the external carotid artery, while the supraorbital artery is a branch of the internal carotid artery. The lymphatic network of the scalp is also unique in that the scalp has no lymph barriers and contains many medium-caliber channels both subdermally and subcutaneously. The lymphatics drain toward the parotid gland, the preauricular area, the upper neck, and the occipital region.

In contrast to the scalp, facial skin is also unique in that it has several distinguishing characteristics on various parts of the face with unique anatomic features providing different functions. For example, the skin around the eyelids is extremely thin with almost no subcutaneous fat. In contrast, the skin around the central part of the face adjacent to the nose and lips is intimately attached to the underlying facial mus-

cles and offers facial expression. Thus, the skin of the central part of the face is mobile, while there are areas of facial skin along the lateral aspect of the nose, the bridge of the nose, and along the preauricular region and temple which are relatively immobile. These unique characteristics of the facial skin have significant surgical implications. Similar to the scalp, the facial skin has a rich blood supply through the facial and superficial temporal arteries. However, unlike the scalp, the facial skin has predictable patterns of lymphatic drainage to preauricular and peri-parotid lymph nodes as well as perivascular facial lymph nodes adjacent to the body of the mandible, eventually draining into the deep jugular chain of lymph nodes.

The most common malignant lesions of the skin of the face and scalp are basal cell carcinomas, squamous cell carcinomas, and melanomas. Occasionally one may see rare lesions such as a keratoacanthoma, Merkel cell tumor, and sweat gland carcinoma. If the extent of the excision is such that a primary closure through an elliptical defect is not possible, then one

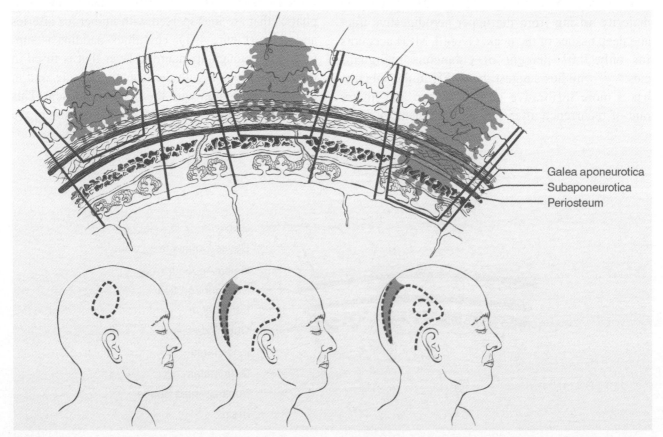

Galea aponeurotica
Subaponeurotica
Periosteum

Figure 4–2. The extent of surgical procedure that would be required for tumors of the scalp depends on the extent and depth of invasion of the tumor.

must consider the applicability of split-thickness or full-thickness skin graft or local, regional or composite microvascular free flaps.

Principles of Treatment

The extent of surgical resection for scalp tumors depends largely upon the depth of infiltration by the tumor. Excision through partial thickness of the scalp can be carried out for superficial tumors while excision through the entire thickness of the scalp including the periosteum may be necessary in deeply infiltrating tumors. On the other hand, tumors that are adherent to or involve the underlying cranium must have removal of the outer table of skull or a through-and-through resection up to and including the dura if necessary. The extent of the surgical procedure that would be required for tumors of the scalp depends on the extent and depth of invasion by the tumor as shown in Figure 4–2.

Small lesions of the skin of the face are excised in the direction of the cleavage planes which are at right angles to the pull of the facial muscles. A brief review of the skin lines of the face is important prior to embarking upon excision of a facial skin lesion. Generally, an elliptical incision is best suited for small lesions. Configuration of the facial skin lines and potential directions for elliptical incisions are shown in Figure 18–4. Remember that the facial skin lines are at right angles to the muscle fibers of the underlying muscles of facial expression (Figure 4–3). By asking the patient to grimace, the line of direction of the long axis for elliptical incision is established. These lines are horizontal on the forehead and around the bridge of the nose and the outer canthus of the eye. Near the cheek the tension lines run obliquely or perpendicularly; near the lips they run radially from the mouth opening, and on the chin they run horizontally on the midline and obliquely perpendicular at the sides. On the sides of the neck, the wrinkles and tension lines run obliquely downward and forward. Horizontal elliptical excision of a small growth of the lower eyelid or the upper eyelid is perfectly suitable, but larger excisions of the lower eyelid performed in this manner result in ectropion. Meticulous attention should be paid to approximation of subcutaneous tissues using absorbable interrupted sutures, and the skin should

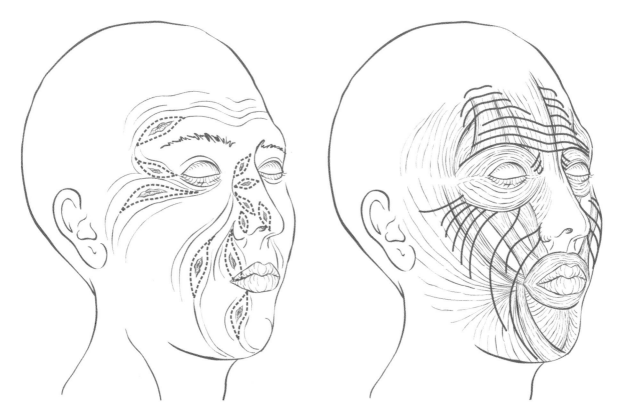

Figure 4–3. Facial skin lines are at right angles to the muscle fibers of the underlying muscles of facial expression.

be closed with fine sutures, which can be removed as early as 4 days postoperatively. Alternatively one may elect to use a subcuticular suture, particularly in the area of the eyelids where the skin is very thin.

Application of split- or full-thickness skin graft is best suited to that part of the face with minimal facial motion such as the lateral aspect of the bridge of the nose or the temple. Similarly, a skin graft can be used in the parotid region because the facial movement in this area is minimal and cosmetic disfigurement is minimal. The most suitable donor sites for obtaining full-thickness skin grafts are from the retroauricular or supraclavicular regions.

Flaps from the immediate neighborhood of the defect are most desirable from both the functional and esthetic points of view. Primary closure of the donor site defect can usually be accomplished with ease by proper planning of local skin flaps. When repair of a surgical defect demands more adequate full-thickness reconstruction, local flaps are best suited for this purpose. The blood supply of facial skin and soft tissues is extremely rich, as the terminal branches of the external carotid artery provide a major source of blood to the facial skin. In addition to this, there is an extensive subdermal anastomotic network, which facilitates the use of several random flaps with relative ease. Some flaps carry an identifiable axial blood supply while others are more random. Examples of axial skin flaps are: nasolabial, glabellar, Mustarde cheek, and temporal forehead; examples of random flaps are: cervical, rhomboid, and bilobed. If local flaps are not suitable, then consideration should be given to regional or distant microvascular free flaps for appropriate repair of large surgical defects in the facial region.

Metastatic dissemination to regional lymph nodes from primary cutaneous malignancies of the scalp and face is infrequent. In general, squamous carcinomas less than 2 cm in diameter have an exceedingly low risk of metastatic potential and therefore elective treatment of regional lymph nodes is not recommended. Lesions larger than 2 cm have a proportionately higher risk of regional lymphatic dissemination. In general, however, elective resection of regional lymphatics does not offer significant therapeutic advantage. Slight improvement in prognosis is observed with elective dissection of regional lymph nodes for intermediate thickness malignant melanomas of cutaneous origin.

Selection of Treatment

Surgery and radiotherapy remain the mainstay of treatment for cutaneous malignancies of the scalp and facial skin. Radiotherapy is particularly of benefit in patients with basal cell carcinomas of the eyelids where surgical resection is likely to result in significant morbidity. Extensive basal cell carcinomas may be treated by radiotherapy under select circumstances with a palliative intent.

Mohs' micrographic surgery is an ideal method to secure histologic clearance of all subdermal and intradermal extensions of cutaneous cancers. It is of particular value in patients with the morphea form of basal cell carcinomas, recurrent basal cell carcinomas adjacent to vital areas of the face, and extensive recurrent skin cancers in previously irradiated fields where the clinical assessment of the extent of disease is suboptimal. On the other hand, this technique is not cost-effective for most patients with small skin cancers, which can be adequately excised surgically with primary repair of the surgical defect.

Selected Cases

Case 1. Excision of Scalp Tumor and Split-thickness Skin Graft

The patient shown in Figure 4–4A has a nodular-pigmented basal cell carcinoma of the scalp measuring approximately 2.5 × 4.5 cm. This skin tumor is freely mobile over the underlying periosteum, so the galea aponeurotica will form the deep margin of the surgical specimen for this tumor.

Although most of the lesion is nodular and protuberant in nature, there is an additional intracutaneous component, which could only be seen after the scalp was shaved. Generally, a margin of at least 1 cm around the lesion is desirable. A fairly thick split-thickness skin graft (1/18,000") is desirable to avoid ulceration and trauma to the scalp. Thin split-thickness skin grafts give a very tight and shiny appearance and are prone to ulceration even with trivial trauma.

The deep surface of the surgical specimen showed galea aponeurotica which was grossly uninvolved by tumor. When the bolster dressing is removed, trimming of crust and clots at the edges of the surgical defect is necessary to keep it clean until full maturation of the grafted area takes place. The patient should be instructed in avoiding direct trauma or injury to this area.

The postoperative appearance of the patient approximately 6 months following surgery shows a 100 percent take of the skin graft (Figure 4–4B). The split-thickness skin graft can be used effectively to provide immediate coverage for defects in the scalp when the periosteum can be preserved.

Case 2. Excision of Scalp Tumor with Advancement Rotation Flap

Surgical excision of tumors in the non-hair-bearing areas of the scalp requires coverage of the surgical defect with tissues that resemble the normal tissues in the area for a satisfactory esthetic appearance. Although split-thickness skin graft can be used to cover such surgical defects, its esthetic appearance is unacceptable. Advancement rotation scalp flaps provide a very satisfactory method of closure of such surgical defects. The defect is covered with the adjacent scalp while the donor site deformity is transferred posteriorly in the hair-bearing area of the scalp which may be either closed primarily or, on occasion, covered with a split-thickness skin graft. Alternatively, large defects of the non-hair-bearing area of the scalp or forehead can be repaired with a radial forearm microvascular free flap.

When surgical excision of a scalp tumor requires excision of the underlying periosteum, then bare bones of the calvaria are exposed. Scalp flaps or microvascular free flaps are the ideal method of coverage of such surgical defects.

The patient shown in Figure 4–5A had a recurrent basal cell carcinoma involving the midline frontal area of the scalp. A local excision was performed for biopsy purposes elsewhere prior to presentation. The intended extent of surgical excision and the outline of the rotation advancement flap are shown in Figure 4–5A. Even though the anticipated surgical defect is relatively small, a large area of the scalp has to be ele-

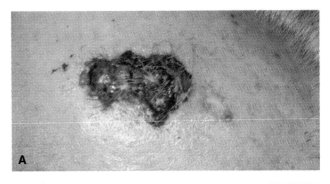

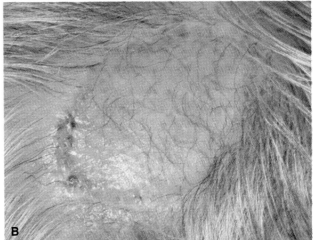

Figure 4–4. *A* A pigmented basal cell carcinoma of the scalp. *B* The defect of surgical excision was reconstructed with a split-thickness skin graft and resulted in an acceptable appearance 6 months postoperatively.

vated because of its inelasticity and consequent inability to provide sufficient mobilization and coverage. The blood supply of this scalp flap is through both the superficial temporal as well as the occipital artery. The flap is advanced anteriorly and rotated inferiorly to cover the surgical defect. Meticulous attention should be paid in the outline of the flap by appropriate measuring of the surgical defect and the rotated scalp flap, keeping the pivot point in mind. A measurement can be taken using 4 × 8 inch gauze, holding one end at the pivot near the external ear and the other extended to the apex of the surgical defect inferomedially. Using that length as a radius, the scalp flap is outlined all the way up to the parieto-occipital region. Thus, if proper measurements are taken, the flap will satisfactorily rotate and cover the surgical defect.

The flap is reflected laterally showing its proximal mobilization up to the vascular pedicle near the pinna. The flap is now rotated both anteriorly and inferiorly to cover the surgical defect (Figure 4–5B and C). The anterior end of the scalp flap should be adequate to match the lower border of the surgical defect.

The postoperative appearance of the patient approximately 7 months following surgery is shown in Figure 4–5D. There is excellent coverage of the surgical defect near the hairline without any significant functional or esthetic deformity.

Advancement rotation scalp flaps are very satisfactory for most defects of the anterior scalp. However, if these defects are of significant size, then primary closure of the donor site is not possible and a split-thickness skin graft would be necessary in the occipital region.

Case 3. Excision and Full-thickness Skin Graft on the Nose

This patient presented with Hutchinson's melanotic freckle (lentigo maligna) on the dorsum of the nose. The desired extent of excision is marked out with a skin marking pen and its dimensions are measured. The ideal donor site is the skin of the supraclavicular region for a defect of this size.

The postoperative appearance of the skin graft in this patient immediately after surgery is shown in Figure 4–6A and 6 months postoperatively in Figure 4–6B. Since sensations on this skin are absent, the

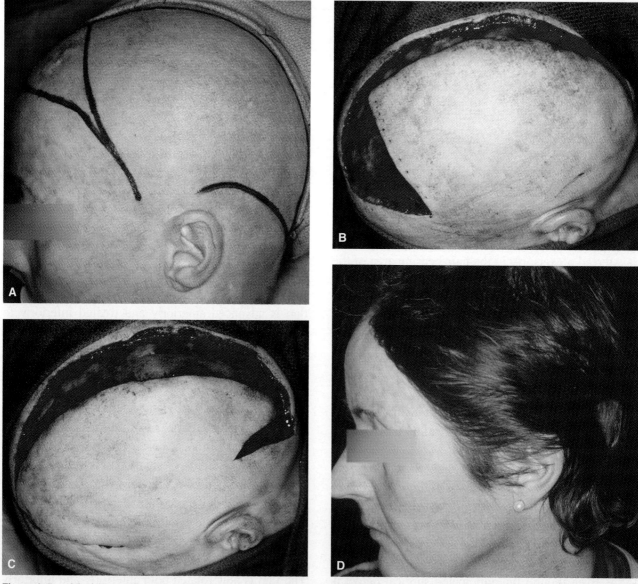

Figure 4–5. *A,* Incisions outlined for excision of a recurrent basal cell carcinoma of the frontal scalp. *B* and *C,* A scalp flap is elevated rotated and advanced into the surgical defect. *D,* Postoperative appearance of the patient 7 months following surgery.

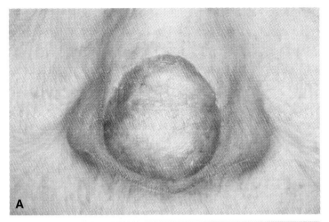

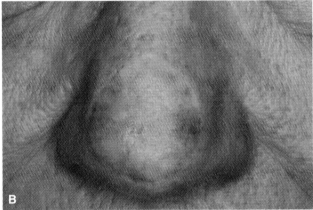

Figure 4–6. *A,* Immediate postoperative appearance of a full-thickness skin graft on the dorsum of the nose. *B,* The same patient 6 months later.

patient must avoid trauma to prevent ulceration and infection. The esthetic result with a full-thickness skin graft is excellent on the lateral aspect of the nose with no specific donor site deformity.

Case 4. Glabellar Flap

This flap is best suited for reconstruction of surgical defects at either the bridge or the upper half of the nose. It is an axial flap, which derives its blood supply mainly from the supratrochlear artery and also from the dorsal nasal branches. The flap can also be used for complex defects of the nasal dorsum with a split-thickness skin graft on its undersurface.

The patient shown here has a basal cell carcinoma involving the skin of the bridge of the nose (Figure 4–7A). The skin is freely mobile over the underlying periosteum. The lesion is excised and flap rotated into place for reconstruction (Figure 4–7B). The skin flap has set well in place with well balanced eye-

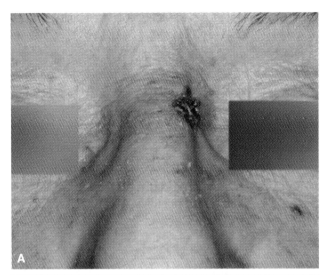

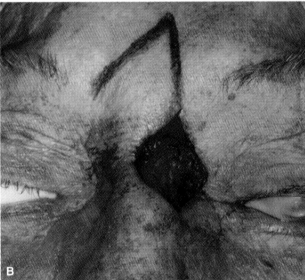

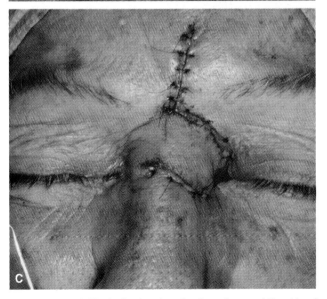

Figure 4–7. *A,* The lesion is a basal cell carcinoma of the skin of the nose. *B,* The defect of surgical excision and outline of the glabellar flap. *C,* The flap is inset and the donor defect is closed primarily.

brows on both sides and satisfactory coverage of the skin and soft-tissue defect at the bridge of the nose. Closure of the donor site leaves an esthetically acceptable midline vertical scar (Figure 4–7C).

A modification of this procedure is an island glabellar flap where the flap is tunneled under an intact bridge of skin at the glabella, keeping its blood supply intact on the vascular pedicle containing the supratrochlear artery and vein. However, elevation of an island flap in this fashion is risky and has very limited application.

Case 5. Nasolabial Flap

The nasolabial flap is an axial flap deriving its blood supply from the nasolabial artery, one of the termi-

nal branches of the facial artery. The width to length ratio can be as much as 1:5 in select circumstances. The nasolabial flap is a highly reliable and very versatile flap. It is generally employed in reconstruction of surgical defects resulting from excision of skin cancers on the side of the nose or the ala of the nose, as well as for full-thickness reconstruction of excised nasal ala, philtrum and columella.

Case 5a. Inferiorly Based Nasolabial Flap

Since the vascular supply of the nasolabial flap is through the nasolabial artery, it would appear logical to have the flap based inferiorly. This flap is ideally suited for small defects of the lateral aspect of the nose in its lower half (Figure 4–8). The elevated dis-

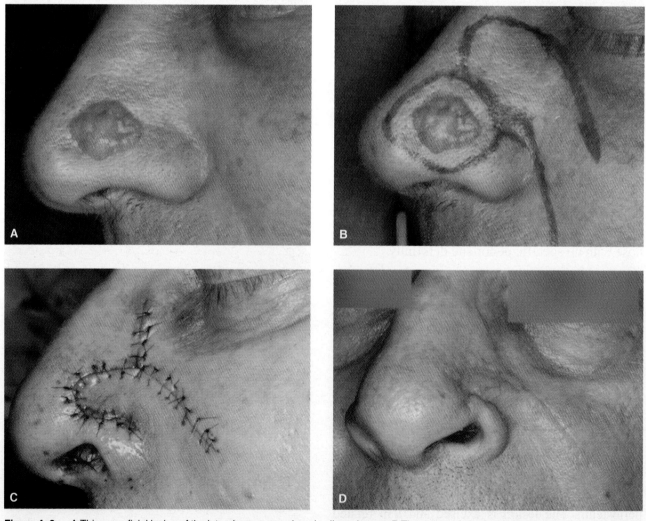

Figure 4–8.   *A,* This superficial lesion of the lateral nose was a basal cell carcinoma. *B,* The extent of surgical excision and in inferiorly based nasolabial flap have been marked out. *C,* Immediate postoperative appearance of the flap set into the surgical defect. The donor defect is closed primarily. *D,* Postoperative appearance of the patient 6 months later.

tal part of the flap is rotated downward and anteriorly to fill the surgical defect. However, the length of a flap used in this way is limited since the skin at the root of the nose near the medial canthus is rather tight and little flexibility is available for closure of the donor site defect.

Edema of the flap and slight duskiness is not unusual on the first postoperative day. Although the flap may look dusky or bluish, its vascularity is guaranteed; the discoloration is usually due to venous congestion, but the arterial blood supply of the flap is usually intact. Satisfactory healing of the skin is achieved in approximately 5 to 7 days. Excessive fat retained on the flap will result in a so-called fat flap, which may require defattening under local anesthesia; but this procedure is not recommended for at least 6 months to a year. If sufficient care is taken to match the thickness of the flap to the thickness of the surgical defect with appropriate excision of excess fat from the flap at the time of the closure, one can avoid a fat flap complication. Postoperative appearance of the patient several months later shows an excellent cosmetic result with essentially very little facial deformity at either the donor site or along the nasolabial skin crease.

Case 5b. Superiorly based Nasolabial Flap Reconstruction for a Complex Defect of the Alar Region

A patient with a recurrent basal cell carcinoma involving the skin of the ala and through the alar cartilage and nasal mucosa into the nasal vestibule is shown in Figure 4–9A. The lesion had previously been treated by electrodesiccation and curettage on two occasions.

The plan of surgical excision requires a through-and-through resection of the ala of the nose including the underlying mucosa, and a superiorly based nasolabial flap is planned for reconstruction of the surgical defect, providing external and inner lining (see Figure 4–9A).

The excision is completed showing a through-and-through defect. The superiorly based nasolabial flap is elevated (Figure 4–9B). The flap is elevated lateral to the nasolabial crease with a generous amount of fat on the undersurface. The tip of the flap is turned in to provide inner lining and the donor defect can be easily approximated primarily.

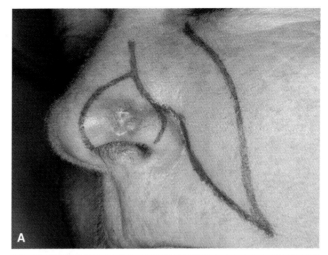
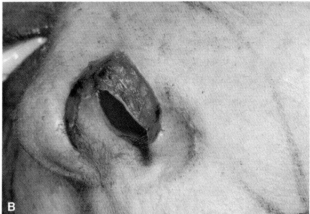
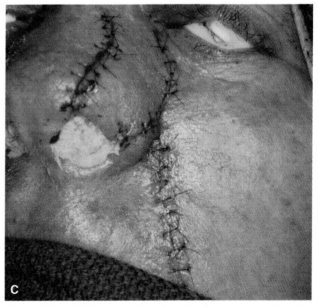

Figure 4–9. *A,* The patient has a basal cell carcinoma of the skin of the nasal ala adherent to the underlying cartilage and mucosa. The extent of surgical excision is outlined along with a superiorly based nasolabial flap. *B,* A composite resection including the skin, cartilage and mucosa resulted in a full-thickness alar defect. *C,* The superiorly based nasolabial flap is elevated and set into the defect. Its tip is turned on to itself to provide inner lining and the donor defect is closed primarily.

The nasolabial flap used in this way is ideal for repair of a complex defect of the alar region of the nose. The flap is folded over itself to replace the free edge of the ala (Figure 4–9C) and is esthetically quite acceptable. Cartilage support is usually not necessary unless the alar defect extends from the tip of the nose to the region of the nasolabial crease.

Case 6. Rhomboid Flap

This versatile geometric flap was described by Limberg, a mathematician. It can be used in many areas of the body and provides a satisfactory closure of surgical defects, particularly in patients with lax skin.

The patient shown in Figure 4–10A was referred having undergone excisional biopsy of a malignant melanoma of the cheek. The scar of previous surgery was widely encompassed in the surgical incisions which were planned to provide access for superficial parotidectomy at the same operation. The rhomboid flap outline should be made in such a way that the donor site closure line will match facial skin lines. A surgical defect of any shape can be converted to a rhomboid, thus allowing design and elevation of this flap. Surgical excision of the recurrent cancer is carried out to include the subcutaneous tissue but remains superficial to the muscular layer. In this particular patient, terminal branches of the facial nerve remain at risk because of their proximity to the deep margin of the surgical specimen. These branches must be preserved by meticulous dissection, unless tumor invasion is demonstrated. A superficial parotidectomy was completed in this patient and the inferiorly based rhomboid flap (Figure 4–10B) was used to reconstruct the defect with an acceptable esthetic result approximately 6 months after surgery (Figure 4–10C).

The rhomboid is a random flap and therefore has limited application for coverage of larger-size defects. It is a highly reliable flap, and when properly planned as to placing the incisions for flap elevation, the eventual esthetic result is excellent.

Case 7. Bilobed Flap

The bilobed flap is a random flap but is excellent for coverage of various surgical defects throughout the

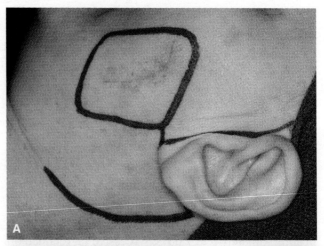

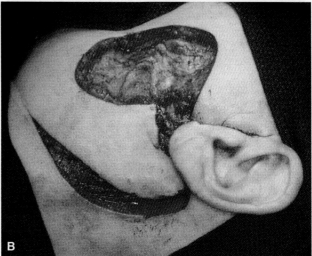

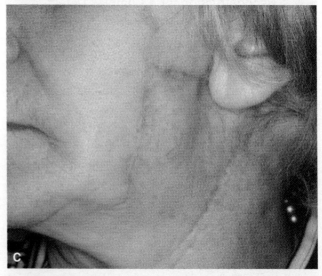

Figure 4–10. *A* The patient had undergone excisional biopsy of a malignant melanoma of the cheek elsewhere. The scar of previous excision was widely encompassed in the surgical incisions which were planned to provide access for a superficial parotidectomy. *B* An inferiorly based cervical Limberg flap has been elevated and the surgical bed of resection shows the branches of the facial nerve preserved. *C* Postoperative appearance of the patient approximately 6 months following surgery.

body. The principle of "borrowing from Peter to pay Paul" is exemplified in the design and elevation of this flap.

The bilobed flap can be used very effectively on defects of the anterior cheek. Surgical defects of the skin and soft tissues of the cheek overlying the zygoma and the buccinator muscle are very well suited for reconstruction using a bilobed flap. The patient shown here has a recurrent malignant melanoma involving the skin and subcutaneous tissues of the left zygomatic region. The area of skin at risk around the tumor which measures approximately 5 cm in diameter is outlined, and the inferiorly based bilobed flap has been planned (Figure 4–11A).

The surgical excision is completed and Figure 4–11B shows the defect, exposing the branches of the facial nerve in the upper part of the surgical field. The bilobed flap is elevated, superficial to the facial musculature but keeping all the subcutaneous fat on the flap. The flap is rotated into the defect and final skin closure is shown in Figure 4–11C.

The postoperative appearance of the patient approximately 2 months following surgery shows satisfactory closure of the surgical defect with an acceptable esthetic result (Figure 4–11D). Bilobed flaps used in this fashion provide a very readily available tool for the closure of sizable skin defects of the cheek. The flap works best in patients who have excess or

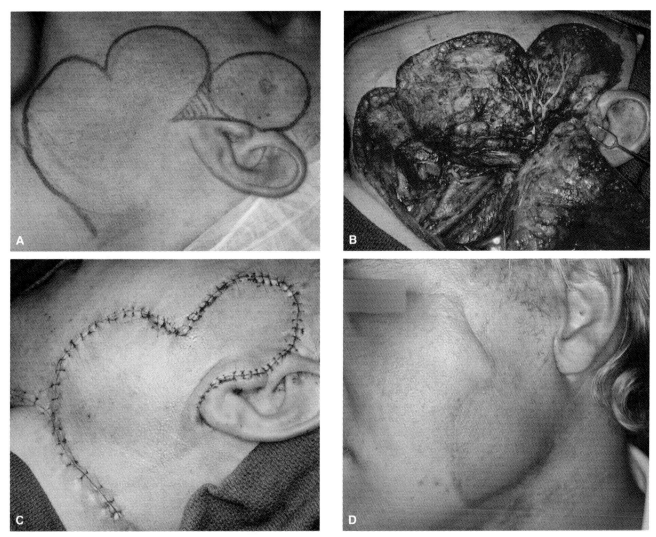

Figure 4–11. *A,* The lesion is a malignant melanoma in the left zygomatic region. A generous area of excision is outlined around the tumor and the inferiorly based bilobed flap is planned. *B,* The primary lesion has been excised in continuity with the superficial parotid lobe and the contents of the upper neck. The branches of the facial nerve have been carefully preserved and are clearly demonstrated in the surgical bed. The bilobed flap has been elevated and retracted laterally. *C,* The bilobed flap is rotated into the surgical defect and sutured into place. *D,* Approximately 2 months later the flap has healed well and has produced an acceptable cosmetic result.

lax skin providing easy rotation of the flap and closure of the donor site deformity, leaving a transverse scar along the upper skin crease in the neck.

Case 8. Mustardé Advancement Rotation Cheek Flap

Skin defects resulting from surgical excision of lesions involving the skin in the infraorbital region and medial part of the cheek are best suited for repair using a Mustardé flap. The major blood supply of this skin flap is from the posterior branches of the facial artery with the wide pedicle of the flap remaining inferiorly.

A patient with a Hutchinson's melanotic freckle (lentigo maligna or in situ melanoma) presenting on the skin of the cheek in the right infraorbital region is shown in Figure 4–12A. The superior margin of the surgical defect and the Mustardé flap are kept as close to the tarsal margin as possible, depending on the location of the lesion and the surgical defect. In this particular patient, the medial border of the defect was aligned to the nasolabial skin crease. The extent of surgical resection depends on the surface dimension, depth, and histology of the primary tumor.

Excision of the tumor is completed, preserving the orbicularis oculi and its nerve supply but carefully excising a generous margin of underlying fat (Figure

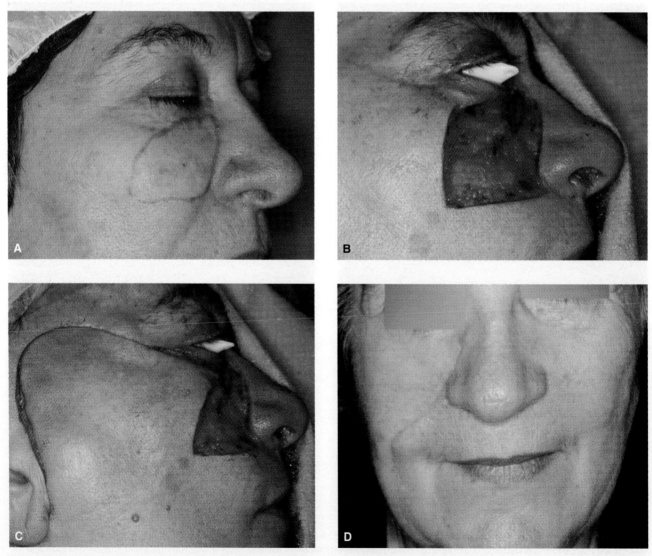

Figure 4–12.   *A,* The area of excision around a superficial pigmented lesion in the right infraorbital region is marked out. *B,* The defect of surgical excision. *C,* A Mustarde-type advancement flap has been elevated to reconstruct the defect. *D,* Postoperative appearance of the patient 3 months later.

4–12B). Skin incision is completed for elevation of the Mustardé flap (Figure 4–12C) and the flap is rotated anteromedially to cover the surgical defect.

The postoperative appearance of the patient approximately 3 months later shows an acceptable esthetic result achieved by this technique (Figure 4–12D).

Case 9. Cervical Flap

Skin defects resulting from excision of lesions of the skin of the chin or the lower part of the face present a problem best handled by reconstruction using a cervical flap. The transverse-oriented cervical flap is a random flap, so the length to which it can be elevated with ease without compromise of blood supply is limited. Generally, a width to length ratio of 1:3 is the maximum that a random flap can tolerate.

A patient with a recurrent nodular basal cell carcinoma involving the skin, soft tissues and the underlying musculature of the chin is shown in Figure 4–13A. A cervical flap is marked out inferior to the proposed surgical defect (Figure 4–13B). Surgical excision in this patient will be carried down to the bone because of the depth of the tumor infiltration, so the cervical flap requires inclusion of the underlying subcutaneous tissue and platysma to provide soft tissue in addition to skin. The resultant donor defect can be easily closed primarily if the orientation of the flap takes advantage of the laxity of the tissues of the neck.

A satisfactory esthetic result can be accomplished in a one-stage procedure for a sizeable defect of the skin of the chin. Minor revision and defatting of the flap can be undertaken at a later stage to enhance the esthetic appearance of the patient.

Case 10. Island Pedicle Flap

Island pedicle flaps with their vascular pedicles can be isolated in various locations in the head and neck area. One of the most versatile and easily available island pedicle flaps is based on the anterior branch of the superficial temporal artery and vein which provides blood supply to the forehead. This flap is elevated from the lateral aspect of the forehead.

Its advantages include fairly regular and identifiable artery and vein, a long vascular pedicle, and thick forehead skin to provide for replacement of excised skin and soft tissues. The color match is also excellent for coverage of facial surgical defects. The disadvantages are that the size of the flap is limited and occasionally it may be hair-bearing. It is important to ensure smooth rotation of the pedicle since a kink in the vascular pedicle of the flap can result in a disaster with complete loss of flap.

A patient with a recurrent basal cell carcinoma who had previous curettage and desiccation as well as surgical excision of this lesion performed elsewhere is shown in Figure 4–14A. The lesion is indurated and adherent to the underlying zygoma.

The plan of surgical excision and repair showing the incision at the site of the primary tumor is shown in Figure 4–14A. The surgical defect shows a through-and-through three-dimensional excision of

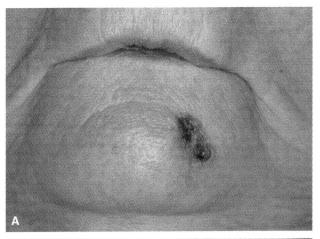
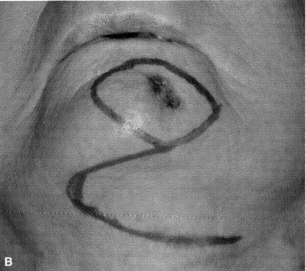

Figure 4–13. *A* The patient has a basal cell carcinoma on the left chin. *B* An area of excision has been outlined around the tumor along with the proposed cervical flap for reconstruction of the defect.

the recurrent basal cell carcinoma (Figure 4–14B). All margins of resection are checked at this point to ensure adequacy of excision.

The island pedicle flap is now isolated with a circular disk of skin from the forehead on the vascular pedicle from the anterior branch of the superficial temporal artery and vein (see Figure 4–14B and C). The flap is elevated, rotated and sutured into place and the donor defect is covered with a split-thickness skin graft.

The postoperative appearance of the patient approximately 2 months after surgery is shown in

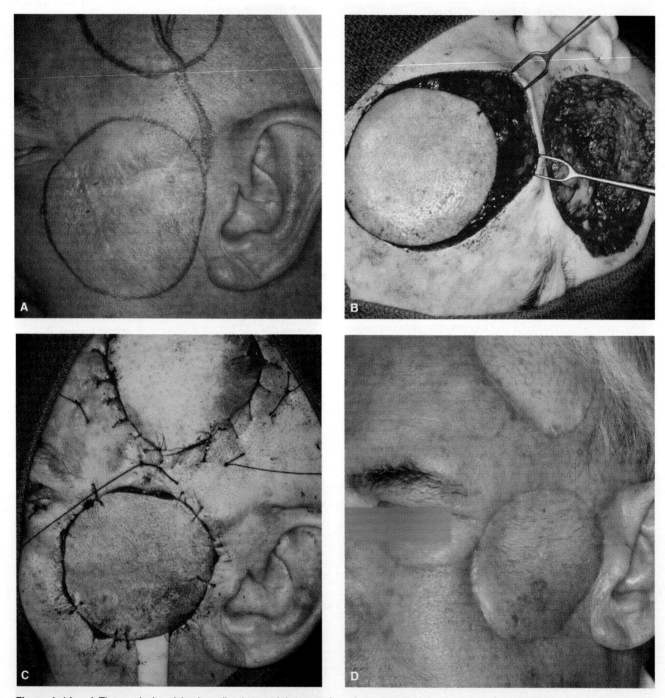

Figure 4–14.   *A,* The surgical excision is outlined around the scar of previous surgery and a corresponding island of skin is marked on the lateral forehead based on the anterior branch of the superficial temporal artery. *B* and *C,* After excision of the primary lesion, the flap is elevated on its vascular pedicle, rotated cauded to fill the surgical defect, and the donor site is skin grafted. *D,* The postoperative appearance of the patient 2 months after surgery.

Figure 4–14D. Although excellent coverage of the surgical defect is obtained, the esthetic result is not as pleasing as one would like to see, due largely to loss of underlying zygoma and masseter muscle, causing lack of soft-tissue support. This in turn causes lack of fullness and a sunken appearance of the cheek.

Island pedicle flaps are excellent for coverage of certain surgical defects resulting from loss of skin and soft tissues in the region of the nose or the side of the cheek. However, extreme caution and skill must be exercised in anticipation of the size of both the surgical defect and the elevated skin flap. Meticulous attention should be paid to extremely careful and skillful dissection and gentle handling of the vascular pedicle, as injury to the vascular pedicle would mean loss of the flap. Those branches of the vessels that are not necessary for the vascularity of the flap are sacrificed, but short stumps of these vessels must be left attached to the main vascular pedicle so that the lumen of the feeding artery and draining vein is not compromised. Similarly, extreme care must be exercised during transport of the flap and its rotation to avoid any kinking or torsion. The island flap generally manifests venous congestion in the first 48 hours, but as long as capillary filling is present the flap will survive.

Case 11. Excision and Repair of a Large Defect of Facial Skin with Myocutaneous Free Flap

Larger defects of the facial skin are best repaired using a free tissue transfer where unlimited quantities of skin and soft tissue are available to repair the surgical defect. The disadvantage of free tissue transfer is that the color match often is not satisfactory and occasionally the tissue may be too bulky.

The patient shown in Figure 4–15A has a locally advanced, fungating squamous cell carcinoma of the preauricular region requiring wide excision, superficial parotidectomy and a neck dissection. A generous portion of the skin in the preauricular region was excised to encompass a three-dimensional resection in continuity with an ipsilateral comprehensive neck dissection (Figure 4–15B). The surgical defect thus created was repaired with a myocutaneous rectus abdominis flap. Postoperative appearance of the patient shows a satisfactory reconstruction of this large surgical defect, although the color match is not ideal (Figure 4–15C).

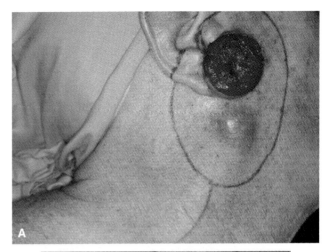

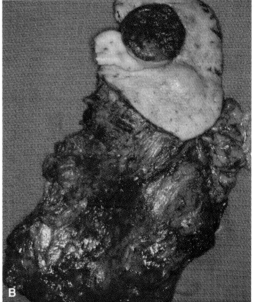

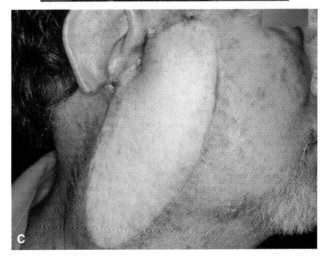

Figure 4–15. *A* Locally advanced squamous cell carcinoma of the right preauricular skin showing extent of surgical excision outlined. *B* The surgical specimen shows the extent of excision of the primary tumor en bloc with the contents of the right neck. *C* The defect was reconstructed using a myocutaneous rectus abdominis flap—seen here 1 month after surgery.

Case 12. Wedge Excision of the External Ear

Malignant tumors of the skin of the external ear often invade the underlying cartilage or perforate through to present on both sides of the external ear. These lesions require a through-and-through excision of a portion of the pinna to remove the tumor

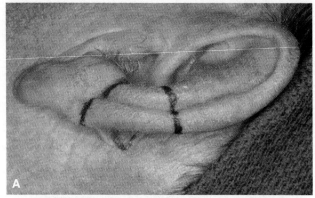

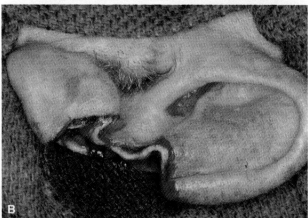

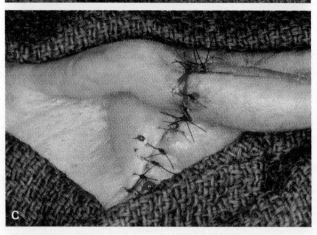

Figure 4–16.   *A,* The patient has a recurrent basal cell carcinoma of the pinna involving the underlying cartilage and presenting mainly on the posterior aspect. A wedge-shaped area of excision has been marked out. *B,* The full-thickness surgical defect showing retraction of the skin edges over the cartilage. *C,* The surgical defect is closed primarily in layers.

satisfactorily. Surgical defects resulting from excision of one-third of the vertical height of the pinna are suitable for primary closure by approximating the edges of the surgical defect. The height of the pinna is reduced, but the esthetic result is acceptable.

The preoperative appearance of the anterior surface of the pinna of a patient with a recurrent basal cell carcinoma involving the underlying cartilage mainly presenting on the posterior aspect is shown in Figure 4–16A. The lesion involves the helix and the underlying cartilage.

A plan of surgical excision is outlined by an incision drawn to resect a wedge of the ear with the apex of the wedge in the retroauricular skin crease (see Figure 4–16A). A similar incision is marked out on the anterior aspect of the pinna so that the apex of the surgical defect meets at approximately the same point both anteriorly and posteriorly. Excision is made with a scalpel in a through-and-through fashion along the pre-drawn skin incision. A wedge of the pinna is excised, including the skin of the anterior aspect, the cartilage beneath as well as the skin of the posterior aspect until the two skin incisions meet at the apex of the wedge. An extra margin of the cartilage is removed to facilitate skin closure. The skin edges usually retract over the cartilage immediately following excision of the tumor (Figure 4–16B).

Wedge excision of the pinna is a very acceptable and satisfactory operative procedure for lesions requiring through-and-through excision of any parts of the external ear. Primary closure is possible for defects not exceeding one-third of the vertical height of the pinna (Figure 4–16C). Larger defects are not suitable for primary closure.

CONCLUSION

Cancers of the skin are the most common human malignancies. Skin cancers include a myriad of tumors, which vary widely in their clinical behavior. The epidemiology, evaluation and treatment of many of the skin cancers is changing, as highlighted in malignant melanoma, where increasing incidence, application of screening techniques, use of molecular markers and advent of novel treatments are changing the clinical course of the disease. An understanding of the biology of each pathologic subtype is required to plan and deliver successful treatment. Surgical extirpation plays an important role in the management forms of many skin cancers and requires an approach that takes into account not only tumor factors, but also achieves a delicate balance with cosmesis and function. The use of adjuvant treatments plays an integral role in management, especially for advanced cancers. A systematic approach to evaluation and treatment is required to optimize outcomes.

REFERENCES

1. Greenlee RT, Hill-Harmon MB, Murray T, Thun M. Cancer statistics, 2001. CA Cancer J Clin 2001;51(1):15–36.

2. Hayes AG, Berry AD. Basal cell carcinoma arising in a fibroepithelial polyp. J Am Acad Dermatol 1993;28(3):493–5.

3. Eads TJ, Chuang TY, Fabre VC, et al. The utility of submitting fibroepithelial polyps for histological examination. Arch Dermatol 1996;132(12):1459–62.

4. Cribier B, Asch P, Grosshans E. Differentiating squamous cell carcinoma from keratoacanthoma using histopathological criteria. Is it possible? A study of 296 cases. Dermatology 1999;199(3):208–12.

5. Netscher DT, Wigoda P, Green LK, Spira M. Keratoacanthoma: when to observe and when to operate and the importance of accurate diagnosis. South Med J 1994;87(12):1272–6.

6. Schwartz RA. The actinic keratosis. A perspective and update. Dermatol Surg 1997;23(11):1009–19.

7. Salasche SJ. Epidemiology of actinic keratoses and squamous cell carcinoma. J Am Acad Dermatol 2000;42(1 Pt 2):4–7.

8. Sloan JB, Jaworsky C. Clinical misdiagnosis of squamous cell carcinoma in situ as seborrheic keratosis. A prospective study. J Dermatol Surg Oncol 1993;19(5):413–6.

9. Marks R. Treatment of keratoses. Australas J Dermatol 1988;29(1):58–9.

10. Hughes BR, Marks R, Pearse AD, Gaskell SA. Clinical response and tissue effects of etretinate treatment of patients with solar keratoses and basal cell carcinoma. J Am Acad Dermatol 1988;18(3):522–9.

11. Marks R, Rennie G, Selwood TS. Malignant transformation of solar keratoses to squamous cell carcinoma. Lancet 1988;1(8589):795–7.

12. Moy RL. Clinical presentation of actinic keratoses and squamous cell carcinoma. J Am Acad Dermatol 2000;42(1 Pt 2):8–10.

13. Dinehart SM. The treatment of actinic keratoses. J Am Acad Dermatol 2000;42(1 Pt 2):25–8.

14. Feldman SR, Fleischer AB Jr, Williford PM, Jorizzo JL. Destructive procedures are the standard of care for treatment of actinic keratoses. J Am Acad Dermatol 1999;40(1):43–7.

15. Bercovitch L. Topical chemotherapy of actinic keratoses of the upper extremity with tretinoin and 5-fluorouracil: a double-blind controlled study. Br J Dermatol 1987;116(4):549–52.

16. Kurwa HA, Yong-Gee SA, Seed PT, et al. A randomized paired comparison of photodynamic therapy and topical 5- fluorouracil in the treatment of actinic keratoses. J Am Acad Dermatol 1999;41(3 Pt 1):414–8.

17. Kurwa HA, Barlow RJ. The role of photodynamic therapy in dermatology. Clin Exp Dermatol 1999;24(3):143–8.

18. Cribier B, Scrivener Y, Grosshans E. Tumors arising in nevus sebaceus: A study of 596 cases. J Am Acad Dermatol 2000;42(2 Pt 1):263–8.

19. Chun K, Vazquez M, Sanchez JL. Nevus sebaceus: clinical outcome and considerations for prophylactic excision. Int J Dermatol 1995;34(8):538–41.

20. Julian CG, Bowers PW. A clinical review of 209 pilomatricomas. J Am Acad Dermatol 1998;39(2 Pt 1):191–5.

21. Geh JL, Wilson GR. Unusual multiple pilomatrixomata: case report and review of the literature. Br J Plast Surg 1999;52(4):320–1.

22. Geh JL, Moss AL. Multiple pilomatrixomata and myotonic dystrophy: a familial association. Br J Plast Surg 1999;52(2):143–5.

23. Bremnes RM, Kvamme JM, Stalsberg H, Jacobsen EA. Pilomatrix carcinoma with multiple metastases: report of a case and review of the literature. Eur J Cancer 1999;35(3):433–7.

24. Duflo S, Nicollas R, Roman S, et al. Pilomatrixoma of the head and neck in children: a study of 38 cases and a review of the literature. Arch Otolaryngol Head Neck Surg 1998;124(11):1239–42.

25. Marenda SA, Otto RA. Adnexal carcinomas of the skin. Otolaryngol Clin North Am 1993;26(1):87–116.

26. Lopansri S, Mihm MC Jr. Pilomatrix carcinoma or calcifying epitheliocarcinoma of Malherbe: a case report and review of literature. Cancer 1980;45(9):2368–73.

27. Green A, Beardmore G, Hart V, et al. Skin cancer in a Queensland population. J Am Acad Dermatol 1988;19(6):1045–52.

28. Biggs PJ, Wooster R, Ford D, et al. Familial cylindromatosis (turban tumour syndrome) gene localised to chromosome 16q12-q13: evidence for its role as a tumour suppressor gene. Nat Genet 1995;11(4):441–3.

29. Gerretsen AL, van der Putte SC, Deenstra W, van Vloten WA. Cutaneous cylindroma with malignant transformation. Cancer 1993;72(5):1618–23.

30. Hammond DC, Grant KF, Simpson WD. Malignant degeneration of dermal cylindroma. Ann Plast Surg 1990;24(2):176–8.

31. Niizuma K. Syringocystadenoma papilliferum: light and electron microscopic studies. Acta Derm Venereol 1976;56(5):327–36.

32. Greer KE, Bishop GF, Ober WC. Nevus sebaceous and syringocystadenoma papilliferum. Arch Dermatol 1976;112(2):206–8.

33. Patrizi A, Neri I, Marzaduri S, et al. Syringoma: a review of twenty-nine cases. Acta Derm Venereol 1998;78(6):460–2.

34. Schepis C, Siragusa M, Palazzo R, et al. Palpebral syringomas and Down's syndrome. Dermatology 1994;189(3):248–50.

35. Ishimura E, Iwamoto H, Kobashi Y, et al. Malignant chondroid syringoma. Report of a case with widespread

metastasis and review of pertinent literature. Cancer 1983;52(10):1966–73.

36. Agrawal V, Gupta RL, Kumar S, et al. Malignant chondroid syringoma. J Dermatol 1998;25(8):547–9.

37. Hong JJ, Elmore JF, Drachenberg CI, et al. Role of radiation therapy in the management of malignant chondroid syringoma. Dermatol Surg 1995;21(9):781–5.

38. Ahluwalia BK, Khurana AK, Chugh AD, Mehtani VG. Eccrine spiradenoma of eyelid: case report. Br J Ophthalmol 1986;70(8):580–3.

39. Beekley AC, Brown TA, Porter C. Malignant eccrine spiradenoma: a previously unreported presentation and review of the literature. Am Surg 1999;65(3):236–40.

40. Tay JS, Tapen EM, Solari PG. Malignant eccrine spiradenoma. Case report and review of the literature. Am J Clin Oncol 1997;20(6):552–7.

41. Evans HL, Su D, Smith JL, Winkelmann RK. Carcinoma arising in eccrine spiradenoma. Cancer 1979;43(5):1881–4.

42. Warkel RL, Helwig EB. Apocrine gland adenoma and adenocarcinoma of the axilla. Arch Dermatol 1978;114(2):198–203.

43. El-Domeiri AA, Brasfield RD, Huvos AG, Strong EW. Sweat gland carcinoma: a clinico-pathologic study of 83 patients. Ann Surg 1971;173(2):270–4.

44. Harari PM, Shimm DS, Bangert JL, Cassady JR. The role of radiotherapy in the treatment of malignant sweat gland neoplasms. Cancer 1990;65(8):1737–40.

45. Mehregan AH, Hashimoto K, Rahbari H. Eccrine adenocarcinoma. A clinicopathologic study of 35 cases. Arch Dermatol 1983;119(2):104–14.

46. Howrey RP, Lipham WJ, Schultz WH, et al. Sebaceous gland carcinoma: a subtle second malignancy following radiation therapy in patients with bilateral retinoblastoma. Cancer 1998;83(4):767–71.

47. Rundle P, Shields JA, Shields CL, et al. Sebaceous gland carcinoma of the eyelid seventeen years after irradiation for bilateral retinoblastoma. Eye 1999;13(Pt 1):109–10.

48. Janjua TA, Citardi MJ, Sasaki CT. Sebaceous gland carcinoma: report of a case and review of literature. Am J Otolaryngol 1997;18(1):51–4.

49. Lindsey WH. Diagnosis & management of cutaneous malignancies of the head & neck. Compr Ther 1997;23(11):724–9.

50. Marks R, Motley RJ. Skin cancer. Recognition and treatment. Drugs 1995;50(1):48–61.

51. Nguyen AV, Whitaker DC, Frodel J. Differentiation of basal cell carcinoma. Otolaryngol Clin North Am 1993;26(1):37–56.

52. Singh B, Bhaya M, Shaha A, et al. Presentation, course, and outcome of head and neck skin cancer in African Americans: a case-control study. Laryngoscope 1998;108(8 Pt 1):1159–63.

53. Buzzell RA. Effects of solar radiation on the skin. Otolaryngol Clin North Am 1993;26(1):1–11.

54. Shumrick KA, Coldiron B. Genetic syndromes associated with skin cancer. Otolaryngol Clin North Am 1993;26(1):117–37.

55. Shockley WW. Special problems associated with carcinoma of the nose. Otolaryngol Clin North Am 1993;26(2):247–64.

56. Barksdale SK, O'Connor N, Barnhill R. Prognostic factors for cutaneous squamous cell and basal cell carcinoma. Determinants of risk of recurrence, metastasis, and development of subsequent skin cancers. Surg Oncol Clin N Am 1997;6(3):625–38.

57. Lo JS, Snow SN, Reizner GT, et al. Metastatic basal cell carcinoma: report of twelve cases with a review of the literature. J Am Acad Dermatol 1991;24(5 Pt 1):715–9.

58. Brown RO, Osguthorpe JD. Management of the neck in nonmelanocytic cutaneous carcinomas. Otolaryngol Clin North Am 1998;31(5):841–56.

59. Westgate SJ. Radiation therapy for skin tumors. Otolaryngol Clin North Am 1993;26(2):295–309.

60. Clark D. Cutaneous micrographic surgery. Otolaryngol Clin North Am 1993;26(2):185–202.

61. Lang PG Jr, Osguthorpe JD. Indications and limitations of Mohs' micrographic surgery. Dermatol Clin 1989;7(4):627–44.

62. Swanson NA, Grekin RC, Baker SR. Mohs' surgery: techniques, indications, and applications in head and neck surgery. Head Neck Surg 1983;6(2):683–92.

63. Haydon RCd. Cutaneous squamous carcinoma and related lesions. Otolaryngol Clin North Am 1993;26(1):57–71.

64. Hochman M, Lang P. Skin cancer of the head and neck. Med Clin North Am 1999;83(1):261–82, xii.

65. Veness MJ, Quinn DI, Ong CS, et al. Aggressive cutaneous malignancies following cardiothoracic transplantation: the Australian experience. Cancer 1999;85(8):1758–64.

66. Wang CY, Brodland DG, Su WP. Skin cancers associated with acquired immunodeficiency syndrome. Mayo Clin Proc 1995;70(8):766–72.

67. Kavouni A, Shibu M, Carver N. Squamous cell carcinoma arising in transplanted skin. Clin Exp Dermatol 2000;25(4):302–4.

68. Frierson HF Jr, Deutsch BD, Levine PA. Clinicopathologic features of cutaneous squamous cell carcinomas of the head and neck in patients with chronic lymphocytic leukemia/small lymphocytic lymphoma. Hum Pathol 1988;19(12):1397–402.

69. McCord MW, Mendenhall WM, Parsons JT, et al. Skin cancer of the head and neck with clinical perineural invasion. Int J Radiat Oncol Biol Phys 2000;47(1):89–93.

70. Kraus DH, Carew JF, Harrison LB. Regional lymph node metastasis from cutaneous squamous cell carcinoma. Arch Otolaryngol Head Neck Surg 1998;124(5):582–7.

71. Medina JE. Malignant melanoma of the head and neck. Otolaryngol Clin North Am 1993;26(1):73–85.

72. Stal S, Loeb T, Spira M. Melanoma of the head and neck. Update and perspective. Otolaryngol Clin North Am 1986;19(3):549–64.

73. Stadelmann WK, McMasters K, Digenis AG, Reintgen DS. Cutaneous melanoma of the head and neck: advances in evaluation and treatment. Plast Reconstr Surg 2000;105(6):2105–26.

74. Harwood AR. Melanomas of the head and neck. J Otolaryngol 1983;12(1):64–9.

75. Johanson CR, Harwood AR, Cummings BJ, Quirt I. 0-7-21 radiotherapy in nodular melanoma. Cancer 1983;51(2):226–32.

76. Harwood AR, Lawson VG. Radiation therapy for melanomas of the head and neck. Head Neck Surg 1982;4(6):468–74.

77. Geara FB, Ang KK. Radiation therapy for malignant melanoma. Surg Clin North Am 1996;76(6):1383–98.

78. Ang KK, Peters LJ, Weber RS, et al. Postoperative radiotherapy for cutaneous melanoma of the head and neck region. Int J Radiat Oncol Biol Phys 1994;30(4):795–8.

79. Ang KK, Byers RM, Peters LJ, et al. Regional radiotherapy as adjuvant treatment for head and neck malignant melanoma. Preliminary results. Arch Otolaryngol Head Neck Surg 1990;116(2):169–72.

80. Kirkwood JM, Ibrahim JG, Sondak VK, et al. High- and low-dose interferon alfa-2B in high-risk melanoma: first analysis of intergroup trial E1690/S9111/C9190. J Clin Oncol 2000;18(12):2444–58.

81. Reeves ME, Coit DG. Melanoma. A multidisciplinary approach for the general surgeon. Surg Clin North Am 2000;80(2):581–601.

82. Spitler LE, Grossbard ML, Ernstoff MS, et al. Adjuvant therapy of stage III and IV malignant melanoma using granulocyte-macrophage colony-stimulating factor. J Clin Oncol 2000;18(8):1614–21.

83. Ravaud A, Bedane C, Geoffrois L, et al. Toxicity and feasibility of adjuvant high-dose interferon alpha-2B in patients with melanoma in clinical oncologic practice. Br J Cancer 1999;80(11):1767–9.

84. Fenn NJ, Horgan K, Johnson RC, et al. A randomized controlled trial of prophylactic isolated cytotoxic perfusion for poor-prognosis primary melanoma of the lower limb. Eur J Surg Oncol 1997;23(1):6–9.

85. Creagan ET, Dalton RJ, Ahmann DL, et al. Randomized, surgical adjuvant clinical trial of recombinant interferon alfa-2A in selected patients with malignant melanoma. J Clin Oncol 1995;13(11):2776–83.

86. Kerin MJ, Gillen P, Monson JR, et al. Results of a prospective randomized trial using DTIC and interferon as adjuvant therapy for stage I malignant melanoma. Eur J Surg Oncol 1995;21(5):548–50.

87. Guida M, Abbate I, Casamassima A, et al. Long-term subcutaneous recombinant interleukin-2 as maintenance therapy: biological effects and clinical implications. Cancer Biother 1995;10(3):195–203.

88. Wallack MK, Sivanandham M, Balch CM, et al. A phase III randomized, double-blind multi-institutional trial of vaccinia melanoma oncolysate-active specific immunotherapy for patients with stage II melanoma. Cancer 1995;75(1):34–42.

89. Meisenberg BR, Ross M, Vredenburgh JJ, et al. Randomized trial of high-dose chemotherapy with autologous bone marrow support as adjuvant therapy for high-risk, multi-node-positive malignant melanoma. J Natl Cancer Inst 1993;85(13):1080–5.

90. Lejeune FJ. Phase III adjuvant studies in operable malignant melanoma [review]. Anticancer Res 1987;7(4B):701–5.

91. Paterson AH, Willans DJ, Jerry LM, et al. Adjuvant BCG immunotherapy for malignant melanoma. Can Med Assoc J 1984;131(7):744–8.

92. Singh B, Har-El G. Merkel cell carcinoma. South Med J 1991;84(10):1285–6.

93. Goepfert H, Remmler D, Silva E, Wheeler B. Merkel cell carcinoma (endocrine carcinoma of the skin) of the head and neck. Arch Otolaryngol 1984;110(11):707–12.

94. O'Brien PC, Denham JW, Leong AS. Merkel cell carcinoma: a review of behaviour patterns and management strategies. Aust N Z J Surg 1987;57(11):847–50.

95. Bourne RG, O'Rourke MG. Management of Merkel cell tumour. Aust N Z J Surg 1988;58(12):971–4.

96. Wong KC, Zuletta F, Clarke SJ, Kennedy PJ. Clinical management and treatment outcomes of Merkel cell carcinoma. Aust N Z J Surg 1998;68(5):354–8.

97. Ott MJ, Tanabe KK, Gadd MA, et al. Multimodality management of Merkel cell carcinoma. Arch Surg 1999;134(4):388–92.

98. Morrison WH, Peters LJ, Silva EG, et al. The essential role of radiation therapy in securing locoregional control of Merkel cell carcinoma. Int J Radiat Oncol Biol Phys 1990;19(3):583–91.

99. Gloster HM Jr, Dermatofibrosarcoma protuberans. J Am Acad Dermatol 1996;35(3 Pt 1):355–74.

100. Gloster HM Jr, Harris KR, Roenigk RK. A comparison between Mohs' micrographic surgery and wide surgical excision for the treatment of dermatofibrosarcoma protuberans. J Am Acad Dermatol 1996;35(1):82–7.

101. Farr HW. Soft part sarcomas of the head and neck. Semin Oncol 1981;8(2):185–9.

102. Stojadinovic A, Karpoff HM, Antonescu CR, et al. Dermatofibrosarcoma protuberans of the head and neck. Ann Surg Oncol 2000;7(9):696–704.

103. Barnes L, Coleman JA Jr, Johnson JT. Dermatofibrosarcoma protuberans of the head and neck. Arch Otolaryngol 1984;110(6):398–404.

104. Singh B, Shaha A, Har-El G. Malignant fibrous histiocytoma of the head and neck. J Craniomaxillofac Surg 1993;21(6):262–5.

105. Singh B, Santos V, Guffin TN Jr, et al. Giant cell variant of malignant fibrous histiocytoma of the head and neck. J Laryngol Otol 1991;105(12):1079–81.

106. Camacho FM, Moreno JC, Murga M, et al. Malignant fibrous histiocytoma of the scalp. Multidisciplinary treatment. J Eur Acad Dermatol Venereol 1999;13(3):175–82.

107. Fanburg-Smith JC, Miettinen M. Angiomatoid "malignant" fibrous histiocytoma: a clinicopathologic study of 158 cases and further exploration of the myoid phenotype. Hum Pathol 1999;30(11):1336–43.

108. Fanburg-Smith JC, Spiro IJ, Katapuram SV, et al. Infiltrative subcutaneous malignant fibrous histiocytoma: a comparative study with deep malignant fibrous histiocytoma and an observation of biologic behavior. Ann Diagn Pathol 1999;3(1):1–10.

5

Oral Cavity Cancer

JAY O. BOYLE, MD
ELLIOT W. STRONG, MD, FACS

Oral cavity cancer is the sixth leading cause of cancer worldwide. In the United States alone, there are over 21,500 oral carcinomas diagnosed each year, and 6,000 Americans die of oral cancer each year.[1] The incidence of oral carcinoma varies throughout the world, with estimates exceeding 40 in 100,000 in parts of France, Southeast Asia, Hungary and Singapore.[2] Thus oral cancer is a major cause of morbidity worldwide. Ninety percent of oral malignancies are squamous cell carcinomas and therefore are the principal topic of this chapter. However, the treatment of some other oral malignancies, like sarcoma and minor salivary gland carcinoma, is also primarily surgical excision, and the surgical principles are applicable to the treatment of these other tumors as well.

The etiology of oral cancer is exposure to carcinogens in tobacco and the tumor-promoting effects of alcohol. Ninety percent of the risk of oral cancer in the United States is directly attributable to smoking.[3] Tobacco smoke and alcohol are synergistic in their carcinogenic effects in the oral cavity. The relative risk of oral cancer for heavy smokers is 7 times that of nonsmokers. The risk for heavy drinkers is 6 times that of nondrinkers. The risk for patients abusing both alcohol and tobacco is 38 times that of those who abstain from both.[4] Chewing tobacco and betel quid also increase the risk of oral cancer.[5] Chronic carcinogen exposure creates a field effect and the entire mucosa of the upper aerodigestive tract is at risk for malignancy in smokers and drinkers.[6] After successful treatment of oral cancer, the risk of a second primary cancer is 3.7 percent per year and increases to 24 percent at ten years.[7] Cessation of alcohol and tobacco exposure reduces the risk of second aerodigestive carcinoma.

Chronic carcinogen exposure causes mucosal cells to acquire genetic abnormalities. When these genetics abnormalities result in the activation of proto-oncogenes and the inactivation of tumor-suppressive genes, the cells may be afforded a growth advantage. Dysregulated proliferation due to aberrant cell cycle control leads to clonal populations of premalignant, genetically abnormal mucosal cells. These populations of cells have a high tendency to accumulate additional genetic abnormalities due to genomic instability. Genomic instability is the result of rapid cell cycling with decreased genomic surveillance, decreased capacity to repair genetic defects and ineffective signalling of apoptosis or programmed cell death. In these cell populations the rate of accumulation of acquired genetic abnormalities increases logarithmically with time.[8]

Eventually these abnormal cells acquire the malignant phenotype in which they lose normal differentiation, invade the basement membrane, become locally destructive, and metastasize regionally or distantly. These cells evade immune surveillance of the body, produce angiogenic factors allowing ingrowth of blood vessels, and become clinical carcinomas.

ANATOMY

The critical functions normally accomplished by oral tissues include articulation of speech, facial expression and cosmesis, respiration, mastication, deglutition, and taste. Ablative surgery for oral cancer removes the malignant tumor en bloc with a margin of normal tissue, and the integrity of functionally important structures is not violated unnecessarily.

The oral cavity is bounded anteriorly by the skin and the vermilion border of the upper and lower lips. The oral cavity extends posteriorly to the circumvallate papillae of the tongue, the junction of the hard and soft palates, and the anterior faucial arch. The tonsil, soft palate and posterior one-third of the tongue are oropharyngeal structures and are not considered in our discussion of the oral cavity. Laterally the oral cavity is bounded by the buccal mucosa.

The oral cavity is divided into the following subsites: the lip, anterior two-thirds of the tongue, floor of mouth, gingiva, retromolar trigone, buccal mucosa, and hard palate (Figure 5–1). Figure 5–2 demonstrates the distribution of oral tumors by subsite. Tumors of different subsites demonstrate distinct clinical behavior.

The lip is a common site of skin cancer. The layers of the lip, from external to internal, include the epidermis, dermis, subcutaneous tissue, the orbicularis oris and attached musculature, the oral submucosa and the oral mucosa. The oral submucosa contains minor salivary glands, copious lymphatic vessels, blood vessels and sensory nerves. The lip is supplied by the labial arteries and veins, which are branches of the facial vessels. The generous lymphatics of the lower lip cross and drain bilaterally to level I nodes of the submental and submandibular triangles. Pre- or post-facial nodes lie anterior and posterior to the facial vessels in the superior aspect of the submandibular triangle and are potential sites of metastasis of lip cancers. Lymphatic channels of the upper lip respect the midline and drain to submandibular, periparotid, or preauricular nodes. The upper lip possesses two peaks forming a "cupid's bow" where the filtrum ascends to the columella of the nasal septum.

The orbicularis oris muscle receives motor innervation from the marginal and buccal branches of the facial nerve and performs a sphincteral function to maintain oral competence and to facilitate articulation of speech. This muscle has many attachments from other muscles of facial expression that elevate and depress the lips. Of clinical importance is the innervation of the depressor anguli oris muscle by the marginal mandibular branch of the facial nerve.

Sensation of the lower lip is provided by the mental nerve, the terminal segment of the alveolar branch of the mandibular division of the trigeminal nerve. The nerve exits the mental foramen of the mandible near the root of the canine tooth. Paresthesia of the chin suggests extensive mandible invasion and inferior alveolar nerve involvement by oral carcinoma.

The anterior two-thirds of the tongue is called the oral or mobile tongue and is bounded posteriorly by the V-shaped line of the circumvallate papillae. Posterior to this line is the base of tongue, which is part of the oropharynx. The oral tongue has ventral and dorsal surfaces. The mucosa of the tongue is simple stratified squamous epithelium with interspersed papillae or taste buds of four morphologies: filiform, foliate, fungiform, and circumvallate.

The tongue is comprised of intrinsic and extrinsic muscles. The intrinsic muscles are arranged in vertical and horizontal fascicles that allow the mobile tongue to change shape and consistency. There are three pairs of extrinsic muscles that provide mobility of the tongue: genioglossus, hyoglossus, and styloglossus. Protrusion of the tongue is primarily accomplished by the action of the genioglossus muscle which originates from the mandibular tubercles on the lingual surface of the arch of the mandible, and inserts diffusely into the substance of the intrinsic musculature on each side of the tongue. The motor supply to the intrinsic and extrinsic tongue muscles is the hypoglossal nerve (CN XII), which exits the skull through its own hypoglossal canal and courses laterally and anteriorly between the external and internal carotid arteries, immediately inferior to the occipital artery.

The sensation of the tongue is supplied by the lingual nerve, a branch of the mandibular division of the

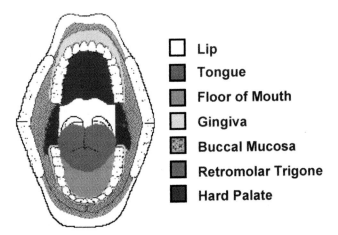

Figure 5–1. Diagram of the oral cavity and subsites.

☐ **Lip**
■ **Tongue**
■ **Floor of Mouth**
☐ **Gingiva**
▨ **Buccal Mucosa**
■ **Retromolar Trigone**
■ **Hard Palate**

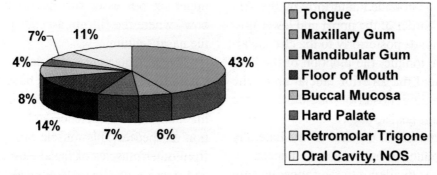

Figure 5–2.   Distribution of oral cancers by subsite. A selected series of cases presenting to the head and neck service of Memorial Sloan-Kettering Cancer Center, New York.

trigeminal nerve (CN V₃). The lingual nerve also transports parasympathetic fibers from the chorda tympani branch of the facial nerve to the submandibular ganglion. The blood supply to the tongue is derived from the paired lingual arteries.

The lymphatic drainage of the tongue begins in a rich submucosal plexus, which may drain bilaterally when lesions approach the midline, the tip, or especially the base of the tongue. Tumors of the lateral mid-tongue drain predictably to the ipsilateral lymph nodes. The first echelon nodes for lesions of the tip include the submental nodes. The lateral and ventral tongue lesions metastasize to submandibular or jugulodigastric nodes while the base of tongue drains to the jugulodigastric and deep jugular nodes. Lesions of the anterior tongue may metastasize directly to the low jugular lymph nodes (level IV) of the neck.

The buccal mucosa lines the lateral oral cavity and blends with the gingiva superiorly and inferiorly and with the retromolar trigone posteriorly. The mucosa is pierced by the Stensen's duct of the parotid gland at the papilla adjacent to the second maxillary molar tooth.

The gingiva consists of thick keratinized mucosa with deep rete pegs and submucosal adherence to the periosteum. The mucosa covers the alveolar processes of the mandible and the maxilla.

The mandible possesses lingual and buccal cortices which envelop cancellous bone, dental sockets, and the mandibular canal transmitting the mandibular vessels and nerves (branch of CN V₃). The mandibular surface is innervated by branches of the lingual and mental nerves while the maxillary sur-

face is innervated by alveolar branches of the second and third divisions of the 5th cranial (trigeminal) nerve.

The retromolar trigone is that portion of adherent keratinized mucosa covering the ascending ramus of the mandible from the third mandibular molar to the maxillary tubercle. It represents the area between the buccal mucosa laterally and the anterior tonsillar pillar medially and posteriorly. Tumors of this small region spread readily to the adjacent mandibular bone, alveolar foramen, masticator space, oropharyngeal tonsil, floor of mouth and base of tongue.

The hard palate lies within the horseshoe shape of the maxillary alveolar process. Keratinized adherent mucosa covers the palatal bone, which is divided into the primary and secondary bony palate. The primary palate consists of the palatal processes of the maxillary bones and represents the premaxilla anterior to the incisive foramen. The secondary palate is made up of the horizontal processes of the L-shaped palatine bones. On the posterior hard palate, near the maxillary second or third molar, are found the greater and lesser palatine foramina which transmit their respective vessels and nerves which are the terminal branches of the sphenopalatine vessels (branches of the internal maxillary artery) and nerves (branches of V₂). Anteriorly, the midline incisive foramen near the incisors transmits the terminal branches of the nasociliary nerve and vessels to supply the primary palate region. Lymphatic drainage of the palate includes the deep jugular chain as well as the retropharyngeal nodes. Anterior lesions may metastasize to pre-vascular facial lymph nodes of the submandibular region.

The floor of the mouth is a soft thin layer of U-shaped mucosa overlying the insertion of the mylohyoid muscle laterally, the hyoglossus muscle medially, and the insertion of the genioglossus muscle anteriorly. It covers the sublingual salivary glands, submandibular (Wharton's) duct, and the lingual nerve. The blood supply is from the lingual vessels. Its lymphatic plexus is copious and drains bilaterally in the midline. The lymphatic drainage patterns include the submental and bilateral submandibular nodes, as well as the ipsilateral jugulodigastric nodes posteriorly.

DIAGNOSIS

The diagnostic evaluation of a patient with oral carcinoma consists of the history and the physical examination, histopathologic tissue diagnosis, and imaging—when indicated.

The clinical history begins with the present illness and includes the duration and location of symptoms such as non-healing ulcer, mass in the oral cavity or neck, pain, bleeding, and any symptoms of cranial nerve deficits. A thorough exploration of the patient's past medical and surgical history, and the review of systems yield operative risk data. A thorough history of etiologic risk factors for squamous carcinomas not only reflects the patient's relative risk of malignancy but also suggests factors that affect the patient's overall health, fitness for surgery and emotional state. Current and distant abuse of tobacco and alcohol are critical factors and may be underreported by the patient. In many parts of the world the use of oral chews ("pan," betel nuts, etc.) is the chief etiologic factor.[9] These may contain tobacco, slaked lime and other irritants and may be retained in the oral cavity nearly constantly. An occupational exposure to heavy metals such as nickel,[10] and previous radiation exposure to head and neck are other important risk factors of head and neck cancer that are elicited in the history.

The social history impacts strongly on the patient's ability to comply with and tolerate treatment and rehabilitation programs, and these issues are resolved during the treatment planning phase. The family history reflects any familial tendencies toward malignant disease and completes the historical data.

A complete examination of the head and neck is performed to assess the precise location and extent of the primary tumor, identify regionally metastatic disease and to rule out multiple primary malignancies. Grossly, the earliest cancers may present as nonulcerous white or red patches. More advanced oral squamous cell carcinomas (SCC) present as mucosal lesions, although occasionally an SCC may present as predominantly submucosal with little or no mucosal involvement. Firm submucosal lesions are often minor salivary gland neoplasms. SCC may be ulcerative and invasive, fungating and exophytic or both (Figure 5–3). They may arise within premalignant lesions such as leukoplakia or erythroplakia. The following characteristics of the lesion should be documented: appearance and character, location, size in centimeters, texture to palpation, mobility, proximity to surrounding structures—especially bone, and the estimated palpable thickness (superficial vs. deeply infiltrating).

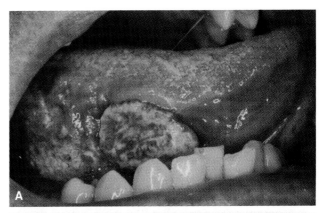

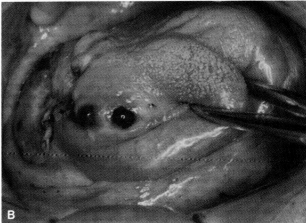

Figure 5–3. *A*, An exophytic lesion involving the right lateral border of the tongue. *B*, An endophytic lesion of the right lateral border of the tongue.

Trismus suggests ominous pterygoid and masticator space involvement. The condition of the dentition should be noted as tumors may, as the first sign, displace or loosen teeth. The distance from the tumor to the mandible and the mobility of the lesion in relation to the mandible are critical elements in determining the management of perimandibular cancers. A complete examination of the cranial nerves is performed, emphasizing sensation over the chin for mandibular nerve deficit, tongue mobility for hypoglossal nerve deficit, facial nerve function, palatal elevation and gag reflex, and function of the accessory nerve. A mirror or a flexible or rigid telescope is needed to document vocal cord mobility and to ensure that no lesions exist in the oropharynx, nasopharynx, endolarynx, and visible hypopharynx. Small lesions of the hypopharynx may only be visible by direct examination under anesthesia with the rigid laryngoscopes.

The neck should be thoroughly palpated for metastatic disease in the nodal groups at risk, and for other abnormalities of the great vessels and the thyroid gland which might impact treatment. Masses of the neck should be measured in centimeters, characterized for site (level), mobility, consistency, skin involvement, and proximity to vital structures. Normal neck structures commonly mistaken for metastatic masses include: the transverse process of C2 in the jugulodigastric region of thin patients, the scalene muscles, a tortuous carotid artery, a carotid aneurysm, a prominent carotid bulb, a cervical rib, and ptotic submandibular glands.

A complete general physical examination should be performed emphasizing the cardiovascular and pulmonary systems, which are commonly abnormal in this oral cancer population. The systemic effects of malnutrition or excessive alcohol intake should also be noted.

The history and physical examination with or without adjunctive imaging and histopathologic tissue diagnosis are sufficient to plan and execute surgical treatment for many patients with oral cancer. However, some patients will benefit from examination under anesthesia including direct palpation with or without biopsy, laryngoscopy, esophagoscopy, and bronchoscopy. The indications for examination under anesthesia include an inadequate assessment of the extent of the disease by history and physical examination and imaging, or the presence of symptoms referable to the trachea, larynx, hypopharynx and esophagus that need endoscopic assessment. It is not cost-effective screening to perform panendoscopy on all patients with head and neck cancer.[11–13] Symptoms suggesting lesions of the trachea, larynx, hypopharynx, or esophagus include: dysphagia, odynophagia, pain, hoarseness, hemoptysis or stridor. A careful history and meticulous head and neck exam is necessary to identify these lesions.

Evaluation of the deep extent of oral cancer often requires the use of imaging modalities. Imaging studies, however, will not adequately identify the superficial mucosal extent of disease, which must be established by visualization, palpation and biopsy. Plain radiographs such as panorex, dental films or a submental occlusal film may demonstrate gross bone involvement but do not show early cortical invasion.

Computed tomography (CT) is the most common modality employed to assess the extent of oral cancers (Figure 5–4). Advantages of CT include good soft-tissue discrimination and vessel identification and excellent definition of bone soft-tissue interfaces. CT scans are readily available and affordable. Cortical destruction and tumor in the alveolar canal and the bone marrow can be seen on CT. Special coronal reconstructions of dedicated mandible CT

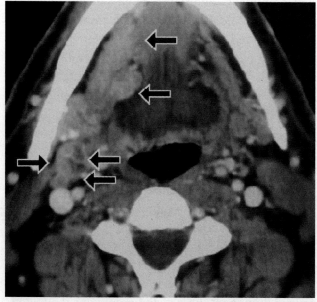

Figure 5–4. CT scan demonstrating an invasive carcinoma in the right half of the tongue with involvement of lymph nodes at level II.

scans (Dentascan) is particularly helpful in imaging the mandible. CT scans of the oral cavity should be combined with neck CT to assess for suspicious subclinical metastatic nodes. Axial and coronal views with bone and soft-tissue windows with contrast from the orbital floor to the base of the tongue as well as axial views of the neck are obtained. Disadvantages of CT scanning include radiation exposure, possible contrast dye sensitivity, dental amalgam interference, difficult positioning for coronal views, and no direct sagittal views.

Compared to CT scanning, magnetic resonance imaging (MRI) offers enhanced soft-tissue discrimination, excellent skull base and CNS assessment, sagittal views, and no radiation exposure (Figure 5–5). Disadvantages are that the examination takes longer, is more expensive, is poorly tolerated by some, and the black signal of bone makes cortical bone abnormalities difficult to see. An experimental imaging modality with promise is positron emission tomographic scanning. Positron emission tomography (PET) is a nuclear medicine study that demonstrates the difference in metabolism of radiolabeled glucose molecules between normal and malignant tissues. The clinical usage of this modality is currently not well-defined, but will likely aid in the diagnosis of recurrent and metastatic lesions.[14]

The appropriate metastatic evaluation of the patient with oral carcinoma is chest radiographs and serum liver function tests. The routine use of CT scanning of the chest, abdomen, and brain, or radionuclide bone scanning to evaluate oral cancer patients is not cost-effective and should be discouraged.

When all of the data from the history, physical examination, biopsy, imaging, and metastatic work-up are available, the tumor is staged according to the AJCC staging system (Table 5–1).

TREATMENT GOALS AND ALTERNATIVES; FACTORS AFFECTING CHOICE OF TREATMENT

The surgeon's goal is complete removal of all cells of the primary tumor and any cancer cells in regional lymph nodes, while preserving the integrity of uninvolved structures. Similarly, the radiotherapist endeavors to damage the abnormal cells

irreparably while sparing the normal tissue. Either modality is effective in controlling early oral carcinomas, but the use of both modalities in combination is necessary to control locally advanced disease. The role of chemotherapy alone in localized disease is palliative. Currently, distantly metastatic disease is incurable but can often be effectively palliated with chemotherapy and radiation.

Treatment choices are best made after considering tumor factors, patient factors and resources factors. Tumor factors include subsite, T stage, N stage, histologic characteristics, endophytic vs. exophytic morphology, and proximity to bone. Patient factors include the patient's age, co-morbidities, convenience, rehabilitation potential, and the patient's wishes. Resource factors include the availability of a well-trained surgeon or radiotherapist with a dedicated interest in head and neck cancer, availability of advanced hardware for the planning and delivery of radiation, and the availability of funds to pay for the treatment.

The mainstay of treatment of early oral cancer is surgery. External beam radiation therapy alone can be effective for some early superficial lesions of the tongue or floor of mouth but sequelae of xerostomia

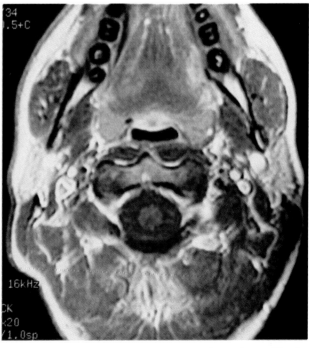

Figure 5–5. A T2N0 squamous carcinoma of the left lateral border of the tongue seen infiltrating the superficial musculature of the tongue on an MRI scan.

and mandible irradiation, and long duration and expense of treatment make radiation a poor choice. Also, bone involvement by oral cancer limits the effectiveness of external beam radiation, so lesions of the gingiva and hard palate are best treated with surgery due to the close proximity of bone and the high incidence of bone invasion. Advantages of surgery for T1 and T2 oral cancer compared to radia-

tion include decreased cost, decreased time of treatment, the generation of a surgical specimen for examination of potential prognostic features and, in some instances, an opportunity to sample the regional clinically negative nodes for occult disease. Advantages of radiation therapy for early lesions are preservation of tissue and no need for general anesthetic.

Advanced T3 and T4 lesions are best treated with a combination of surgery and radiation therapy. Improvement in locoregional control of advanced oral cancer is attributable to the addition of postoperative radiation.[15,16]

Brachytherapy can sometimes be employed for oral cancers (especially tumors of the tongue) utilizing after-loading catheters.[17] However, resection of small lesions is usually simpler and less morbid, and surgery followed by radiation is more appropriate for treating the large volume T3 or T4 lesion. Close proximity of the tumor to the mandible, complex surface anatomy, and uncertainty of the tumor margins are tumor factors that also limit use of brachytherapy for oral cavity cancers. Tumors of the oral cavity are poorly responsive to traditional organ sparing approaches combining either sequential or concomitant chemotherapy and radiation therapy. The control rates for oral cavity cancers using these regimens are the lowest of all head and neck sites.[18] Chemotherapy alone for oral cavity cancers is palliative. While some complete clinical responses can be obtained, they are not durable. Preoperative chemotherapy for oral cancers is usually not helpful because adequate resection margins do not shrink with the clinical response of the tumor. Studies show that microscopic tumor foci exist where previous gross tumor has been shrunken by chemotherapy treatment. It is therefore not ordinarily possible to reduce the extent of surgical resection and the morbidity of oral cancer surgery by tumor shrinkage with preoperative chemotherapy.[19]

It is important that all head and neck cancer patients and their cases be discussed in a multimodality treatment conference setting to insure appropriate management.

SURGICAL TREATMENT

Most patients with oral cancer are in their fifth to seventh decades of life with a history of tobacco and

Table 5–I. UICC/AJCC STAGING SYSTEM FOR ORAL CANCER

Primary Tumor
(T)
TX   Primary tumor cannot be assessed
T0   No evidence of primary tumor
Tis Carcinoma in situ
T1   Tumor 2 cm or less in greatest dimension
T2   Tumor more than 2 cm but not more than 4 cm in greatest dimension
T3   Tumor more than 4 cm in greatest dimension
T4   Tumor (lip) invades adjacent structures (eg, through cortical bone, tongue, skin of neck) Tumor (oral cavity) invades adjacent structures (eg, through cortical bone, into deep [extrinsic] muscle of tongue, maxillary sinus, skin)

Regional Lymph Nodes
(N)
NX   Regional lymph nodes cannot be assessed
N0   No regional lymph node metastasis
N1   Metastasis in a single ipsilateral lymph node, 3 cm or less in greatest dimension
N2   Metastasis in a single ipsilateral lymph node, more than 3 cm but not more than 6 cm in greatest dimension; or in multiple ipsilateral lymph nodes, none more than 6 cm in greatest dimension; or in bilateral or contralateral lymph   nodes, none more than 6 cm in greatest dimension
  N2a Metastasis in single ipsilateral lymph node more than 3 cm but not more than 6 cm in greatest dimension
  N2b Metastasis in multiple ipsilateral lymph nodes, none more than 6 cm in greatest dimension
  N2c Metastasis in bilateral or contralateral lymph nodes, none more than 6 cm in greatest dimension
N3   Metastasis in a lymph node more than 6 cm in greatest dimension

Distant Metastasis
(M)
MX   Presence of distant metastasis cannot be assessed
M0   No distant metastasis
M1   Distant metastasis

Stage Grouping

Stage	T	N	M
Stage 0	Tis	N0	M0
Stage I	T1	N0	M0
Stage II	T2	N0	M0
Stage III	T3	N0	M0
	T1	N1	M0
	T2	N1	M0
	T3	N1	M0
Stage IV	T4	N0	M0
	T4	N1	M0
	Any T	N2	M0
	Any T	N3	M0
	Any T	Any N	M1

alcohol abuse, and therefore warrant preoperative clearance by the patient's medical doctor, a cardiologist, and/or an anesthesiologist prior to surgery. All patients require preoperative chest radiographs, EKG, CBC and blood chemistry evaluation.

A significant portion of oral cancer patients will present in the malnourished state due to odynophagia or alcoholism. The malnourished patient will not withstand aggressive surgical and postoperative radiation treatment without complications. For this reason, preoperative nutritional support should be considered for patients with weight loss greater than 10 percent of body weight and those with low serum albumin. The benefits of 2 or 3 weeks of enteral feeding supplementation, to place the patient in a positive nitrogen balance, outweigh the risk of treatment delay in these patients. Nasogastric tube placement is the most common route of enteral supplementation. However, if patients require significant cancer resection, complex reconstruction, postoperative radiation therapy and extended swallowing rehabilitation, the temporary placement of a gastrostomy tube is safe and well-tolerated. The benefits of consistent nutrition and hydration during treatment and rehabilitation cannot be overemphasized.[20]

In patients with oral cancer undergoing general anesthesia, the management of the airway is the responsibility of both the surgeon and the anesthesiologist. Preoperative communication and preparation are critical. Patients may be difficult to orally intubate due to trismus, hemorrhage, or tumor bulk, and the presence of the oral endotracheal tube may interfere with the resection. The appropriate solution is nasal intubation with or without flexible fiberoptic nasopharyngoscopic guidance. Another option for airway management is preoperative tracheostomy under local anesthetic. In the event of an airway emergency the surgeon must be prepared to secure a surgical airway via cricothyroidotomy or an emergent tracheostomy. This must be performed within minutes of desaturation to prevent anoxic brain injury or cardiac arrest.

Similarly, postoperative airway management is critical to safe surgery of the oral cavity. Indications for tracheostomy after oral cancer surgery include: (1) the anticipation of significant postoperative edema of the pharynx, floor of the mouth or the base of the tongue, (2) a significant risk of postoperative hemorrhage, (3) the presence of any bolster or other aspiratable dressing material, (4) pre-existing pulmonary disease or obstructive sleep apnea, or the simultaneous operation or compromise of the nasal airway, and (5) the need for frequent endotracheal suctioning or ventilation support.

The anesthetist should be instructed to avoid paralyzing agents if nerve stimulators are to be used to help identify motor nerves. Also, fluid overload should be avoided in oral cancer cases. Patients undergoing head and neck surgeries have a decreased need for intraoperative fluid replacement, compared to patients undergoing abdominal surgeries of similar duration. This is due to less third spacing of fluid and less insensate losses of fluid in head and neck cases compared to abdominal cases.

Management of Leukoplakia

During the carcinogenic process, some abnormal clonal populations of mucosal cells form clinical premalignant lesions. These are manifested as leukoplakia or erythroplakia. Leukoplakias are common lesions in smokers and patients with a previous history of head and neck cancer. These are also noted in patients without heavy carcinogenic exposure. In general, dysplastic leukoplakia should be treated while lesions harboring only hyperplasia and hyperkeratosis may be observed. Clinical characteristics of lesions suggesting the presence of dysplasia include large size, tongue or floor of the mouth location, red color, friability, and the patient's prior history of oral cancer or dysplasia. It should be emphasized that any lesion which is red or red-speckled (erythroplakia) is of the highest risk for dyplasia or carcinoma and should be biopsied.

Treatment of dysplastic leukoplakia is generally surgical. While the vitamin A analogue isotretinoin (13 *cis*-retinoic acid or Accutane™) has been shown to be effective in the treatment of dysplastic oral leukoplakia, most lesions will recur after therapy has been stopped and many patients do not tolerate the mucocutaneous toxicity of isotretinoin treatment. [21,22]

Small dysplastic leukoplakia lesions may be easily excised in the office under local anesthesia with millimeter margins. All excised leukoplakia should be submitted for histopathologic assessment. Laser excision of oral leukoplakias can also be accomplished with good hemostasis and little tissue reaction.[23] Other treatment options for leukoplakia include destruction by electrodesiccation, and cryotherapy with liquid nitrogen. Local recurrence is common and occurs in up to one-third of cases.[24]

SURGERY FOR ORAL CANCER

The lip is the most common site for oral cancer. It is usually considered separately from cancers of other oral subsites as it behaves more like skin cancer. It occurs in sun-exposed surfaces and more commonly on the lower lip than upper lip. It is usually diagnosed early due to bleeding and a visible ulcer. Large lesions may rarely invade the mandible or the mental nerve and foramen.

T1 and T2 lesions are usually cured by wedge resection of the lip with primary closure, (Figure 5–6) although primary radiation therapy is also highly effective. Large T3 or T4 lesions require resection of involved tissues, bilateral upper neck dissections, complex reconstruction, and postoperative radiation therapy.

Depending on the size of the mouth and the presence of dentition, up to 50 percent of the lower lip can be resected and closed primarily in three layers with care to close the orbicularis oris muscle securely. Re-approximation of the vermilion line is important cosmetically. If greater than 40 to 50 percent of the lip is to be resected an Abbe or Estlander lip switch reconstruction borrows lip tissue from the normal upper lip. Karapandzic advancement flaps can also be useful for large lip reconstructions.[25] Free flap reconstruction is sometimes necessary but always inferior cosmetically and functionally due to the lack of orbicularis oris function and difficulty with commissure reconstruction.[26]

The anterior two-thirds of the tongue is the most common site of primary lesions accounting for 40 percent of oral cancers. Most malignancies occur on the lateral borders and ventral surface but are occasionally confined to the tip or the dorsum. Even small lesions of the oral tongue are visible and usually symptomatic, so oral tongue lesions tend to present in earlier stages: 37 percent stage I, 34 percent stage II, 21 percent stage III, and 8 percent stage IV.[27]

Tongue cancer may spread along the mucosal surface to involve the floor of the mouth and the mandible, or the oropharynx, or it may spread by deep invasion between muscle fascicles which offer little resistance to tumor spread (Figure 5–7). It is

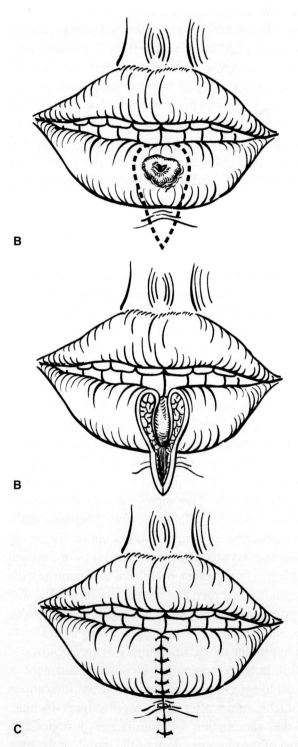

B

B

C

Figure 5—6. *A* to *C,* Wedge resection of lower lip carcinoma with primary closure in layers.

Peroral resection is the most common approach for T1 and T2 lesions of the oral tongue (Figure 5–8). A partial glossectomy is easily performed using electrocautery to maximize hemostasis. A 1 to 1.5 cm margin of normal tongue tissue is maintained in all dimensions, and both visual assessment and palpation of the tongue guide the resection. Intraoperative margin specimens for frozen section are taken with a scalpel to minimize cautery artifact. Resection can be performed with a carbon dioxide laser. Whenever feasible, the resection is planned in a transverse wedge fashion. Intraoperative frozen sections of the margins are mandatory. The defect of a partial glossectomy is closed in the horizontal direction causing a foreshortening of the tongue. The appearance and function after horizontal closure are excellent. This is preferable to a longitudinal closure, which results in a thin pointed tongue. The size and the extent of the tumor will determine the orientation of the resection.

For many T2 and T3 oral tongue tumors, and for any sized tumor in the posterior portion of the tongue or floor of mouth, the mandibulotomy approach provides the exposure required to perform an oncologically sound resection. The low morbidity of paramedian mandibulotomy is always preferred to the poor visualization and inadequate assessment

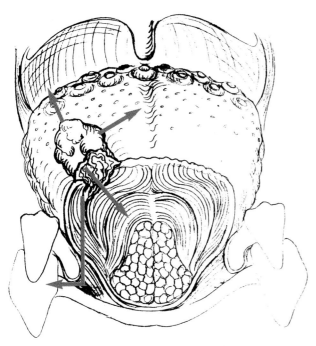

Figure 5–7. The anatomical routes of spread of oral tongue cancer.

easy to underestimate the deep extension of tongue tumors and great care should be exercised to take more than 1 cm cuff of normal tongue musculature as the margin of surgical resection. The midline raphe of the tongue does not provide any substantial resistance to tumor spread for lesions approaching or crossing the midline.

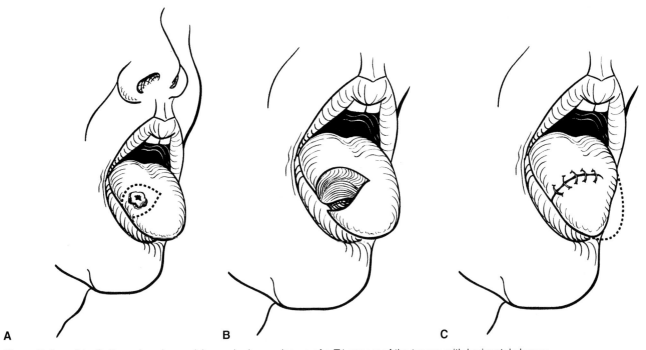

A   B   C

Figure 5–8.   *A* to *C*, Peroral wedge excision and primary closure of a T1 cancer of the tongue with horizontal closure.

of the deep and posterior margins that result from inappropriate peroral excision.[28,29] In addition, the majority of these patients benefit from staging elective supraomohyoid neck dissection, which provides the neck exposure needed for the mandibulotomy approach (Figure 5–9).

This procedure begins with elective supraomohyoid or modified radical neck dissection, in which the skin and muscle flaps of the neck are raised exposing the lower border of the mandible. The floor of the mouth is exposed via the submandibular triangle. Next the lower lip splitting incision is performed. The vermilion border is marked to ensure accurate realignment, and the lip is split sharply in the midline and connected with the anterior extent of the neck incision. The periosteum of the mandible is left undisturbed while the soft tissues of the lip and cheek are elevated to identify and preserve the mental nerve. The gingival mucosa and periosteum are incised at the mandibulotomy site anterior to the mental foramen and lateral to the insertion of the digastric muscle. The cut is planned either between the lateral incisor and the canine tooth, or directly through the root of a lateral incisor tooth that is extracted. Cuts between tooth roots may damage both roots and both teeth may be lost subsequently. Prior to performing the bone cut, the 4-hole reconstructive plates for the lateral and inferior margin of the mandible are molded and the screw holes drilled to ensure accurate realignment. The cut is performed at right angles to the alveolar ridge and angled 45 degrees anteriorly below the tooth roots for better stabilization. Taking care to avoid the lingual nerve, the floor of mouth

mucosa and mylohyoid muscles are divided posteriorly up to the anterior tonsillar pillar, and one centimeter from the medial aspect of the mandible.[28] Appropriate tumor resection is performed through the exposure thus provided (Figure 5–10).

The reconstruction requires the floor of mouth incision to be closed in layers, and the bone reapproximated with the preformed plates and screws (Figure 5–11). The lip is closed meticulously in three layers with attention to the orbicularis oris muscle and the exact apposition of the vermilion border. The best reconstructive options for partial and hemiglossectomy are primary horizontal closure if the defect is not too large, or free flap reconstruction. Other options include closure by secondary intention, split-thickness skin grafting and pedicled flaps. After large resections of the oral tongue, patients require speech and swallowing therapy for functional recovery.

Every effort should be made to achieve negative margins with the initial resection. Intraoperative positive frozen-section margins in tongue surgery significantly reduce local control and survival, even when additional resection and ultimately negative frozen and permanent sections are obtained.[30] When intraoperative positive frozen sections occur it reflects a tumor biology that is more invasive and aggressive than is estimated by the surgeon and thus warrants consideration of postoperative radiation therapy.

Final histopathology report of margins may show foci of premalignant change, carcinoma in situ (CIS), close surgical margins (less than 5 mm) or the presence of microscopic foci of invasive cancer. The presence of any of these findings at the surgical mar-

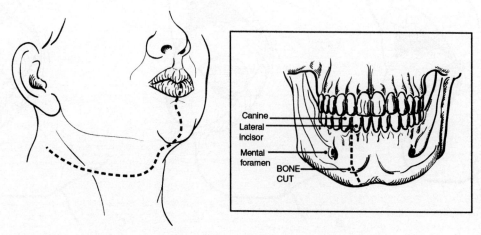

Figure 5–9. The mandibulotomy approach to tumors of the posterior oral cavity.

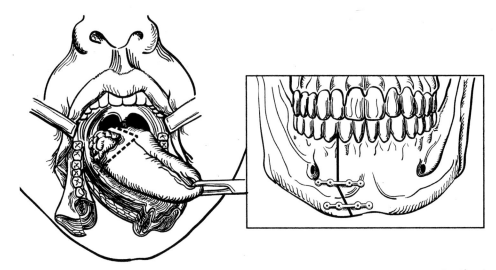

Figure 5–10. The mandibulotomy approach to tumors of the posterior oral cavity. Biplane fixation of the mandible is necessary.

gin increases the risk of local recurrence twofold, and significantly increases the mortality from oral cancers. Any of these histologic findings suggest a role for postoperative radiation therapy.[31,32]

Early tongue cancers demonstrate occult spread to the cervical lymph nodes in 20 to 30 percent of cases. The frequency of metastasis is related to the T stage and depth of invasion of tongue cancers. Increasing T stage correlates with increasing incidence of metastatic disease. A depth of invasion by tongue cancer of greater than 5 mm is associated with an increased incidence of occult metastasis.[33] Tumor depth greater than 2 mm is correlated with significantly lower sur-

vival and control of disease in the neck. In a study of early staged cancers of the tongue and floor of the mouth, the 5-year survival of patients with thin lesions was greater than 95 percent, while survival of patients with thick lesions was less than 80 percent, regardless of T stage (Table 5–2).[34] An appreciation of tumor depth can aid in the decision to perform elective neck dissection. Except for oral cancers less than 2 mm thick, all early staged oral cancer patients should receive elective supraomohyoid neck dissection (SOHND). On the other hand, elective radiotherapy to the neck should be employed if radiation therapy is the treatment selected for the primary tumor.

Survival after treatment for tongue cancers has improved over the last 15 years, due to the use of combined modality treatment for advanced disease, and the aggressive treatment of the neck in early stage disease. Franceschi reported 5-year survival of 82 percent for patients treated between 1978 and 1987 with stage I and II disease and 49 percent for

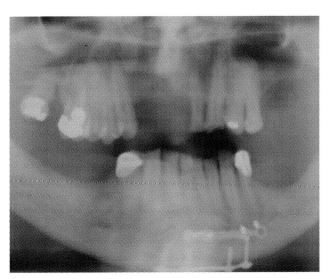

Figure 5–11. The mandibular osteotomy is fixed using miniplates which provide accurate dental occlusion, and stability.

Table 5–2. THICKNESS OF ORAL CANCER PREDICTS SURVIVAL AND TREATMENT FAILURE		
Tumor Thickness	5-year Disease Specific Survival (%)	Treatment Failure (%)
< 2mm	97	2
2–8mm	83	45
>8mm	65	

Data from Spiro RH, et al. Predictive value of tumor thickness in squamous cacinoma confined to the tongue and floor of the mouth. Am J Surg 1986,152:345–50.

stage III and IV disease. These are improvements over the survival rates in their experience from the period 1967 to 1978 (Figure 5–12).[27]

The floor of the mouth is the second most common subsite accounting for 20 percent of oral cancers. Due to its dependent location, carcinogens may pool in the floor of mouth leading to high rates of cancer. Because of the small size of this area, floor of the mouth lesions often extend to involve the tongue and the mandibular gingiva. The size distribution of floor of mouth cancers at the time of diagnosis is 30 percent T1, 37 percent T2, 19 percent T3, and 14 percent T4.[28] Forty-one percent of patients present with regional neck metastasis, and micrometastases are identified histologically in 17 percent of elective neck dissection specimens. Of all treatment failures, 21 percent recur locally, 37 percent recur in the neck and 29 percent at both sites. Staging elective supraomohyoid neck dissection is appropriate for all but very superficial T1 lesions of the floor of the mouth, and bilateral staging neck dissection is indicated for midline lesions. Finally, survival for floor of mouth lesions is 88 percent, 80 percent, 66 percent, and 32 percent for disease of stages I to IV respectively.[35]

Because of the frequent involvement of the mandible by floor of the mouth tumors, management of the mandible is an important aspect of planning resections of the floor of the mouth. The key clinical question is: does the mandible require resection, and if so how much—the periosteum, a marginal mandibular resection or a segmental resection? Management of the mandible depends on the lesion's proximity to the mandible, whether the mandible is dentate or edentulous, the degree of atrophy of the alveolar ridge, whether the mandible has been irradiated, and whether there is mandibular invasion.

Historically, a segmental mandibular resection was often performed not only for bone involvement by cancer, but also to accomplish a monobloc resection of the primary carcinoma with cervical lymph nodes. It was incorrectly presumed that lymphatics from the oral cavity passed through the periosteum of the mandible to the neck and that in-transit metastasis could be resected with the mandible. The elegant histologic work of Marchetta and colleagues[36,37] has conclusively demonstrated that the lymphatic drainage of the tongue and floor of mouth

does not pass through the mandibular periosteum nor through the substance of the mandible.

An additional advantage to routine mandibular resection in decades past was improved access and visualization of oral cancers. However, the morbidity and reconstructive challenges of segmental mandibulectomy led surgeons to reconsider the indications for this procedure, and to explore the possibility of partial-thickness mandibular resections. In these procedures only the alveolar ridge and/or the lingual plate of the mandible is resected (marginal mandibulectomy), and the inferior alveolar artery and nerve and the continuity of the mandibular arch are spared. In order to justify the oncologic soundness of marginal mandibulectomy, studies were undertaken to understand the routes of invasion and spread of cancer in the mandible. The results allow a rational approach to management of the mandible in oral cancer.

McGregor and colleagues have reported that the primary route of SCC invasion of the edentulous mandible is through cortical deficiencies of the occlusal surface of the bone.[38] The route of spread in the dentate nonirradiated mandible is via the tooth sockets, and the presence of teeth is a relative barrier to tumor infiltration. Also, the dentate mandible has a greater height from the floor of the mouth than does the edentulous mandible due to the resorption of the alveolar ridge after tooth loss. Therefore, tumors of the floor of the mouth must advance farther up the gingival mucosa to reach the occlusal

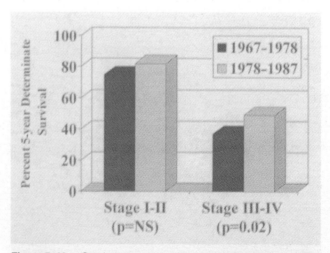

Figure 5–12.   Graph demonstrating improved survival in tongue cancer from the years 1967 through 1978 to the years 1978 through 1987. Data from Franceschi et al. Improved survival in the treatment of squamous carcinoma of the oral tongue. Am J Surg 1993;166:360–5.

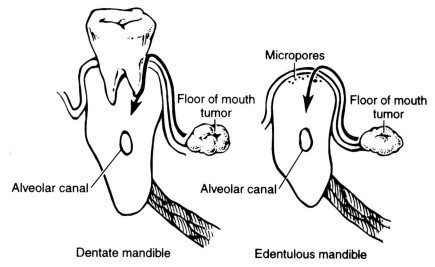

Figure 5–13. The routes of spread of oral cancer to the mandible in the dentate and edentulous mandible.

surface of the dentate mandible than the edentulous mandible (see Figure 5–13).

Cancer invasion of the *irradiated* mandible occurs not only through the occlusal surface but also directly through cortical bone of other surfaces.[39] This suggests the loss of barrier function of the periosteum after irradiation.

In both radiated and nonirradiated mandibles, the spread of squamous carcinoma within the cancellous bone is generally directed inferiorly toward the inferior alveolar nerve canal. Brown and colleagues reported that the early phase of mandibular invasion is erosive and that this phase progresses to an infiltrative phase as the depth of invasion increases.[40] In the histologic studies by McGregor and McDonald, tumor spread proximally and distally within the cancellous bone of the mandible was observed to be no farther than 5 mm beyond the region of overlying soft-tissue involvement, suggesting that a 5 to 10 mm bony margin, beyond the extent of the soft-tissue tumor, is oncologically sound.[40] On the other hand, invasion of the alveolar canal by oral cancer allows extensive perineural spread. By this route, disease can travel distally or proximally to the skull base, but does not tend to seed the bone along the course of the nerve or form skip lesions. Invasion of the ramus via the body of the bone occurs readily, especially in the irradiated mandible.[41]

With these principles in mind, one can develop a rational approach to management of the mandible in oral carcinoma. Because the dentate mandible is relatively resistant to cancer infiltration by adjacent lesions, marginal resection of the alveolar ridge and/or the lingual plate, sparing the alveolar artery, is sometimes acceptable treatment for disease in proximity to the bone. First, the proximity of the tumor is assessed by observation, palpation, and by CT scan if the lesion is fixed to the bone. If the tumor is greater than 1 cm away from the bone, then no mandible resection is needed. If the tumor is less than 1 cm from the mandible, then a marginal resection of the mandible will ensure 1 cm margins. If the tumor involves the gingival mucosa and the periosteum without clinical or radiologic evidence of cortical or cancellous bone involvement, then a marginal resection of the mandible is satisfactory, because any subclinical bone involvement is likely to be localized to the alveolar process. If the tumor is fixed to the occlusal surface with clinical or radiologic evidence of cortical or cancellous bone involvement, then a segmental resection is performed because, once the occlusal cortex is breached, there is no barrier to the vertical spread of tumor through cancellous bone to the alveolar canal. Totsuka and colleagues published studies showing that marginal mandibular resection was safe for some tumors with minimal gross bone invasion if there was a histologically "expansive" rather than "infiltrative" pattern of invasion. However, this pattern of invasion was not readily predictable based on radiographic findings.[42,43]

When extensive involvement of the cancellous bone is noted, the alveolar nerve must be assessed by frozen section, and further resection along the course of the nerve to the inferior alveolar foramen, the mental foramen, or the skull base is considered.

Contraindications to marginal resection of the mandible include gross involvement of the cortical or cancellous bone of the mandible, inability to preserve the inferior alveolar artery, significant resorption of the mandible—suggesting very thin and weak residual bone, a previously irradiated mandible, and cancer abutting the mandible on more than two surfaces.

Small T1 lesions that are 1 cm from the mandible are amenable to wide local excision via the peroral approach. This is easier in the edentulous patient due to better visualization. The mucosal margin is at least one centimeter. The deep margin is just below the sublingual salivary gland for superficial lesions. Wharton's duct may be ligated, but the authors prefer to reroute the duct to the posterior edge of the resection if the submandibular gland is not resected in the neck dissection. Caution is taken to identify and preserve the uninvolved branches of the lingual nerve as anesthesia of the tip of the tongue will result from their sacrifice. Small defects may be closed primarily but many can be allowed to granulate and heal by secondary intention. A split-thickness skin graft is an excellent reconstruction for small defects in the floor of mouth that expose the mylohyoid muscle.

Excision of small lesions of the floor of the mouth may require local resection with en bloc marginal resection of the mandible (Figure 5–14).[44] This may be accomplished via a peroral approach. The mucosal and soft-tissue excision is left attached to the mandible, the extraction of teeth at sites of alveolar cuts is performed, and the bone cuts are performed with the sagittal saw and ultra-thin blades. Smooth cuts rather than right-angle cuts are favored to evenly distribute forces of mastication and pre-

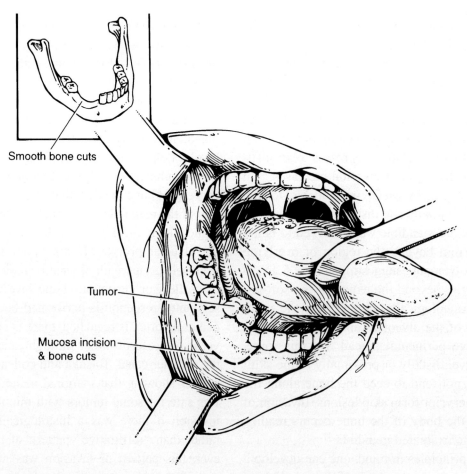

Smooth bone cuts

Tumor

Mucosa incision & bone cuts

Figure 5–14.   Resection of floor of the mouth cancer with marginal mandibulectomy.

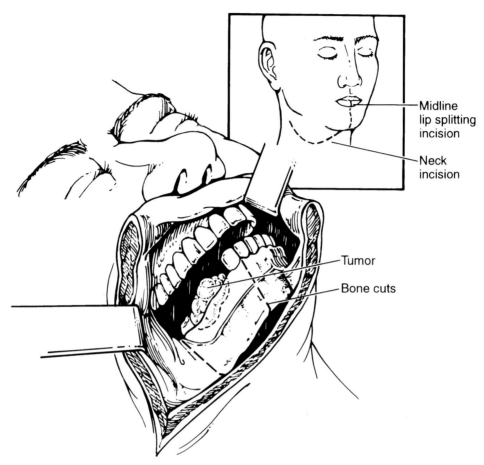

Figure 5–15. Segmental resection of the mandible through a lower cheek flap approach for a large floor of the mouth carcinoma with gross mandibular bone involvement.

vent subsequent fractures. When the dentate mandible is encroached upon by tumor at the lingual plate only, a vertical partial mandibular resection can be accomplished using the tooth roots as the vertical plane of resection. The related teeth are extracted and the right-angle saw blade is used to resect only the lingual plate, exercising caution to preserve the alveolar artery. Elective or therapeutic neck dissection improves the exposure of the lower mandible. The specimen is delivered en bloc. The resulting defects of the floor of the mouth and the mandible can be left to granulate, however mucosal advancement flaps or a split-thickness skin graft can often close these defects well.[45,46]

Most T3 and T4 floor of mouth cancers require extended local resections including partial glossectomy or a segmental mandibular resection, which is performed through a lower lip splitting incision and a lower cheek flap exposure (Figure 5–15). The mental nerve is sacrificed. An elective or therapeutic neck dis-

section is always indicated in surgical treatment of large floor of the mouth tumors and this provides good inferior exposure for the resection of the mandible. Tooth extractions and gingival mucosal incisions are then performed. Mandibular reconstruction plates may be pre-bent and screw holes drilled. With the soft-tissue portion of the tumor well defined and protected, the bone cuts are performed with the sagittal saw and the specimen removed en bloc, often with the neck specimen attached as well.[44] A frozen-section assessment of the alveolar nerve is prudent. Reconstruction of lateral mandibular defects with reconstruction plates or free bone grafts requires excellent soft-tissue coverage with myocutaneous flaps although the failure rate is 50 percent. Exposure of reconstruction plates used for anterior arch reconstruction approaches 100 percent. The free tissue transfer of fibula with attached muscle and skin is the state of the art reconstruction for large composite resections, especially when the anterior arch is involved.

An alternative surgical approach to T3 and T4 floor of the mouth lesions that do not require segmental mandibular resection is the transcervical pull-through procedure.[47] The primary tumor specimen is delivered into the neck with or without marginal mandibular resection. Bilateral upper neck dissections are usually performed. If necessary a marginal or lingual plate resection of the mandible is accomplished. The remaining soft-tissue attachments to the mandible, including the mylohyoid muscles, are divided and the oral contents delivered inferiorly into the neck. This provides good visualization of the tumor for the remainder of the soft-tissue resection. It is critical that the oral tissues are properly re-suspended and that the remaining extrinsic tongue musculature is appropriately attached to the mandible for postoperative swallowing function.

Maxillary and mandibular gingival lesions are often reported in the literature together as gingival lesions. Surgically, lesions of the mandibular gingiva and retromolar trigone are similar and will be discussed together. Lesions of the maxillary gingiva are surgically similar to those of the hard palate and so these two subsites will subsequently be addressed.

Three-quarters of gingival lesions involve the mandibular alveolus and one-quarter involve the maxillary alveolus. A report of 283 mandibular alveolar lesions from Memorial Sloan-Kettering Cancer Center showed the distribution of these primary tumors to be 30 percent T1, 48 percent T2, 17 percent T3 and 11 percent T4.[48] Only 5 percent were resected without bone, 32 percent were amenable to marginal resection and 63 percent required segmental bone resection. Local recurrence was 25 percent when the mandible was initially involved with tumor. Occult neck metastasis was found in only 6 of 107 elective radical neck dissections, indicating a low incidence of occult neck disease compared to tumors of other subsites of the oral cavity. Staging elective supraomohyoid neck dissection is indicated for T2 or larger lesions in conjunction with segmental mandibular resection. Five-year survival for all alveolar cancers was 77 percent stage I, 70 percent stage II, 42 percent stage III, and 24 percent stage IV.

Overholt[49] reviewed the M.D. Anderson Hospital experience of 155 mandibular alveolar lesions and determined that parameters affecting local control and survival were: size greater than 3 cm, bone involvement, and positive surgical margins. As discussed above, marginal mandibular resection is appropriate for periosteal involvement and segmental resection indicated when the cortical bone is involved with cancer.

Peroral wide local resection with marginal mandibular resection can be performed for smaller lesions, while segmental resection requires lip splitting incision and lower cheek flap elevation as described previously.

Tumors of the retromolar trigone occur with a disproportionately high frequency considering the small surface area (Figure 5–16). Fifteen percent of oral cancers occur in the retromolar trigone. This site is difficult to assess clinically because of its posterior location, mucosal irregularity, small area, and visual interference by the dentition. Trismus, if present, may also inhibit the examination, and is indicative of pterygoid involvement. Retromolar lesions are relatively difficult to treat because they spread early to deep structures such as the ascending ramus of the mandible, pterygoid muscles, the masticator space, and the skull base. Another avenue of local spread is the foramen of the inferior alveolar nerve into the ramus of the mandible. Tumor may also spread proximally along the perineurium or within the nerve to the trigeminal ganglion and the CNS. Surgical access to this region is challenging. Bone resection is nearly always indicated, and recurrence is difficult to diagnose.

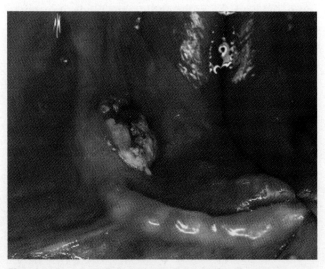

Figure 5–16.   An exophytic lesion in the retromolar trigone.

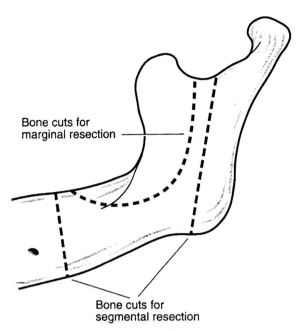

Figure 5–17. Bone cuts for marginal and conservative segmental resections of the mandibular ramus and body.

The peroral approach to the retromolar region is rarely satisfactory due to the posterior location of the trigone and the necessity for bone resection since the periosteum or bone is usually involved with cancer. Often a segmental resection of the ascending ramus of the mandible and part of the pharynx is necessary. Mandibular rim resection of the molar alveolus and the ascending ramus of the mandible is acceptable for small lesions without gross bony involvement. Marginal mandibular resection of the ascending ramus through the open mouth is not satisfactory.

If bone is grossly involved by clinical or imaging evaluation, then segmental resection of the ramus and/or body is required. If superficial involvement of the molar alveolus or ascending ramus is identified, then conservative segmental mandibular resection sparing the condyle and a posterior strut of ascending ramus is satisfactory bone resection.[41] Cuts are performed through the mandibular notch and the coronoid process (Figure 5–17). The alveolar foramen and nerve are included in the resection. Intraoperatively, a frozen-section margin on this nerve is important. Assessment of the superior extent of the disease, including the coronoid process of the mandible, the temporalis muscle, maxillary tubercle, masticator space, and pterygomaxillary space is necessary. Marginal resection of the maxil-

lary alveolus or partial maxillectomy may be necessary if they are involved with cancer.

Soft-tissue reconstruction with primary closure, or healing by secondary intention over the retromolar trigone is occasionally satisfactory. Posteriorly-based buccal mucosal random-pattern rotational flaps, soft palate, tongue, and masseter muscle flaps are all described for this area. The need for thin tissue here suggests an advantage for skin grafting and radial forearm free flap reconstructions. If the ramus is sacrificed, a bulkier pectoralis pedicled flap may cover reconstructive hardware but tends to pull inferiorly with time. The excellent bone stock of the fibular free flap is detracted from by its association with bulky muscle, and variable survival of the overlying skin paddle. It is infrequent today that a lateral mandibular defect is left unreconstructed, but this defect is tolerated well by many patients and it allows easier assessment of the region for recurrence. Defects that are small, posterior and occur in the edentulous patient are tolerated well.

Carcinomas of the hard palate (Figure 5–18) and upper alveolus are relatively uncommon, accounting for 10 percent of oral cancers,[50] except in areas of Southeast Asia where reverse smoking is practiced.[51] In the United States, carcinoma of the hard palate is only half as common as carcinoma of the soft palate[52,53] and carcinoma of the maxillary alveolar ridge is only one-third as common as carcinoma of the mandibular alveolar ridge.[48] These areas are lined with adherent keratinized mucosa, which pro-

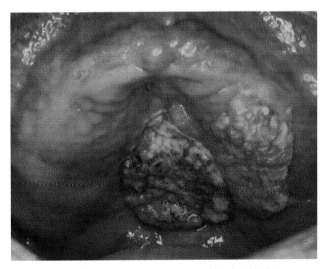

Figure 5–18. Squamous cell carcinoma of the hard palate.

vides protection from the trauma of mastication, and may provide relative protection of the basal nuclei from the effects of carcinogens.

Histologically, carcinomas of the upper alveolar ridge are nearly all squamous cell carcinomas, but up to one-third of hard palate cancers are of minor salivary gland origin.[54] In contrast to squamous cell carcinomas, palatal minor salivary gland tumors are often submucosal masses rather than ulcerative or fungating mucosal lesions. Kaposi's sarcoma can be seen on the hard palate of patients with acquired immunodeficiency syndrome. Malignant melanoma of the oral cavity, while rare, occurs most frequently on the palate.

Lesions of the maxillary alveolar ridge are symptomatic, thus allowing early diagnosis. Eighty-two percent of maxillary alveolar ridge carcinomas are T1 or T2 at the time of diagnosis, and 86 percent are N0.[48] Palatal carcinomas tend to be larger when diagnosed but only 13 percent have regional metastases when diagnosed.[49] The presence of regional metastases to the neck or locally advanced disease decreases 5-year survival from approximately 70 percent to approximately 30 percent.[53]

Surgery is the treatment of choice for cancer of the maxillary alveolus and the hard palate, and it is frequently necessary to resect periosteum and bone in order to ensure an adequate margin. The mucosa and the underlying periosteum are fused in this region forming a mucoperiosteum. Invasive carcinomas of this area frequently involve the periosteum or the underlying bone, thus reducing the effectiveness of primary radiation therapy for these lesions. However, postoperative radiation therapy for aggressive minor salivary gland malignancies or advanced squamous carcinoma is recommended.[54,55]

T1 and T2 lesions may be amenable to peroral wide local excision with resection of the involved mucoperiosteum and usually the underlying bone. Mucosal incisions are performed with electrocautery, allowing a 1 cm margin of normal tissue. Teeth are extracted at the osteotomy sites, and bony cuts are performed with an oscillating saw. Many small defects granulate well and close by secondary intention. Primary closure is usually not possible due to the immobility of the surrounding adherent mucosa. A posteriorly-based buccal mucosa flap

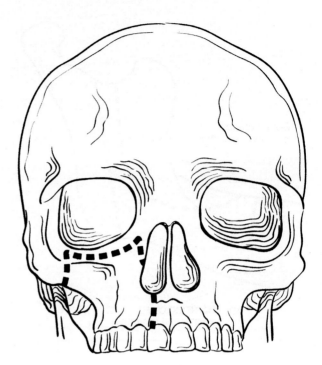

Figure 5–19.   Bone cuts for subtotal maxillectomy preserving the inferior orbital rim and floor of the orbit.

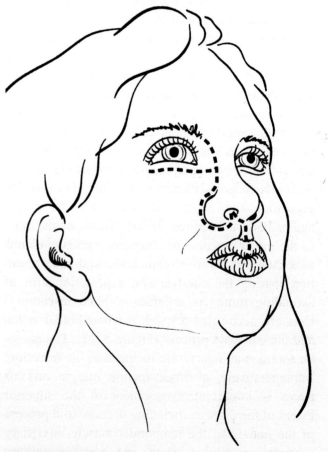

Figure 5–20.   The Weber-Ferguson incision and its subciliary and brow extensions for maxillectomy.

with random blood supply is effective in closing lateral palatal and alveolar defects. A flap of the palatal mucoperiosteum, based on the greater palatine artery in the posterior aspect of the hard palate, can be rotated to cover a small defect, and the donor site left to granulate or be skin grafted. If the nasal and antral mucosa are intact after the resection, the oral defect can be closed with a local flap with a low risk of oronasal fistula formation.

T3 or T4 cancers with invasion of the maxillary antrum or nasal cavity often require partial or subtotal maxillectomy. Advanced lesions invade the nasal cavity, maxillary sinus, the pterygomaxillary space, pterygoid plates and skull base. T3 and T4 cancers requiring subtotal maxillectomy (preservation of the infraorbital rim and floor of the orbit) (Figure 5–19) need exposure via an extended Weber-Ferguson incision and an upper cheek flap for maximum exposure (Figure 5–20), or exposure via the midface degloving approach. A midface degloving approach provides excellent exposure for anterior lesions involving the lower maxilla and nasal cavity bilaterally without any external incisions, but superior exposure is limited above the orbital rim.[56,57] After the exposure is obtained, the soft-tissue cuts and dental extractions are performed as needed. Alveolar cuts should be made through the sockets of extracted teeth and not between them. This allows good bony support for the remaining teeth that will bear considerable forces from dental rehabilitation. The following cuts are performed using the oscillating saw: (1) from the lateral maxillary wall to the infraorbital rim preserving the latter, (2) from the infraorbital rim to the nasal cavity through the lacrimal fossa, (3) from the nasal cavity through the alveolar ridge, and (4) through the hard palate (see Figure 5–19). The remaining cuts are the lateral nasal wall cut, which joins the lacrimal cut to the nasopharynx using a thin osteotome and Mayo scissors, and finally the posterior cut. The posterior cut is performed only after all other aspects of the maxilla are freed. This is because significant bleeding can occur from the pterygoid venous plexus and the internal maxillary artery after this cut is performed. The expedient removal of the specimen and prompt packing of the maxillectomy defect are necessary to adequately control bleeding. The final cut is made anterior to the pterygoid plates if the posterior wall of the antrum is not involved, and posterior to the pterygoid plates if the posterior wall and the pterygomaxillary space are involved with cancer. The cut is made using a curved osteotome and the heavy curved Mayo scissors under palpation guidance with cognizance of the proximity of the internal carotid artery in the deep aspect of the parapharyngeal space, and the apex of the orbit superomedially. Hemostasis is obtained, the lacrimal sac is tacked open with chromic suture and/or the lacrimal duct cannulated with silastic tubing, and the cavity is skin grafted. The graft is supported by packing with xeroform gauze, which is supported by a preformed dental obturator that is wired to the remaining maxillary teeth or the alveolar bone.

Only rarely is total maxillectomy (including the orbital rim and floor) or radical maxillectomy (including orbital exenteration) necessary for oral cavity cancers.

REHABILITATION

The rehabilitation of function after oral surgery is a critical element in effective oral cancer surgery. After major oral resections the patients need rehabilitation of speech, swallowing, dentition and mastication as well as cosmesis. This process is best accomplished in a multidisciplinary environment which include the head and neck surgeons, plastic surgeons, speech and language therapists, nurses, dentists, prosthodontists and oral and maxillofacial surgeons.

Perhaps the most important element of rehabilitation is optimizing the patient's resection and reconstruction at the time of surgery. While the oncologic soundness of the tumor resection must not be compromised for functional reasons, neither should excessive resection of uninvolved soft tissue, nerve or bone be performed. Whenever oncologically possible, preservation of the hypoglossal, lingual and mental nerves should be attempted. Gentle handling of tissues, hemostasis, and obliteration of dead space are general principles of surgery which should be adhered to. This, in combination with antiseptic preparation of the oral cavity preoperatively and the use of perioperative antibiotics, may reduce inflammation and improve healing and reduce scar tissue formation, which will tend to maximize postoperative function.

Reconstruction of oral defects after ablative surgery is critical for oral rehabilitation. Perhaps the most important advance in head and neck surgery in the last 15 years has been the safe and effective use of free tissue transfer for reconstruction. Free tissue transfer techniques now allow the excellent reconstruction of the mandible, skin, and mucosa of the oral cavity. Bone flaps from the fibula, iliac crest and scapula are available to the reconstructive surgeon. Soft tissue from the radial forearm, lateral arm, trapezius, rectus abdominis and other sites provide vascularized, nonirradiated soft tissue for reconstructive purposes. It is clear that the appropriate use of these reconstructive tissues has dramatically improved the functional outcome of oral cancer patients. They should be employed whenever necessary. Adequate reconstruction of the mandibular arch, and soft tissues of the tongue and floor of mouth will significantly increase the likelihood of acceptable speech and swallowing after major oral cavity cancer surgery.

Rehabilitation of swallowing after oral cavity surgery is important. Swallowing can be divided into the preparation phase, the oral phase and the pharyngeal phase. Oral cavity surgery impacts most on the preparatory phase and the oral phase. The preparatory phase of swallowing begins with lubrication of the food bolus by saliva. This is impaired when pre- or postoperative radiation therapy is employed. Significant xerostomia results in the majority of irradiated patients. The xerostomia significantly limits the types and consistencies of food that can be swallowed. Most patients with oral cavity radiation require frequent sips of water to maintain moisture and liquid to wash down the food at mealtimes. One experimental strategy to try to limit xerostomia is to use a salivary gland protectant such as Salagen (pilocarpine hydrochlonde) during radiation. The benefit of Salagen™ is not yet proven and it is contraindicated in the presence of coronary artery disease. Amifostine is approved for the prevention of radiation-induced xerostomia. It is not widely used. A number of preparations are marketed for xerostomia but are not superior to water for the majority of patients.

Mastication is critical to an effective preparatory phase of swallowing. Certainly the quality and quantity of the teeth are important for mastication. Mastication requires intact sensation of the dentition, gingiva, tongue and buccal mucosa, and intact motor function of the hypoglossal nerve for tongue musculature, the facial nerve for oral competence and the third division of the trigeminal nerve for buccinator function. This combination of sensory and motor functions allows the food to be kept in the plane of the molars without biting the soft tissues.

Continuity of the mandibular arch provides great advantage for mastication. However, a patient with a segmental defect of the body of the mandible can frequently masticate some foods satisfactorily. Occasionally a guide plane prosthesis is helpful to maximize occlusion of the teeth in a patient with a lateral mandible defect. These guide plane prostheses help overcome the deviation of the mandible to the resected side from the unopposed action of the intact contralateral pterygoids. An unreconstructed defect of the anterior mandible is uncommon today. This defect will prohibit mastication of solids and patients will tolerate no more than a puréed diet. The combination of poor mastication, swallowing, speech and articulation, cosmetic defect and oral incompetence makes the anterior mandibular arch defect something to be avoided in almost every circumstance. The oral preparatory phase of swallowing can also be inhibited by trismus, which is common after surgery and/or irradiation of the posterior oral cavity and oropharynx.

The oral phase of swallowing consists of preparation of the food bolus followed by presentation to the oropharynx, where the swallowing reflex is initiated during the oropharyngeal phase. The oral phase is volitional. Preparation of the bolus is accomplished by the tongue, cheek, teeth and palate. After mastication and lubrication, the bolus is then propelled to the oropharynx by elevation of the tongue against the hard palate. When the bolus is sensed in the oropharynx the reflexive portion of the oropharyngeal phase of swallowing is initiated. Tongue elevation can be restricted due to either loss of tissue volume or motor function after surgery. Patients with near total glossectomy can be sometimes well rehabilitated with a palatal drop prosthesis, which lowers the level of the hard palate so that the residual tongue tissue can articulate with it to propel the bolus posteriorly (Figure 5–21).

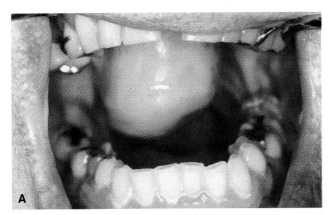

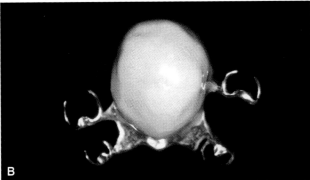

Figure 5–21. *A*, Patient with poor tongue mobility with a palatal drop prosthesis in place. *B*, Palatal drop prosthesis.

The oral prosthodontist plays a critical role in the rehabilitation of swallowing after oral cancer treatment. The proper number and quality of teeth and their alignment can be restored by maxillary and/or gingival dentures. After resection of the maxilla or hard palate, a dental obturator to cover the oro-antral and oronasal fistulae is necessary for swallowing without nasal regurgitation (Figure 5–22). Patients with large maxillary defects can attain excellent functional results with an obturator. For defects of the soft palate, dysphagia due to nasal regurgitation, hyponasal speech and difficulty with articulation of speech sounds, an obturator with a nasopharyngeal bulb is effective in minimizing nasal regurgitation and improving hyponasal speech. The bulb is properly positioned in the nasopharynx articulating with the posterior pharyngeal wall at the prominence of the body of C2, allowing the remainder of the soft palate to seal off the nasopharynx during swallowing (Figure 5–23).

Osseointegrated implants are an important advance in oral rehabilitation. If adequate bone stock exists, titanium posts can be placed in a multi-

staged process and the ingrowth of healthy bone into and around the implants results in a very secure foundation for oral prostheses.[58] Osseointegrative implants can be placed in fibula free flap reconstructions of the mandible after the healing and removal of the fibula fixation hardware (Figure 5–24). Osseointegrative implants should be avoided in the atrophic edentulous mandible especially after

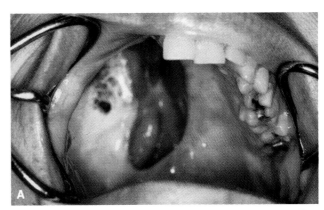

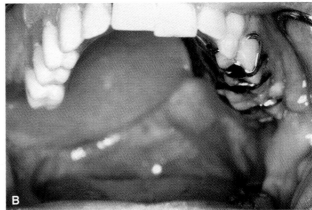

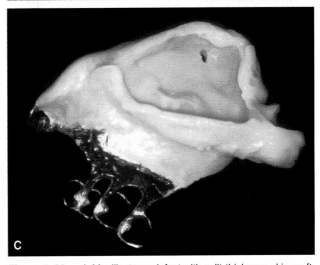

Figure 5–22. *A*, Maxillectomy defect with split-thickness skin graft. *B*, Prosthesis in place. *C*, Prosthesis.

radiation. Osseointegration can also be utilized effectively for external fixation of cosmetic prostheses after extended surgery for oral cavity cancer, which includes soft tissues of the face. It is important for the patient's rehabilitation that they have an acceptable cosmetic appearance in public.

Many patients benefit from evaluation and therapy by certified speech and swallowing therapists.

They can often recommend exercises for the articulation of speech and can help both the patient and prosthodontist to optimize prostheses and to recommend alternative methods of phoneme formation.[59] Patients with significant resections of the lips, maxilla, tongue and palate will often benefit from speech therapy.

Speech and swallowing therapists can also help improve swallowing in patients who have undergone oral surgery.[60] A modified barium swallow under fluoroscopic observation by a radiologist and a speech therapist may be helpful diagnostically.[61] From this study, abnormalities of mastication, bolus preparation and bolus presentation of the oropharynx can be observed and studied frequently from this data. Strategies for improved function can be devised and taught to the patient and exercises implemented. Accompanying abnormalities of the pharyngeal phase of swallowing can also be diagnosed. Based on

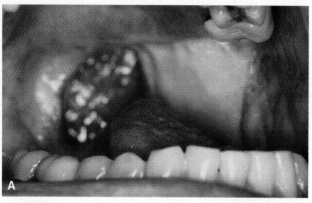

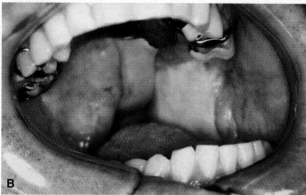

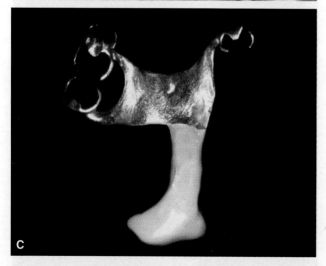

Figure 5–23 *A,* Soft palate defect after surgical resection and free flap reconstruction of the lateral pharyngeal wall. *B,* Prosthesis in place. *C,* The nasopharyngeal bulb prosthesis.

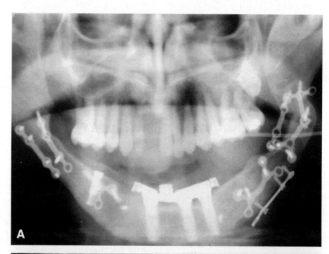

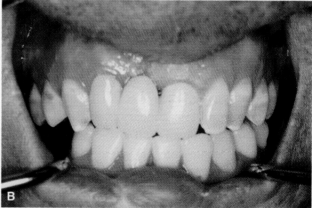

Figure 5–24. *A,* Panorex of osseointegrated implants in the anterior and right lateral aspects of a fibula free flap reconstruction of the mandible. *B,* The prosthesis in place.

the clinical findings and the modified barium swallow, therapists can also suggest optimal consistencies, and temperatures of food that can be best managed.

Consultation with a trained nutritionist with experience in treating head and neck cancer patients is essential to provide patients with information and suggestions regarding optimal foods to maintain a balanced nutrition within the patient's consistency restrictions. Patients with impaired oral function risk nutritional deficiency unless an appropriately varied diet is maintained. Many patients benefit from prepared commercial supplements, which are formulated specifically as a balanced diet. Some patients may subsist on liquid dietary supplements alone, while the majority benefit from regular foods as tolerated with additional dietary supplements as needed. Nearly any everyday food can be puréed with liquid in a blender and drunk. Patients should be weighed frequently in the postoperative period to monitor for weight loss. Supplemental tube feeding may be necessary while the patient is relearning swallowing.

Members of the rehabilitation team must educate the oral cancer patient regarding oral hygiene. Teeth brushing and fluoride treatments should be done at least twice daily. The patient should perform these fluoride treatments at home regularly using molded dental trays. Patients with post-radiation xerostomia require frequent sips of water, and may benefit from sialagogues such as lozenges or chewing gum; however it is critical that these be sugar free as the risk of caries is dramatically increased after radiation treatment. All patients with impaired oral function should be instructed to cleanse the oral cavity after eating. This may involve simple rinsing with water or saline solution or irrigation with a hanging bag and warm saline solution. Reconstruction flaps with skin lining the oral cavity may require frequent brushing to eliminate accumulated skin debris and sometimes trimming of the hair growing on the skin flaps is necessary for patient comfort and to decrease the adherence of food. Reconstructive flaps that have been irradiated no longer grow hair. Mouth washes, which contain alcohol, should be avoided as they dry the tissues and cause burning and discomfort. Normal saline or saline with bicarbonate of soda is preferred. Successful oral rehabilitation after oral cancer surgery requires a dedicated team of specialists working together. Each can contribute significantly toward the rehabilitation of speech, swallowing and appearance of the oral cancer patient.

SEQUELAE, COMPLICATIONS AND THEIR MANAGEMENT

Complications can be minimized by appropriate preoperative evaluation including medical cardiology and anesthesia consultation as indicated. Since the majority of oral cancer patients are elderly, many will have significant co-morbidities which need assessment, diagnosis or intervention prior to, or after, surgery. A preoperative medical evaluation is recommended for all patients over the age of 60 regardless of their health status. Routine preoperative testing should screen for previously undiagnosed major organ diseases and should consist of at least a preoperative chest radiograph, serum tests of renal and hepatic function and electrocardiography. Patients in negative nitrogen balance due to poor nutrition would be considered for a nasogastric feeding tube placement and several weeks of nutritional therapy prior to surgery. Properly selected patients should have a low incidence of major complications.[62]

The most common complications after oral surgery are wound related. The excellent blood supply to the oral cavity helps to ensure good healing of soft tissues and to resolve infection. Careful surgical technique can help to minimize complications. It is important to handle tissues atraumatically, avoid excessive char from electrocautery, observe careful hemostasis, obliterate any dead spaces and to minimize bacteria colony counts by gentle antiseptic preoperative preparation and copious irrigation with saline with or without antibiotics. Careful techniques of closure will help to minimize postoperative wound complications. Closure under tension should be avoided, especially of an irradiated tissue. Separate suture layers of muscle and mucosa should be performed. Oral wounds closed by primary intention will heal best. Many oral lesions will granulate well over several days to several weeks. Skin grafts can be helpful but are frequently lost when placed over mobile surfaces or directly over cortical bone. Any exposed bone or cartilage in the oral cavity will lead to granulation tissue formation and delay of healing.

Obviously carious or infected teeth should be removed at the time of surgery. Twenty-four hours of IV antibiotics, initiated at least 1 hour prior to surgery, may help to reduce the wound infection rate.

Other intraoperative measures to decrease complications include consideration of procedure duration to minimize the time of general anesthesia. Judicious intraoperative use of crystalloid will prevent postoperative complications of fluid overload. Insensate fluid loss in oral cavity surgery is significantly less than in abdominal surgery, which results in a lower requirement of intravenous fluid for oral cavity surgery patients than for abdominal surgery patients.

Postoperative management impacts significantly on complications of oral surgery. Aggressive oral irrigation should begin on the first day of the surgery. It should be accomplished with normal saline or normal saline and bicarbonate of soda solution in hanging irrigation bags or via compressed air-sprayer.

Major systemic complications are uncommon in oral cavity surgery. Cardiopulmonary complications occur due to pre-existing co-morbidities, the physiologic stress of surgery and fluid overload. Respiratory complications such as pneumonia can be minimized by appropriate early mobilization and the use of sequential compression devices, and careful observation for aspiration of liquids. Due to early mobilization, oral cavity cancer patients rarely suffer from deep venous thrombosis (DVT) or pulmonary embolism, however, immobilized patients should be placed on appropriate DVT prophylaxis, such as subcutaneous heparin or sequential compression devices.[63]

The majority of wound complications will heal with aggressive cleansing and infection control. Management of co-morbidities, such as diabetes mellitus, malnutrition and hypothyroidism, in order to maximize wound healing is critical. Poor healing or a persistent oral cutaneous fistula may result from the presence of a foreign body such as hardware, non-absorbable suture or sequestered bone. Persistent or recurrent tumor must be ruled out by biopsy in any non-healing wound after oral cancer surgery. The frequency, complexity and duration of wound complications are greater in the irradiated patient.

In summary, the incidence of major complications in oral cancer surgery can be minimized by appropriate patient selection, preoperative evaluation, meticulous technique and appropriate postoperative care.

OUTCOMES AND FUNCTION

Outcomes in oral cavity surgery may be divided into survival and functional outcomes. Five-year survival rates for early (T1 and T2) oral cancers are reported to be in the 70 to 90 percent range. In all head and neck sites, the presence of metastatic nodes to the neck decreases the survival by 50 percent. Five-year survival for patients with stage IV disease, especially with bulky or bilateral lower neck metastases, is less then 20 percent.[27]

In resectable stage III and stage IV tumors with N0 or N1 disease, 5-year survival has been increased to the 50 to 60 percent range by the aggressive addition of postoperative radiation therapy.[15,16] With improved local control rates a higher percentage of deaths are due to distant disease and second primary carcinomas rather than from uncontrolled locoregional disease.

Factors that predict survival of oral cancer patients are low T stage, low N stage, low overall stage, and the absence of significant co-morbidities. While the study of the molecular genetics of oral cancer is rapidly evolving, there are currently no molecular markers which have been shown to predict survival in head and neck cancer patients in large prospectively gathered series. It is however likely that in the next several years valid molecular markers will be developed which can predict tumor behavior, response to surgical and non-surgical treatment and patient survival rates.

Functional outcomes for surgery for early oral cancers is excellent. It is rare for patients to suffer significant loss of speech and swallowing function after surgical resection for T1 or T2 lesions. Even large T2 lesions of the tongue rehabilitate extremely well due to the plasticity of the tongue as well as its good blood supply, copious sensory innervation and the presence of intact musculature. Over 6 to 12 months, the patients invariably find dramatic improvement in articulation of speech sounds, mastication and swallowing. Aggressive and appropriate rehabilitation with speech and swallowing therapy and prosthodontics is critical to these results.

With increasing volumes of resected tissue, functional outcomes diminish. Tissues impacting most on function include tongue muscle, hypoglossal nerve, lingual nerve, anterior mandibular arch, and soft palate. When extensive or multiple resections of the above structures are undertaken for advanced disease, patient function may be poor even with the most advanced reconstructive and rehabilitative techniques. Despite improvements in postoperative function attributed to free flap reconstruction, the degree of coordination of motor and sensory function necessary for good oral function cannot be attained with the current technology. These patients are gastrostomy tube-dependent and speak poorly. Xerostomia from oral radiation therapy and trismus from surgery or radiation are also factors that can dramatically compromise function.

REFERENCES

1. Landis SH, Murray T, Bolden S, Wingo PA. Cancer statistics, 1999. CA Cancer J Clin 1999;49:8–31.
2. Cancer epidemiology and prevention. 2nd ed. New York: Oxford University Press; 1999.
3. Shopland DR, Eyre HJ, Pechacek TF. Smoking-attributable cancer mortality in 1991: is lung cancer now the leading cause of death among smokers in the United States? J Natl Cancer Inst 1991;83:1142–8.
4. Blot WJ, McLaughlin JK, Winn DM, et al. Smoking and drinking in relation to oral and pharyngeal cancer. Cancer Res 1988;48:3282–7.
5. Mahale A, Saranath D. Microsatellite alterations on chromosome 9 in chewing tobacco-induced oral squamous cell carcinomas from India. Oral Oncol 2000;36:199–206.
6. Slaughter DP, Southwick HW, Smejkal J. "Field cancerization" in oral stratified squamous epithelium. Cancer 1953;5:963–8.
7. Day GL, Blot WJ. Second primary tumors in patients with oral cancer. Cancer 1992;70:14–9.
8. Califano J, van der Reit P, Westra W, et al. Genetic progression model for head and neck cancer: implications for field cancerization. Cancer Res 1996;56:2488–92.
9. Chen YK, Huang HC, Lin LM, Lin CC. Primary oral squamous cell carcinoma: an analysis of 703 cases in southern Taiwan. Oral Oncol 1999;35:173–9.
10. Sunderman FW Jr, Morgan LG, Andersen A, et al. Histopathology of sinonasal and lung cancers in nickel refinery workers. Ann Clin Lab Sci 1989;19:44–50.
11. Benninger MS, Enrique RR, Nichols RD. Symptom-directed selective endoscopy and cost containment for evaluation of head and neck cancer. Head Neck 1993;15:532–6.
12. Shaha AR, Hoover EL, Mitrani M, et al. Synchronicity, multicentricity, and metachronicity of head and neck cancer. Head Neck Surg 1988;10:225–8.
13. Hordijk GJ, Bruggink T, Ravasz LA. Panendoscopy: a valuable procedure? Otolaryngol Head Neck Surg 1989;101:426–8.
14. Hanasono MM, Kunda LD, Segall GM, et al. Uses and limitations of FDG positron emission tomography in patients with head and neck cancer. Laryngoscope 1999;109:880–5.
15. Vikram B, Strong EW, Shah JP, Spiro R. Failure at the primary site following multimodality treatment in advanced head and neck cancer. Head Neck Surg 1984;6:720–3.
16. Vikram B, Strong EW, Shah JP, Spiro R. Failure in the neck following multimodality treatment for advanced head and neck cancer. Head Neck Surg 1984;6:724–9.
17. Rudoltz MS, Perkins RS, Luthmann RW, et al. High-dose-rate brachytherapy for primary carcinomas of the oral cavity and oropharynx. Laryngoscope 1999;109:1967–73.
18. Wolf GT, Forastiere A, Ang K, et al. Workshop report: organ preservation strategies in advanced head and neck cancer—current status and future directions. Head Neck 1999;21:689–93.
19. Schuller DE, Metch B, Stein DW, et al. Preoperative chemotherapy in advanced resectable head and neck cancer: final report of the Southwest Oncology Group. Laryngoscope 1988;98:1205–11.
20. Williams EF III, Meguid MM. Nutritional concepts and considerations in head and neck surgery. Head Neck 1989;11:393–9.
21. Lotan R. Retinoids and chemoprevention of aerodigestive tract cancers. Cancer Metastasis Rev 1997;16:349–56.
22. Hong WK, Endicott J, Itri LM, et al. 13-cis-retinoic acid in the treatment of oral leukoplakia. N Engl J Med 1986;315:1501–5.
23. White JM, Chaudhry SI, Kudler JJ, et al. Nd:YAG and CO_2 laser therapy of oral mucosal lesions. J Clin Laser Med Surg 1998;16:299–304.
24. Schoelch ML, Sekandari N, Regezi JA, Silverman S Jr. Laser management of oral leukoplakias: a follow-up study of 70 patients. Laryngoscope 1999;109:949–53.
25. Hamilton MM, Branham GH. Concepts in lip reconstruction. Otolaryngol Clin N Am 1997;30:593–606.
26. Cordeiro PG, Santamaria E. Primary reconstruction of complex midfacial defects with combined lip- switch procedures and free flaps. Plast Reconstr Surg 1999;103:1850–6.
27. Franceschi D, Gupta R, Spiro RH, Shah JP. Improved survival in the treatment of squamous carcinoma of the oral tongue. Am J Surg 1993;166:360–5.
28. Spiro RH, Gerold FP, Shah JP, et al. Mandibulotomy approach to oropharyngeal tumors. Am J Surg 1985;150:466–9.
29. Spiro RH, Gerold FP, Strong EW. Mandibular "swing" approach for oral and oropharyngeal tumors. Head Neck Surg 1981;3:371–8.
30. Scholl P, Byers RM, Batsakis JG, et al. Microscopic cutthrough of cancer in the surgical treatment of squamous carcinoma of the tongue. Prognostic and therapeutic implications. Am J Surg 1986;152:354–60.
31. Loree TR, Strong EW. Significance of positive margins in oral cavity squamous carcinoma. Am J Surg 1990;160:410–4.
32. Looser KG, Shah JP, Strong EW. The significance of "positive" margins in surgically resected epidermoid carcinomas. Head Neck Surg 1978;1:107–11.

33. Fukano H, Matsuura H, Hasegawa Y, Nakamura S. Depth of invasion as a predictive factor for cervical lymph node metastasis in tongue carcinoma. Head Neck 1997;19: 205–10.

34. Spiro RH, Huvos AG, Wong GY, et al. Predictive value of tumor thickness in squamous carcinoma confined to the tongue and floor of the mouth. Am J Surg 1986;152: 345–50.

35. Shaha AR, Spiro RH, Shah JP, Strong EW. Squamous carcinoma of the floor of the mouth. Am J Surg 1984;148: 455–9.

36. Marchetta FC, Sako K, Murphy JB. The periosteum of the mandible and intraoral carcinoma. Am J Surg 1971;122: 711–3.

37. Marchetta FC, Sako K, Badillo J. Periosteal lymphatics of the mandible and intraoral carcinoma. Am J Surg 1964;108: 505–7.

38. McGregor IA, MacDonald DG. Spread of squamous cell carcinoma to the nonirradiated edentulous mandible—a preliminary report. Head Neck Surg 1987;9:157–61.

39. McGregor AD, MacDonald DG. Routes of entry of squamous cell carcinoma to the mandible. Head Neck Surg 1988;10:294–301.

40. Brown JS, Browne RM. Factors influencing the patterns of invasion of the mandible by oral squamous cell carcinoma. Int J Oral Maxillofac Surg 1995;24:417–26.

41. McGregor AD, MacDonald DG. Patterns of spread of squamous cell carcinoma to the ramus of the mandible. Head Neck 1993;15:440–4.

42. Totsuka Y, Usui Y, Tei K, et al. Results of surgical treatment for squamous carcinoma of the lower alveolus: segmental vs. marginal resection. Head Neck 1991;13:114–20.

43. Totsuka Y, Usui Y, Tei K, et al. Mandibular involvement by squamous cell carcinoma of the lower alveolus: analysis and comparative study of histologic and radiologic features. Head Neck 1991;13:40–50.

44. Shaha AR. Marginal mandibulectomy for carcinoma of the floor of the mouth. J Surg Oncol 1992;49:116–9.

45. Schramm VL Jr, Myers EN. Skin grafts in oral cavity reconstruction. Arch Otolaryngol 1980;106:528–32.

46. Schramm VL Jr, Johnson JT, Myers EN. Skin grafts and flaps in oral cavity reconstruction. Arch Otolaryngol 1983; 109:175–7.

47. Stanley RB. Mandibular lingual releasing approach to oral and oropharyngeal carcinomas. Laryngoscope 1984;94: 596–600.

48. Soo KC, Spiro RH, King W, et al. Squamous carcinoma of the gums. Am J Surg 1988;156:281–5.

49. Overholt SM, Eicher SA, Wolf P, Weber RS. Prognostic factors affecting outcome in lower gingival carcinoma. Laryngoscope 1996;106:1335–9.

50. Petruzzelli GJ, Myers EN. Malignant neoplasms of the hard palate and upper alveolar ridge. Oncology 1994;8:43–8.

51. Reddy CR. Carcinoma of hard palate in India in relation to reverse smoking of chuttas. J Natl Cancer Inst 1974;53: 615–9.

52. Ratzer ER, Schweitzer RJ, Frazell EL. Epidermoid carcinoma of the palate. Am J Surg 1970;119:294–7.

53. Evans JF, Shah JP. Epidermoid carcinoma of the palate. Am J Surg 1981;142:451–5.

54. Chung CK, Rahman SM, Constable WC. Malignant salivary gland tumors of the palate. Arch Otolaryngol 1978;104: 501–4.

55. Kovalic JJ, Simpson JR. Carcinoma of the hard palate. J Otolaryngol 1993;22:118–20.

56. Casson PR, Bonanno PC, Converse JM. The midface degloving procedure. Plast Reconstr Surg 1974;53:102–3.

57. Price JC, Holliday MJ, Johns ME, et al. The versatile midface degloving approach. Laryngoscope 1988;98:291–5.

58. Marx RE, Morales MJ. The use of implants in the reconstruction of oral cancer patients. Dent Clin N Am 1998; 42:177–202.

59. Fletcher SG. Speech production following partial glossectomy. J Speech Hear Disord 1988;53:232–8.

60. Logemann JA. Rehabilitation of the head and neck cancer patient. Semin Oncol 1994;21:359–65.

61. Logemann JA. Role of the modified barium swallow in management of patients with dysphagia. Otolaryngol Head Neck Surg 1997;116:335–8.

62. Sessions RB, Hudkins C. Complications of surgery of the oral cavity. In: Eisele DW, editor. Complications in head and neck surgery. Baltimore: Mosby; 1993. p.218–22.

63. Lowry JC. Thromboembolic disease and thromboprophylaxis in oral and maxillofacial surgery: experience and practice. Br J Oral Maxillofac Surg 1995;33:101–6.

6

Tumors of the Oropharynx

SNEHAL G. PATEL, MD, FRCS

JATIN P. SHAH, MD, FACS

It has been estimated that there will be about 8,400 new cases and 2,100 deaths from pharyngeal cancer in the United States during 2001.[1] The majority of tumors of this region are squamous cell carcinomas that are related to chronic abuse of tobacco and alcohol. The critical location of this part of the pharynx at the crossroads between the respiratory and digestive tracts means that tumors involving the oropharynx are prone to alter swallowing, speech and breathing. Treatment planning for these tumors must therefore be guided not only by disease-free survival statistics but also by the functional outcome of each therapeutic approach.

ANATOMY

The oropharynx extends from the level of the hard palate above to the hyoid bone below (Figure 6–1). On a practical basis, this region may be divided into the palatine arch consisting of the soft palate, uvula and the anterior faucial pillar, and the oropharynx proper[2] as tumors of the arch tend to be less virulent than those arising at other subsites. For the purpose of tumor classification, however, 4 main anatomical subdivisions are described (Table 6–1).

The anterior wall of the oropharynx is formed by the base or posterior third of the tongue bounded anteriorly by the v-shaped line of circumvallate papillae. Numerous lymphatic aggregates give the base of the tongue its characteristic nodularity, a normal feature that may cause great difficulty in the diagnosis of early lesions of this region. Lymphatics from the tongue base course downward toward the hyoid bone where they pierce the pharyngeal wall to drain into the upper deep cervical chain or level II nodes. The jugulodigastric lymph node, the largest of these nodes, is frequently the first to be involved by metastatic tumor followed by those at levels III and IV. Disruption of normal lymphatic channels by the presence of a tumor or surgery to the neck may result in aberrant patterns of spread to levels I and V,

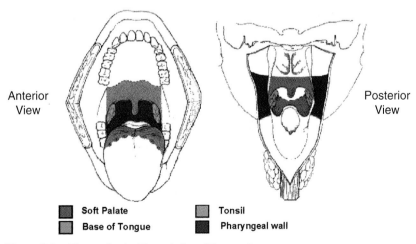

Anterior View

Posterior View

■ Soft Palate   ■ Tonsil

■ Base of Tongue   ■ Pharyngeal wall

Figure 6-1. The anatomical boundaries of the oropharynx.

Table 6–1. ANATOMICAL SUBDIVISIONS OF THE OROPHARYNX
Anterior wall (glossoepiglottic area)
Tongue posterior to the circumvallate papillae (base of tongue)
Vallecula excluding the lingual surface of the epiglottis
Lateral wall
Tonsil
Tonsillar fossa and faucial pillars
Glossotonsillar sulcus
Posterior wall
Superior wall
Inferior surface of the soft palate
Uvula

or to the contralateral side of the neck. Crossover patterns of lymphatic drainage have been demonstrated and tumors involving or growing close to the midline exhibit bilateral nodal involvement in approximately one-third of patients.

The lateral wall of the oropharynx includes the tonsil, the tonsillar fossae, the faucial pillars and more posteriorly, the lateral pharyngeal wall that blends into the posterior wall. Immediately lateral to the lateral pharyngeal wall lies the inverted cone-shaped parapharyngeal space with its base at the temporal bone and its apex at the greater cornu of the hyoid bone. This potential space contains several important neurovascular structures such as the carotid artery, the internal jugular vein, the sympathetic chain, and cranial nerves IX through XII (Figure 6–2). Involvement of this space not only results in cranial nerve deficits and trismus, but also provides tumors access to the base of skull superiorly or the neck inferiorly.

The tonsil is the largest aggregation of lymphoid tissue in Waldeyer's ring and is characterized by deep crypts in which squamous carcinomas may arise without causing obvious surface ulceration. The tonsils have a rich lymphatic network that drains directly through the pharyngeal wall into the upper deep cervical (jugulodigastric) nodes. Lymph node metastasis is less frequent from primary tumors of the tonsillar pillars compared to tumors of the tonsillar fossa. Lesions of the posterior tonsillar pillar are more likely to metastasize to the spinal accessory and upper posterior triangle nodes. Metastatic squamous carcinoma deposits involving nodes from an asymp-

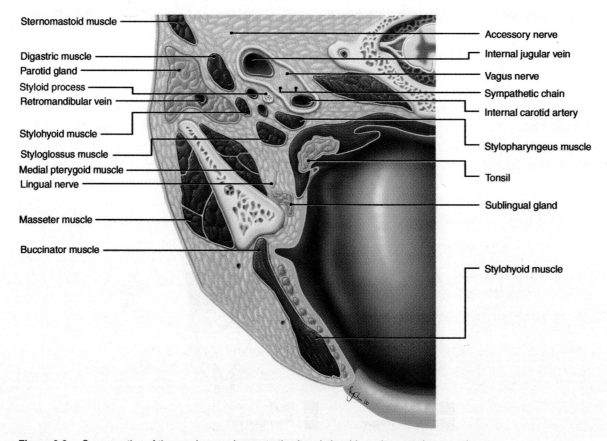

Figure 6-2.   Cross-section of the oropharynx demonstrating its relationship to the parapharyngeal space.

tomatic, small tonsillar primary have a tendency to undergo cystic degeneration. Fine needle aspiration of the cystic mass may draw fluid that is often acellular or non-diagnostic, prompting local excision of the mass with a mistaken diagnosis of branchial cyst. Lymphatics from the upper part of the lateral wall drain to the retropharyngeal nodes, of which the only constant one is the node of Rouvière situated close to the skull base between the internal carotid artery and the lateral wall of the pharynx.

The posterior pharyngeal wall extends from the level of the hard palate and Passavant's ridge superiorly to the level of the hyoid bone inferiorly where it becomes continuous with the hypopharynx. In contrast to other areas of the oropharynx, the mucosa is smooth and contains only occasional small aggregates of lymphoid tissue. The primary echelons of drainage from posterior pharyngeal wall tumors are the retropharyngeal nodes and the nodes at levels II and III. The risk of lymph node metastasis ranges from 25 percent for T1 lesions to over 75 percent for T4 tumors.[3]

The roof of the oropharynx is formed by the curved arch of the inferior surface of the soft palate and the uvula in the midline. Tumors of the soft palate drain lymph to the upper jugulodigastric and the retropharyngeal nodes. About a third of patients present with clinically positive neck nodes and involvement of the tonsillar fossa increases this risk. Occult nodal metastases occur in 16 percent of patients, and about 15 percent of patients who have a midline primary lesion will have bilateral or contralateral neck metastases.[4]

CLINICAL PRESENTATION AND DIAGNOSIS

Small tumors at certain sites, such as the crypts of the tonsils, the glossotonsillar sulci and the tongue base rarely produce symptoms and are not always easy to detect. When present, the initial symptoms of oropharyngeal cancer are often vague and non-specific, leading to a delay in diagnosis. Consequently, the overwhelming majority of patients present with locally advanced tumors.

Presenting symptoms may include sore throat, foreign-body sensation in the throat, altered voice or referred pain to the ear that is mediated through the glossopharyngeal and vagus nerves. Over two-thirds of patients present with a neck lump. As the tumor grows and infiltrates locally, it may cause progressive impairment of tongue movement which affects speech and swallowing, and necrosis and secondary infection may result in foul breath or even hemorrhage.

All patients must undergo a complete and thorough clinical examination of the upper aerodigestive tract and the neck, including fiberoptic nasolaryngoscopy. Most aspects of the pharynx and larynx can be readily assessed in the office with a flexible endoscope under topical anesthetic, but areas such as the pharyngoglossoepiglottic folds and the posterior surface of the soft palate may be difficult. The visual extent of the tumor is often misleading, and accurate assessment must include bimanual palpation of the tumor. Particular note must be taken of the inferior limit and circumferential extent of the tumor, its superior extent towards the nasopharynx, and mobility of structures at or below the level of the hyoid. Advanced tumors that cause trismus may be better assessed under a general anesthetic. Morphologically, a squamous cell carcinoma may present either as an exophytic (Figure 6–3) or ulcerative (Figure 6–4) lesion. Tumors of the minor salivary glands may present as smooth, lobulated swellings without surface ulceration (Figure 6–5), and malignant lymphomas typically cause nodular enlargements in the tonsil or tongue base.

Direct involvement of the XIIth nerve with the tumor, or infiltration from a metastatic neck node results in paralysis that is manifested by wasting of the ipsilateral tongue with deviation to that side on protrusion. Involvement of the glossopharyngeal and vagus nerves near the skull base must be suspected when there is impaired movement of the soft palate and ipsilateral vocal cord paralysis respectively. Similarly, involvement of the inferior alveolar nerve (impaired sensation over the anterior chin which is the sensory distribution of the mental nerve) and the lingual nerve in the infratemporal fossa (altered sensations over the lateral part of the tongue) are ominous signs that indicate locoregionally advanced disease.

Fine-needle aspiration cytology (FNAC) of any suspicious node in the neck at the initial consultation

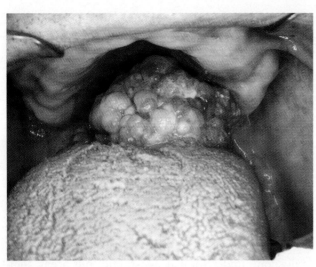

Figure 6-3.   An exophytic lesion of the base of the tongue.

generally allows the clinician to establish tissue diagnosis in patients in whom the primary tumor is not readily visible. Occasionally, aspiration of cystic fluid from a necrotic metastatic node may give a false-negative result. The false-negative rate can be reduced somewhat by completely removing cyst fluid and repeating FNA of any residual solid mass. A complete and detailed head and neck exam must

be complemented by appropriate imaging studies in these cases to rule out an obvious mucosal primary lesion before an open biopsy of a suspicious neck node is attempted.

Apart from the obvious advantages of CT and MRI in detection of subclinical nodal disease, imaging can also provide other information that may be vital to treatment planning. The controversy about the superiority of one imaging modality over the other seems unwarranted because both CT and MRI have their specific advantages, and may be used to complement each other based on the specific information required for making accurate treatment decisions. As a general rule, MRI enables superior distinction of tumor from muscle and other soft tissue while CT is better at imaging cortical bone. Gadolinium-enhanced MRI has also been shown to reliably demonstrate invasion along nerves. Both CT and MRI are effective in evaluating neck metastases, but accurate prediction of invasion of structures such as the carotid sheath and prevertebral fascia is usually not possible until direct assessment at surgery. Imaging may identify retropharyngeal nodes that are ordinarily out of bounds to palpation. Imaging is also especially valuable in assessing the neck in obese patients or those with a thick neck. Assessment of the post-radiotherapy or postsurgical neck is unreliable because differentiation between

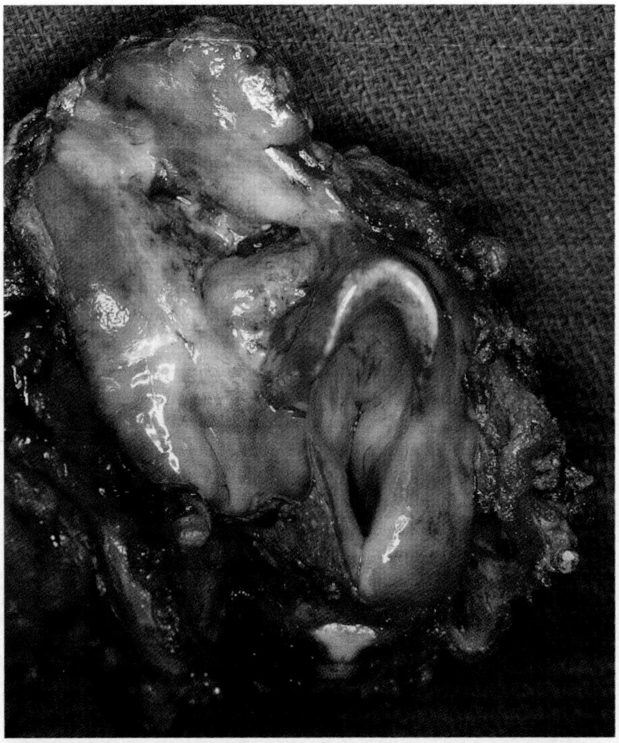

Figure 6-4.   An infiltrating, ulcerative lesion of the base of the tongue.

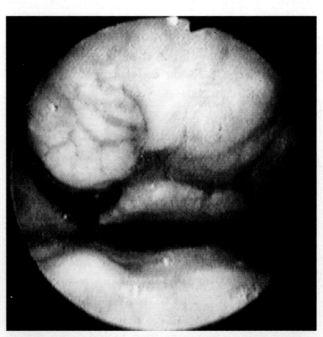

Figure 6-5.   An endoscopic view of a minor salivary gland tumor of the base of the tongue.

tumor, edema, inflammation and fibrosis is difficult. [18]FDG-PET scanning[5] may be the most sensitive technique currently available for these situations. The role of imaging in the detection of early mandibular invasion remains questionable, and a meticulous evaluation under anesthetic has been shown to be more reliable in assessing bony involvement.[6] A preoperative Panorex (orthopantomogram) may be necessary to assess the state of the dentition prior to instituting radiotherapy. Radiologic imaging, however, is essential to treatment planning if a mandibulotomy or any form of mandibular resection is planned. Dynamic contrast imaging using videofluoroscopy provides vital information on the functional aspects of deglutition and protection of the airway, both pre- and postoperatively. It is also a useful aid for prescribing speech and swallowing exercises. A plain radiograph of the chest helps screen for metastatic carcinoma, synchronous bronchial primary and coexisting acute or chronic pulmonary disease. Further investigation with chest CT scan, pulmonary function tests or bronchoscopy is generally merited based only on the patient's symptoms or an abnormal chest film.

A detailed examination and biopsy under general anesthetic may be the only accurate method of assessing the extent of tumors such as those of the tongue base that may be in a submucosal location. It may be prudent to use this opportunity to carry out dental extractions in patients with poor dentition who will require radiation therapy in order to minimize delay in treatment. The information collected by clinical, endoscopic and radiologic examination is then collated and used to assign a TNM stage to each individual tumor.

Pathology

Tumors of the oropharynx may arise from any of its constituent tissues, but the vast majority of epithelial tumors are squamous cell carcinomas. As there is a higher concentration of lymphoid tissue in this region, the incidence of lymphomas is considerably higher compared to other sites in the upper aerodigestive tract. The minor salivary glands of the soft palate, uvula and base of tongue can be the site of salivary gland tumors. Other rarer entities include soft tissue sarcomas and metastases from distant sites.

Squamous Cell Carcinoma

In common with squamous cancers at other upper aerodigestive sites, chronic abuse of tobacco is the most important etiologic factor, and alcohol abuse may potentiate its carcinogenic effect synergistically. Other factors such as genetic, environmental and dietary influences also play a part, and may explain some of the geographic variations in incidence. The disease is more common in men than in women (2.5:1) and is most frequently seen between the sixth and seventh decades of life. Premalignant lesions such as leukoplakia and erythroplakia do not seem to have the same significance in predisposition for oropharyngeal cancer as they do for squamous carcinoma of the oral cavity.

The most common sites for carcinoma in the oropharynx are the base of the tongue and the tonsil, while tumors of the soft palate and posterior wall are less common (Figure 6–6). Most squamous cancers initially expand along the mucosal surface and eventually invade the deeper structures, spreading along fascial planes and neurovascular structures. The base of the tongue is an exception because tumors tend to invade its musculature early, resulting in decreased mobility or fixation of the tongue and nodal metastasis. The anterior surface of the soft palate is affected more frequently than its posterior surface and delineation of the lesion from leukoplakia and keratinization may be difficult in heavy smokers. Tumors of the pharyngeal wall are commonly associated with extensive submucosal spread and so-called skip lesions.

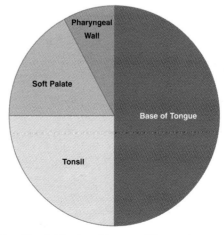

Figure 6-6. Site distribution of tumors of the oropharynx.

The majority of patients present with locoregion-ally-advanced tumors (Figure 6–7). Between 30 and 80 percent of patients develop nodal metastases at some stage of their disease (Table 6–2) and various characteristics of the primary tumor may be responsible.[7] Tumors arising in areas of rich lymphatics such as the tongue base and tonsillar fossae have a high risk of metastatic nodal disease at presentation compared with those in other areas such as the soft palate and anterior faucial pillar.[8] Levels II, III and IV are at greatest risk of metastasis. Involvement of levels I and V is rare (1.4% each) in the clinically N0 neck but the risk is higher (12.6% for level I and 9.7% for level V) in the clinically positive neck. Level V involvement occurs only in presence of metastasis at other levels and isolated skip metasta-sis to level I is also extremely rare (0.4%).[9] Although the risk of nodal involvement is generally propor-tional to the size of the primary tumor, early-stage oropharyngeal tumors, especially those of the tonsil and tongue base, can give rise to massive nodal dis-ease. The grade of the primary lesion does not seem to influence the risk of nodal metastases. Risk fac-tors for bilateral nodal metastases include tumors of the base of tongue or soft palate, tumors approach-ing or involving the midline, and alteration of the cervical lymphatics either by tumor or treatment (previous surgery, or irradiation or both).

Distant metastases, most often to the lungs, bones and liver, occur in up to 20 percent of patients with oropharyngeal tumors. The majority of these patients have active locoregional disease, primary or recurrent, at the time of detection of metastases.

Table 6–2. NODAL METASTASES IN OROPHARYNGEAL CARCINOMA		
Site	Node Positive (%)	Bilateral Nodes (%)
Base of tongue	78	34
Tonsil	76	21
Soft palate	44	19
Anterior faucial pillar	45	7
Posterior wall	37	—

Patients with oropharyngeal tumors, especially pos-terior pharyngeal wall tumors[10] are at high risk to develop second and subsequent primary tumors.

Lymphoepithelioma or undifferentiated carci-noma of nasopharyngeal type (UCNT) is a variant of squamous cell carcinoma that is characterized by an increased propensity to metastasize and by its extreme radiosensitivity. While the squamous com-ponent of the tumor may be extremely undifferenti-ated, a non-neoplastic lymphocytic infiltrate often permeates widely throughout the tumor. Nodal metastases consist of squamous cells similar to those of the primary tumor and usually lack the reac-tive lymphoid component of the primary tumor.

Lymphoma, especially the non-Hodgkin's type, accounts for about 8 percent of oropharyngeal tumors.[11] The tonsil and base of tongue are the most frequently involved sites and B-cell lym-phoma is the most common type. Although the lesion arises in the submucosa, it can ulcerate the mucosa and present like a squamous cancer. An adequate biopsy specimen must be submitted to avoid confusion with lymphoid hyperplasia. If a lymphoma is suspected, the clinician must have the foresight to consult the pathologist and submit fresh tissue for special studies which may include immunohistochemical stains, flow cytometry, and molecular genetic techniques.

Salivary gland tumors arise from the minor salivary glands of the soft palate and tongue base, and account for about 5 percent of oropharyngeal tumors.[12] The majority of these tumors are malig-nant and adenoid cystic carcinoma is the most com-mon histologic variant. As with other sites in the head and neck, the tumor has a tendency to spread along nerve sheaths in the perineural lymphatics and metastasizes late to lymph nodes, lung and bone. Although the short-term prognosis for these tumors

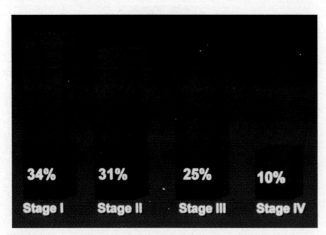

Figure 6-7. Stage distribution of oropharyngeal tumors.

is excellent, eventually about 60 to 80 percent of patients die from or with metastatic disease.

TREATMENT GOALS AND TREATMENT ALTERNATIVES

General Principles

Treatment of tumors of the oropharynx has the potential to cause significant functional deficit, and the optimal treatment plan must strike a balance between minimum functional derangement and long-term disease-free survival. Surgery or radiation therapy, alone or in combination, are currently accepted as standard treatment for oropharyngeal cancer. Other modalities such as chemotherapy must be considered experimental and are generally reserved for patients with advanced or recurrent disease that is not amenable to conventional therapy

Locoregional control and survival for patients with early tumors (T1-2) is equivalent with surgery or radiation therapy. The decision to choose one form of therapy over the other must weigh the expectation of disease control against the perceived functional outcome of treatment. In selected instances when a small primary tumor presents with advanced nodal disease, a so-called bimodality approach using neck dissection followed by radiation to the primary site and neck may provide the best functional results without compromising locoregional control. Advanced lesions (stages III and IV) are best treated using combined therapy with radical surgery followed by postoperative radiation. Choosing optimal treatment for T3 to T4 tumors of the base of the tongue is more difficult because radical surgery generally involves loss of a significant part of the tongue and possibly the larynx. Due consideration must therefore be given to the option of organ preservation, using a combination of chemotherapy and radiation, when laryngectomy is required for surgical excision of the tumor. Curative treatment may not be feasible for patients with very advanced or disseminated disease, and palliative therapy may be the only option.

Optimal management of the patient's disease hinges on close multidisciplinary cooperation between the surgeon, radiation oncologist and medical oncologist. Specialist medical consultations and appropriate investigations must be ordered for patients suffering from diabetes, or cardiovascular, pulmonary or other medical problems. The process of rehabilitation must begin before treatment is instituted, and successful rehabilitation depends on involvement of all the individuals who will be responsible for postoperative care of the patient, eg, the maxillofacial prosthodontist, nursing staff, speech therapists, nutritionists, physical therapists and social workers.

Factors Affecting Choice of Treatment

Although a variety of interrelated factors must be considered as guidelines when choosing the appropriate treatment, on a practical basis, the treatment must be tailored to the individual patient.

Tumor Factors

Small, superficial lesions in accessible sites such as the soft palate or tonsil are easily treated by peroral surgical excision with minimal functional deficit. On the other hand, patients with advanced tumors of the base of the tongue who require total glossectomy with or without laryngectomy may benefit from nonsurgical treatment, reserving surgery for salvage. Lesions with well-defined borders can be accurately resected, but if the margins are diffuse or the lesion exists within "unstable" mucosa, radiation therapy is usually the better option. Lymphoepitheliomas and lymphomas are exquisitely sensitive to radiation while other tumors such as those of minor salivary gland origin are not. Endophytic, deeply ulcerative lesions are best treated with surgery and postoperative radiation therapy, as these tumors respond poorly to primary radiation and the results of surgical salvage are dismal.[13]

Patient Factors

Performance status and comorbidity are important factors that affect outcome of treatment. Although aggressive therapy may be technically feasible, poor performance status or significant comorbidity may preclude safe delivery of treatment. The patient's preference, ability and willingness to cope with the treatment and its functional consequences may also influence the decision. The presence of advanced dental and alveolar disease has the potential to delay and complicate radiation therapy. Surgical excision may be the preferred option in such patients even if the tumor would ordinarily be amenable to radiation therapy. Logistic problems and social factors must also be considered and the input of the social worker and the family may be invaluable.

Functional Outcome and Long-term Sequelae

The functional deficit that is expected to result from a proposed treatment is a useful parameter to help make the choice when one or more options are known to produce equivalent locoregional control. For instance, both surgical excision and primary radiotherapy can be expected to control early lesions equally well. Surgery for an easily resectable tumor results in minimal functional deficit and may be preferred over radiation therapy that invariably has irreversible effects such as xerostomia and loss of taste. In addition, long-term sequelae of radiation such as the risk of second tumors must be considered, especially in younger patients. Conversely, when surgical excision requires sacrifice of structures such as the tongue or larynx, due consideration must be given to organ-sparing nonsurgical approaches.

Surgical Treatment

Successful outcome after surgery should provide the patient with durable locoregional control of the disease and minimal functional deficit. This depends on meticulous planning with accurate mapping of both surface and deep extent of the tumor. The anatomic extent of the surgical defect must be anticipated in all dimensions, and the need for reconstructive effort considered prior to surgery.

The approach chosen must afford good exposure, both for accurate and complete resection of the lesion but also for reconstruction of the defect. Incisions must be planned to provide optimal access while minimizing cosmetic defects. Appropriate modifications may be required when treating individuals who have had previous radiation therapy or surgery. The following is a general description of the commonly used approaches to tumors of the oropharynx, but obviously the one used for a particular patient will depend as much on the factors described as the surgeon's individual preference.

Transoral excision may be appropriate for very select, small, superficial cancers with well-defined margins located in the anterior portion of the oropharynx. Early tumors of the tonsils, faucial arches and the soft palate may be safely resected using either diathermy or transoral endoscopic laser, and a discontinuous neck dissection may be combined if indicated.[14] The resultant mucosal defect may be closed primarily, skin-grafted or left to epithelialize. All other tumors that require resection of bone, or those that are located more posteriorly, mandate more extensive access.

Anterior (supra- or transhyoid) pharyngotomy has been used to approach selected small lesions of the tongue base, posterior pharyngeal wall and for low-grade salivary gland tumors.[15] The oropharynx is accessed by either transecting or excising the hyoid bone (transhyoid approach) or displacing it inferiorly (suprahyoid approach) (Figure 6–8). After resection of the tumor inferiorly from the neck, the resultant defect is closed primarily. The main drawbacks of the procedure are that the vallecula is entered blindly and access is very limited.

A **lateral pharyngotomy** approach may be used for small lesions of the posterior and posterolateral pharyngeal walls. The oropharynx is entered through the mucosa of the superior aspect of the pyriform sinus after carefully retracting the superior laryngeal nerve. Exposure, however, is limited superiorly by the lower border of the mandible, and this approach is applicable in only selected instances.

The **anterior midline labiomandibuloglossotomy** approach (Figure 6–9) may be used to resect locally limited lesions of the base of the tongue. Through a midline lip-splitting incision, a median mandibulotomy is carried out and the tongue is bisected anteriorly in its relatively avascular midline to access the region of the base. After resection of the tumor, the surgical defect is closed primarily and the bisected halves of the anterior tongue are sutured back in layers, usually resulting in excellent postop-

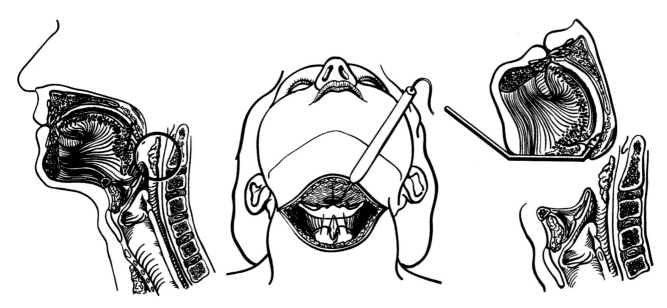

Figure 6-8. Suprahyoid pharyngotomy.

erative function. The operation is, however, not advisable if excision of the tumor is likely to result in a substantial soft-tissue defect with a tongue remnant of doubtful viability.

The **mandibulotomy approach with paralingual extension**, the so-called mandibular swing provides the best exposure for resection of most tumors of the oropharynx.[16] The site of the mandibular osteotomy directly influences the exposure obtained at surgery and the functional results of the procedure. Table 6–3 describes the salient features of the 3 types of mandibulotomy that have been in common use. We prefer to use the paramedian mandibulotomy when extensive access is required to the oropharynx. This operation causes minimal disrup-

tion of the anatomy of the region and results in fewer functional deficits postoperatively as compared to the other two types of osteotomy.

For a paramedian mandibulotomy, the lower lip is split in the midline and the incision carried over into the ipsilateral gingivolabial sulcus to just beyond the canine tooth. Bilateral flaps are raised for a short distance, dissecting in the plane above the periosteum and taking care to limit dissection to the point where the mental nerve exits the mental foramen. We prefer to use an angled osteotomy (Figure 6–10) that creates a single notch and provides good stability with very little risk of fracture. An oscillating power saw with the thinnest available blades is essential for accurate bony cuts and to prevent

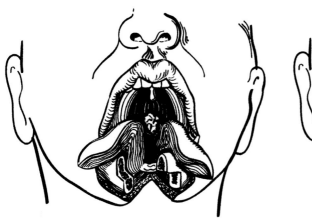
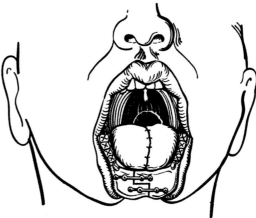

Figure 6-9. Anterior midline labiomandibuloglossotomy.

Table 6–3. SALIENT FEATURES OF THE 3 TYPES OF MANDIBULAR OSTEOTOMY			
	Lateral	Median	Paramedian
Site of osteotomy	Through the body/angle of mandible	In the midline	Between lateral incisor and canine
Exposure	Limited	Good	Good
Dental extraction	May be necessary	One central incisor	Not required
Inferior alveolar nerve and vessels	Must be transected	Can be spared	Can be spared
Division of genial muscles	Not required	Inevitable	Not required-only the mylohyoid needs division
Mechanical stability	Poor due to unequal pull of muscles on the two mandibular segments	Good	Good
Fixation of osteotomy	May require intermaxillary fixation which interferes with maintenance of postoperative oral hygiene	Miniplates or stainless steel wire	Miniplates or stainless steel wire
Postoperative radiation therapy	Osteotomy lies within the lateral portal—increased risk of complications	Lies outside the lateral portal—safe	Lies outside the lateral portal—safe

excessive bone loss. The vertical limb of the osteotomy is carried down to a level just beyond the dental apices between the lateral incisor and canine teeth, and the cut is then angled medially. This is possible without extracting the teeth or exposing or damaging their roots because of their diverging configuration (see Figure 6–10). After the osteotomy is complete, the mucosa and muscles of the floor of the mouth are incised posteriorly right up to the anterior pillar of the soft palate. The floor-of-mouth incision must be placed more toward the tongue than the alveolus so that there is an adequate mucosal cuff attached to the alveolus. This step is vitally important to accurate watertight closure of the incision. The lingual nerve and the styloglossus muscle cross

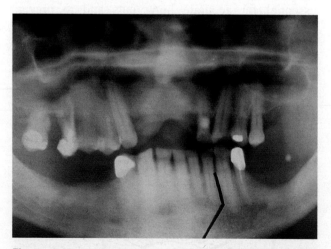

Figure 6-10. A paramedian osteotomy can be safely sited between the lateral incisor and the canine teeth to avoid damage or exposure of the dental roots.

the field, and once they are transected the mandible can be swung out laterally to expose the oropharynx (Figure 6–11).

After resection of the tumor and reconstruction of the defect, the mandibulotomy can be fixed using either stainless steel wires or miniplates with comparable stability.[17] Pre-localizing the fixation drill holes on the intact mandible, before the osteotomy cuts are actually made, and fixation in more than one plane are probably more important to accurate dental occlusion and stability than the actual mode of fixation itself. If miniplates are preferred, 2 plates are used across the osteotomy, one on the anterior surface and the other is contoured to fit the inferior edge of the mandible (Figure 6–12). Slight discrepancies in dental occlusion tend to correct themselves spontaneously as the fracture site matures and moulds to the stresses of chewing postoperatively. The lip and neck incisions are then closed in layers over suction drains as usual.

The base of the tongue may be difficult to assess for the extent of a tumor due to its normal nodularity—careful palpation is vital to ensure adequate margins as excision proceeds. Advanced tumors of the tongue are associated with diffuse infiltration, and surgical margins have been reported positive by some authors in as many as one-quarter of the cases.[18] Frozen-section evaluation of the margins and the base of excision can therefore only minimize the chances of incomplete resection. Partial glossectomy may be oncologically adequate for limited

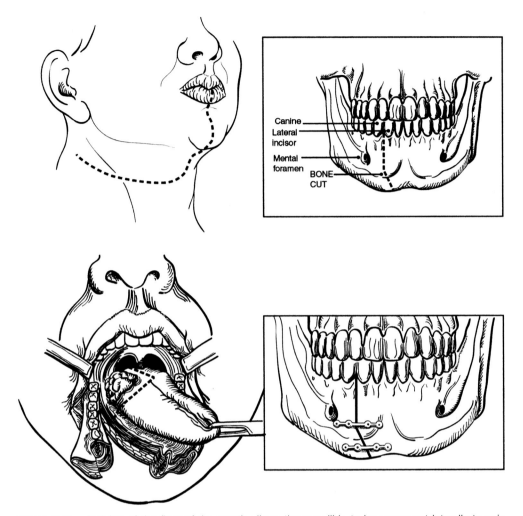

Figure 6-11. Incision of the floor of the mouth allows the mandible to be swung out laterally to gain access to the tumor in the oropharynx.

tumors of the base of the tongue, and postoperative functional outcome depends upon the orientation of the resection, the volume of tongue resected, the method of repair, as well as the mobility, sensitivity and the shape of the tongue remnant. Substantial defects of the tongue must therefore be adequately and appropriately reconstructed (Figure 6–13).

Access to posterior pharyngeal wall lesions may require transhyoid or lateral pharyngotomy, median labiomandibular glossotomy or paramedian mandibulotomy. Early lesions rarely involve the prevertebral fascia and the intervening avascular retropharyngeal space usually provides a good plane of cleavage during surgical dissection. Superficial lesions that involve only part of the pharyngeal circumference can be excised safely while preserving the larynx.[19] Reconstruction of the defect requires thin, pliable tissue such as a split-thickness skin graft or a free radial forearm flap. For more advanced tumors, resectability depends on ascertaining that the under-

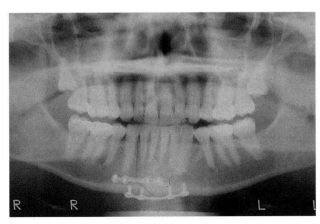

Figure 6-12. The two halves of the mandible are secured in place using miniplates at the end of the procedure.

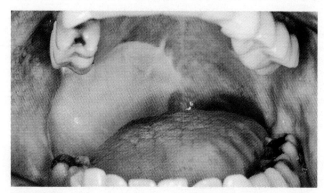

Figure 6-13. Free radial flap reconstruction of the surgical defect after partial resection of the soft palate, and tonsil.

lying prevertebral fascia is not involved, a question that is most often resolved only at surgical exploration. Locally advanced pharyngeal wall tumors that involve a substantial portion of the circumference usually require a total laryngopharyngectomy with restoration of pharyngeal continuity using free jejunal transfer or other reconstructive options.

As described above, the mandibulotomy approach provides excellent access to all sites within the oropharynx, and there can be no excuse for resecting the uninvolved mandible solely to gain access to the tumor. Tonsillar or lateral pharyngeal wall tumors that abut against the periosteum of the mandible need marginal resection of the ascending ramus of the mandible (Figure 6–14). More advanced tumors are resected by combining soft-tissue resection en bloc with mandibulectomy, the so-called commando operation (Figure 6–15). Appropriate bony recon-

struction of segmental mandibular defects combined with osseointegrated dental implants is necessary for restoration of useful masticatory function.

Early lesions at some sites such as the soft palate and the posterior pharyngeal wall are at low risk for nodal metastases, and the clinically negative neck in these patients may be safely observed. In all other patients, elective treatment of the N0 neck must be considered. In general, if the primary tumor is treated with radiation therapy, the neck is included in the fields, and if surgical treatment is chosen for the primary, a selective neck dissection is carried out. The uninvolved neck in well-lateralized lesions of the tonsil and tongue may be treated unilaterally, but both sides need treatment in lesions approaching or involving the midline. Dissection of levels II, III and IV generally encompasses the majority of nodes at risk in the clinically N0 neck. Grossly suspicious nodes should be subjected to frozen-section analysis and the dissection extended to include the remaining levels as appropriate. Clinically involved nodes require a comprehensive neck dissection including

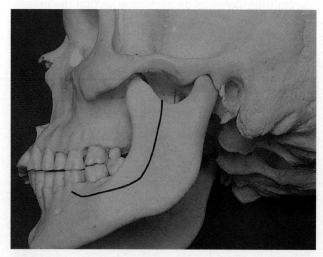

Figure 6-14. Marginal resection of the ascending ramus of the mandible.

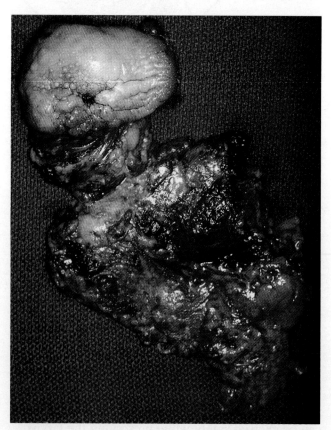

Figure 6-15. Composite resection of an advanced base of tongue tumor including the mandible: the "commando" operation.

all 5 nodal levels, and a modified radical neck dissection preserving the spinal accessory nerve is the procedure of choice. Bilaterally involved nodes are treated with simultaneous or staged bilateral neck dissection. Postoperative radiation therapy is given for the usual indications, based on adverse features of either the primary or the neck nodes.

Locally advanced oropharyngeal tumors can cause considerable difficulty during endotracheal intubation, mainly by obstructing visualization of the larynx, but also because invasion of the pterygoid muscles may result in trismus. Although fiberoptic endoscope-guided endotracheal intubation is an option, it may be safer to perform a preliminary tracheostomy under local anaesthetic. Patients who have had significant surgical resection and reconstruction require a temporary tracheostomy to protect the airway in the postoperative period. A cuffed, low-pressure high-volume tracheostomy tube minimizes aspiration in the early postoperative period. Apart from the ability to tolerate plugging of the tube, factors such as the efficacy of deglutition, the extent of aspiration and the performance status of the patient generally determine when postoperative decannulation of the tracheostomy can be safely undertaken.

Deeply invasive tumors only need to breach the hyoepiglottic ligament to gain access to the pre-epiglottic space (Figure 6–16) from where they can spread to involve the framework of the larynx. Complete excision of such lesions requires either partial supraglottic or total laryngectomy in addition to excision of the base of the tongue.

For practical purposes, major soft-tissue defects of the oropharynx can be divided into those that require thin, pliable flaps for resurfacing and those that need bulkier myocutaneous flaps to provide volume. The posterior pharyngeal wall is an example of the former, and is best resurfaced using either a split skin graft or a free radial forearm flap. On the other hand, substantial defects of areas including the base of the tongue and tonsillar region need reconstruction with bulkier myocutaneous flaps such as the pectoralis major or the latissimus dorsi pedicled flaps or a composite free flap. Pedicled myocutaneous flaps are generally used to reconstruct partial circumference defects of the pharynx while circum-

ferential defects are best restored using microvascular jejunal transfer or gastric pull-up. Restoration of mandibular continuity after segmental resection using free-tissue transfer with secondary osseointegrated dental implants has the potential for resulting in excellent cosmesis and function, and this complex issue has been discussed in other chapters.

Ancillary procedures such as cricopharyngeal myotomy, laryngeal suspension and palatal augmentation may help improve functional results after major glossectomy. Patients who have had major oropharyngeal resection and reconstruction, and those scheduled for postoperative radiation therapy generally require prolonged nutritional support, and a percutaneous endoscopic gastrostomy must be considered at the time of the operation.

NONSURGICAL TREATMENT

Treatment of early tumors of the oropharynx using radiation therapy has been reported to be equally effective as surgical excision[20] with the advantage of "superior function." Even for tumors of the base of the tongue[21] where the functional results have been

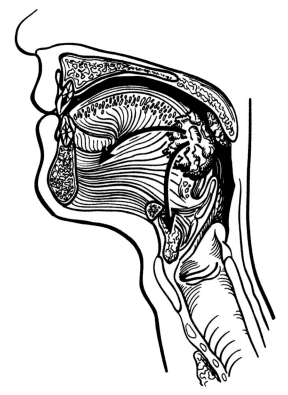

Figure 6-16. Invasion of the preepiglottic space from a tumor of the base of the tongue.

assessed, this "advantage" of radiation over surgery is largely assumed due to selection bias of favorable lesions. There is no prospective randomized trial for cancer of the base of the tongue comparing the two modalities with respect to tumor control and functional assessment. In general, superficial and exophytic lesions are best treated by radiotherapy, and deeply infiltrating lesions are best treated by surgery followed with postoperative radiotherapy. Surgical treatment of small lesions at most other sites, with the probable exception of the soft palate, produces very little functional deficit, in contrast to radiation therapy that almost invariably causes irreversible xerostomia and loss of taste, with the potential risk of dental decay and radionecrosis.

For more advanced tumors, initial treatment with nonsurgical "organ-sparing" approaches have recently come into vogue and concurrent chemoradiation therapy seems to hold promise.

Radiation Therapy

Conventional techniques have delivered radiation using external beam therapy, brachytherapy or a combination of both. More recent advances include altered fractionation schedules, radiation combined with chemotherapy or other sensitizers, and the use of accurately targeted beams with three-dimensional treatment planning or intensity-modulated radiotherapy. Important considerations in the delivery of radiation therapy include determination of adequate treatment volume (initial portals), reduction of portals at the appropriate doses (shrinking fields), design of neck portals, boosting the site of the primary tumor, and hyperfractionation. Radiation portals are designed to include adequate margins around the primary tumor as well as the neck nodes, especially the retropharyngeal nodes which may be involved in as many as 50 percent of patients with stage III and IV tumors.[22] Tumors in sites such as the tongue base in selected patients can be effectively boosted using interstitial brachytherapy.[23] Treatment using more than one daily fraction, or hyperfractionation,[24] and the use of the radiation sensitizer nimorazole[25] have been reported to have an advantage over conventional regimes.

Except for well-lateralized lesions of the tonsil, most other tumors require the use of parallel opposed portals. Depending on the risk of occult nodal metastases, the entire neck may need to be irradiated even if there is no clinical evidence of metastases. For patients presenting with clinically palpable nodal disease, bilateral neck treatment is recommended based on the relatively high risk of contralateral nodal metastases. Except for very radiosensitive tumors such as undifferentiated carcinoma, especially of the nasopharyngeal type, planned neck dissection, either before or after radiotherapy to the primary tumor is advisable for the majority of patients with significant neck disease.

Postoperative radiotherapy is indicated for large or infiltrating primary tumors, high-risk features of the primary tumor such as lymphatic or vascular invasion, close or positive surgical margins, multiple nodal involvement or extracapsular spread from nodal metastasis. A dose of 60 Gy is generally delivered to the primary site and involved nodal areas, and areas of residual disease are boosted to higher doses of up to 70 Gy using either electron beam therapy or brachytherapy catheters. The opposite uninvolved side of the neck in patients with unilateral nodal disease is electively irradiated to a dose of 50 Gy based on the high risk of contralateral metastases.

Role of Chemotherapy and Organ-preserving Approaches

Although numerous randomized trials have failed to demonstrate any survival benefit for neoadjuvant or sequential chemotherapy schedules, the major spin-off of the neoadjuvant approach was the observation that function of important structures such as the larynx and tongue could be preserved without compromising local control or survival.[26] More recently, the radiosensitizing effects of chemotherapy have been exploited in designing concurrent chemoradiation protocols, and 3-year local control rates of 64 percent were achieved at the Memorial Sloan-Kettering Cancer Center (MSKCC) for a subset of patients with oropharyngeal tumors treated with concomitant chemoradiation and delayed accelerated fractionation.[27] For the surgeon, there are several considerations in operating on patients who have persistent or residual disease after nonsurgical treatment. Apart from the technical difficulties and risks associated with surgery in previously treated patients, assessment of the margins of the tumor may be extremely difficult and unreliable, especially in tumors of the base of the tongue. Although well-planned nonsurgical therapy has the potential to preserve function, it must also be emphasized that these approaches require special multidisciplinary expertise and experience, and their current use should generally be restricted to specialized head and neck units or to a clinical trial setting.

SEQUELAE, COMPLICATIONS AND THEIR MANAGEMENT

Although modern anesthetic and surgical technique has greatly increased the safety of surgery for oropharyngeal tumors, careful planning and meticulous technique are vital to successful outcome. The most common complications of surgery arise due to difficulties associated with inadequate exposure and the failure to anticipate the need for reconstruction. Incisions must be planned to take previous surgery and/or radiation into consideration. It is important to resist the temptation to close a borderline surgical defect primarily as any tension or tightness almost always results in a breakdown of the suture line with all its attendant complications such as fistula, infection and major vessel erosion. Poor surgical technique and inappropriate reconstruction are also likely to result in narrowing of the lumen and/or outlet of the neo-pharynx causing difficulties in swallowing. In addition, inadequate clearance and pooling of saliva predisposes to aspiration and pulmonary complications. Conservative measures to improve the situation (such as dilation) are generally inappropriate and almost always ineffective, and corrective reconstructive surgery can be extremely difficult. Aspiration of saliva, especially during the early postoperative period, is a common but generally transient consequence of surgery. Most patients overcome these initial problems with appropriate rehabilitative therapy, and long-term aspiration is usually a result of poor surgical planning and inadequate or inappropriate reconstruction. Complications such as postoperative bleeding and hematoma, wound breakdown, and chyle fistulae can follow neck dissection. Expert postoperative nursing care should minimize the complications associated with poor oral hygiene, nasogastric feeding tubes, tracheostomy tubes, deep vein thrombosis, and decubitus ulcers.

Mucositis during radiation therapy can be severe enough to affect swallowing and nutritional intake, requiring institution of tube feeding to prevent significant weight loss. In some patients, this may prolong the course of radiation or even force it to be abandoned with adverse prognostic effect. Decreased mucus secretion combined with an increase in viscosity cause symptoms such as dry mouth and a sticky throat, depending on the fields of radiation. Xerostomia and loss of taste sensation are however not as severe as those after radiation for oral cavity tumors because uninvolved oral mucosa and one parotid can be safely shielded. Desquamation of the skin of the neck may cause painful ulceration and may delay completion of therapy. The incidence of soft-tissue complications such as fibrosis and radionecrosis has decreased significantly with modern radiotherapy techniques, but may still have a devastating impact on the patient's quality of life. In addition, persistent or new ulceration at the site of the primary tumor may make it impossible to rule out residual tumor or recurrence. Osteoradionecrosis of the mandible is a particularly difficult problem to treat, but its development can be largely prevented by a few simple precautions. Almost all bone necrosis occurs around diseased teeth within the radiation fields, and it is vital that dental and alveolar disease be adequately treated before radiation is commenced. Brachytherapy using interstitial implants runs the risk of producing major hemorrhage that may require surgical control. Complications such as soft tissue and bone necrosis are more common after implants, but appropriate treatment selection combined with good nursing care can minimize the risk. Combining chemotherapy with radiation to treat locally advanced tumors can result in severe toxicity and a higher-than-usual rate of treatment-related mortality.

REHABILITATION AND QUALITY OF LIFE

Although appropriate reconstructive measures can minimize the effect on function, rehabilitation is often a prolonged and painstaking process that requires a great deal of patience. Successful rehabilitation depends on close multidisciplinary cooperation between the surgeon, the speech therapist, the prosthodontist, the dietitian, the nursing staff and the physiotherapist. Cessation of high-risk activity such as smoking and alcohol abuse must be emphasized.

Quality of life and functional issues are now recognized as important outcome measures of treatment but data on these is largely retrospective and subjective. There is however, objective proof that even nonsurgical treatments that are delivered with the purpose of organ preservation can cause functional problems. Problems are especially associated with eating dysfunction[28] and pain control, but the quality of vocal function may also suffer.[29] Quality-of-life measures need to be undertaken prospectively, preferably using pretreatment function as a baseline, and carrying out long-term longitudinal assessments using devices that are simple to use and which take cultural differences into account. It is also vital that quality-of-life assessments are reported in conjunction with survival statistics to allow meaningful interpretation.

Long-term follow-up of these patients is essential for monitoring locoregional recurrence, distant metastases and second primary tumors. Periodic clinical examination must be combined with the judicious use of imaging and biopsy under anesthetic in suspicious cases.

OUTCOMES AND RESULTS OF TREATMENT

As discussed above, outcome measures must include evaluation of function as well as control of tumor and survival statistics. Unfortunately, most series have reported only limited information that is based on retrospective assessment. The following is a compilation of results of treatment for tumors involving each of the individual subsites within the oropharynx.

Carcinoma of the Base of the Tongue

The results of primary irradiation in recently reported series of base-of-tongue carcinomas treated by external beam radiotherapy alone are listed in Table 6–4 and those for external beam with brachytherapy are listed in Table 6–5.

Table 6–4. 2-YEAR ACTUARIAL LOCAL CONTROL RATES FOR EXTERNAL BEAM RADIOTHERAPY OF CARCINOMA OF THE BASE OF TONGUE

Author	No. of Patients	T1 (%)	T2 (%)	T3 (%)	T4 (%)
Jaulerry[37]	166	96	57	45	23
Fein[38]	107	90	92	76	40
Henk[49]	33	–	78	72	–

Surgery is equally effective in controlling early lesions of the base of the tongue. Although a retrospective report has shown that radiation therapy provides a better post-treatment performance status than surgery for both early as well as advanced tumors,[21] there are no prospective randomized comparisons of the oncologic and functional results in the literature of surgery versus radiation alone or combined treatment. Table 6–6 lists the survival rates and functional results after surgical treatment of base-of-tongue tumors as reported in recent literature. The stagewise survival rates after treatment for cancer of the base of the tongue are shown in Table 6–7.

Carcinoma of the Tonsil

Table 6–8 lists the local control rates after radical radiation therapy for tonsillar carcinoma. Local recurrence rates are, however, unacceptable for more advanced disease that has spread to involve the base of the tongue (47%) or the lateral pharyngeal wall (33%).[30] Although surgical resection is not commonly used for early tumors of the tonsil, excellent control rates have been reported for such a policy.[31]

Surgery combined with postoperative radiation is generally recommended for locally advanced lesions but there are advocates of radical irradiation, reserving surgery for salvage.[32] Some authors[33] have shown a survival benefit for combination therapy in the treatment of advanced tonsillar carcinoma while others[34] could not demonstrate any advantage in

Table 6–5. RESULTS OF COMBINED EXTERNAL BEAM AND BRACHYTHERAPY FOR CARCINOMA OF THE BASE OF TONGUE

Author	No. of Patients	2-Year Local Control (%)	5-Year Survival (%)
Harrison[23]	36	87.5	87.5
Crook[39]	48	75	50
Puthawala[40]	70	83	33

Table 6–6. SURVIVAL AND FUNCTIONAL RESULTS AFTER SURGICAL TREATMENT OF BASE OF TONGUE TUMORS

Author	No. of Patients	Survival (%)	Total Glossectomy (%)	Mandibular Resection (%)	Impaired Swallowing (%)	"Useful" Speech (%)	Severe Aspiration (%)	Concomitant / Interval Laryngectomy (%)
Weber[18]	n=27	51 at 2 years	27	—	56	92	11	0 / 8
Ruhl[41]	n=54	41 at 5 years	54	—	—	—	—	—
Razack[42]	n=45	20 at 5 years	45	49	69	84	37	40 / 13
Gehanno[43]	n=80	65 at 1 year	80	—	49	39	—	—
Kraus[44]	n=100	65 at 5 years	—	14	—	—	—	20

treating stage III and IV disease using a combined modality approach. Table 6–9 lists the stage-wise survival of patients treated for tonsillar carcinoma.

Carcinoma of the Posterior Pharyngeal Wall

The staging of posterior pharyngeal wall tumors is often difficult because most lesions transgress 2 separate anatomical regions that have their own distinct

Table 6–7. STAGE-WISE SURVIVAL RATES IN PATIENTS TREATED FOR CARCINOMA OF THE BASE OF THE TONGUE

Author	Follow-up (yrs)	Stage I (%)	Stage II (%)	Stage III (%)	Stage IV (%)
Thawley[45]	5	50	44	45	28
Weber[18]	5	100	72	50	30
Barrs[46]	3	68	55	55	11
Kraus[44]	5	77	77	64	59
Foote[47]	5	60	48	76	20–35*

* Tumors were staged based on the American Joint Committee on Cancer, 1988 recommendations.

Table 6-8. LOCAL CONTROL RATES AFTER RADICAL RADIOTHERAPY FOR CARCINOMA OF THE TONSILLAR FOSSA

Author	No. of Patients	T1 (%)	T2 (%)	T3 (%)	T4 (%)
Bataini[48]	465	90	84	64	47
Fein[38]	200	87	79	71	44
Henk[49]	52	100	58	76	–

rules for tumor staging: oropharyngeal tumors are classified by size while hypopharyngeal tumors are classified according to the number of sites involved. Combined with their relative rarity, this makes retrospective comparisons of treatment modalities unreliable and difficult.

Radiation therapy alone has limited effectiveness in treatment mainly because of the technical difficulty in delivering adequate doses to tissue in close proximity to the spinal cord, but also because these tumors are not very radiosensitive.

Surgical treatment of these tumors is prone to a high incidence of local failure which ranges between 30 and 40 percent.[3,10] Local recurrence increases from 16 percent for stage I to 63 percent for stage IV, and only about 40 percent of patients are successfully salvaged. Table 6–10 shows a list of studies that have reported the results of treatment of posterior pharyngeal wall tumors.

Carcinoma of the Soft Palate

Primary irradiation controls early lesions effectively but local control rates for T3 and T4 tumors are 45 and 25 percent respectively, and the results of salvage surgery in these patients are poor.[35] Overall 5-year survival rates range from 80 to 90 percent for stage I and II tumors and 30 to 60 percent for stage III and IV lesions[36] (Table 6–11).

Table 6–9. RESULTS OF TREATMENT OF TONSILLAR CARCINOMA

Author	No. of Patients	Follow-up (yrs)	Stage I (%)	Stage II (%)	Stage III (%)	Stage IV (%)
Perez[50]	218	3	76	40	42	25
Spiro[34]	117	3	89	83	58	49
Dasmahapatra[33]	174	5	83	72	23	15
Amornmarn[51]	185	5	100	73	52	21
Mizono[52]	171	5	92	77	56	29
Givens[53]	104	5	93	57	27	17

Table 6–10. RESULTS OF TREATMENT OF POSTERIOR PHARYNGEAL WALL CARCINOMA

Author	No. of Patients	Treatment*	Follow-up (yrs)	Survival (%)
Wang[54]	36	R	3	25
Pene[55]	131	S, R	5	3
Marks[56]	51	R±C	3	14
Schwaab[57]	24	C+R	3	60
			5	25
Jaulerry[58]	98	R	3	30
			5	14
Spiro[10]	78	S±R	2	49
			5	32

*R = radiation, S = surgery, C = chemotherapy

Table 6–11. RESULTS OF TREATMENT FOR CARCINOMA OF THE SOFT PALATE

Author	No. of Patients	Treatment*	Follow-up (yrs)	Survival (%)
Esche[59]	43	I±R	3	81
			5	64
Keus[60]	146	R	3	59
			5	53
Leemans[61]	52	S, R, C, L	5	77
Medini[62]	24	R	3	81

* I = interstitial implant, R = external radiation, S = surgery, C = chemotherapy, L = laser resection.

SUMMARY

The results of treatment of tumors of the oropharynx need to be evaluated not only in terms of survival, but also the functional outcome after treatment. Newer modalities such as concurrent chemoradiation appear promising and will add to the options available to clinicians in achieving optimal outcome.

REFERENCES

1. Greenlee RT, Hill-Harman MB, Murray T, Thun M. Cancer Statistics, 2001. CA Cancer J Clin 2001;51:15–36.
2. Rhys Evans PH. Tumours of the oropharynx and lymphomas of the head and neck. In: Kerr AG, editor. Scott-Brown's oto-laryngology, Volume 5, 6th Ed. London: Butterworth; 1997.
3. Guillamondegui OM, Meoz R, Jesse RH. Surgical treatment of squamous cell carcinoma of the pharyngeal walls. Am J Surg 1978;136:474–6.
4. Lindberg RD, Barkley HT, Jesse RH, Fletcher GH. Evolution of the clinically negative neck in patients with squamous cell carcinoma of the faucial arch. Am J Roentgenol Radium Ther Nucl Med 1971;111:60–5.
5. McGuirt WF, Greven K, Williams D, et al. PET scanning in head and neck oncology: a review. Head Neck 1998; 20:208–15.
6. Jones AS, England J, Hamilton J, et al. Mandibular invasion in patients with oral and oropharyngeal squamous carcinoma. Clin Otolaryngol 1997;22:239–45.
7. Shah JP. Patterns of cervical lymph node metastasis from squamous carcinomas of the upper aerodigestive tract. Am J Surg 1990;160:405–9.
8. Lindberg RD. Distribution of cervical lymph node metastases from squamous cell carcinoma of the upper respiratory and digestive tracts. Cancer 1972;29:1446–50.
9. Candela FC, Kothari K, Shah JP. Patterns of cervical node metastases from squamous carcinoma of the oropharynx and hypopharynx. Head Neck 1990;12:197–203.
10. Spiro RH, Kelly J, Vega AL, et al. Squamous carcinoma of the posterior pharyngeal wall. Am J Surg 1990;160:420–3.
11. Stell PM, Nash JRG. Tumours of the oropharynx. In: Kerr A, editor. Scott-Brown's otolaryngology. 5th ed., London: Butterworth; 1987.
12. Spiro RH, Koss LG, Hajdu SI, Strong EW. Tumours of minor salivary gland origin: a clinicopathologic study of 492 cases. Cancer 1973;31:117–29.
13. Rodriguez J, Point D, Brunin F, et al. Surgery of the oropharynx after radiotherapy. Bull Cancer Radiother 1996;83: 24–30.
14. Eckel HE, Volling P, Pototschnig C, et al. Transoral laser resection with staged discontinuous neck dissection for oral cavity and oropharynx squamous cell carcinoma. Laryngoscope 1995;105:53–60.
15. Zeitels SM, Vaughan CW. Suprahyoid pharyngotomy for oropharynx cancer including the tongue base. Arch Otolaryngol Head Neck Surg 1991;117:757–60.
16. Spiro RH, Gerold FP, Shah JP, et al. Mandibulotomy approach to oropharyngeal tumours. Am J Surg 1985;150:466–9.
17. Shah JP, Kumarawamy SV, Kulkarni V. Comparative evaluation of fixation methods after mandibulotomy for oropharyngeal tumours. Am J Surg 1993;166:431–4.
18. Weber R, Gidley P, Morrison W, et al. Treatment selection for carcinoma of the base of tongue. Am J Surg 1990;160: 415–9.
19. Lydiatt WM, Kraus DH, Cordeiro PG, et al. Posterior pharyngeal carcinoma resection with larynx preservation and radial forearm free flap reconstruction: a preliminary report. Head Neck 1996;18:501–6.
20. Parsons JT, Mendenhall WM, Million RR, et al. The management of primary cancers of the oropharynx: combined treatment or irradiation alone? Semin Radiat Oncol 1992;2:142–8.
21. Harrison LB, Zelefsky MJ, Armstrong JG, et al. Performance status after treatment for squamous cell cancer of the base of tongue—a comparison of primary radiation therapy versus primary surgery. Int J Radiat Oncol Biol Phys 1994;30:953–7.
22. Hasegawa Y, Matsuura H. Retropharyngeal node dissection in cancer of the oropharynx and hypopharynx. Head Neck 1994;16:173–80.
23. Harrison LB, Zelefsky M, Sessions RB, et al. Base-of-tongue cancer treated with external beam irradiation plus brachytherapy. Radiology 1992;184:267–70.
24. Horiot JC, le Fur T, N'Guyen C, et al. Hyperfractionation compared with conventional radiotherapy in oropharyngeal carcinoma. Eur J Cancer 1990;26:779–80.
25. Overgaard J, Hansen HS, Overgaard M, et al. A randomized double-blind phase III study of nimorazole as a hypoxic radiosensitizer of primary radiotherapy in supraglottic

larynx and pharynx carcinoma. Results of the Danish Head and Neck Cancer Study (DAHANCA) protocol 5-85. Radiother Oncol 1998;46:135–46.

26. Pfister DG, Harrison LB, Strong EW, et al. Organ-function preservation in advanced oropharynx cancer: results with induction chemotherapy and radiation. J Clin Oncol 1995;13:671–80.

27. Harrison LB, Raben A, Pfister DG, et al. A prospective phase II trial of concomitant chemotherapy and radiotherapy with delayed accelerated fractionation in unresectable tumors of the head and neck. Head Neck 1998;20:497–503.

28. List MA, Haraf D, Siston A, et al. A longitudinal study of quality of life and performance in head and neck cancer patients on a concomitant chemo-radiotherapy protocol (Abstract 248). Proceedings of the 4th International Conference on Head and Neck Cancer; Toronto, Canada. 1996.

29. Orlikoff RF, Kraus DH, Pfister DG, et al. Assessment and rehabilitation of vocal function in nonsurgically treated head and neck cancer patients (Abstract 791). Proceedings of the 4th International Conference on Head and Neck Cancer; Toronto, Canada. 1996.

30. Tong D, Laramore GE, Griffen TW, et al. Carcinoma of the tonsil region: results of external irradiation. Cancer 1982;49:2009–14.

31. Remmler D, Medina JE, Byers RM, et al. Treatment of choice for squamous cell carcinoma of the tonsillar fossa. Head Neck Surg 1985;7:206–11.

32. Mendenhall W, Parsons J, Cassisi N, et al. Squamous cell carcinoma of the tonsillar area treated with radical irradiation. Radiother Oncol 1987;10:23–30.

33. Dasmahapatra K, Mohit-Tabatabai M, Rush B, et al. Cancer of the tonsil: improved survival with combination therapy. Cancer 1986;57:451–5.

34. Spiro JD, Spiro RH. Carcinoma of the tonsillar fossa: an update. Arch Otol Head Neck Surg 1989;115:1186–9.

35. Amdur RJ, Mendenhall WM, Parsons JT, et al. Carcinoma of the soft palate treated with irradiation: analysis of results and complications. Radiother Oncol 1987;9:185–94.

36. Weber RS, Peters LJ, Wolf PS, Guillamondegui O. Squamous cell carcinoma of the soft palate, uvula and anterior faucial pillar. Otolaryngol Head Neck Surg 1988;99:16–23.

37. Jaulerry C, Rodriguez J, Brunin F, et al. Results of radiation therapy in carcinoma of the base of tongue: the Curie Institute experience with about 166 cases. Cancer 1991;67:1532–8.

38. Fein DA, Lee RW, Amos WR, et al. Oropharyngeal carcinoma treated with radiotherapy: a 30-year experience. Int J Radiat Oncol Biol Phys 1996;34:289–96.

39. Crook J, Mazeron JJ, Marinello G, et al. Combined external irradiation and interstitial implantation for T1 and T2 epidermoid carcinomas of the base of tongue: the Creteil experience (1971–1981). Int J Radiat Oncol Biol Phys 1988;14:105–14.

40. Puthawala AA, Nisar Syed AM, Eads DL, et al. Limited external beam and interstitial ^{192}iridium irradiation in the treatment of carcinoma of the base of tongue: a ten-year experience. Int J Radiat Oncol Biol Phys 1988;14:839–48.

41. Ruhl CM, Gleich LL, Gluckman JL. Survival, function and quality of life after total glossectomy. Laryngoscope 1997;107:1316–21.

42. Razack MS, Sako K, Bakamjian VY, Shedd DP. Total glossectomy. Am J Surg 1983;146:509–11.

43. Gehanno P, Guedon C, Barry B, et al. Advanced carcinoma of the tongue: total glossectomy without total laryngectomy. Review of 80 cases. Laryngoscope 1992;102:1369–71.

44. Kraus DH, Vastola AP, Huvos AG, Spiro RH. Surgical management of squamous cell carcinoma of the base of the tongue. Am J Surg 1993;166:384–8.

45. Thawley SE, Simpson JR, Marks JE, et al. Preoperative irradiation and surgery for carcinoma of the base of the tongue. Ann Otol Rhinol Laryngol 1983;92:485–90.

46. Barrs DM, DeSanto LW, O'Fallo WM. Squamous cell carcinoma at the tonsil and tongue-base regions. Arch Otolaryngol 1979;105:479–85.

47. Foote RL, Olsen KD, Davis DL, et al. Base of tongue carcinoma: patterns of failure and predictors of recurrence after surgery alone. Head Neck 1993;15:300–7.

48. Bataini JP, Asselain B, Jaulerry CH, et al. A multivariate primary tumour control analysis in 465 patients treated by radical radiotherapy for cancer of the tonsillar region: clinical and treatment parameters as prognostic factors. Radiother Oncol 1989;14:265–77.

49. Henk JM. Results of radiotherapy for carcinoma of the oropharynx. Clin Otolaryngol 1978;3:37–43.

50. Perez CA, Purdy JA, Breaux SR, et al. Carcinoma of the tonsillar fossa: a non-randomized comparison of preoperative radiation and surgery and irradiation alone: long-term results. Cancer 1982;50:2314–22.

51. Amornmarn R, Prempree T, Jaiwatana J, Wizenberg MJ. Radiation management of carcinoma of the tonsillar region. Cancer 1984;54:1293–9.

52. Mizono GS, Diaz RF, Fu KK, Boles R. Carcinoma of the tonsillar region. Laryngoscope 1986;96:240–4.

53. Givens CD, Johns ME, Cantrell RW. Carcinoma of the tonsil: analysis of 162 cases. Arch Otolaryngol 1981;107:730–4.

54. Wang CC. Radiotherapeutic management of carcinoma of the posterior pharyngeal wall. Cancer 1971;27:894–6.

55. Pene F, Avedian V, Eschwege F, et al. A retrospective study of 131 cases of carcinoma of the posterior pharyngeal wall. Cancer 1978;42:2490–3.

56. Marks JE, Freeman RB, Lee F, Ogura JH. Pharyngeal wall cancer: an analysis of treatment results, complications and patterns of failure. Int J Radiat Oncol Biol Phys 1978;4:587-93.

57. Schwaab G, Vandenbrouck C, Luboinski B, Rhys Evans P. Les carcinomes de la paroi posteriure du pharynx traites par chirurgie premiere. J Eur Radiother 1983;4:175–9.

58. Jaulerry C, Brunin F, Rodriguez J, et al. Carcinomas of the posterior pharyngeal wall. Experience of the Institut Curie. Analysis of the results of radiotherapy. Ann Otolaryngol Chir Cervicofac 1986;103:559–63.

59. Esche BA, Haie CM, Gerbaulet AP, et al. Interstitial and external radiotherapy in carcinoma of the soft palate and uvula. Int J Radiat Oncol Biol Phys 1988;15:619–25.

60. Keus RB, Pontvert D, Brunin F, et al. Results of irradiation in squamous cell carcinoma of the soft palate and uvula. Radiother Oncol 1988;11:311–7.

61. Leemans CR, Engelbrecht WJ, Tiwari R, et al. Carcinoma of the soft palate and anterior tonsillar pillar. Laryngoscope 1994;104:1477–81.

62. Medini E, Medini A, Gapany M, Levitt SH. External beam radiation therapy for squamous cell carcinoma of the soft palate. Int J Radiat Oncol Biol Phys 1997;38:507–11.

7

Cancer of the Nasopharynx

SUZANNE L. WOLDEN, MD

Nasopharyngeal carcinoma is rare in the United States, with an annual incidence of 0.6 per 100,000 people. The incidence in Southern China is 50 times higher than in the United States.[1] Native people of North Africa, the Middle East, Alaska, and Malaysia have an intermediate risk. The peak incidence for this cancer occurs in the fourth to fifth decade of life but it may occur in children and in the elderly. The male to female ratio is 2 to 3:1.

The etiology of nasopharynx cancer is thought to be multifactorial with genetic, viral, dietary, and environmental influences. A genetic predisposition has not been explicitly demonstrated but data from China show common human leukocyte antigen (HLA) patterns among some patients with the disease.[2] The Epstein-Barr virus (EBV) has been closely associated with cancer of the nasopharynx. Molecular studies have shown evidence of EBV infection of malignant epithelial cells within a majority of tumor specimens.[3] Clinical correlation confirms that many patients have elevated antibody titers to EBV that subsequently decrease with effective treatment of the cancer. A diet high in salted fish, especially during childhood, has been implicated as a risk factor among Southern Chinese.[4] Salted fish contains a known carcinogen, dimethylnitrosamine. Cigarette smoking also appears to be a weak risk factor.[5]

ANATOMY

The nasopharynx is a hollow passageway, lined by mucosa, that serves to connect the nasal cavity to the oropharynx (Figure 7–1). It is bounded anteriorly by the posterior nasal choanae and nasal septum. The floor is formed by the superior surface of the soft palate and is in communication with the oropharynx at the level of the uvula. The posterior wall of the nasopharynx lies anterior to the first 2 cervical vertebrae, pre-vertebral and buccopharyngeal fascia, superior pharyngeal constrictor muscles and the pharyngeal aponeurosis. The roof is formed by the basisphenoid and basioccipital bones of the skull base. The lateral walls lie medial to the maxillopharyngeal space, pterygoid plates, and parapharyngeal space. The eustachian tube orifices enter the nasopharynx in the lateral walls and each is surrounded by a cartilaginous protuberance called the torus tubarius. A recess behind the torus tubarius, Rosenmüller's fossa, is the most common location for cancers to arise.

Cancers of the nasopharynx have multiple routes for local spread. Tumors commonly extend into the nasal cavity, oropharynx, parapharyngeal space and skull base. The sphenoid sinus is more commonly invaded than the ethmoid or maxillary sinuses. The orbit, cervical vertebrae and pterygoid structures may be involved in advanced disease. Invasion of the clivus occurs frequently. Tumors may extend through the foramen lacerum, ovale, or spinosum to the cavernous sinus, potentially involving cranial nerves (CN) II to VI. Less commonly, tumors may invade the cranium through the carotid canal, jugular foramen, or hypoglossal canal.

Branches of the external carotid artery provide blood supply to the nasopharynx while venous drainage is through the pharyngeal plexus, to the internal jugular vein. Nerve supply is provided by branches of cranial nerves V_2, IX, and X, as well as sympathetic nerves. The nasopharynx has a rich

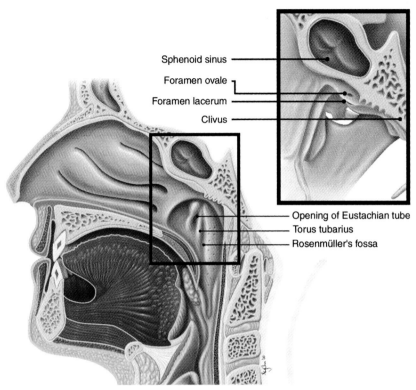

Sphenoid sinus
Foramen ovale
Foramen lacerum
Clivus

Opening of Eustachian tube
Torus tubarius
Rosenmüller's fossa

Figure 7–1. Mid-sagittal section of the nasopharynx and surrounding structures. Inset demonstrating the relationship of the nasopharynx to foramina of the skull base.

lymphatic network with multiple pathways for drainage. The first echelon lymph nodes are in the parapharyngeal and retropharyngeal space. The highest paired lymph nodes in this chain are named the nodes of Rouvière. Drainage to the jugular chain may occur by way of the parapharyngeal lymph nodes or by direct channels. A separate direct pathway leads to lymph nodes of the spinal accessory chain, in the posterior triangle. Further drainage may occur to the contralateral neck and down the cervical chains to the supraclavicular lymph nodes.

Diagnosis

Presenting symptoms may include a neck mass, epistaxis, nasal obstruction, a change in voice quality, pain, otalgia, decreased hearing, or cranial neuropathies. Approximately 85 percent of patients have cervical adenopathy and 50 percent have bilateral neck involvement.[6] Serous otitis media may occur due to eustachian tube obstruction. Cranial nerve VI is most frequently affected but multiple cranial nerves may be involved. Common combined neurologic findings are described as petrosphenoid or Jacod's syndrome (CN II to VI) and Villaret's syndrome (CN IX to XII and sympathetic nerves). The former may result from intracranial extension to the cavernous sinus and the latter may occur when nerves are invaded in the retropharyngeal space. Symptoms of advanced tumors may also include trismus, dysphagia, and proptosis. Distant metastatic disease is detected in 3 percent of patients at diagnosis but may occur in up to 50 percent of patients during the course of the disease.[7–9] The most common sites of hematogenous spread are the lungs, bones and liver.

The diagnosis of nasopharynx cancer is made by biopsy, preferably of the primary tumor. A variety of neoplasms may arise within the nasopharynx, including lymphomas and sarcomas. This chapter is restricted to epithelial carcinomas, categorized by the World Health Organization (WHO) into 3 histologic types. Type I is described as keratinizing squamous cell carcinoma and Type II is non-keratinizing. Type III, undifferentiated carcinoma, is the most common subtype.[10] The term lymphoepithelioma is often used to describe epithelial carcinomas with a rich infiltrate of benign lymphocytes.

A complete work-up includes a history and physical examination, including visualization of the nasopharynx by endoscopy or mirror examination. Magnetic resonance imaging (MRI) and/or computerized tomography (CT) of the skull base, nasopharynx and neck is necessary to determine the extent of disease (Figure 7–2). Every patient should have a chest radiograph, complete blood count, urinalysis, biochemical profile, including liver and kidney function tests, and serum IgA titers to the EBV viral capsid antigen. Prior to treatment with radiotherapy, patients require a dental evaluation. Bone scan and CT scan of the lungs or liver should be done if there is reason to suspect metastases because of symptoms or results of standard tests. Positron emission tomography (PET) scan is a new imaging modality that may prove to be useful in some clinical situations.[11]

Numerous staging systems for nasopharynx cancer have been used throughout the world. The Ho system has been used for decades in China and has been prognostically validated.[12] The American Joint Committee on Cancer/Union Internationale Contre Cancer (AJCC/UICC) staging classification was modified in 1997 to incorporate features of the Ho system. The AJCC/UICC system typically used in the United States and the western world is outlined in Table 7–1.[13]

Treatment Goals and Treatment Alternatives—The Role of Multidisciplinary Treatment

Cure is the goal of treatment for most patients without distant metastases. Prognosis depends upon disease stage, histology, and biological factors such as degree of angiogenesis.[9,14–16] Palliation of symptoms is a secondary goal for patients with curable disease and a primary goal for patients with distant metastatic disease. Palliative approaches range from supportive care to chemotherapy, radiation therapy and, rarely, surgical intervention.

The optimal management of nasopharynx cancer requires multidisciplinary collaboration. A head and neck surgeon often makes the diagnosis and performs the necessary biopsies. The patient should be referred to a radiation oncologist as soon as the diagnosis is established, as radiotherapy is the foundation of curative treatment. A medical oncologist should

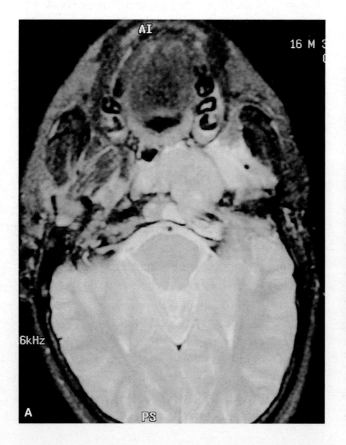

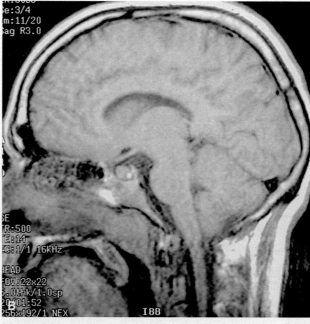

Figure 7–2. Magnetic resonance images (MRI) of an advanced nasopharyngeal cancer. *A,* Axial T2-weighted image with fat suppression demonstrating a large, left-sided nasopharynx tumor with parapharyngeal extension and skull base invasion. *B,* Sagittal T1-weighted image of the same tumor.

Table 7–1. 1997 AJCC/UICC NASOPHARYNGEAL CANCER STAGE CLASSIFICATION	
T Stage	**Primary Tumor Extent**
T1	Confined to the nasopharynx
T2	Extends to oropharynx or nasal cavity
2a	Without parapharyngeal extension
2b	With parapharyngeal extension
T3	Invades bones or paranasal sinuses
T4	Involvement of cranial nerves, intracranial contents, infratemporal fossa, hypopharynx or orbit

N Stage	**Lymph Node Disease**
N0	No lymph node metastases
N1	Unilateral lymph node(s) ≤ 6 cm
N2	Bilateral lymph nodes ≤ 6 cm
N3	Metastases in lymph nodes
3a	Greater than 6 cm
3b	With extension to the supraclavicular fossa

M Stage	**Distant Metastases**
M0	Absent
M1	Present

Stage Group	T Stage	N Stage	M Stage
I	T1	N0	M0
IIA	T2a	N0	M0
IIB	T2b	N0	M0
	T1–T2b	N1	M0
III	T3	N0–1	M0
	T1–T3	N2	M0
IVA	T4	N0–2	M0
IVB	T1–4	N3	M0
IVC	T1–4	N0–3	M1

Data from: L. Sobin and C. Wittekind, editors, UICC, TNM classification of malignant tumors. 5th ed. New York: Wiley-Liss; 1997.

However, the standard of care for patients with advanced locoregional disease has recently changed in the United States. Despite a number of negative trials of neoadjuvant and post-radiation chemotherapy,[17–19] a large Head and Neck Intergroup Trial (#0099) was conducted in the United States to study the effect of concurrent and adjuvant chemotherapy with radiotherapy.[20] Patients with 1992 AJCC Stage III and IV (but M0) disease were randomized to receive 70 Gy radiation therapy alone, or the same radiotherapy with 3 cycles of concurrent cisplatin chemotherapy followed by 3 cycles of cisplatin and 5-fluorouracil. Patients in the combined modality arm enjoyed a significant improvement in 3-year progression-free survival (69% vs. 24%, p< 0.001) and overall survival (76% vs. 46%, p < 0.001) over patients treated with radiotherapy alone.

Patients with stage II cancers according to the 1997 AJCC criteria were previously classified as stage III in the 1992 system and would have been eligible for the Intergroup trial. For this reason, it is recommended that patients with 1997 AJCC stage II to IVB disease receive combined modality therapy. Based on current data, patients with stage I tumors should be managed with radiotherapy alone and those with stage IVC disease should be treated with chemotherapy, adding radiation for palliation of local symptoms.

also be consulted because the role of chemotherapy is increasing in the treatment of this disease. Other important members of the multidisciplinary team include the radiologist, pathologist, and dentist. Specialized nurses, dieticians, occupational therapists and counselors may also provide useful services.

Factors Affecting Choice of Treatment

Because of anatomical constraints and the radiosensitivity of carcinoma of the nasopharynx, primary surgical resection is not indicated. Radiation therapy is the principal treatment modality for curative therapy and may also be used to palliate local symptoms. Chemotherapy has been studied as an adjuvant to primary radiotherapy and serves as systemic treatment for patients with disseminated disease.

The basic treatment of nasopharynx cancer has consisted of radiation therapy alone for many years.

Surgical Treatment

The role of surgery in nasopharynx cancer is limited. Surgical biopsy is necessary to establish the diagnosis. Neck dissection is indicated only if there is evidence of residual disease in cervical lymph nodes following treatment with radiotherapy with or without chemotherapy. Nasopharyngectomy is a challenging procedure that may be performed by highly specialized surgeons in selected patients with limited residual or recurrent disease within the nasopharynx.[21]

Nonsurgical Treatment

Effective radiotherapy requires careful simulation and treatment planning. The patient generally lies supine while the head is immobilized with the neck extended using a headrest and customized mask. A tongue blade is inserted to depress the tongue away from the palate, and palpable lymph nodes are outlined with wires. The most common field arrangement consists of opposed lateral fields to encompass the primary tumor and upper neck (Figure 7–3). A third, anterior field is matched below the lateral fields to treat the lower cervical and supraclavicular lymph nodes. The larynx is generally shielded and care must be taken to avoid overlapping fields on the spinal cord. The treatment design must be individualized for each patient, depending upon disease distribution and stage. CT or MRI scans should be used to define the gross tumor volume and this should be expanded by 1 to 2 cm to define the planning target volume. It is important to adequately treat the skull base and anterior as well as posterior cervical lymph nodes.

Radiation therapy is most often delivered with a linear accelerator in fractions of 1.8 to 2 Gy per day. Various accelerated fractionation regimens have also been used.[22,23] A shrinking field technique is used to give a range of doses to various regions. For instance, the optic nerves and spinal cord should be blocked from photon irradiation after a dose of 40 to 45 Gy. The posterior neck may then be treated to the appropriate total dose with electron beams. Electively treated nodal regions should receive doses of

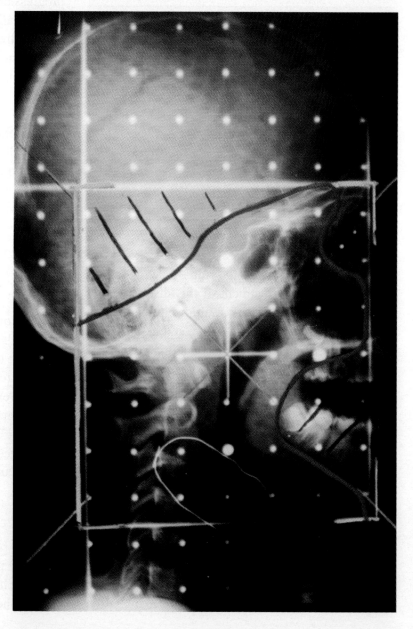

Figure 7–3.   Initial lateral simulation film for a patient with a stage T3 nasopharyngeal cancer invading the skull base. The cavernous sinuses, posterior ethmoid sinuses and skull base are included in the treatment field. The eyes and oral cavity are shielded. A palpable lymph node is marked with a wire. The field should be reduced during the course of therapy to prevent overdosing critical structures such as the optic nerves, optic chiasm, brain stem, and spinal cord. Treatment fields must be customized for each patient based on the extent of disease.

45 to 54 Gy. The portals may then be reduced to treat the primary tumor and gross adenopathy to total doses in the range of 65 to 75 Gy.

The appropriate radiation dose for an individual patient is derived by balancing the likelihood of achieving local control with the risks of radiation toxicity. Large tumors may require higher doses than small tumors. In general, several retrospective studies have shown improved local control using cumulative doses of ≥ 70 Gy.[24–26] Yan and colleagues conducted a study randomizing patients with residual disease after a dose of 70 Gy to receive a boost to 90 Gy or no additional treatment.[27] Local failure was significantly lower for patients receiving the boost but there was an increase in radiation toxicity.

A variety of techniques exist for delivering higher doses of radiation to the nasopharynx while minimizing the dose to critical structures such as the brainstem, optic nerves, mandible, temporal lobes, and inner ears. Intracavitary brachytherapy is a traditional technique whereby radiation sources are placed within the nasopharynx (Figure 7–4).[28,29] Alternative external beam techniques have also been used and this approach has been aided by the development of CT scan planning.[30] Newer technologies for boosting this region include stereotactic radiosurgery and intensity modulated radiotherapy (IMRT) as demonstrated in Figure 7–5.[31,32]

Nasopharynx cancer responds to a wide variety of chemotherapy agents. The most commonly used

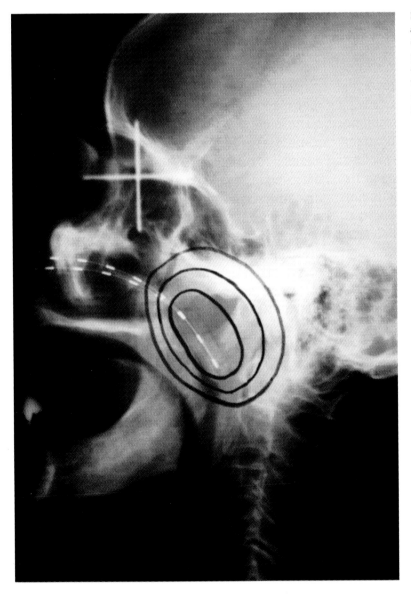

Figure 7–4. Verification film for a patient receiving an intracavitary brachytherapy boost for a stage T1 nasopharyngeal cancer. Radioactive sources are placed in catheters within the nasopharynx. In this case, the applicator has a thin metal shield inferiorly to allow relative sparing of the soft palate. The dose distribution is represented by the colored lines: red = 29 Gy, blue = 10 Gy, and brown = 5 Gy.

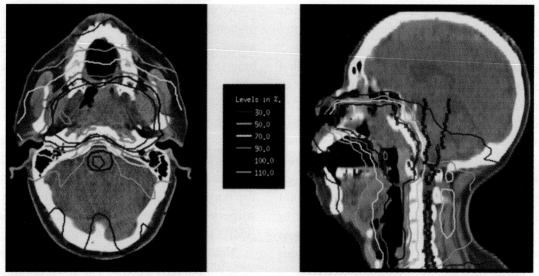

Figure 7–5. Axial and sagittal views of an intensity modulated radiotherapy (IMRT) plan for a stage T3 nasopharynx cancer. Seven beam angles are used in this case. Isodose curves are labeled by color. The target volume consists of the gross tumor plus a margin and is covered by the 100 percent dose level. The brain stem receives less than 50 percent of the prescribed dose.

regimen for patients with advanced disease in the United States includes cisplatin and 5-fluorouracil, based on the Head and Neck Intergroup study.[20] Patients should have measurement of creatinine clearance, an electrocardiogram, and an audiogram to ensure that they are appropriate candidates before starting this chemotherapy. Cisplatin 100 mg/m^2 is generally given on days 1, 22, and 43 during radiotherapy, with appropriate hydration and supportive care. Following chemoradiotherapy, patients receive 3 cycles of cisplatin 80 mg/m^2 and 5-fluorouracil 1000 mg/m^2/day (96-hour infusion) every 4 weeks.

Local recurrence after primary radiotherapy may be managed with re-irradiation or nasopharyngectomy in selected cases.[33,34] A discussion of these techniques is beyond the scope of this chapter. Regional nodal recurrence in the neck may be managed with a neck dissection. Most patients with locoregional recurrence and those with distant metastases should be offered systemic chemotherapy.

Sequelae, Complications, and their Management

The acute side effects of radiotherapy are significant and are increased when concurrent chemotherapy is given. Nearly all patients will experience a radiation skin reaction, mucositis, xerostomia, altered taste,

weight loss, and fatigue.[14] In cases where patients cannot maintain a reasonable oral intake, a feeding tube may be placed to ensure that they receive adequate nutrition. Cisplatin chemotherapy may also cause nausea and suppression of blood counts. The addition of adjuvant 5-fluorouracil may prolong mucositis. The mucosa of the nasopharynx becomes dry following treatment, causing formation of synechiae and crusted mucus. This can interfere with physical examination but may be minimized by instructing patients to perform regular nasal irrigations and to use humidifiers.

Most of the acute effects of radiotherapy resolve within 1 to 2 months. However, the majority of patients will have some degree of permanent xerostomia, dental problems, skin hyperpigmentation, and soft-tissue fibrosis.[35] Efforts to reduce long-term xerostomia include the use of radioprotectors such as amifostine or salivary stimulants such as pilocarpine.[36,37] Meticulous dental care and daily fluoride therapy are effective in minimizing the risk of serious dental complications. Approximately one-third of patients will eventually develop hypothyroidism. This is usually subclinical and detected by annual screening with thyroid function tests. Thyroid hormone replacement should be prescribed in this setting. Chronic serous otitis media occurs in approximately 15 percent of patients and may be managed with placement of myringotomy tubes. Radiation effects, along with cisplatin ototoxicity, could cause permanent hearing loss. Therefore, patients should be monitored with follow-up audiograms.[9]

More serious complications of radiotherapy include severe trismus and osteoradionecrosis (5 to 10% of patients).[35] Options for management of these problems are limited but include stretching exercises for the former, and antibiotics as well as hyperbaric oxygen for the latter. Extensive necrosis with bone sequestration will require surgical intervention. Pituitary dysfunction is rarely reported but may occur in younger patients, necessitating hormonal therapy. Fortunately, devastating neurologic complications of radiotherapy occur in less than 1 percent of patients in this country.[14,15] These include carotid artery stenosis, brain necrosis, blindness, cranial neuropathies and spinal myelitis. Neurologic complications are generally irreversible but may be prevented with careful radiation treatment planning. Radiation-induced second malignancies are rare but may include salivary gland neoplasms, skin cancers, sarcomas, meningiomas and thyroid cancers.

Rehabilitation and Quality of Life

Scientific studies of quality of life following treatment for nasopharynx cancer are lacking. The aforementioned acute and long-term toxicities of treatment, as well as direct effects of the cancer are certainly expected to impact quality of life. The specific interventions mentioned for each of the side effects help with rehabilitation. In addition, some patients may require physical therapy or nutritional counseling to restore an optimal level of function. Patients may also benefit from short or long-term psychological counseling after enduring difficult therapy for this life-threatening illness.

Outcomes

Data regarding local and regional control as well as survival comes from retrospective series using radiation alone (Tables 7–2, 7–3 and 7–4). Overall outcomes in the United States have been substantially improved by the addition of chemotherapy (excluding stage I cancers) to radiotherapy. In the previ-

ously described study published by Al-Sarraf and colleagues, combined modality therapy resulted in a 3-year actuarial progression-free survival of 69 percent and overall survival of 78 percent. Long-term follow-up of patients receiving chemoradiotherapy will be necessary to confirm the survival advantage and to assess complication rates.

The majority of patients (52%) experiencing a failure will do so in the first year after therapy.

Table 7–2. LOCAL CONTROL OF NASOPHARYNX CANCER BY STAGE WITH RADIOTHERAPY*

Author	No. of Patients	T1	T2	T3	T4
Hoppe[14]	82	87	94	68	44
Perez[26]	143	85	75	67	40
Lee[40]	4128	80	81	75–82	59–78
Sanguineti[41]	378	87	75	63	55
Wang[42]	259	72		66	49
Vikram[24]	107	74		100	63

* Based on staging prior to 1997 AJCC revisions.

Table 7–3. REGIONAL CONTROL OF NASOPHARYNX CANCER BY STAGE WITH RADIOTHERAPY*

Author	No. of Patients	N0	N1	N2	N3
Hoppe[14]	82	96	92	87	89
Mesic[15]	238	100	90	88	82
Perez[26]	143	82	86	72	
Wang[42]	259	62	63	67	

* Based on staging prior to 1997 AJCC revisions.

Table 7–4. ACTUARIAL FIVE-YEAR SURVIVAL FOR PATIENTS TREATED WITH RADIOTHERAPY ALONE FOR NASOPHARYNX CANCER, ACCORDING TO T AND N STAGE*

Author	No. of Patients	T1	T2	T3	T4
Hoppe[14†]	82	76	68	55	0
Wang[42‡]	259	65		58	42
		N0	N1	N2	N3
Hoppe[14†]	82	78	70	42	39
Wang[42‡]	259	63	63	56	
Chu[9**]	80	42	27	52	27

* Based on staging prior to 1997 AJCC revisions.
† Disease-free survival.
‡ Disease-specific survival.
** Overall survival.

Within 5 years, 90 percent of relapses are apparent but occasional recurrences more than 10 years from treatment are reported.[38] The prognosis following disease recurrence is better for patients with no distant metastases, limited disease extent, and an interval of at least 2 years since primary therapy.[39]

REFERENCES

1. Lee AW, Poon YF, Foo W, et al. Retrospective analysis of 5037 patients with nasopharyngeal carcinoma treated during 1976–1985: overall survival and patterns of failure. Int J Radiat Oncol Biol Phys 1992;23:261–70.

2. Simons MJ, Wee GB, Goh EH, et al. Immunogenetic aspects of nasopharyngeal carcinoma. IV. Increased risk in Chinese of nasopharyngeal carcinoma associated with a Chinese- related HLA profile (A2, Singapore 2). J Natl Cancer Inst 1976;57:977–80.

3. Liebowitz D. Nasopharyngeal carcinoma: the Epstein-Barr virus association. Semin Oncol 1994;21:376–81.

4. Ho JH. An epidemiologic and clinical study of nasopharyngeal carcinoma. Int J Radiat Oncol Biol Phys 1978;4:183–98.

5. Lin TM, Yang CS, Tu SM, et al. Interaction of factors associated with cancer of the nasopharynx. Cancer 1979;44:1419–23.

6. Lindberg RD. Distribution of cervical lymph node metastases from squamous cell carcinoma of the upper respiratory and digestive tracts. Cancer 1972;29:1446.

7. Ahmad A, Stefani S. Distant metastases of nasopharyngeal carcinoma: a study of 256 male patients. J Surg Oncol 1986;33:194-7.

8. Bedwinek JM, Perez CA, Keys DJ. Analysis of failures after definitive irradiation for epidermoid carcinoma of the nasopharynx. Cancer 1980;45:2725–9.

9. Chu AM, Flynn MB, Achino E, et al. Irradiation of nasopharyngeal carcinoma: correlations with treatment factors and stage. Int J Radiat Oncol Biol Phys 1984;10:2241–9.

10. International histological classification of tumors. Histological typing of upper respiratory tract tumors. World Health Organization 19:32, 1978.

11. Greven KM, Williams DW, Keyes JWJ, et al. Positron emission tomography of patients with head and neck carcinoma before and after high dose irradiation. Cancer 1994;74:1355–9.

12. Teo PM, Leung SF, Yu P, et al. A comparison of Ho's, International Union Against Cancer, and American Joint Committee stage classifications for nasopharyngeal carcinoma. Cancer 1991;67:434–9.

13. AJCC Cancer Staging Manual 5th ed. Fleming ID, Cooper J, Henson DE, et al. Philidelphia: Lippincott-Raven; 1997.

14. Hoppe RT, Goffinet DR, Bagshaw MA. Carcinoma of the nasopharynx. Eighteen years' experience with megavoltage radiation therapy. Cancer 1976;37:2605–12.

15. Mesic JB, Fletcher GH, Goepfert H. Megavoltage irradiation of epithelial tumors of the nasopharynx. Int J Radiat Oncol Biol Phys 1981;7:447–53.

16. Fu KK. Prognostic factors of carcinoma of the nasopharynx. Int J Radiat Oncol Biol Phys 1980;6:523–6.

17. Chan AT, Teo PM, Leung TW, et al. A prospective randomized study of chemotherapy adjunctive to definitive radiotherapy in advanced nasopharyngeal carcinoma [see comments]. Int J Radiat Oncol Biol Phys 1995;33:569–77.

18. Chua DT, Sham JS, Choy D, et al. Preliminary report of the Asian-Oceanian Clinical Oncology Association randomized trial comparing cisplatin and epirubicin followed by radiotherapy versus radiotherapy alone in the treatment of patients with locoregionally advanced nasopharyngeal carcinoma. Asian-Oceanian Clinical Oncology Association Nasopharynx Cancer Study Group. Cancer 1998;83:2270–83.

19. Rossi A, Molinari R, Boracchi P, et al. Adjuvant chemotherapy with vincristine, cyclophosphamide, and doxorubicin after radiotherapy in local-regional nasopharyngeal cancer: results of a 4-year multicenter randomized study. J Clin Oncol 1988;6:1401–10.

20. Al-Sarraf M, LeBlanc M, Giri PG, et al. Chemoradiotherapy versus radiotherapy in patients with advanced nasopharyngeal cancer: phase III randomized Intergroup study 0099. J Clin Oncol 1998;16:1310–7.

21. Fee WEJ, Roberson JBJ, Goffinet DR. Long-term survival after surgical resection for recurrent nasopharyngeal cancer after radiotherapy failure. Arch Otolaryngol Head Neck Surg 1991;117:1233–6.

22. Ang KK, Peters LJ, Weber RS, et al. Concomitant boost radiotherapy schedules in the treatment of carcinoma of the oropharynx and nasopharynx. Int J Radiat Oncol Biol Phys 1990;19:1339–45.

23. Wang CC. Accelerated hyperfractionation radiation therapy for carcinoma of the nasopharynx. Techniques and results. Cancer 1989;63:2461–7.

24. Vikram B, Mishra UB, Strong EW, et al. Patterns of failure in carcinoma of the nasopharynx: I. Failure at the primary site. Int J Radiat Oncol Biol Phys 1985;11:1455–9.

25. En-Pee Z, Pei-Gun L, Kuang-Long C, et al. Radiation therapy of nasopharyngeal carcinoma: prognostic factors based on a 10-year follow-up of 1302 patients. Int J Radiat Oncol Biol Phys 1989;16:301–5.

26. Perez CA, Devineni VR, Marcial-Vega V, et al. Carcinoma of the nasopharynx: factors affecting prognosis. Int J Radiat Oncol Biol Phys 1992;23:271–80.

27. Yan JH, Xu GZ, Hu YH, et al. Management of local residual primary lesion of nasopharyngeal carcinoma: II. Results of prospective randomized trial on booster dose. Int J Radiat Oncol Biol Phys 1990;18:295–8.

28. Chang JT, See LC, Tang SG, et al. The role of brachytherapy in early-stage nasopharyngeal carcinoma. Int J Radiat Oncol Biol Phys 1996;36:1019–24.

29. Wang CC. Improved local control of nasopharyngeal carcinoma after intracavitary brachytherapy boost. Am J Clin Oncol 1991;14:5–8.

30. Kutcher GJ, Fuks Z, Brenner H, et al. Three-dimensional photon treatment planning for carcinoma of the nasopharynx. Int J Radiat Oncol Biol Phys 1991;21:169–82.

31. Verhey LJ. Comparison of three-dimensional conformal radiation therapy and intensity-modulated radiation therapy systems. Semin Radiat Oncol 1999;9:78–98.

32. Cmelak AJ, Cox RS, Adler JR, et al. Radiosurgery for skull base malignancies and nasopharyngeal carcinoma. Int J Radiat Oncol Biol Phys 1997;37:997–1003.

33. Chua DT, Sham JS, Kwong DL, et al. Locally recurrent nasopharyngeal carcinoma: treatment results for patients with computed tomography assessment. Int J Radiat Oncol Biol Phys 1998;41:379–86.

34. Hsu MM, Ko JY, Sheen TS, et al. Salvage surgery for recurrent nasopharyngeal carcinoma. Arch Otolaryngol Head Neck Surg 1997;123:305–9.

35. Lee AW, Law SC, Ng SH, et al. Retrospective analysis of nasopharyngeal carcinoma treated during 1976–1985: late complications following megavoltage irradiation. Br J Radiol 1992;65:918–28.

36. Rieke JW, Hafermann MD, Johnson JT, et al. Oral pilocarpine for radiation-induced xerostomia: integrated efficacy and safety results from two prospective randomized clinical trials. Int J Radiat Oncol Biol Phys 1995;31:661–9.

37. McDonald S, Meyerowitz C, Smudzin T, et al. Preliminary results of a pilot study using WR-2721 before fractionated irradiation of the head and neck to reduce salivary gland dysfunction. Int J Radiat Oncol Biol Phys 1994;29:747–54.

38. Lee AW, Foo W, Law SC, et al. Recurrent nasopharyngeal carcinoma: the puzzles of long latency. Int J Radiat Oncol Biol Phys 1999;44:149–56.

39. Pryzant RM, Wendt CD, Delclos L, et al. Re-treatment of nasopharyngeal carcinoma in 53 patients. Int J Radiat Oncol Biol Phys 1992;22:941–7.

40. Lee AW, Law SC, Foo W, et al. Nasopharyngeal carcinoma: local control by megavoltage irradiation. Br J Radiol 1993;66:528–36.

41. Sanguineti G, Geara FB, Garden AS, et al. Carcinoma of the nasopharynx treated by radiotherapy alone: determinants of local and regional control [see comments]. Int J Radiat Oncol Biol Phys 1997;37:985–96.

42. Wang CC. Carcinoma of the nasopharynx. In: Wang CC, editor. Radiation therapy for head and neck neoplasms. 3rd ed. New York: John Wiley & Sons, Inc.; 1997. p. 257–80.

8

The Larynx: Advanced Stage Disease

JOHN F. CAREW, MD

Of the 295,000 cases of cancer of the head and neck accrued by the National Cancer Data Base over a 10-year period, larynx was the most common site accounting for more than 20 percent of all head and neck cancers.[1] Squamous cell carcinoma which arises from the mucosa lining the larynx accounted for over 90 percent of all cancers in this site.[2] In one of the larger studies of patients with larynx cancer, 40 percent of patients presented with advanced stage disease (stage III or IV).[2] Despite the use of aggressive multimodality treatment in patients with advanced stage cancer of the larynx, overall survival for these patients ranges from 42 to 77 percent.[2–14] As mentioned in the section on early stage disease, other neoplasms such as lymphomas, minor salivary gland tumors, mucosal melanomas and sarcomas may affect this site, although large series evaluating these specific pathologies at this site are lacking in the literature. Unless otherwise specified, squamous cell carcinomas of the larynx will be the subject of this chapter.

The larynx performs several unique and vital functions related to phonation, breathing and swallowing, and the treatment of patients with neoplasms of this organ requires consideration of these critical functions. Specifically, the impact of therapeutic options on both the extent as well as the quality of life needs to be taken into account. As this section focuses on advanced cancer of the larynx, most treatment options involve multimodality therapy in the form of either chemotherapy and radiation therapy or surgery and radiation therapy. The critical decision, which continues to evolve, is selecting the appropriate treatment for each individual patient.

Additionally, the optimal treatment plan which combines chemotherapy and radiation therapy with regards to timing (sequential vs. concomitant), radiation fractionation, chemotherapeutic agents and adjuvants remains undefined. In this section, the diagnosis, treatment and outcome of patients with advanced cancer of the larynx will be presented.

ANATOMY

While the basic anatomy of the larynx already has been described in the section on early larynx cancer, this section will highlight the critical points relevant to treating patients with advanced cancers of the larynx. The majority of larynx cancers are found in the glottic region (56%) followed by the supraglottic region (41%), while tumors of the subglottic region are relatively infrequent (1 to 2%) (Figure 8–1).[2,15] It is important to realize that tumors in these different regions of the larynx have different clinical behaviors. Supraglottic tumors, for example, have a much higher rate of occult and bilateral metastasis than glottic primaries.[10,16] The regional lymph nodes of the neck in patients with advanced stage supraglottic tumors and clinically negative necks must therefore be addressed in treatment planning.

The connective tissue barriers which lie between the mucosa and cartilaginous skeleton of the larynx, namely the conus elasticus and quadrangular membrane, are critical to the understanding of patterns of spread and clinical behavior of advanced cancers of the larynx (Figure 8–2). These membranes provide a barrier to the spread of cancer but are often breached

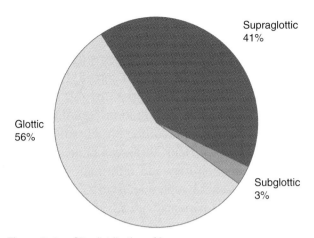

Figure 8–1. Site distribution of larynx cancers.

by advanced tumors (Figure 8–3).[17] Once a tumor has broken through these boundaries, it can spread into the soft tissues of the neck as well as vertically within the larynx.

Two regions that are deep to the quadrangular membrane and conus elasticus are the preepiglottic and paraglottic space. Advanced tumors often enter these spaces when they transgress these connective tissue barriers within the larynx and thus enter a compartment where further spread is less hindered. The preepiglottic space is bounded by the thyrohyoid membrane anteriorly, the valleculae superiorly, the epiglottis posteriorly and the hyoid inferiorly. This space is commonly involved by local spread of supraglottic tumors. Once this space is involved, a supraglottic tumor is staged as a T3.[18] Tumors

involving this area can then spread into the soft tissues of the neck via the foramen in the thyrohyoid membrane or inferiorly via the paraglottic space. In some patients, however, a connective tissue barrier separates the preepiglottic and paraglottic space.[19]

The paraglottic space is the compartment which is bounded by the thyroid lamina laterally, the conus elasticus medially-inferiorly and the quadrangular membrane and preepiglottic space medially-superiorly. Loose connective tissue and adipose tissue lying between thyroid lamina and the connective tissue membranes of the larynx occupy this space. This area is most commonly involved by advanced glottic tumors. Once this compartment is entered, tumors can spread relatively freely in a superior and inferior direction, as well as outside the confines of the larynx via the cricothyroid membrane or the preepiglottic space. Involvement of this space frequently results in decreased vocal fold movement.

Cancers of the larynx can be classified as advanced (stage III or IV) either by virtue of an advanced primary tumor or by the presence of regional lymph node metastasis. When regional lymph node metastases are present they are described by their location, number and size. The location of the lymph nodes is described by levels in the neck as illustrated in the chapter on neck metastasis. Levels II, III and IV are at highest risk for lymph node metastasis from cancers in the larynx.

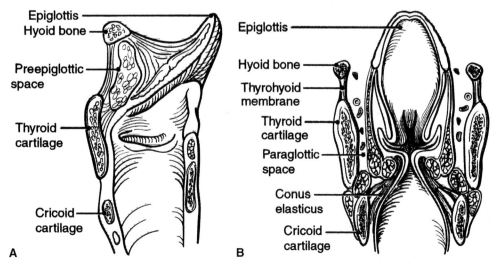

Figure 8–2. *A,* Sagittal section of larynx demonstrating the preepiglottic and *B,* coronal section of larynx demonstrating the paraglottic space.

Diagnosis

Patients with advanced glottic cancers will present with symptoms similar to patients with early glottic cancers. As listed earlier these include hoarseness or a change in the quality of voice, odynophagia, halitosis or otalgia. Not suprisingly the more ominous symptoms, such as hemoptysis, dysphagia, airway compromise and neck mass are more common in advanced stage disease. Additionally, the supraglottic and subglottic lesions tend to be less symptomatic and their insidious growth results in a high percent of patients presenting with advanced stage disease.

As mentioned earlier, adequate examination of the larynx by use of the laryngeal mirror or a rigid telescope or fiberoptic flexible nasopharyngoscope is essential to staging and treatment planning (Figure 8–4).[20] Critical in this evaluation is assessment of the epicenter of the tumor, vocal fold mobility, extra-laryngeal involvement and regional lymph nodes in the neck. Although early tumors are often adequately assessed by history and physical exam alone, appropriate evaluation of advanced lesions usually requires radiographic imaging to ascertain the depth of the tumor involvement, preepiglottic space extension, paraglottic extension, cartilage involvement and extra-laryngeal spread. High-resolution CT scans with thin cuts through the larynx usually give adequate information regarding these aspects (Figure 8–5).[21] Additionally, in patients with necks which are difficult to assess clinically, radiographic evaluation may add information in establishing the regional lymph node status.

The staging of patients with advanced cancers of the larynx is outlined in Table 8–1.[18] As with other sites in the head and neck, the complex anatomy in this region makes accurate staging challenging. At times, the location of the lesion appears to carry more weight than the tumor burden. For example, a relatively small tumor on the posterior aspect of the larynx which involves the post-cricoid area will be stage T3, while a bulky tumor replacing the aryepiglottic fold, epiglottis and spilling down the medial wall of the pyriform sinus will be staged a T2 as long as the vocal cord remains mobile. While survival has been related to both T stage and N stage, it

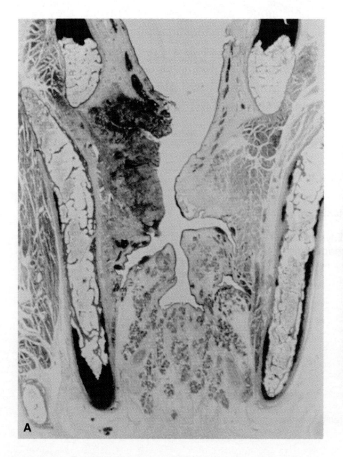

A

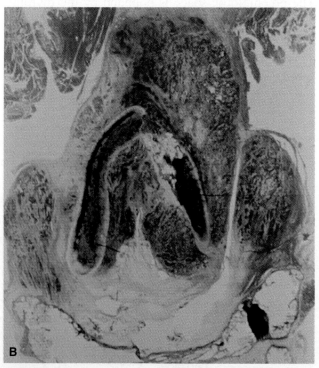

B

Figure 8–3.   Whole organ sections showing tumor involving the preepiglottic and paraglottic space.

is most profoundly affected by the nodal status of the patient.[2,10,11] It has long been known that regional lymph node involvement in head and neck cancer patients decreases survival by approximately 50 percent.[10,11] The present staging system of the American Joint Committee for Cancer (AJCC) groups both patients with locally advanced tumors (T3N0) and patients with regional lymph node metastasis (T1-3N1) together into stage III.[18] This may arbitrarily group 2 subsets of patients together who have vastly different prognoses. Both the stage as well as the nodal status must thus be considered when interpreting results from the treatment of larynx cancer.

Just as there are ominous symptoms in patients with advanced cancer of the larynx, there are also several physical findings that are harbingers of clin-

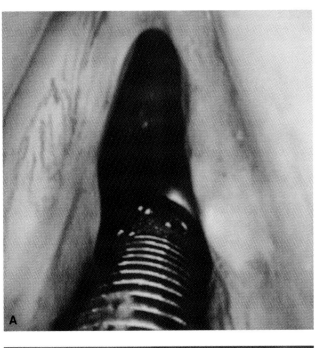
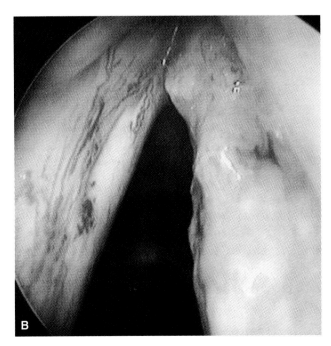
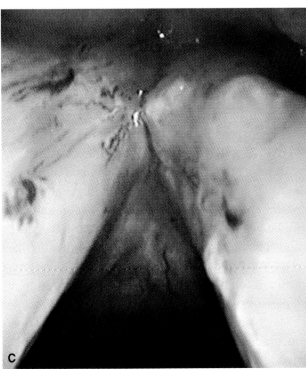
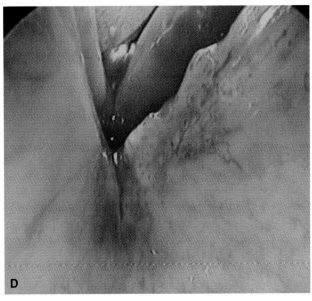

Figure 8–4.   Endoscopic view and assessment of a laryngeal cancer using the A-0°; B-30°; C-70°; D-120° telescopes.

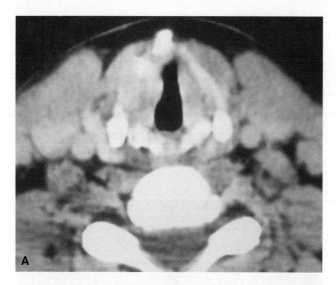

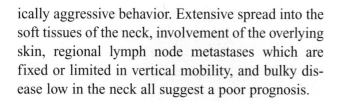

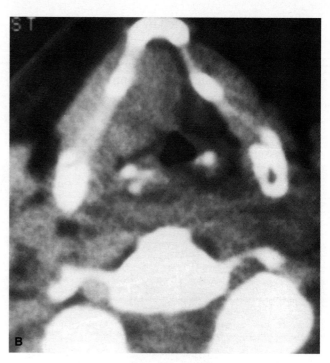

Figure 8–5. *A,* Axial CT of advanced laryngeal primary tumor demonstrating paraglottic involvement and cartilage destruction but without extension into the soft tissues of the neck. *B,* Axial CT of advanced laryngeal primary tumor demonstrating cartilage destruction and extension into the soft tissues of the neck.

ically aggressive behavior. Extensive spread into the soft tissues of the neck, involvement of the overlying skin, regional lymph node metastases which are fixed or limited in vertical mobility, and bulky disease low in the neck all suggest a poor prognosis.

Treatment Goals and Treatment Alternatives–The Role of Multidisciplinary Treatment

In the last 2 decades, 5-year survival of patients with laryngeal cancer has not changed dramatically.[22] Maximizing survival, therefore, continues to be the ultimate goal in treating patients with advanced stage larynx cancer. Recently, however, due to the lack of improvement in survival, significant efforts have been made to improve the quality of life in these patients. Paramount to this is preservation of a functional larynx. Toward this goal, treatment options have been formulated with the hopes of increasing laryngeal preservation without sacrificing survival. Multimodality treatment paradigms, in the form of chemotherapy, radiotherapy and surgical salvage, has emerged as a viable treatment option allowing anatomical preservation of the larynx without decreasing survival.[3] Now that a method of laryngeal preservation has been established, future

goals in treatment are directed at increasing both the rate of laryngeal preservation and survival.

Factors Affecting Choice of Treatment

Factors affecting choice of treatment can be divided into patient factors and tumor factors. As demonstrated in multiple clinical trials, survival is statistically equivalent in selected patients with advanced cancer of the larynx who are treated with either chemotherapy and radiation therapy or surgery and radiation therapy.[3,6,7,9,23–25] Given this, patients who wish to utilize a treatment paradigm that may preserve their larynx, such as chemotherapy and radiation therapy, should be given this nonsurgical option. Alternatively, there is a cohort of patients who are of the mindset that they would rather have all cancer removed and would prefer surgery and radiation therapy, understanding that their ability to communicate will be significantly affected. Finally, any patient who is considering chemotherapy and radiation therapy as a treatment option must be reliable and must enroll a multidisciplinary team experienced in treating patients with advanced cancer of the larynx.

Many tumor factors also contribute to the decision process in determining the optimal treatment for each patient. If a tumor or lymph node metastasis shows ominous clinical signs suggesting unresectability, then certainly a surgical option should not be contemplated and consideration given to chemotherapy and radiation therapy.[26,27] A clinical situation which is interesting but infrequent arises when a patient presents with an early stage primary lesion and clinically apparent regional lymph node metastasis. In this situation several treatment options exist. If the primary lesion is best treated by radia-

tion therapy, one could consider a comprehensive neck dissection followed by radiation therapy to the primary site and the neck. Alternatively, if the primary lesion is best treated by a surgical approach, one could consider a partial laryngectomy and neck dissection with the addition of adjuvant radiation therapy as indicated based on pathologic findings.

Of the most important factors in deciding the optimal treatment are the characteristics of the primary tumor. Tumors which are endophytic, show extensive cartilage invasion, involve the soft tissues of the neck, or involve the airway to such an extent that a tracheostomy is required, often demonstrate aggressive clinical behavior and respond poorly to treatment. Whether these patients fare better in a surgical treatment arm as opposed to a nonsurgical plan has yet to be substantiated in a randomized prospective trial. The ideal treatment in these patients, therefore, remains controversial. In such patients, aggressive early surgical intervention will improve the chances for locoregional control and thus improve the quality of life that would otherwise be significantly deteriorated with persistent or recurrent disease. Early aggressive surgical intervention may not improve survival or risk of distant metastasis, but would certainly offer avoidance of airway obstruction, asphyxiation or intractable pain.

Surgical Treatment

In the majority of patients with advanced primary tumors of the larynx, the surgical treatment consists of a total laryngectomy. It should be remembered, however, that partial laryngectomy and conservational surgical procedures which preserve the function of the larynx may be options in selected patients. As discussed in the section on early larynx cancer, vertical partial, supraglottic partial and supracricoid partial laryngectomies can be performed in carefully selected patients. In patients with advanced lesions, however, the more extensive partial laryngectomies are utilized more frequently and even more selectively. These procedures, although categorized in broad terms such as near-total laryngectomy or supracricoid partial laryngectomy with cricohyoidopexy, are usually individually designed to adequately encompass each patient's

Table 8-1. AJCC STAGING OF CARCINOMA OF THE LARYNX

Supraglottis

T1: Tumor limited to one subsite of the supraglottis with normal vocal cord mobility
T2: Tumor invades mucosa of more than one adjacent subsite of the supraglottis or glottis or region outside the supraglottis (eg, mucosa of the base of tongue, valleculae, medial wall of pyriform sinus) without fixation of the larynx
T3: Tumor limited to the larynx with vocal cord fixation and/or invades any of the following: postcricoid area, preepiglottic tissues
T4: Tumor invades through the thyroid cartilage, and/or extends into the soft tissues of the neck, thyroid and/or esophagus

Glottis

T1: Tumor limited to the vocal cord(s) (may involve anterior or posterior commissure) with normal vocal cord mobility
    T1A: Tumor limited to one vocal cord
    T1B: Tumor involves both vocal cords
T2: Tumor extends to the supraglottis and/or subglottis, and/or with impaired vocal cord mobility
T3: Tumor limited to the larynx with vocal cord fixation
T4: Tumor invades through the thyroid cartilage and/or extends to other tissues beyond the larynx (eg, trachea, soft tissues of the neck, including thyroid, pharynx)

Subglottis

T1: Tumor limited to the subglottis
T2: Tumor extends to the vocal cord(s) with normal or impaired mobility
T3: Tumor limited to the larynx with vocal cord fixation
T4: Tumor invades through the cricoid or thyroid cartilage and/or extends to other tissues beyond the larynx (eg, trachea, soft tissues of the neck, including thyroid, esophagus)

Neck

N0: No regional lymph node metastasis
N1: Ipsilateral lymph node metastasis ≤ 3 cm
N2: Lymph node metastasis in a single ipsilateral lymph node > 3 cm and ≤ 6 cm, or in multiple lymph nodes none more than 6 cm (including bilateral nodal metastasis)
    N2A: Lymph node metastasis in single ipsilateral lymph node > 3 cm and ≤ 6 cm
    N2B: Lymph node metastasis in multiple ipsilateral lymph nodes all ≤ 6 cm
    N2C: Lymph node metastasis in bilateral or contralateral lymph nodes all ≤ 6 cm
N3: Lymph node metastasis > 6 cm

particular tumor while sparing as much functional tissue as oncologically feasible (Figure 8–6).[28–31]

Appropriate management of the neck is critical to maximizing survival in patients with advanced cancer of the larynx. The treatment of the neck depends in part on the treatment of the primary. If the primary is to be treated by surgical means, then an elective dissection of the lymph nodes at risk should be planned in the clinically negative neck. For a glottic lesion, the ipsilateral levels II to IV should be cleared, while for a supraglottic lesion, bilateral levels II to IV are at risk and should be dissected. If there is clinically apparent lymph node metastasis in the neck and the primary is to be treated by surgery, then a comprehensive neck dissection (levels I to V) should be performed.

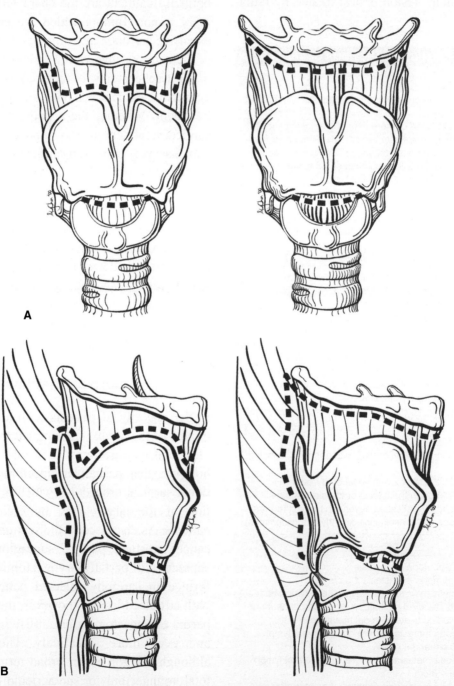

Figure 8–6. Schematic diagram of two well-described voice-preserving, extended laryngeal procedures: *A*, supracricoid laryngectomy with cricohyoidoepiglottopexy and *B*, supracricoid laryngectomy with cricohyoidopexy (dotted lines represent line of surgical excision).

Alternatively, if a patient with a clinically negative neck is to be treated by chemotherapy and radiation therapy to the primary lesion, the neck at risk should also be treated electively by radiation therapy. A somewhat more controversial situation exists if there is a clinically positive neck and the primary is to be treated by chemotherapy and radiation therapy. The options that exist include performing a comprehensive neck dissection prior to chemotherapy/radiation therapy, performing a planned comprehensive or selective neck dissection after chemotherapy/ radiation therapy or assessing response following chemotherapy/radiation therapy and performing appropriate neck dissection based on response. At this time, data is lacking to substantiate an advantage in any of these approaches and all are acceptable.

Nonsurgical Treatment

The appreciation of the psychosocial consequences of total laryngectomy has been the impetus for the development of treatment options which could preserve the larynx of patients with advanced stage larynx cancer. In the early 1990s, a prospective, randomized trial of patients treated at Veterans Affairs Hospitals with stage III and stage IV squamous cell carcinoma of the larynx, comparing conventional treatment of surgery and postoperative radiotherapy, with induction chemotherapy followed by radiotherapy was performed.[3] In this study, patients in the chemotherapy-radiation therapy (chemo/RT) arm who did not display at least a 50 percent response to induction chemotherapy, or who showed persistent or recurrent disease following radiation, were salvaged with surgery. This landmark study demonstrated survivals which were not statistically different between treatment arms (68%), and allowed 64 percent of patients within chemo/RT arms to preserve their larynx.[3] With the results of the Veterans Affairs Larynx Cancer Study Group (VALCSG) trial, the combination of induction chemotherapy and radiation therapy has emerged as a treatment option which allows preservation of the larynx in nearly two-thirds of patients. Since this trial, many other studies have been performed to confirm chemo/RT as an effective treatment for patients with advanced larynx cancer.[6,7,9,23–25,32]

Sequelae, Complications and their Management

Surgery and Radiotherapy

The complications associated with total laryngectomy can be divided into acute and chronic. The acute complications include those related to surgery and general anesthesia. These include bleeding, infection, pneumonia and fistula. The most troublesome of these is the pharyngocutaneous fistula. The fistula rate following total laryngectomy remains relatively high, ranging from 8 to 22 percent.[33–35] Appropriate treatment of a pharyngocutaneous fistula requires early recognition and then wide opening of the wound with appropriate wound care. The patient should stop all oral intake and an alternative route of alimentation should be established. If significant carotid exposure is seen, then consideration should be given to coverage with a regional flap to afford carotid protection, especially in the setting of previous radiation therapy. Often the fistula will close spontaneously with aggressive wound care. In those cases where it does not, local, regional and even free flaps may be used to obtain closure.

The most common chronic complication of total laryngectomy is stricture formation with dysphagia. It is crucial to rule out recurrent tumor whenever a patient develops new dysphagia or worsening dysphagia. This is usually best evaluated by endoscopy with direct visualization of the mucosa of the neopharynx. Preoperative esophagrams are often helpful in defining the location and extent of stricture. If a stricture is seen, it can usually be dilated, although repeated treatments are often required. Ultimately, if a stricture is unresponsive to these conservative measures, consideration can be given to free tissue transfer to reconstruct an adequate neopharynx.

The early sequelae of radiation therapy relate primarily to the acute tissue reactions with characteristic skin changes and mucositis. These are managed symptomatically with oral hygiene and topical medications. The late sequelae of radiation therapy include skin changes, xerostomia and, very rarely, chondroradionecrosis of the laryngeal skeleton. Xerostomia is treated symptomatically with oral hygiene and humidification. In severe cases where chondroradionecrosis profoundly impairs swallowing and breathing, a total laryngectomy may need to be performed to restore the ability to swallow.

Chemotherapy and Radiotherapy

Treatment protocols using chemo/RT to preserve organ function have successfully demonstrated their ability to anatomically preserve the larynx without compromising survival. One aspect of these protocols that is often underappreciated is the functional capacity of the retained organs. Few investigators have clearly documented the functional sequelae of chemotherapy and radiation therapy. Recently, Lazarus retrospectively studied patients being treated with chemotherapy and radiation therapy and found that 40 percent had swallowing difficulties.[36] Clinical evidence of disorders in the pharyngeal phase of swallowing has been demonstrated in patients who have undergone chemotherapy and radiation therapy for tumors of the upper aerodigestive tract. Specifically, reduced laryngeal closure, reduced laryngeal elevation and reduced posterior tongue base movement relative to age-matched controls has been documented.[36] Certainly, patients who successfully undergo chemo/RT treatments to preserve their larynx have a much improved quality of life relative to patients requiring total laryngectomy.[37] Nevertheless, it should be realized that anatomic preservation does not always result in functional preservation. Very rarely, total laryngectomy is performed in order to restore the ability to swallow when a larynx is incompetent and nonfunctional but clinically free of cancer.

In addition to functional sequelae, chemotherapy (specifically when given in combination with radiation therapy) has some definite toxicities. Toxicity from induction chemotherapy has prevented 7 to 18 percent of patients from receiving a full course of chemotherapy.[3,4,6,8] Even mortality, as a result of chemotherapy and radiation-related toxicity, has been reported to range from 0.6 to 6 percent.[3,5–9,25]

Rehabilitation and Quality of Life

In the past, conventional treatment of advanced stage laryngeal cancer consisted of surgery and postoperative external beam radiation. Surgical resection of the majority of advanced stage laryngeal lesions con-

sisted of total laryngectomy with the resultant deleterious effects on deglutition, phonation and the creation of a permanent tracheostoma. The psychosocial consequences of total laryngectomy have been well studied.[14,37–39] Not suprisingly, quality of life measurements and psychosocial indicators are significantly affected by total laryngectomy. Although techniques for voice rehabilitation have improved, studies have shown that the psychosocial effects of laryngectomy are as much related to loss of voice as they are to other factors such as the necessity of a permanent tracheostoma.[14,38,39] When the patients treated in the Veterans Affairs Laryngeal Cancer Study Group were evaluated, an improved long-term quality of life was seen in the cohort who were randomized to chemotherapy and radiation therapy compared to those treated by surgery and radiation therapy.[37] Interestingly, this difference was primarily related to freedom from pain, better emotional well-being and lower levels of depression rather than the preservation of the ability to speak.

Nevertheless, several methods are available to rehabilitate the ability of a patient to communicate following total laryngectomy. Many patients are able to acquire esophageal speech, in which air is swallowed and then used to create a voice. Approximately 2 decades ago a significant advance in the rehabilitation of patients with laryngectomies took place when the tracheoesophageal puncture was developed.[40] This is a relatively minor procedure where a fistula is created between the trachea and esophagus (Figure 8–7). A prosthesis with a one-way valve is placed into this fistula, which allows the creation of a lung powered voice. In the motivated patient, this voice can be quite good.

Outcomes and Results of Treatment

Historically, surgery in the form of total laryngectomy followed by adjuvant postoperative radiation therapy has been the standard treatment for most patients with advanced stage cancer of the larynx.[10–12,41,42] Additionally, selected patients with advanced stage larynx cancer have been treated with definitive radiation therapy alone.[13,42,43] The results of these treatments are summarized in Table 8–2 with 5-year survival ranging from 54 to 91 percent.[10–13,41–43]

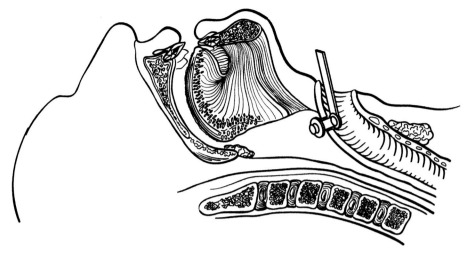

Figure 8–7. Schematic diagram of tracheoesophageal puncture (TEP).

More recently, chemotherapy/radiation therapy has evolved as an effective treatment for advanced stage cancer of the larynx. A summary of results from the various studies evaluating chemo/RT in the treatment of patients with advanced stage laryngeal cancer, with the goal of larynx preservation, are listed in chronologic order in Table 8–3.[3–9,25] In all but one study, more than 90 percent of patients evaluated had stage III or IV disease. Most studies included only those patients who would have required a total laryngectomy if treated by conventional means with surgery and postoperative radiotherapy. Treatment results for patients treated with chemo/RT in these studies are fairly consistent with 2-year survival ranging from 50 to 77 percent, lar-

ynx preservation rates ranging from 64 to 79 percent, locoregional failure rates ranging from 20 to 33 percent and distant failure rates ranging from 8 to 21 percent.[3–9,25] It should be noted, however, that only one of these studies was limited only to patients with laryngeal primaries,[3] while the remainder of the studies included patients with hypopharynx, oropharynx, oral cavity and even paranasal sinuses as sites of primary tumors.[4–9,25] The majority of these studies that included non-laryngeal sites did so because surgical treatment of the primary would have required total laryngectomy. The data presented

Table 8–2. RESULTS OF CONVENTIONAL TREATMENT OF ADVANCED CARCINOMA OF THE LARYNX

Author	Year	No.	Type of Therapy	Stage III/IV (%)	5 yr Survival (%)
Kirchner[12]	1977	308	S/RT	100	54–56*
Harwood[13]	1979	353	RT	54	70
Harwood[43]	1983	410	RT	66	57
Yuen[41]	1984	192	S	100	77
		50	S/RT	100	91
Mendenhall[42]	1992	100	RT	100	74
		65	S±RT	100	63
Nguyen[11]	1996	116	S/RT	100	68
Myers[10]	1996	65	S±RT	100	62†

Survival rates refer to disease-free survival when available, otherwise they refer to overall survival.
* study included both laryngeal and non-laryngeal sites.
S = Surgery; RT = Radiation therapy; † 2-year survival.

Table 8–3. RESULTS OF TREATMENT OF ADVANCED CARCINOMA OF THE LARYNX UTILIZING CHEMOTHERAPY AND RADIATION THERAPY

Author	Year	No.	Type of Therapy	Stage III/IV (%)	2 yr. Survival (%)
Jacobs[4]	1987	30	C/RT	100	52*
Demard[5]	1990	50	C/RT	64	74* (Response rate)
Veterans Affairs Larynx Group[3]	1991	166	C/RT	100	68
		166	S/RT	100	68*
Pfister[6]	1991	13	C/RT	98	77*
Karp[7]	1991	14	C/RT	92	50*
Urba[8]	1994	8	C/RT	93	75*
Clayman[9] (includes data from Shirinian)[25]	1995	26	C/RT	96	68*
		52	S/RT	96	81*

Survival rates refer to disease-free survival when available, otherwise they refer to overall survival.
* Study included both laryngeal and non-laryngeal sites. C = chemotheapy; S = surgery; RT = radiation therapy.

in this table refers, whenever possible, to the subset of patients with laryngeal primaries, although this information was not always available.

In several of these aforementioned studies, single modality therapy in the form of definitive radiotherapy was utilized and yielded disease-specific survivals similar to those seen with the combination of induction chemotherapy and radiation therapy.[3–9,13,25,42,43] Although the selected cohort of patients who received radiation therapy alone had less stage IV and node-positive patients, the contribution of chemotherapy to these larynx preservation protocols remains undetermined. While previous randomized prospective trials have not included a radiation therapy-only arm, an ongoing prospective randomized trial has included a radiation therapy-only arm, to address this question. This phase III trial has 3 treatment arms including: (1) radiotherapy alone, (2) sequential chemotherapy and radiotherapy and (3) concomitant chemotherapy and radiotherapy. Data from this study will help to further define the optimal treatment for patients with advanced larynx cancer. Additionally, 2 studies have recently been published which compared radiotherapy alone to concurrent chemotherapy (cisplatin/5-fluorouracil) and radiotherapy in patients with locoregionally-advanced squamous cell carcinoma of the head and neck.[44,45] In these studies, between 36 and 56 percent of patients had either laryngeal or hypopharyngeal primaries. In both studies, a statistically significant increase in 3-year relapse-free survival was seen in the concurrent chemo/RT arm as compared to the RT-alone arm (p < 0.004[44] and p < 0.03[45]).

The debate also continues regarding the optimal fractionation of radiation therapy, chemotherapeutic agents, and optimal timing of chemotherapy and radiation therapy (sequential vs. concomitant). Protocols with accelerated fractionation of radiotherapy and plans using concomitant chemotherapy and radiotherapy have been investigated. It has been postulated that part of the cause of increased locoregional failures seen with chemo/RT protocols result from an accelerated tumor cell repopulation during the prolonged course of treatment.[46,47] Clinical and experimental evidence suggest that tumor cell populations, after a lag period of several weeks, will decrease their doubling time and increase their rate of regrowth after the commencement of cytotoxic treatment, regardless of whether it is chemotherapy or radiation therapy.[46,47] A longer treatment time will therefore result in high rates of failure.[48]

In order to minimize these problems, investigators have evaluated accelerated radiotherapy regimens and concomitant chemo/RT protocols. In the past, accelerated (twice a day) courses of radiation therapy have improved 3-year local control of advanced laryngeal tumors (T3-4) from 26 to 59 percent (p < 0.0001).[48,49] These gains in local control are not accomplished without cost with regards to treatment related morbidity. In this study, although the larynx was anatomically preserved, its function was profoundly impaired in a subset of patients, and significant long-term treatment related morbidity was seen in one-quarter of patients. Additionally, all patients in this series undergoing salvage surgery after radiotherapy experienced major wound complications.[50] Ultimately a benefit in local or regional control or survival was not seen, although the power of this study was limited.

Another method of shortening treatment time, decreasing the effects of accelerated tumor cell repopulation and improving results involves the use of concomitant chemotherapy and radiation therapy. Prior studies using concomitant chemotherapy and radiation in advanced stage head and neck cancer have shown promising results with regard to locoregional control, organ preservation and survival.[51,52] Prospective randomized trials assessing the benefit of concomitant chemotherapy and radiation therapy as it applies to advanced stage laryngeal cancer, however, are limited. As mentioned earlier, a randomized prospective trial comparing sequential to concomitant chemotherapy and radiation therapy is currently underway.

Additionally, randomized prospective studies comparing sequential chemotherapy and radiation therapy to concomitant chemo/RT in patients with unresectable tumors of the head and neck have been reported.[27,53] While an improvement in locoregional control was seen in the concomitant arm in the larger study,[53] neither study showed a difference in overall survival.[27,53] At this time, neither accelerated fraction radiation therapy nor concomitant chemo/RT have conclusively demonstrated a benefit in treating advanced stage laryngeal cancer relative to induction chemotherapy followed by conventional fraction radiation therapy. For this reason, along with the potential for treatment related morbidity, it remains investigational at this time.

Finally, novel treatment strategies continue to evolve which intend to further improve the survival and functional outcome in patients with advanced cancer of the larynx. One such unique strategy utilizes the high-dose intra-arterial cisplatin with a systemic neutralizing agent along with conventional radiation therapy.[54] In this study, where the majority of patients had stage IV disease (86%) and clinically involved regional lymph nodes (79%), a major response rate was seen in 95 percent of patients. Nine of 10 patients retained their larynx and 2-year disease-specific survival was 76 percent. It should be noted that 3 of the 42 patients experienced central nervous system complications as a result of catherization of the carotid system. Nevertheless, this remains a promising option and a novel approach in the treatment of advanced laryngeal cancer.

CONCLUSION

The treatment of patients with advanced cancers of the larynx has changed dramatically over the last 2 decades. While anatomic preservation of the larynx can now be achieved in a large fraction of patients, overall survival remains unchanged. The continued optimization of multimodality treatment paradigms along with the incorporation of biological markers, novel treatment approaches, novel chemotherapeutic agents and innovative biologic and gene transfer techniques will hopefully further increase our ability to improve survival in these patients.

REFERENCES

1. Hoffman HT, Karnell LH, Funk GF, et al. The National Cancer Data Base report on cancer of the head and neck. Arch Otolaryngol Head Neck Surg 1998;124(9):951–62.
2. Shah JP, Karnell LH, Hoffman HT, et al. Patterns of care for cancer of the larynx in the United States. Arch Otolaryngol Head Neck Surg 1997;123(5):475–83.
3. Induction chemotherapy plus radiation compared with surgery plus radiation in patients with advanced laryngeal cancer. The Department of Veterans Affairs Laryngeal Cancer Study Group [see comments]. N Engl J Med 1991;324(24):1685–90.
4. Jacobs C, Goffinet DR, Goffinet L, et al. Chemotherapy as a substitute for surgery in the treatment of advanced resectable head and neck cancer. A report from the Northern California Oncology Group. Cancer 1987;60(6):1178–83.
5. Demard F, Chauvel P, Santini J, et al. Response to chemotherapy as justification for modification of the therapeutic strategy for pharyngolaryngeal carcinomas. Head Neck 1990;12(3):225–31.
6. Pfister DG, Strong E, Harrison L, et al. Larynx preservation with combined chemotherapy and radiation therapy in advanced but resectable head and neck cancer. J Clin Oncol 1991;9(5):850–9.
7. Karp DD, Vaughan CW, Carter R, et al. Larynx preservation using induction chemotherapy plus radiation therapy as an alternative to laryngectomy in advanced head and neck cancer. A long-term follow-up report. Am J Clin Oncol 1991;14(4):273–9.
8. Urba SG, Forastiere AA, Wolf GT, et al. Intensive induction chemotherapy and radiation for organ preservation in patients with advanced resectable head and neck carcinoma. J Clin Oncol 1994;12(5):946–53.
9. Clayman GL, Weber RS, Guillamondegui O, et al. Laryngeal preservation for advanced laryngeal and hypopharyngeal cancers. Arch Otolaryngol Head Neck Surg 1995;121(2):219–23.
10. Myers EN, Alvi A. Management of carcinoma of the supraglottic larynx: evolution, current concepts, and future trends. Laryngoscope 1996;106(5 Pt 1):559–67.
11. Nguyen TD, Malissard L, Theobald S, et al. Advanced carcinoma of the larynx: results of surgery and radiotherapy without induction chemotherapy (1980–1985): a multivariate analysis. Int J Radiat Oncol Biol Phys 1996;36(5):1013–8.
12. Kirchner JA, Owen JR. Five hundred cancers of the larynx and pyriform sinus. Results of treatment by radiation and surgery. Laryngoscope 1977;87(8):1288–303.
13. Harwood AR, Hawkins NV, Beale FA, et al. Management of advanced glottic cancer. A 10-year review of the Toronto experience. Int J Radiat Oncol Biol Phys 1979;5(6):899–904.
14. Harwood AR, Rawlinson E. The quality of life of patients following treatment for laryngeal cancer. Int J Radiat Oncol Biol Phys 1983;9(3):335–8.
15. Dahm JD, Sessions DG, Paniello RC, Harvey J. Primary subglottic cancer. Laryngoscope 1998;108(5):741–6.
16. Levendag P, Sessions R, Vikram B, et al. The problem of neck relapse in early stage supraglottic larynx cancer. Cancer 1989;63(2):345–8.
17. Meyer-Breiting E, Burkhardt A. Tumours of the larynx: Histopathology and clinical inferences. New York (NY): Springer-Verlag; 1988.
18. Oliver H. Beahrs OH. Manual for staging of cancer/ American Joint Commission on Cancer. Philadelphia (PA): JB Lippincott Co; 1997.
19. Reidenbach MM. The paraglottic space and transglottic cancer: anatomical considerations. Clin Anat 1996;9(4):244–51.
20. Cummings CW, Fredrickson JM, Harker LA, et al. Otolaryngology—head & neck surgery: St. Louis (MO): Mosby-Year Book, Inc.; 1998.
21. Som PM, Curtin HD. Head and neck imaging. St. Louis (MO): Mosby-Year Book, Inc.; 1996.

22. Landis SH, Murray T, Bolden S, Wingo PA. Cancer statistics, 1999 [see comments]. CA Cancer J Clin 1999;49(1): 8–31, 1.

23. Pfister D, Armstrong J, Strong E, et al. A matched pair analysis of cisplatin/5-fluorouracil versus other cisplatin based regimens as induction chemotherapy for larynx preservation treatment. Proceedings of the American Society of Clinical Oncology 1993;12:280.

24. Pfister D, Harrison L, Kraus D, et al. Larynx preservation: does induction cisplatin based chemotherapy compromise the delivery of concomitant chemotherapy with radiation therapy. Proceedings of the American Society of Clinical Oncology 1994;13:292.

25. Shirinian MH, Weber RS, Lippman SM, et al. Laryngeal preservation by induction chemotherapy plus radiotherapy in locally advanced head and neck cancer: the M. D. Anderson Cancer Center experience. Head Neck 1994; 16(1):39–44.

26. Harrison LB, Raben A, Pfister DG, et al. A prospective phase II trial of concomitant chemotherapy and radiotherapy with delayed accelerated fractionation in unresectable tumors of the head and neck. Head Neck 1998;20(6):497–503.

27. Pinnaro P, Cercato MC, Giannarelli D, et al. A randomized phase II study comparing sequential versus simultaneous chemo-radiotherapy in patients with unresectable locally advanced squamous cell cancer of the head and neck. Ann Oncol 1994;5(6):513–9.

28. Laccourreye H, Laccourreye O, Weinstein G, et al. Supracricoid laryngectomy with cricohyoidopexy: a partial laryngeal procedure for selected supraglottic and transglottic carcinomas. Laryngoscope 1990;100(7):735–41.

29. Laccourreye H, Menard M, Fabre A, et al. [Partial supracricoid laryngectomy. Techniques, indications and results]. Ann Otolaryngol Chir Cervicofac 1987;104(3):163–73.

30. Laccourreye O, Salzer SJ, Brasnu D, et al. Glottic carcinoma with a fixed true vocal cord: outcomes after neoadjuvant chemotherapy and supracricoid partial laryngectomy with cricohyoidoepiglottopexy. Otolaryngol Head Neck Surg 1996;114(3):400–6.

31. Pearson BW. Subtotal laryngectomy. Laryngoscope 1981; 91(11):1904–12.

32. Clark JR, Busse PM, Norris CM Jr, et al. Induction chemotherapy with cisplatin, fluorouracil, and high-dose leucovorin for squamous cell carcinoma of the head and neck: long-term results. J Clin Oncol 1997;15(9):3100–10.

33. Soylu L, Kiroglu M, Aydogan B, et al. Pharyngocutaneous fistula following laryngectomy. Head Neck 1998;20(1):22–5.

34. Shemen LJ, Spiro RH. Complications following laryngectomy. Head Neck Surg 1986;8(3):185–91.

35. Parikh SR, Irish JC, Curran AJ, et al. Pharyngocutaneous fistulae in laryngectomy patients: the Toronto Hospital experience. J Otolaryngol 1998;27(3):136–40.

36. Lazarus CL, Logemann JA, Pauloski BR, et al. Swallowing disorders in head and neck cancer patients treated with radiotherapy and adjuvant chemotherapy. Laryngoscope 1996;106(9 Pt 1):1157–66.

37. Terrell JE, Fisher SG, Wolf GT. Long-term quality of life after treatment of laryngeal cancer. The Veterans Affairs Laryngeal Cancer Study Group. Arch Otolaryngol Head Neck Surg 1998;124(9):964–71.

38. Maas A. A model for quality of life after laryngectomy. Soc Sci Med 1991;33(12):1373–7.

39. DeSanto LW, Olsen KD, Perry WC, et al. Quality of life after surgical treatment of cancer of the larynx. Ann Otol Rhinol Laryngol 1995;104(10 Pt 1):763–9.

40. Singer MI. Blom ED. Tracheoesophageal puncture: A surgical prosthetic method for post laryngectomy speech restoration. Third International Symposium on Plastic Reconstructive Surgery of the Head and Neck, 1979.

41. Yuen A, Medina JE, Goepfert H, Fletcher G. Management of stage T3 and T4 glottic carcinomas. Am J Surg 1984; 148(4):467–72.

42. Mendenhall WM, Parsons JT, Stringer SP, et al. Stage T3 squamous cell carcinoma of the glottic larynx: a comparison of laryngectomy and irradiation. Int J Radiat Oncol Biol Phys 1992;23(4):725–32.

43. Harwood AR, Beale FA, Cummings BJ, et al. Supraglottic laryngeal carcinoma: an analysis of dose-time-volume factors in 410 patients. Int J Radiat Oncol Biol Phys 1983;9(3):311–9.

44. Wendt TG, Grabenbauer GG, Rodel CM, et al. Simultaneous radiochemotherapy versus radiotherapy alone in advanced head and neck cancer: a randomized multicenter study. J Clin Oncol 1998;16(4):1318–24.

45. Adelstein DJ, Saxton JP, Lavertu P, et al. A phase III randomized trial comparing concurrent chemotherapy and radiotherapy with radiotherapy alone in resectable stage III and IV squamous cell head and neck cancer: preliminary results. Head Neck 1997;19(7):567–75.

46. Withers HR, Taylor JM, Maciejewski B. The hazard of accelerated tumor clonogen repopulation during radiotherapy. Acta Oncol 1988;27(2):131–46.

47. Bourhis J, Wilson G, Wibault P, et al. Rapid tumor cell proliferation after induction chemotherapy in oropharyngeal cancer. Laryngoscope 1994;104(4):468–72.

48. Fowler JF, Lindstrom MJ. Loss of local control with prolongation in radiotherapy. Int J Radiat Oncol Biol Phys 1992;23(2):457–67.

49. Wang CC, Blitzer PH, Suit HD. Twice-a-day radiation therapy for cancer of the head and neck. Cancer 1985;55(9 Suppl):2100–4.

50. Eisbruch A, Thornton AF, Urba S, et al. Chemotherapy followed by accelerated fractionated radiation for larynx preservation in patients with advanced laryngeal cancer. J Clin Oncol 1996;14(8):2322–30.

51. Adelstein DJ, Saxton JP, Van Kirk MA, et al. Continuous course radiation therapy and concurrent combination chemotherapy for squamous cell head and neck cancer. Am J Clin Oncol 1994;17(5):369–73.

52. Glicksman AS, Wanebo HJ, Slotman G, et al. Concurrent platinum-based chemotherapy and hyperfractionated radiotherapy with late intensification in advanced head and neck cancer. Int J Radiat Oncol Biol Phys 1997;39(3):721–9.

53. Taylor SG, Murthy AK, Vannetzel JM, et al. Randomized comparison of neoadjuvant cisplatin and fluorouracil infusion followed by radiation versus concomitant treatment in advanced head and neck cancer. J Clin Oncol 1994;12(2):385–95.

54. Robbins KT, Fontanesi J, Wong FS, et al. A novel organ preservation protocol for advanced carcinoma of the larynx and pharynx. Arch Otolaryngol Head Neck Surg 1996;122(8):853–7.

9

The Larynx: Early Stage Disease

WILLIAM M. LYDIATT, MD, FACS
DANIEL D. LYDIATT, DDS, MD, FACS

The American Cancer Society estimated that in the United States there would be 10,600 cases of laryngeal carcinoma diagnosed in 1999, and 4,200 deaths.[1] This accounts for 0.9 percent of cancers from all sites and 0.8 percent of all cancer deaths. Laryngeal carcinoma makes up 1 to 2 percent of cancers worldwide, and the incidence is increasing (Figure 9–1). Spain has one of the highest rates in the world with Basque and Navarra regions reaching a rate of 20 cases per 100,000 persons. There is also a very high incidence in France, Italy, and Poland.[2] Men are affected 4 times more frequently than women in the United States and up to 10 times more frequently in other countries.[2] This ratio is higher for glottic cancer than supraglottic. Recently, the ratio

has decreased in several countries, including the United States, and is thought to be due to an increased incidence in women. Age at diagnosis ranges from the second to tenth decade, with the seventh the most common. Over 90 percent of all laryngeal cancers are squamous cell carcinoma, which will be the primary focus of this chapter. Other histologic types include lymphoma, spindle-cell carcinoma, neuroendocrine carcinoma, minor salivary gland carcinomas, mucosal melanoma, and various sarcomas. Metastatic lesions and direct extension of thyroid carcinoma are other rare possibilities.

Early laryngeal carcinoma is an excellent paradigm for examining the role of competing and complementary therapies. While we will define early

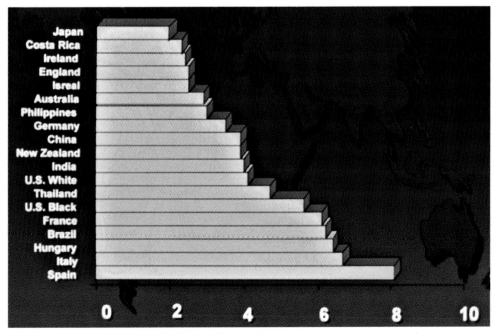

Figure 9–1. Bar graph of world incidence of laryngeal cancer.

stage as stage I (T1N0M0) and II (T2N0M0), there is controversy about what constitutes early laryngeal cancer. Ferlito and colleagues point out that early laryngeal cancer is more accurately called minimally invasive cancer without muscle or cartilage invasion.[3] Most T2 and many T1 cancers of the larynx have more extensive invasion. Stage I glottic cancer with only superficial invasion may be best treated endoscopically, while a bulky stage I lesion will require more aggressive resection or radiation therapy. We will discuss therapeutic options and their rationale with respect to stage and site later in this chapter.

ANATOMY

Embryologically, the larynx begins as a slit-like groove in the pharyngeal floor. Anterior to this slit the epiglottis develops from the ventral ends of the third and fourth branchial arches. Lateral to this swelling the arytenoids develop from the sixth branchial arches. The ventral fourth and fifth arches form the laryngeal cartilages.[4] The supraglottic larynx develops from the buccopharyngeal anlage and the glottic (each side unilaterally) and subglottic portions from the tracheopulmonary anlage.[5] The lymphatics follow this pattern with areas above the ventricle, (the junction of the supraglottic and glottic larynx), draining superiorly through the thyrohyoid membrane and areas below the ventricle draining inferiorly through the cricothyroid membrane to regional lymph nodes.[5,6] This embryology forms the rationale for the vertical partial laryngectomy, and the supraglottic horizontal laryngectomy. The need for bilateral neck dissections in most supraglottic laryngectomies is based on the midline development of the epiglottis and consequent bidirectional lymphatic flow. If neck dissection is indicated for a lesion of the true vocal cord, unilateral dissections are usually adequate based on this embryology. The marked edema seen after supraglottic laryngectomies for radiotherapy failure results in part from the lymphatic differences between the arytenoids (sixth arch) and the remainder of the larynx (fourth and fifth arches). Conversely, surgical salvage by a vertical partial laryngectomy after failed radiation therapy is possible due to this embryology.

The larynx is also divided roughly along embryologic lines for staging purposes (Figure 9–2). The supraglottic larynx is composed of the epiglottis, aryepiglottic folds, arytenoids, and false cords. The glottis consists of the true vocal cords, and the anterior and posterior commissures. The subglottis involves the remaining portion of the larynx to the inferior border of the cricoid cartilage.[7]

Intralaryngeal barriers to tumor spread consist of ligaments, fibroelastic membranes, and perichondrium.[5] The conus elasticus (triangular membrane) has a base that attaches to the thyroid and cricoid cartilages and an apex that attaches to the vocal process of the arytenoid and the vocal ligament. The conus elasticus, along with the vocal ligament, may limit early invasive cancer and make it amenable to conservative treatment.[5] The paraglottic space is the area between the conus elasticus and the perichondrium of the thyroid ala and is occupied by the thyroarytenoid muscle. This space may also limit spread of early true vocal cord cancer.

Whole organ sections have failed to consistently demonstrate a barrier between the supraglottic and glottic larynx. Cancer tends to remain confined

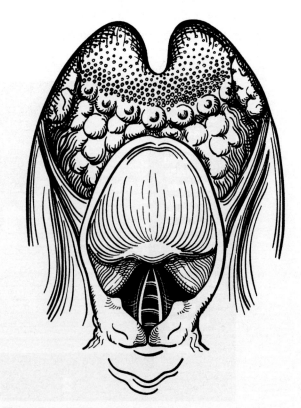

Figure 9–2. Anatomic diagram of the larynx.

between these embryologic areas. Cancer of the supraglottic larynx tends to invade anteriorly into the preepiglottic space, and recurrences after supraglottic laryngectomy are much more common at the base of the tongue than the anterior commissure.[5,8]

Diagnosis

Risk Factors

The most important risk factor for squamous cell carcinoma of the larynx is tobacco.[9–13] It is also the primary preventable risk factor, accounting for 90 to 95 percent of glottic and supraglottic carcinomas. Other factors increasing its carcinogenic potential are hand-rolled versus commercially produced cigarettes, black versus blond tobacco, number of cigarettes smoked per day, number of years of smoking, and constant daily smoking versus intermittent smoking.[2,14] Alcohol is a significant cofactor with tobacco in supraglottic carcinoma—creating a more than additive risk[13,15,16] (Figure 9–3). Alcohol is an independent risk factor as well.

A diet deficient in fruits and vegetables increases the risk of laryngeal cancer and, conversely, one rich in fruits and vegetables may be preventive.[17,18] Exactly which compounds in this diet are protective remain elusive. Occupational exposures which appear relevant include diesel fumes, mists containing sulfuric acid, coal dust, and machining fluids.[2,19,20] The role of human papillomavirus (HPV) as a causative agent in laryngeal cancer has been investigated, and while the type of cancer associated with HPV appears more aggressive and there is a higher than expected rate of paired incidence of cervical cancer, a causative role has not been proved.[21,22] Finally, family history appears to be relevant beyond the obvious link with smoking.[23]

Presenting Signs and Symptoms

The diagnosis of laryngeal carcinoma should be considered when hoarseness is present for more than 2 to 3 weeks. Glottic carcinoma presents early with hoarseness due to vocal cord involvement. Other signs of glottic carcinoma are hemoptysis, airway embarassment—especially with exertion, halitosis, and the so-called hot potato voice. Cancers of the supraglottic larynx generally present later due to a lack of symptoms in the early stages. Common signs and symptoms include difficulty swallowing, otalgia, and odynophagia. Following the history, the next step in diagnosis is a careful examination of the larynx by a qualified specialist.

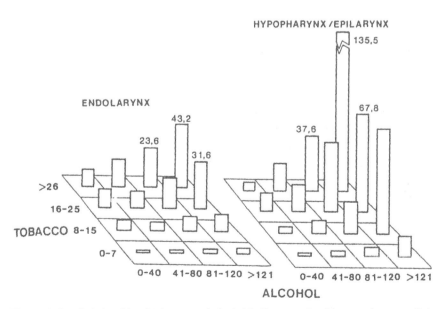

Figure 9–3. Relationship of tobacco and alcohol to the genesis of laryngeal cancer. Data from Tuyns AJ, et al. Cancer of the larynx/hypopharynx, tobacco and alcohol: IARC international case-control study in Turin and Varese (Italy), Saragoza and Navarra (Spain), Geneva (Switzerland) and Calvados (France). Int J Cancer 1988;41:483–91.

A laryngeal mirror provides an excellent panoramic view of the larynx, oropharynx and hypopharynx in most people. A flexible or rigid endoscope provides an alternate view which can be done in the office (Figures 9–4A and B). By having the patient perform a Valsalva's maneuver, the pyriform sinuses can often be examined in better detail. These studies may be videotaped for documentation or a more sophisticated stroboscopic examination can be done to document dysfunction from the tumor. The neck must be carefully palpated for adenopathy. Chest radiography and liver function tests will suffice for a metastatic survey in the absence of any systemic complaints. A computed tomography scan provides detail of cartilage invasion but should be reserved for those cases when management would be changed—

as in the case of large lesions or fixed vocal cords. Biopsies can be done in the clinic or in the operating room at the time of direct laryngoscopy.

TREATMENT GOALS AND TREATMENT ALTERNATIVES—THE ROLE OF MULTIDISCIPLINARY TREATMENT

The primary treatment objective is control of the cancer. Recent quality of life surveys highlight the importance of cure, since recurrence of cancer significantly reduces the quality of life. It appears that patients adapt quite well to lifestyle modifications resulting from treatment sequelae.[24] Important secondary objectives include a serviceable voice and the ability to swallow without aspiration.

Factors Affecting Choice of Treatment

Tumor Factors

Squamous cell carcinoma accounts for over 90 percent of all laryngeal cancers. Specific tumor parameters include mobility of the vocal cord, anterior commissure involvement, depth of cord invasion, extent of lesion on the cords (ie, T1A or T1B), and proximity of a supraglottic lesion to the anterior commissure (Table 9–1). Exophytic tumors tend to respond to radiation better than endophytic tumors and have a more favorable prognosis.[25] Poorly-differentiated tumors tend to metastasize more readily than well-differentiated tumors (see Table 9–1).

Patient Factors

Patient factors such as occupation, mental status, health status and wishes of the patient all guide treatment decisions. General medical condition is critical to the assessment process, particularly pulmonary function. Vocal quality may be more important to a person that uses their voice as part of their livelihood,

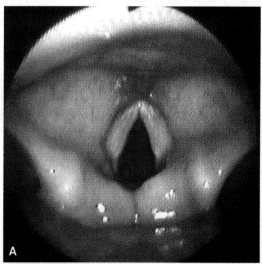

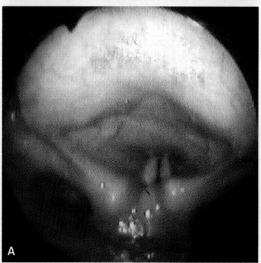

Figure 9–4. *A*, Larynx during quiet breathing. *B*, Larynx during phonation.

Table 9–1. TUMOR FACTORS
Mobility of vocal cord
Anterior commissure involvement
Depth of cord invasion
Extent of tumor involvement of cord
Proximity of supraglottic cancer to commissure
Differentiation of tumor
Exophytic vs. endophytic

Table 9–2. PATIENT FACTORS
Patient wishes
Medical condition
Occupation
Distance from treatment facilities
Mental status of patient

Table 9–3. HEALTH CARE FACTORS
Team approach to treatment
Skills of surgeon and radiation oncologist
Modern radiation facilities
Availability of support services

and radiation may provide a better voice than a partial laryngectomy. Treatment time of 6 to 7 weeks and long-distance travel to the radiation facility may cause the patient to favor surgery over radiation therapy (Table 9–2).

Health Care Factors

Optimal therapeutic skills in oncologic laryngeal surgery, radiotherapy with modern radiation facilities and medical oncology are essential. A multidisciplinary planning conference is also valuable in negating the natural bias shown to exist with physicians recommending the type of treatment they perform.[26] For stage I and II laryngeal cancer, multimodality therapy is usually not indicated and every effort should be made to use single modality treatment whenever possible. Support services for speech and swallowing therapy, dental oncology, psychosocial, emotional, occupational and vocational rehabilitation are also important to a comprehensive therapeutic team (Table 9–3).

Surgical Treatment

This chapter will discuss the most common approaches to stage I and II laryngeal cancers. Each procedure is predicated on an accurate evaluation to determine extent of disease. An exhaustive breakdown of each of the modifications on these standard operations is beyond the scope of this text.

Vertical Partial Laryngectomy

Cancers that arise on the true vocal cord with limited involvement of the anterior commissure (Figure 9–5) or arytenoid can be resected with a vertical partial laryngectomy. The majority of the ipsilateral thyroid cartilage, the true vocal cord, and portions of the subglottic mucosa and false vocal cord are removed (Figures 9–6 to 9–8). The strap muscles are closed over the defect and can be used to form a "pseudocord." A tracheotomy is generally left in place for 3 to 7 days. Anterior commissure involvement can be addressed using a

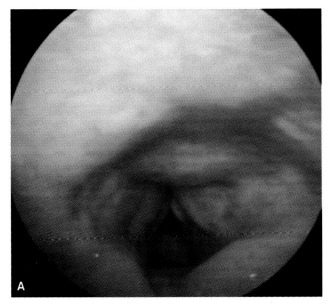
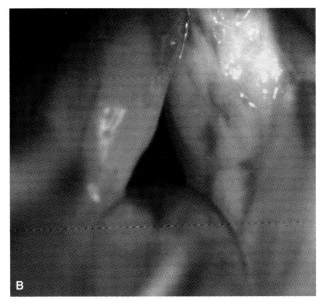

Figure 9–5. *A,* Clinical photo of glottic squamous cell carcinoma that had failed external beam radiation therapy. *B,* Endoscopic examination confirms the suitability of the lesion for vertical partial laryngectomy.

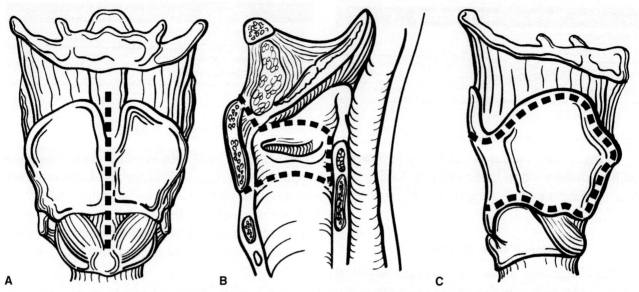

Figure 9–6. *A,* A midline thyrotomy is used to access the larynx when the anterior commissure is uninvolved by tumor. *B,* Cut section of the larynx demonstrating the extent of mucosal resection in a vertical partial laryngectomy. *C,* External view showing resection of the thyroid ala.

fronto-lateral partial laryngectomy. Voice quality and airway are not as reliable with this operation which extends the resection to the contralateral cord including the anterior commissure. Contraindications include tumor involvement of the posterior or interarytenoid area, subglottic extension of greater than 10 mm, and poor medical condition or pulmonary reserve.

Supraglottic Laryngectomy

A supraglottic laryngectomy removes the epiglottis, hyoid bone, thyrohyoid membrane, upper half of the thyroid cartilage and the supraglottic mucosa. The vallecula is transected superiorly, the ventricles inferiorly, and the aryepiglottic folds laterally (Figures 9–9 to 9–13). Thus most stage I and II tumors of the laryngeal surface of the epiglottis and false vocal cords can be removed. Margins are close, however, and it appears that 2 to 3 mm of normal mucosa inferiorly is adequate to prevent local recurrence.[27] Clo-

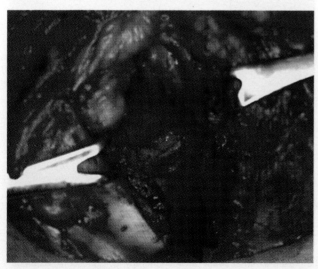

Figure 9–7. Surgical exposure for vertical partial laryngectomy.

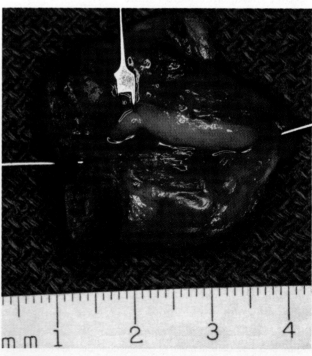

Figure 9–8. Vertical partial laryngectomy, excised specimen.

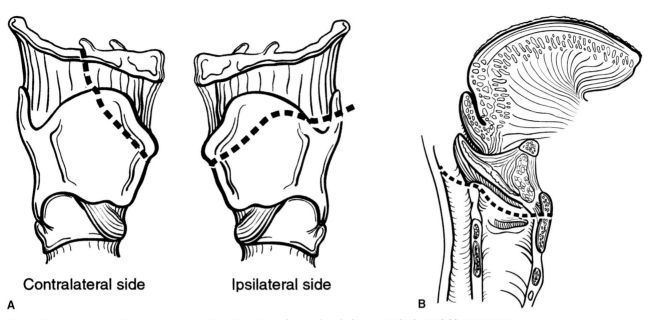

Contralateral side   **Ipsilateral side**

A   **B**

Figure 9–9. *A*, and *B*, Diagram demonstrating the extent of resection during supraglottic partial laryngectomy.

sure is performed by approximating the base of tongue to the lower half of the thyroid cartilage and closing the posterior false vocal cord mucosa to the medial pyriform sinus mucosa. A temporary tracheotomy is required. Elective neck dissections can be done without significant functional deficits occurring. Extensions of this operation have been proposed for more advanced disease. Relative contraindications include tumor involvement of the interarytenoid area, pyriform sinus apex, anterior commissure and preepiglottic space, and poor pulmonary reserve or general medical condition. Supraglottic laryngectomy is usually not appropriate in irradiation failures, although exceptions exist.[28]

Supracricoid Subtotal Laryngectomy with Cricohyoidoepiglottopexy

The supracricoid subtotal laryngectomy with cricohyoidoepiglottopexy (SCSL with CHEP) has gained

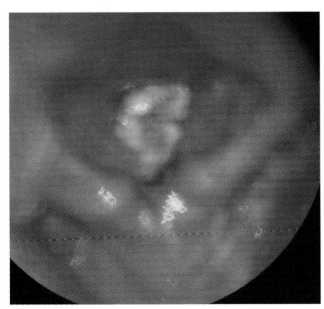

Figure 9–10. Clinical photo of supraglottic carcinoma.

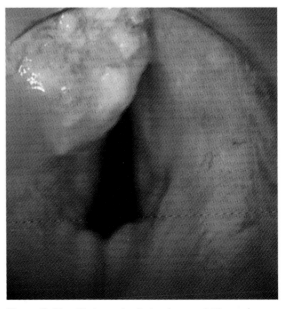

Figure 9–11. Endoscopic photo of supraglottic carcinoma.

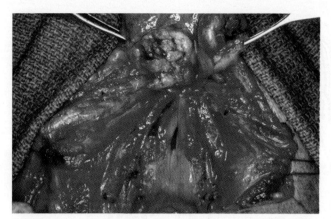

Figure 9–12.   Surgical exposure for supraglottic partial laryngectomy.

popularity over the past decade, particularly in Europe. SCSL involves removing the entire thyroid cartilage and paraglottic space followed by reconstruction using the epiglottis, hyoid bone, cricoid cartilage and tongue[29] (Figures 9–14 to 9–16). A temporary tracheotomy and feeding tube is required. SCSL has been advocated for T1B glottic carcinoma with or without anterior commissure involvement, T1A with anterior commissure involvement, T1 glottic carcinoma with associated areas of severe dysplasia, or unilateral or bilateral T2 glottic carcinoma. It can be extended to include the epiglottis as well. One arytenoid can be removed for a margin but the operation should not be used if the cord is fixed. Contraindications include poor pulmonary reserve, extensive anterior commissure involvement, and sub-

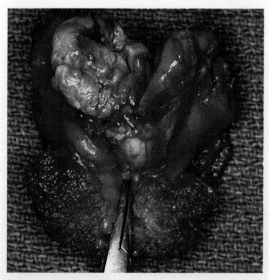

Figure 9–13.   Surgical specimen from supraglottic partial laryngectomy.

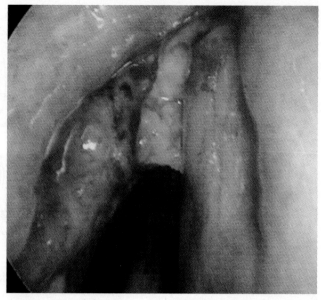

Figure 9–14.   Endoscopic view of tumor amenable to supracricoid subtotal laryngectomy.

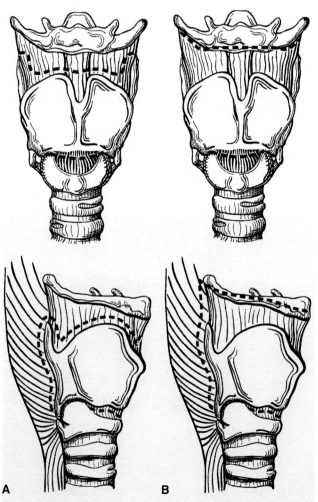

A   B

Figure 9–15.   *A,* and *B,* Diagram of supracricoid subtotal laryngectomies.

glottic extension below 10 mm. This procedure can be successfully performed after radiation failure.

Endoscopic Resection

Endoscopic management of premalignant, stage I and some stage II laryngeal carcinomas can be done using an operative microscope, appropriate laryngoscope and microlaryngoscopy instruments (Figure 9–17). The CO_2 laser can be easily attached to facilitate excision or ablation of appropriate lesions. Lesions that are on the suprahyoid epiglottis, aryepiglottic fold, true vocal cords, or other areas perpendicular to the laryngoscope are readily removed.[30] Surgery is performed as an outpatient procedure in most cases. Reports of endoscopic surgery for more extensive lesions have been reported but have not gained widespread popularity in the United States.[30,31]

Elective Neck Dissection

Elective treatment of cervical lymph node metastasis is generally recommended when the risk of occult disease is around 15 to 20 percent. Candela and colleagues demonstrated that the nodal groups at risk from laryngeal cancer are at levels II, III and IV.[32] Level I was rarely involved in isolation and level V was never involved alone. This tends to support the removal of levels II, III and IV, the so-called jugular node dissection or lateral neck dissection,

for elective neck treatment[33] (Figure 9–18). Spiro and colleagues concluded that this dissection should extend at least 2 cm lateral to the jugular vein to adequately sample the nodes at risk.[34]

Nonsurgical Treatment

Radiation is the primary nonsurgical treatment for stage I and II laryngeal cancer. Chemotherapy plays a very small role except in certain bulky T2 tumors which would require a total laryngectomy for resection. The role of combination therapy involving chemotherapy and radiation will be discussed extensively in the next chapter.

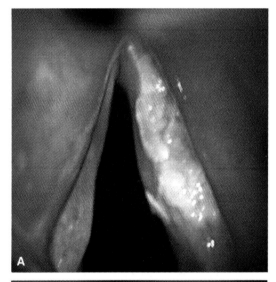

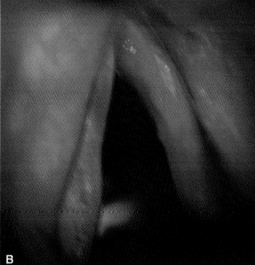

Figure 9–17.   *A,* Endoscopic view of a right-sided T1 vocal cord lesion amenable to endoscopic excision. *B,* Endoscopic view after resection of the lesion.

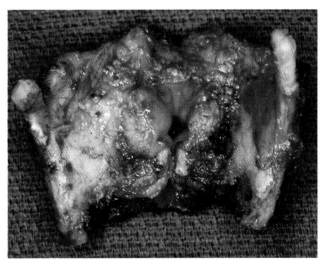

Figure 9–16.   Surgical specimen from supracricoid subtotal laryngectomy.

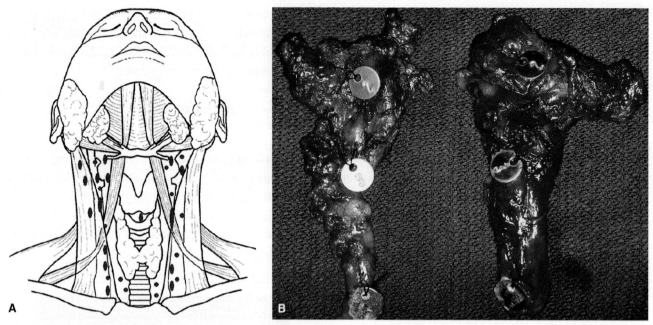

Figure 9–18. *A,* Bilateral jugular node dissection encompasses lymph nodes at levels II, III and IV. *B,* Lymph node bearing specimen from a bilateral jugular node dissection.

Sequelae, Complications and their Management

Conservation Laryngeal Surgery

Almost all patients who undergo a vertical partial laryngectomy will be decannulated and thus able to take all nutrition by mouth within the first month. Voice is generally adequate for lung powered conversation but has a breathy quality. Complications generally depend on the extent of surgical resection.[35] Acute complications include wound infection, fistula formation, and glottic incompetence with aspiration. Granulation formation may require repeat laser removal which can be performed as an outpatient procedure. Stenosis is a more difficult problem and may necessitate long-term tracheal cannulation.

Most patients will have an element of postoperative aspiration following supraglottic partial laryngectomy. The degree and severity generally relates to the extent of resection and the health of the patient. Aspiration pneumonia is infrequent, ranging from 1 to 8 percent, and rarely requires completion total laryngectomy.[36–39] Tracheotomy decannulation occurred at a median of 15 days following surgery in a study reported by Soo and colleagues.[37] Patients undergoing radiation therapy postoperatively required the tracheotomy longer in all studies. Wound complications ranged from 5 to 15 percent and consisted of wound infections and fistulae.[38,39] None required operative intervention. Voice quality is generally judged to be good but depends on whether postoperative radiation will be needed.

Endoscopic procedures tend to be less invasive and therefore have fewer complications. The risk of aspiration depends on the extent of tissue resection and the location of the tumor. Rarely a patient may require a tracheotomy. Most patients can begin oral feeding within several days. General anesthetic and dental complications are seen rarely.

Mendenhall and colleagues reported on a series of 129 patients undergoing radiation therapy for supraglottic cancer: 67 had T1 or T2 lesions, and severe complications were seen in 6 percent of cases.[40] Similar to surgical series, higher stage disease tended to have higher complication rates. Airway edema requiring permanent tracheotomy occurred in approximately 3 percent of cases.[40] Other potential but infrequent complications include cartilage necrosis, soft-tissue necrosis with potential bleeding and major artery rupture, aspiration pneumonia and dysphagia. Dysphagia, mucositis and xerostomia increase with the wider fields employed for supraglottic tumors.

Accelerated fractionation results in more acute side effects. The long-term side effects are less clear.

The major complication rates are similar between surgery and radiation therapy. Generally, surgery has more immediate complications while radiation has a combination of acute and chronic effects.

Rehabilitation and Quality of Life

The most important factors in determining good quality of life are control of the cancer and improved survival. Only treatments with equivalent survival should be compared. For stage I and II glottic cancer, surgery and radiation have equivalent local control and survival statistics. Recent studies tend to indicate that communication and swallowing disorders cause a reduction in quality of life.[41] De Graeff and colleagues demonstrated that a temporary deterioration in functioning occurred following radiation for laryngeal carcinoma and was worse for T2 patients than for T1.[42] Despite worsening sense of taste and smell, dry mouth and tenacious saliva, emotional functioning and mood were actually improved at 6 to 12 months following treatment. Coping mechanisms appear to play a role in this apparent paradox. Psychologic counseling may further augment these coping mechanisms.[43]

No prospective randomized trial exists comparing surgery and radiation therapy with respect to voice quality or quality of life. Isolated voice analysis tends to show approximately equivalent results for endoscopic treatment and radiation for superficial lesions. For more bulky disease, radiation appears to result in better voice quality than partial laryngeal surgery. Similar stage supraglottic cancers have more treatment related sequelae for all modalities. Swallowing disorders are more frequent following all treatments for supraglottic cancer than for glottic. No comparison between surgery and radiation exists with respect to swallowing disorders post-treatment. While communication skills are important to quality of life, a provocative study suggests that even total laryngectomy does not result in permanent reduction in quality of life, demonstrating the remarkable adaptability of our patients and the importance of rendering them disease free.[24]

OUTCOMES AND RESULTS OF TREATMENT

Carcinoma in Situ

Irradiation or microsurgical excision (with or without a laser) of localized lesions can provide local control rates of 50 to 90 percent[44-48] (Table 9–4). Murty and colleagues reported 75 percent local control with microsurgery.[44] Twenty-five percent of the patients formed a glottic primary and were subsequently managed with radiotherapy. One of these patients failed and died of local failure. Nguyen and colleagues employed both surgical excision and radiation therapy and found a 50 percent initial control with surgery and an overall control of 75 percent including reoperation.[45] Surgical failures were all salvaged with radiation. All patients treated with irradiation maintained local control. Overall, both groups had a 100 percent local control rate. Mahieu and colleagues reported a 97 percent local control rate using laser excision of carcinoma in situ (CIS) and T1A glottic cancer.[46] One patient was salvaged with irradiation alone and one also required a total laryngectomy. Laryngeal irradiation also gives excellent local control with results of 85 to 100 percent.[44,45,47] Anterior commissure involvement by carcinoma in situ is associated with a higher rate of transformation to invasive carcinoma although this may represent undetected disease extent.[48]

Table 9-4. TREATMENT COMPARISONS FOR CIS				
Type of Therapy	Initial Primary Control (%)	Overall Local Control (%)	Survival (%)	Larynx Intact (%)
Surgery	50–97	97–100	97–100	97–100
Radiation	85–100	97–100	95–100	85–100

Table 9–5. TREATMENT COMPARISON FOR T1 AND T2 GLOTTIC CARCINOMA				
Type of Therapy	Primary Local Control (%)	Overall Local Control (%)	Survival (%)	Larynx Intact (%)
Surgery	50–90	83–100	87–97	87–100
Radiation	70–85	85–95	85–95	87

Voice quality following surgical excision is somewhat dependent on the amount of tissue removed and is definitely related to the mechanism of phonation. Anterior commissure involvement and resection results in a worse vocal quality.[49] Generally, vocal quality is judged to be good in the majority of patients using either modality. Both modalities cause subsequent abnormalities seen by video stroboscopy. Sixty-eight percent of patients with microlaryngoscopy and laser resection had a normal strobe examination and 81 percent were judged to have a normal or near-normal voice.[45] Normal vocal quality was perceived in 75 percent of patients following radiation for carcinoma in situ of the glottis.[47] Abnormalities were described on complete voice analysis in maximum vocal intensity, dynamic vocal intensity range, jitter, and mean fundamental frequency.[50]

Outpatient surgery for in situ laryngeal disease costs approximately one-third as much as a course of radiation.[51] Even if more than one operation is required, surgical therapy is probably more cost effective. Since surgery can be repeated if necessary more readily than irradiation, it is our preferred option for most laryngeal carcinoma in situ.

Use of various chemotherapeutic options to cause regression of existing lesions and prevention of subsequent lesions is an attractive option. Currently, little evidence exists to make these a standard of care. We would encourage entering patients into protocols investigating this therapy.

Glottic Carcinoma

The overall survival of T1 and T2 glottic lesions is excellent (Table 9–5). Most deaths are due to comorbid disease or second primaries. We will therefore concentrate on local control and quality of voice in our analysis of the literature. The results for micro-excision of glottic carcinomas are excellent. Local control rates with or without use of the laser are 92 to 100 percent.[45,51,52] A substantial number of patients require re-excision, ranging from 10 percent to over 50 percent. The average number of procedures was 2 in a study by Myers et al.[51] Surgical salvage included partial and total laryngectomy or irradiation which improved local control to 97 to 100 percent. Voice preservation was achieved in 92 to 100 percent of patients as well.[45,51,52] Voice quality

following laser resection is comparable to radiation in selected cases.[53] Cordectomy, either open or endoscopic, also results in local control of 90 to 95 percent.[54] However, when a cordectomy is required, voice is poor and functional results are probably superior with radiotherapy.[55]

Results of partial laryngectomy for T1 and T2 glottic cancers demonstrate local control rates ranging from 83 to 90 percent.[37,53,56–59] Voice preservation occurred in approximately 88 to 95 percent of cases. However, vocal quality is inferior when compared to radiation.[37] Overall determinate survival at 5 years was 87 to 97 percent.[37,56–58] Soo and colleagues found that margin status and differentiation were the most important factors in predicting survival.[37] Others have found anterior commissure involvement to predict a worse local control and outcome.[56]

Radiation therapy resulted in local control rates of 85 to 100 percent for T1 and 70 to 85 percent for T2 lesions.[60–64] Surgical salvage involved both partial and total laryngectomy with overall voice preservation rates of approximately 87 percent.[64] Local control after surgical salvage was generally in the 85 to 95 percent range. Factors which influenced outcome were not consistent across all reports. Anterior commissure involvement was not consistently as important as an adverse factor. Use of 4MV or 6MV also did not appear significant.[62] Lower doses and longer treatment times were associated with local failure, however.[60,64,65] Hyperfractionation for certain T2 tumors may provide improved local control.[63,66] The use of re-irradiation has also been advocated by some for radiation failures.[67]

Vertical partial laryngectomy may remain an option following irradiation failure, thus preserving a lung powered voice.[68–70] We found complication rates are comparable to patients without a prior history of irradiation. We did not see an increase in

Table 9–6. TREATMENT COMPARISON FOR T1 AND T2 SUPRAGLOTTIC CARCINOMA				
Type of Therapy	Initial Local Control (%)	Overall Local Control (%)	Survival (%)	Larynx Intact (%)
Surgery	90–100	90–100	85–95	85–97
Radiation	58–85	82–96	76–90	77–96

length of hospitalization, time to decannulation or number of swallowing problems.[68] Supracricoid partial laryngectomy can also be performed following selected cases of irradiation failure.[71]

We prefer microsurgical removal for selected superficial lesions not involving cordectomy, due to the excellent local control, good voice quality and reduced expense. We treat most stage I and II glottic cancers with irradiation, preferring hyperfractionation for larger tumors and reserving surgical salvage for failures. In cases where the patient prefers surgery or cannot take time to travel for daily radiation treatments, or in selected cases of anterior commissure involvement, partial laryngectomy remains an excellent option.

Supraglottic Carcinoma

Results of surgical therapy for stage I and II lesions are sometimes difficult to interpret as most reports use T characterization rather than stage (Table 9–6). Neck control impacts survival in these patients and often is not adequately reported. Overall control rates are in the range of 70 to 85 percent using either surgery or radiation therapy.[8,40,72] Surgery tends to show better local control rates in general. Carl and colleagues reported a 58 percent 5-year local control rate for T1 supraglottic lesions using 4MV radiation with lateral opposed fields to a dose of 60 Gy.[73] This was improved to 82 percent with surgical salvage. The report of Spriano and colleagues illustrates a comparison between surgery and radiotherapy quite well.[36] Over a 10-year period, 166 cases of stage I and II supraglottic carcinoma were treated for cure. Sixty-six patients received conservation surgery and 100 received either conventional or hyperfractionated radiation therapy (median 67 Gy, range 64 Gy to 72 Gy). Surgery resulted in a local recurrence rate of 5 percent. This is comparable to other surgical series of early lesions with local failure rates of 0 to 10 percent.[74,75] On the other hand, a 23 percent local failure rate was observed with radiotherapy, but the data did suggest that hyperfractionation may yield results comparable to surgery. Ultimate local control after total laryngectomy was accomplished in all but one surgical patient and half of the irradiation failures giving a total of 98 percent and 89 percent local control for surgery and radiation, respectively. It must be pointed out that this is not a randomized trial and a probable bias exists against radiation therapy. Overall, voice preservation was 95 percent for surgery and 77 percent for radiation therapy. Disease-specific survival was 88 percent and 76 percent for surgery and irradiation, respectively. These findings are compatible with most reported series. Using radiation therapy, Mendenhall reported local control in 47 of 55 patients (85%) with T1 and T2 cancers.[40] More recent series of accelerated fractionation schemes suggest, however, that local control is improved over once-a-day fractionation. Nakfoor and colleagues reported local control rates of 96 percent and 85 percent for T1 and T2 supraglottic tumors.[76] They reported overall local control with surgical salvage as 96 percent and 93 percent with a voice preservation rate of 96 percent and 80 percent for T1 and T2 tumors, respectively.

In summary, it appears that surgery yields better local control and a higher rate of voice preservation in appropriately selected individuals. However, the quality of voice is generally inferior in patients requiring partial laryngectomy compared to radiotherapy. It must be emphasized that no prospective randomized trial exists. The role of accelerated fractionation is still evolving. Neck failure remains an ominous occurrence.

Elective Treatment of the Neck

For stage I and II glottic cancer, there is a very low risk of cervical lymph node metastasis. The rate of positivity ranges from 1 to 8 percent in most series.[77,78] Given this low rate of occult metastasis, there is little role for elective neck treatment either surgically or with radiation therapy.

On the other hand, neck relapse remains a significant cause of failure in patients with supraglottic cancer. The anatomy of the supraglottic larynx with its rich lymphatics, coupled with the difference in biologic behavior helps account for the high rate of cervical metastasis. Levendag and colleagues found a 35 percent rate of nodal disease either upon elective dissection or subsequent relapse in a series of stage I and II supraglottic cancers.[79] Gregor found that patients with lesions centrally located involving both sides of the supraglottis frequently had bilateral neck disease.[80] If the lesion was strictly on one side, no contralateral metastasis occurred. On the other hand, Weber and colleagues felt bilateral selective neck dissections improved regional control.[81] Both of the later 2 studies examined all stages, so extrapolation may be hazardous to early stage disease. Complications of bilateral selective neck dissection are not significantly increased over those of unilateral dissection.[38] Given the risk of disease and its morbidity, it appears that elective neck dissection is warranted when surgery is expected to be the only treatment. Bilateral lateral neck dissection should be considered for midline lesions and larger unilateral lesions.[36,81] Weber and colleagues did not show improved control by adding radiation therapy to patients with positive neck nodes. From studies of other sites, however, it appears that regional control can be achieved in the N0 neck using either radiation or neck dissection.[36,82] Elective treatment of the lymphatics at risk is warranted in most stage I and II supraglottic cancers. In general, the same modality chosen for the primary should be used to treat the neck. We feel postoperative radiation should be strongly considered for patients with multiple positive neck nodes, and/or extracapsular extension.[37]

REFERENCES

1. Greenlee RT, Hill-Harmon MB, Murray T, Thun M. Cancer statistics, 2001. CA Cancer J Clin 2001;51:15–36.
2. Cattaruzza MS, Maisonneuve P, Boyle P. Epidemiology of Laryngeal Cancer. Eur J Cancer 1996; 32B(5):293–305.
3. Ferlito A, Carbone A, DeSanto LW, et al. Early cancer of the larynx: the concept as defined by clinicians, pathologists, and biologists. Ann Otol Rhinol Laryngol 1996;105: 245–50.
4. Gray SW, Skandalakis JE. The larynx. In: Embryology for surgeons: The embryologic basis for the treatment of congenital defects. Philadelphia (PA): W.B. Saunders Co.; 1972. p.283–5.
5. Kirchner JA. Spread and barriers to spread of cancer within the larynx. In: Silver CE, editor. Laryngeal cancer. New York (NY): Thieme Medical Publishers; 1991. p.7.
6. Johner CM. The lymphatics of the larynx. Otolaryngol Clin North Am 1970;3:4439–50.
7. AJCC Cancer Staging Manual. 5th ed. Philadelphia (PA): Lippincott-Raven; 1997. p.41–3
8. Bocca E. Supraglottic cancer. Laryngoscope 1975;85:1318–26.
9. Parkin DM, Pisani P, Lopex AD, Masuyer E. At least one in seven cases of cancer is caused by smoking. Global estimates for 1985. Int J Cancer 1994;59(4):494–504.
10. Franceschi S, Talamini R, Barra S, et al. Smoking and drinking in relation to cancers of the oral cavity, pharynx, larynx, and esophagus in Northern Italy. Cancer Res 1990;50:6502–7.
11. Muscat JE, Wynder EL. Tobacco, alcohol, asbestos and occupational risk factors for laryngeal cancer. Cancer 1992; 69:2244–51.
12. Maier H, Gewelke U, Dietz A, Heller WD. Risk factors of cancer of the larynx: results of the Heidelberg case-control study. Otolaryngol Head Neck Surg 1992;107(4):577–82.
13. Maier H, Dietz A, Gewelke U, et al. Tobacco and alcohol and the risk of head and neck cancer. Clin Invest Med 1992;70(3-4):320–7.
14. La Vecchia C, Bidoli E, Barra S, et al. Types of cigarettes and cancers of the upper digestive and respiratory tract. Cancer Causes Control 1990;1:69–74.
15. Zatonski W, Becker H, Lissowska J, Wahrendorf J. Tobacco, alcohol and diet in the aetiology of laryngeal cancer: a population-based case-control study. Cancer Causes Control 1991;2:3–11.
16. Blot WJ. Alcohol and cancer. Cancer Res 1992; 52(7 Suppl): S2119–S123.
17. Boyle P, Macfarlane GJ, Zheng T, et al. Recent advances in epidemiology of head and neck cancer. Curr Opin Oncol 1992;4:471–7.
18. Guo X. A case-control study of the etiology of laryngeal cancer in Liaoning Province. Chung Hua Erh Pi Yen Hou Ko Tsa Chih 1993;28(4):219–21.
19. Sathiakumar N, Delzell E, Amoateng-Adjepong Y, et al. Epidemiologic evidence on the relationship between mists containing sulfuric acid and respiratory tract cancer. Crit Rev Toxicol 1997;27(3):233–51.
20. Eisen EA, Tolbert PE, Hallock MF, et al. Mortality studies of machining fluid exposure in the automobile industry. III: A case-control study of larynx cancer. Am J Ind Med 1994;26(2):185–202.
21. Clayman GL, Stewart MG, Weber RS, et al. Human papilloma virus in laryngeal and hypopharyngeal carcinomas. Relationship to survival. Arch Otolaryngol Head Neck Surg 1994;120:743–8.
22. Spitz MR, Sider JG, Schantz SP, Newell GR. Association between malignancies of the upper aerodigestive tract and uterine cervix. Head Neck 1992;14:347–51.
23. Foulkes WD, Brunet JS, Kowalski LP, et al. Family history of cancer is a risk factor for squamous cell carcinoma of the head and neck in Brazil: a case-control study. Int J Cancer 1995;63(6):769–73.
24. Deleyiannis FWB, Weymuller EA, Coltrera MD, Futran N. Quality of life after laryngectomy: are functional disabilities important? Head Neck 1999;21:319–24
25. Thompson LDR, Wenig BM, Heffner DK, Gnepp DR. Exophytic and papillary squamous cell carcinomas of the larynx: a clinicopathologic series of 104 cases. Otolaryngol Head Neck Surg 1999;120:718–24.
26. O'Sullivan B, Mackillop W, Gilbert R, et al. Controversies in the management of laryngeal cancer: results of an international survey of patterns of care. Radiother Oncol 1994;31(1):23–32.
27. Bocca E, Pignataro O, Mosciaro O. Supraglottic surgery of the larynx. Ann Otol Rhinol Laryngol 1968;77:1005–10.
28. Parsons JT, Mendenhall WM, Stringer SP, et al. Salvage surgery following radiation failure in squamous cell car-

cinoma of the supraglottic larynx. Int J Radiat Oncol Biol Phys 1995;32:605–9.

29. Laccourreye H, Laccourreye O, Weinstein G, et al. Supracricoid laryngectomy with cricohyoidoepiglottopexy: a partial laryngeal procedure for glottic carcinoma. Ann Otol Rhinol Laryngol 1990;99:421–6.

30. Zeitels SM, Koufman JA, Davis RK, Vaughn CW. Endoscopic treatment of supraglottic and hypopharynx cancer. Laryngoscope 1994;104:71–8.

31. Iro H, Waldfahrer F, Altendorf-Hofmann A, et al. Transoral laser surgery of supraglottic cancer: follow-up of 141 patients. Arch Otolaryngol Head Neck Surg 1998;124: 1245–50.

32. Candela FC, Shah J, Jaques DP, Shah JP. Patterns of cervical node metastases from squamous carcinoma of the larynx. Arch Otolaryngol Head Neck Surg 1990;116:432–5.

33. Robbins KT, Median JE, Wolfe GT, et al. Standardizing neck dissection terminology. Arch Otolaryngol Head Neck Surg 1991;117:601–5.

34. Spiro RH, Gallo O, Shah JP. Selective jugular node dissection in patients with squamous carcinoma of the larynx or pharynx. Am J Surg 1993;166:399–402.

35. Yonkers AJ. Complications of conservation surgery of the laryngopharynx. Laryngoscope 1983;93:314–7.

36. Spriano G, Antognoni P, Piantanida R, et al. Conservative management of T1–T2N0 supraglottic cancer: a retrospective study. Am J Otolaryngol 1997;18:299–305.

37. Soo KC, Shah JP, Gopinath KS, et al. Analysis of prognostic variables and results after supraglottic partial laryngectomy. Am J Surg 1988;156:301–5.

38. Weber PC, Johnson JT, Myers EN. Impact of bilateral neck dissection on recovery following supraglottic laryngectomy. Arch Otolaryngol Head Neck Surg 1993;11:61-4.

39. Lee NK, Goepfert H, Wendt CD. Supraglottic laryngectomy for intermediate-stage cancer: U.T.M.D. Anderson Cancer Center experience with combined therapy. Laryngoscope 1990;100:831–6.

40. Mendenhall WM, Parsons JT, Stringer SP, et al. Carcinoma of the supraglottic larynx: a basis for comparing the results of radiotherapy and surgery. Head Neck 1990;12:204–9.

41. McDonough EM, Varvares MA, Dunphy FR, et al. Changes in quality of life scores in a population of patients treated for squamous cell carcinoma of the head and neck. Head Neck 1996;18:487–93.

42. De Graeff A, de Leeuw RJ, Ros WJG, et al. A prospective study on quality of life of laryngeal cancer patients treated with radiotherapy. Head Neck 1999;21:291–6.

43. Hammerlid E, Persson LO, Sullivan M, Westin T. Quality of life effects of psychosocial intervention in patients with head and neck cancer. Otolaryngol Head Neck Surg 1999;120:507–16.

44. Murty GE, Diver JP, Bradley PJ. Carcinoma in situ of the glottis: radiotherapy or excision biopsy? Ann Otol Rhinol Laryngol 1993;102:592–5.

45. Nguyen C, Naghibzadeh B, Black MJ, et al. Carcinoma in situ of the glottic larynx: excision or irradiation? Head Neck 1996;18:225–8.

46. Mahieu HF, Patel P, Annyas AA, van der Laan T. Carbon dioxide laser vaporization in early glottic carcinoma. Arch Otolaryngol Head Neck Surg 1994;120:383–7.

47. Smitt MC, Goffinet DR. Radiotherapy for carcinoma in situ of the glottic larynx. Int J Radiat Oncol Biol Phys 1993;28:251–5.

48. Myssiorek D, Vambutas A, Abramson AL. Carcinoma in situ of the glottic larynx. Laryngoscope 1994;104:463–7.

49. Sittel C, Eckel HE, Eschenburg C. Phonatory results after laser surgery for glottic carcinoma. Otolaryngol Head Neck Surg 1998;119:418–24.

50. Dagli AS, Mahieu HF, Festen JM. Quantitative analysis of voice quality in early glottic laryngeal carcinomas treated with radiotherapy. Eur Arch Otorhinolaryngol 1997;254:78–80.

51. Myers EN, Wagner RL, Johnson JT. Microlaryngoscopic surgery for T1 glottic lesions: a cost-effective option. Ann Otol Rhinol Laryngol 1994;103:28–30.

52. Thomas JV, Olsen KD, Neel HB III, et al. Recurrences after endoscopic management of early (T1) glottic carcinoma. Laryngoscope 1994;104:1099–104.

53. McGuirt WF, Blalock D, Koufman JA, et al. Comparative voice results after laser resection or irradiation of T1 vocal cord carcinoma. Arch Otolaryngol Head Neck Surg 1994;120:951–5.

54. Olsen KD, Thomas JV, DeSanto LW, Suman VJ. Indications and results of cordectomy for early glottic carcinoma. Otolaryngol Head Neck Surg 1993;108:277–82.

55. Rydell R, Schalen L, Fex S, Elner A. Voice evaluation before and after laser excision vs. radiotherapy of T1A glottic carcinoma. Acta Otolaryngol Stockh 1995;115:560–5.

56. Rucci L, Gallo O, Fini-Storchi O. Glottic cancer involving anterior commissure: surgery vs. radiotherapy. Head Neck 1991;13:403–10.

57. Johnson JT, Myers EN, Hao SP, Wagner RL. Outcome of open surgical therapy for glottic carcinoma. Ann Otol Rhinol Laryngol 1993;102:752–5.

58. Kaiser TN, Sessions DG, Harvey JE. Natural history of treated T1N0 squamous carcinoma of the glottis. Ann Otol Rhinol Laryngol 1989;98:217–9.

59. Ton-Van J, Lefebvre JL, Stern JC, et al. Comparison of surgery and radiotherapy in T1 and T2 glottic carcinomas. Am J Surg 1991;162:337–40.

60. Franchin G, Minatel E, Gobitti C, et al. Radiation treatment of glottic squamous cell carcinoma stage I and II: analysis of factors affecting prognosis. Int J Radiat Oncol Biol Phys 1998;40:541–8.

61. Le QTX, Fu KK, Droll S, et al. Influence of fraction size, total dose, and overall time on local control of T1–T2 glottic carcinoma. Int J Radiat Oncol Biol Phys 1997;39:115–26.

62. Foote RL, Grado GL, Buskirk SJ, et al. Radiation therapy for glottic cancer using 6-MV Photons. Cancer 1996;77:381–6.

63. Fein DA, Mendenhall WM, Parsons JT, Million RR. T1T2 squamous cell carcinoma of the glottic larynx treated with radiotherapy: a multivariate analysis of variables potentially influencing local control. Int J Radiat Oncol Biol Phys 1993;25:605–11.

64. Burke LS, Greven KM, McGuirt WT, et al. Definitive radiotherapy for early glottic carcinoma: prognostic factors and implications for treatment. Int J Radiat Oncol Biol Phys 1997;38:37–42.

65. Barton MB, Morgan G, Smee R, et al. Does waiting time affect the outcome of larynx cancer treated by radiotherapy? Radiother Oncol 1997;44:137–41.

66. Spector JG, Sessions DG, Chao KS, et al. Management of stage II (T2N0M0) glottic carcinoma by radiotherapy and conservation surgery. Head Neck 1999;21:116–23.

67. Wang CC, McIntyre J. Re-irradiation of laryngeal carcinoma—techniques and results. Int J Radiat Oncol Biol Phys 1993;26:783–5.

68. Lydiatt WM, Shah JP, Lydiatt KM. Conservation surgery for recurrent carcinoma of the glottic larynx. Am J Surg 1996;172:662–4.

69. DelGaudio JM, Fleming DJ, Esclamado RM, et al. Hemilaryngectomy for glottic carcinoma after radiation therapy failure. Arch Otolaryngol Head Neck Surg 1994;120:959–63.

70. Lavey RS, Calcaterra TC. Partial laryngectomy for glottic cancer after high-dose radiotherapy. Am J Surg 1991;162:341–4.

71. Laccourreye O, Weinstein G, Naudo P, et al. Supracricoid partial laryngectomy after failed laryngeal radiation therapy. Laryngoscope 1996;106:495–8.

72. Ogura JH, Sessions DG, Spector GJ. Conservation surgery for epidermoid carcinoma of the supraglottic larynx. Laryngoscope 1975;85:1808–18.

73. Carl J, Andersen LJ, Pedersen M, Greisen O. Prognostic factors of local control after radiotherapy in T1 glottic and supraglottic carcinoma of the larynx. Radiother Oncol 1996;39:229–33.

74. Burstein FD, Calcaterra TC. Supraglottic laryngectomy: series report and analysis of results. Laryngoscope 1985;95:833–6.

75. DeSanto LW. Early supraglottic cancer. Ann Otol Rhinol Laryngol 1990;99:593–7.

76. Nakfoor BM, Spiro IJ, Wang CC, et al. Results of accelerated radiotherapy for supraglottic carcinoma: a Massachusetts General Hospital and Massachusetts Eye and Ear Infirmary experience. Head Neck 1998;20:379–84.

77. Daly CJ, Strong EW. Carcinoma of the glottic larynx. Am J Surg 1975;130:489–93.

78. Hawkins NV. The treatment of glottic carcinoma: an analysis of 800 cases. Laryngoscope 1975;85:1485–93.

79. Levendag P, Sessions R, Vikram B, et al. The problem of neck relapse in early stage supraglottic larynx cancer. Cancer 1989;63:345–8.

80. Gregor RT, Oei SS, Hilgers FJM, et al. Management of cervical metastases in supraglottic cancer. Ann Otol Rhinol Laryngol 1996;105:845–50.

81. Weber PC, Johnson JT, Myers EN. The impact of bilateral neck dissection on pattern of recurrence and survival in supraglottic carcinoma. Arch Otolaryngol Head Neck Surg 1994;120:703–6.

82. Chow JM, Levin BC, Krivit JS, Applebaum EL. Radiotherapy or surgery for subclinical cervical node metastases. Arch Otolaryngol Head Neck Surg 1989;115:981–4.

83. Tuyns AJ, Esteve J, Raymond L, et al. Cancer of the larynx/hypopharynx, tobacco and alcohol: IARC international case-control study in Turin and Varese (Italy), Saragoza and Navarra (Spain), Geneva (Switzerland) and Calvados (France). Int J Cancer 1988;41:483–91.

10

Cancer of the Hypopharynx and Cervical Esophagus

DANIEL J. KELLEY, MD

The management of malignant neoplasms of the hypopharynx and cervical esophagus remains difficult despite recent advances in surgical techniques as well as multidisciplinary treatment programs. Many patients present at a later age with advanced disease due to the occult nature of associated symptoms. The disease process and treatment often affect adjacent structures, such as the larynx. Regardless of the type of therapy employed, high recurrence rates, poor survival, and significant alterations in speech and swallowing function are a common experience for patients with malignancies in these anatomic sites. Despite these frustrations, patients are potentially curable and should be offered regimens that carefully consider morbidity and outcome within the context of the patient's overall medical condition.

ANATOMY

Malignant neoplasms of the hypopharynx and cervical esophagus are often discussed within the same context because of their anatomic proximity and similar clinical behavior. The pharynx is a muscular tube that extends from the base of the skull to the esophagus.[1] It is arbitrarily divided into the nasopharynx, oropharynx and hypopharynx based on anatomic landmarks, although it is a continuous structure. The hypopharynx extends from the floor of the vallecula to the inferior border of the cricoid cartilage and is intimately associated with the larynx. It is continous with the oropharynx superiorly and the cervical esophagus inferiorly.

Within the hypopharynx, there are three anatomic subsites which are used to assess tumor stage. The *pyriform sinus* extends from the pharyngoepiglottic fold to the upper end of the esophagus at the lower border of the cricoid cartilage.[2] The medial extent of the pyriform sinus includes the aryepiglottic folds, arytenoid, and cricoid cartilages and its lateral border is the inner surface of the thyroid cartilage.[2] The *post-cricoid region* extends from the level of the arytenoid cartilages and connecting folds to the inferior border of the cricoid cartilage. Finally, the *posterior pharyngeal wall* is bounded superiorly by the floor of the vallecula superiorly and inferiorly by the inferior border of the cricoid cartilage.[2]

The walls of the pharynx consist of five layers from medial to lateral: mucosa, submucosa, pharyngobasilar fascia, muscular layer, and buccopharyngeal fascia.[1] The *mucous membrane* consists of columnar epithelium and is ciliated in some areas.[1] The *submucosa* contains many small veins forming a venous plexus, mucous and minor salivary glands, and lymphoid tissue.[1] The *pharyngobasilar fascia* is attached superiorly to the skull base and fills the gaps between constrictor muscles within the pharynx.[1] The muscular layer at the level of the hypopharynx consists of the *inferior constrictor*, while the middle and superior constrictor form the more superior aspects of the pharynx. Finally, the *buccopharyngeal fascia* forms the outer layer of the pharynx.[1] It is continuous with the visceral fascia of the esophagus and acts as the anterior boundary of the retropharyngeal space.[1]

The blood supply to the hypopharynx includes the *ascending pharyngeal* branch of the external carotid artery, the *ascending palatine and tonsillar* branches of the facial artery (external carotid artery) and the *descending pharyngeal and palatine* branches of the internal maxillary artery (external carotid artery).[1] A plexus of veins located adjacent to the pharyngobasilar fascia drains into the internal jugular vein from the hypopharynx.[1] Lymphatic fluid from the hypopharynx drains into retropharyngeal, jugular, and deep cervical lymph nodes.[1] The pharyngeal branch of the vagus nerve provides motor innervation and the glossopharyngeal nerve provides sensory perception of the hypopharynx. Branches of the superior cervical sympathetic ganglion combine with branches of the glossopharyngeal and vagus nerve to form the *pharyngeal plexus*, which provides additional innervation to the hypopharynx.

The esophagus is a mucosa-lined muscular tube that serves as a conduit between the pharynx and the stomach. For the purposes of classification, staging, and reporting of cancer cases, it is divided into the following subsites: cervical, upper thoracic, mid-thoracic, and lower thoracic.[2] Approximately 5 percent of cases of esophageal carcinoma arise within the cervical esophagus.[3] The cervical esophagus extends from the inferior border of the cricoid cartilage to the thoracic inlet.[2] The wall of the esophagus is comprised of an inner mucosa of squamous epithelium, a prominent submucosa, a muscular layer and an adventitia without serosa.[2,4] The submucosa contains mucous glands, blood and lymphatic vessels, and a plexus of nerves.[4] The muscular layer contains an inner circular layer surrounded by an outer longitudinal layer.[4] Although the lower two-thirds of the esophagus is composed of smooth muscle, the most proximal end is exclusively striated and the remainder is mixed.[5]

The blood supply to the cervical esophagus comes from the inferior thyroid arteries. Branches of the thoracic aorta and bronchial arteries supply the thoracic portion. The cervical esophagus is innervated by cranial nerves IX and X, the cranial root of the spinal accessory nerve as well as sympathetic and parasympathetic fibers.[4] The recurrent laryngeal nerve innervates the upper cervical esophageal muscles and contributes to the innervation of the cricopharyngeus muscle.[6] As many as 8 to 14

branches of the recurrent laryngeal nerve are distributed along the esophagus and trachea.[7] Lymphatics from the submucosa drain into paratracheal lower deep cervical and superior mediastinal lymph nodes.

The *upper esophageal sphincter* (UES) is located at the junction of the hypopharynx and cervical esophagus. It is composed of three muscles: inferior pharyngeal constrictor (IPC), cricopharyngeus (CP) and cervical esophagus (CE).[6] The CP is strategically located between the pharynx and esophagus and is responsible for the high-pressure zone of the UES.[8] All three muscles contract to maintain tone in the UES, but only the CP relaxes in response to physiologic stimulus.[9] These muscles also differ based on the pattern of motor end plates, proportion of fast- and slow-twitch muscle fibers, and their innervation. These differences suggest different roles during swallowing. The physiologic low-pressure zone of the cervical esophagus is composed of equal amounts of striated and smooth muscle, and is located about 5 cm from the proximal portion of the cricopharyngeus muscle.[5] Esophageal distension, pharyngeal pressure and inflation of the lungs contract the CP and UES via vago-vagal and glossopharyngo-vagal reflexes.[9] The UES or CP also contracts with arousal or with changes in posture.[9] These reflexes, along with the elastic properties of the CP, contribute to the generation of tone in the CP and UES.

DIAGNOSIS

Risk factors for the development of hypopharyngeal and cervical esophageal carcinoma include chronic alcohol and tobacco use, older age, geographic location, and family history of upper aerodigestive tract cancers.[10] Environmental exposure to polycyclic aromatic hydrocarbons, asbestos, and welding fumes may increase the risk of pharyngeal cancer.[11] Nutritional deficiencies and infectious agents (especially papillomavirus and fungi) also play a significant role.[10] Chronic irritation of the esophagus appears to participate in the process of carcinogenesis, particularly in patients with thermal and/or mechanical injury, achalasia, esophageal diverticulum, chronic lye stricture, or who have undergone radiation therapy.[10] Plummer-Vinson syndrome, characterized by dysphagia, iron-deficiency anemia and esophageal webs, as well as celiac disease, tylosis and scleroderma are associated with hypopharynx and cervical esophagus cancer.[12]

The principal signs and symptoms of carcinoma of the hypopharynx and cervical esophagus are dysphagia, hoarseness, odynophagia, neck mass and weight loss. Patients are typically older and may also complain of unexplained oropharyngeal bleeding, hemoptysis or hematemesis. Referred otalgia, mediated via the tympanic branch of the glossopharyngeal nerve (Jacobson's nerve), is a frequent presenting complaint.[13] Of these symptoms, the most frequent is odynophagia in over half of patients.[13] Dysphagia may be the first sign of recurrence and can precede clinically detectable recurrent tumors by several months.[14] The most common site of origin of malignancies within the hypopharynx is the pyriform sinus (Figure 10–1).[13] Seventy percent of patients either present with or develop neck metastases during their course of treatment.[15] Tumors have extended beyond the hypopharynx in the majority of patients at initial presentation (Figure 10–2).[13] The hypopharynx and cervical esophagus are also common occult primary sites in patients with a diagnosis of metastatic squamous carcinoma of the neck (excluding the supraclavicular fossa) from an occult primary tumor.

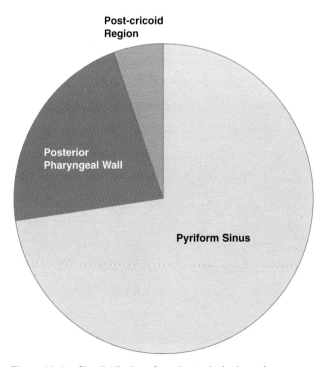

Figure 10–1. Site distribution of carcinoma in the hypopharynx.

Patients who are referred for evaluation of these symptoms require a complete medical history and careful physical examination. A thorough head and neck examination is critical to accurate assessment and staging. Most patients can be examined with a flexible laryngoscope under topical anesthesia (Figure 10–3 and 10–4). The extent of disease at the primary site, the status of lymph nodes in the neck, and evaluation for metastatic disease are vital to appropriate treatment planning. Endoscopic examination of the primary site under anesthesia with biopsy remains the definitive procedure to establish the diagnosis and accurately assess the primary tumor.

The most common histology in patients with hypopharynx and cervical esophagus cancer is squamous cell carcinoma. The physical appearance of these lesions can be confused with benign lesions, such as necrotizing sialometaplasia and ectopic gastric mucosa. Other less common histologies include neuroendocrine carcinomas, extrapulmonary bronchogenic carcinoma, typical and atypical carcinoid tumors, adenocarcinoma and adenosquamous carcinoma, basosquamous cell carcinoma, and lymphoepithelioma. Invasion of the aerodigestive tract by papillary adenocarcinoma of the thyroid occurs in 1 to 6.5 percent of cases and may manifest as a hypopharyngeal or cervical esophageal lesion.[16]

The indications for routine oral panendoscopy for the detection of second primary malignancies shows a significant geographic variation which is not based on differences in patient or tumor characteristics.[17] There is substantial disagreement in the literature about the value of endoscopic screening for synchronous tumors. The incidence of second primary malignancy of the upper aerodigestive tract varies from 3 percent to 15 percent, and the majority of tumors are detected within 2 years of initial presentation.[18] Second primary malignancies are more common in patients with hypopharynx and esophageal carcinoma relative to other head and neck sites.[18] A higher detection rate is reported for patients undergoing routine panendoscopy.[18] Others recommend routine interval endoscopic intervention within 2 years of treatment for optimum detection of second primary cancers. Critics of routine screening esophagoscopy and bronchoscopy point out the low yield, potential for increased morbidity, questionable

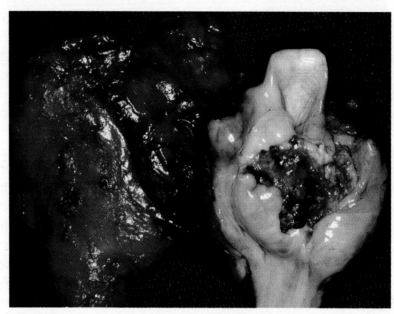

Figure 10–2.   Squamous cell carcinoma of the postcricoid region.

impact on expected survival and outcome and high cost in support of their position.[19] Therefore, the decision regarding routine panendoscopy in the evaluation of hypopharynx and cervical esophagus cancer is currently left to the discretion of the clinician.

The combination of clinical exam and computed tomography (CT) scan is more accurate than physical exam alone in the evaluation of the primary site and neck with tumors of the hypopharynx (Figure 10–5).[20] Open neck exploration is superior to CT when evaluating pre-vertebral muscle invasion by squamous cell carcinoma.[21] Of the radiographic criteria used to evaluate laryngeal involvement, sclerosis of the thyroid cartilage is the most sensitive and extralaryngeal tumor and erosion is the most specific.[22] Computed tomography and magnetic resonance

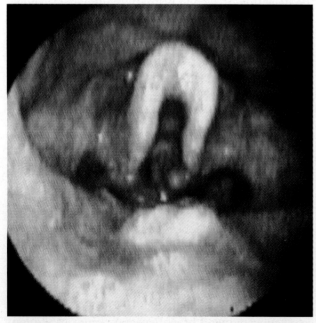

Figure 10–3.   Fiberoptic endoscopic appearance of a carcinoma of the posterior phyaryngeal wall.

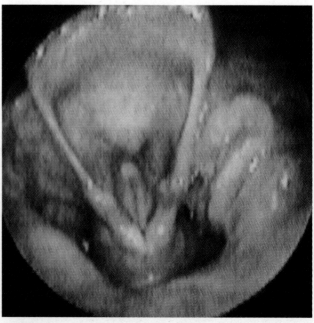

Figure 10–4.   Flexible endoscopic appearance of a carcinoma of the pyriform sinus.

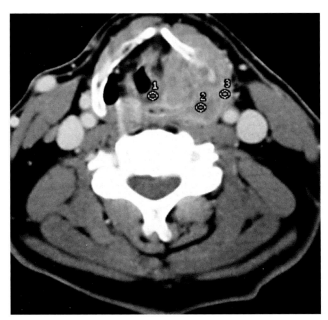

Figure 10–5. CT scan demonstrating invasion of the thyroid cartilage from a carcinoma of the left pyriform sinus.

imaging (MRI) are comparable in the radiologic evaluation of the neck for regional lymph node metastases relative to clinical exam.[23] Diagnostic imaging can also provide information about submucous tumor extension and cartilage involvement, leading to upstaging in many cases. MRI tends to be superior to CT in predicting tumor invasion and is valuable in the selection of candidates for conservation surgery.[24] Any patient considered for chemoradiation protocols should undergo baseline CT as lesions that are reduced by 50 percent or less at 4-month follow-up CT are highly suspicious for treatment failure.[25]

Patients who present at an advanced stage are at increased risk for distant metastases. The hypopharynx has the highest incidence of distant metastases (60%) relative to other head and neck sites. The lung is the most common site of distant metastases (80%), followed by mediastinal nodes (34%), liver (31%), and bone (31%).[26] The standard initial evaluation for distant metastases includes a chest radiograph and serum chemistries. Chest radiographs have an approximate sensitivity and specificity of 50 percent and 94 percent, respectively, for the detection of pulmonary metastases.[27] Elevated serum levels of alkaline phosphatase are highly specific for the presence of bone metastases, but the sensitivity is low (20%).[27] Although serum liver function tests assess hepatic function, abnormal values are found in almost half of patients with head and neck cancer, due to chronic alcohol use, and therefore are of little value in identifying patients with liver metastases during initial assessment.[28] Moderate elevation of liver function tests does not always require further investigation to exclude hepatic metastases.[28] In general, a chest CT should be obtained with an abnormal chest x-ray, a bone scan in the event of an elevated alkaline phosphatase or patient symptoms, and either an ultrasound or CT/MRI scan of the liver when significant elevation of liver function tests is present, depending on tumor stage and associated co-morbidities.[27]

Positron emission tomography (PET) is a new imaging technique which provides absolute and comparable quantitative data on tumor metabolism before and after chemotherapy. Radiolabeled fluorodeoxyglucose (FDG) is used to measure metabolic activity. As tumor cells consume more glucose relative to surrounding normal cells, a difference in signal intensity can be identified. The presence of PET activity correlates with pathologic findings in patients with head and neck cancer.[29] Elevated or rising PET activity after radiation therapy strongly suggests persistent or recurrent disease that may not be detected by CT or MRI. Patients with hypopharynx or cervical esophagus cancer who are candidates for chemoradiation protocols should undergo PET scans as part of their preoperative evaluation.

Although gender and performance status do not correlate with treatment outcome, certain clinical and histologic parameters have prognostic implications for patients with hypopharyngeal or cervical esophageal squamous cell carcinoma. Perineural invasion, vascular invasion, positive nodal status, extracapsular spread, contralateral, bilateral or fixed nodes, level IV to V positive nodes, and N2 disease are all significant predictors of lower survival, higher incidence of neck recurrences, greater risk of distant metastases, and poorer outcome.[30] Cervical esophageal carcinomas are notorious for extensive submucosal spread, increasing the risk of positive margins following resection. Disease extension outside the cervical esophagus is present in more than 75 percent of patients.[31] Tracheal invasion and vocal cord paralysis occur in up to one-third of patients and is associated with significantly decreased survival.[31]

TREATMENT GOALS AND ALTERNATIVES

The goals of treatment for this patient population are: (1) cure with preservation of function or (2) palliation with minimal morbidity. As a general rule, surgery followed by irradiation is considered the standard treatment for cancer of the hypopharynx and cervical esophagus. Surgical resection for advanced stage primary tumors (T3 or T4) typically requires laryngectomy as part of the procedure. Improved 5-year survival rates have been achieved for patients with hypopharyngeal cancer using combined surgical resection and postoperative radiation therapy, compared with single modality treatment.[32] Poor pathologic features following resection, such as close or positive mucosal margins, nerve invasion, positive lymph nodes, or largest lymph node > 3 cm are indications for adjuvant treatment. Postoperative radiation therapy has been shown to decrease the rates of local and regional recurrence, including peristomal recurrence.[33]

The role of chemotherapy for patients with head and neck cancer has historically been limited to palliation. However, chemotherapy in the management of these tumors has evolved in the last decade from palliation to primary combined-modality treatment.[34] Current clinical data supports a role for chemotherapy as part of a combination treatment for cure in patients with advanced hypopharynx cancer requiring total laryngectomy.[34] In fact, the European Organization for Research and Treatment of Cancer (EORTC) has now accepted the use of induction chemotherapy followed by radiation as the new standard treatment in its future phase III larynx preservation trials for carcinoma of the hypopharynx.[35] Survival rates for complete responders are similar to patients treated surgically, although larynx preservation is achieved in only 30 percent of these patients.[36]

Induction or concomitant platinum-based chemotherapy provides notable response rates and allows the prediction of radiosensitivity in those patients who respond to chemotherapy. Side effects include mucositis, cutaneous reactions, neutropenia, thrombocytopenia, sepsis and death.[37] Planned neck dissection is recommended in some treatment plans for all patients with N2+ neck disease and salvage surgery is performed for residual or recurrent locoregional disease.[37] Despite initial tumor responses, neoadjuvant chemotherapy and organ preservation protocols do not offer improved long-term locoregional control or survival.[38] This treatment approach requires a motivated, compliant patient, careful monitoring, close interdisciplinary cooperation among oncologists, and should be administered as part of an approved local, regional, or national protocol.[36]

The survival of patients with carcinoma of the cervical esophagus remains poor in spite of multimodality treatment and technical improvements in surgical resection and reconstruction.[39] The standard operative procedure is laryngopharyngoesophagectomy and reconstruction with regional musculocutaneous flaps, gastric pull-up, or free tissue transfer of jejunum or radial forearm fasciocutaneous flap. The mean survival following diagnosis is measured in terms of months, and 5-year survival rates approach 12 percent. In view of these results, some clinicians do not feel that laryngectomy is justified in these patients. However, unlike hypopharynx cancer, there is currently no prospective randomized clinical trial data comparing chemoradiation protocols to standard surgical therapy for patients with carcinoma of the cervical esophagus. Therefore, multimodality nonsurgical treatment options are more limited for these patients.

Factors Affecting Choice of Treatment

Age

In general, advanced age is not a major contraindication to treatment for head and neck cancer. Survival rates for patients over 75 years of age are comparable to other age groups.[40] However, the site-specific survival for patients older than 75 years with hypopharyngeal or cervical esophageal carcinoma is approximately 10 percent with many patients eliminated from treatment consideration due to associated medical conditions.[41] In view of the anticipated poor prognosis of hypopharyngeal carcinoma in the elderly, some clinicians recommend that treatment should be directed towards palliation without surgery whenever possible.[40]

Associated Medical Conditions

As hypopharynx and cervical esophagus cancer typically occur in older patients, associated medical conditions are often present and should be included when considering treatment options. Although patients with weight loss more than 10 percent during the 6 months before surgery are at greater risk for the occurrence of major postoperative complications, cachexia and malnutrition are not contraindications to treatment due to improvements in nutritional assessment and delivery via enteral and hyperalimentary routes.[42] Anemia should be corrected prior to treatment as hematologic side effects from chemotherapy are common and anemia is a negative prognostic factor in some studies of squamous cell carcinoma of the head and neck.[43] Medical contraindications to surgery are based on the preoperative assessment of anesthetic risk. Eligibility criteria for investigational nonsurgical chemoradiation protocols include adequate performance status as well as reasonable hematologic, hepatic, renal and cardiovascular function.

Past Medical/Surgical History

Previous gastrointestinal surgery is not a contraindication for reconstruction following laryngopharyngoesophagectomy requiring gastric pull-up or free jejunal graft for reconstruction.[44] Previous chemotherapy is not an absolute contraindication to medical therapy, but previous exposure to platinum compounds makes significant responses less likely. Repeat external irradiation or brachytherapy are poor options for patients who have received prior radiotherapy to the head and neck.

TNM Stage

Relative contraindications to surgical resection of hypopharynx and cervical esophagus cancer include invasion of pre-vertebral fascia, the presence of distant metastases, and carotid involvement by either the primary or regional lymph nodes.[45] Conservation surgery (partial laryngopharyngectomy) is indicated for early stage (T1 to T2) lesions in patients who can tolerate some degree of chronic aspiration. Contraindications to medical treatment include ineligibility for protocols based on medical evaluation, and inability to tolerate radiation therapy or chemotherapy. Many patients now undergo pretreatment placement of percutaneous endoscopic gastrostomy

(PEG) tubes because of pre- and post-treatment problems with dysphagia. Avoiding preoperative tracheotomy and the addition of thyroidectomy, paratracheal lymph node dissection and tracheal resection to the procedure can decrease the risk of peristomal recurrence following laryngopharyngoesophagectomy. Postoperative radiotherapy to the stoma and superior mediastinum will help minimize recurrence around the tracheostoma.[46]

Treatment of the associated lymph node groups should be included as part of the management of these disease sites as there is a high rate of regional lymph node metastases. Retropharyngeal adenopathy is common with pharyngeal wall cancers and has a negative impact on neck control and ultimate survival.[47] Patients with clinically palpable neck disease (N1 to N3), histologic evidence of metastatic nodal disease, extracapsular spread, and three or more positive lymph nodes are at greater risk of developing failure at distant sites and should have an extensive evaluation for distant metastatic disease.[48] Neck dissections in patients with clinically negative necks and/or radiotherapy should include lymph node levels II, III, and IV in both necks during treatment due to a high incidence of bilateral disease.[49] Patients with palpable nodes N2 or greater should be offered a comprehensive neck dissection. Planned radiotherapy, either as part of a chemoradiation protocol or following surgical resection, should be included as part of the management of these cancers.

SURGICAL TREATMENT

Resection

The difficulty in surgical treatment of advanced carcinoma of the hypopharynx and cervical esophagus arises from the common requirement for laryngectomy as part of the procedure. The larynx is removed because of direct or submucosal tumor extension and significant risk of chronic or life-threatening aspiration. Histopathologic studies of hypopharyngeal cancer have shown that assessment of the extent of laryngeal disease based on endoscopic findings in the hypopharynx is inaccurate.[50] Therefore, laryngeal conservation surgery for hypopharynx cancer risks a high incidence of positive margins. However, for the rare patient who presents with early-stage hypopharyngeal disease, laryngeal preservation surgery can be performed with excellent functional results.[51] Endoscopic pharyngectomy is possible for small lesions that are easily accessible through an operating laryngoscope. Partial pharyngectomy for posterior pharyngeal or small lateral pharyngeal lesions can be approached through a lateral or transhyoid pharyngotomy.[52]

Partial laryngopharyngectomy (PLP) is indicated for lesions of the pyriform sinus that invade the lateral hypopharyngeal wall and consists of resecting half the larynx and half the hypopharynx (Figure 10–6). The lesion should be confined to the ipsilateral pyriform sinus, aryepiglottic fold, arytenoid eminence and paraglottic space at the level of the false vocal fold. The hyoid bone, thyroid ala, arytenoid cartilage, epiglottis, aryepiglottic fold, arytenoid eminence and false fold are removed on the affected side. Hemi- and supra-cricoid laryngopharyngectomy can be performed for hypopharynx tumors involving the aryepiglottic fold, and anterior, medial, and lateral wall of the pyriform sinus.[53] The surgical specimen includes the ipsilateral half of the hypopharynx, larynx, and cricoid ring (Figure 10–7). Contraindications to these procedures include invasion of the pyriform sinus apex or post-cricoid region, invasion of the posterior pharyngeal wall, and vocal cord paralysis.

Pearson's near-total laryngectomy with permanent tracheopharyngeal shunt (NTL-PTPS) has been used successfully by a limited number of clinicians with good locoregional control rates and infrequent aspiration.[54] Lung-powered "shunt" speech is acquired in many patients following this procedure. The major disadvantage of partial laryngopharyngectomy is an inability to predict postoperative speech and swallowing function, although newer reconstructive techniques may improve outcome.[55]

Many patients are not amenable to partial laryngeal or pharyngeal surgery and require total laryngectomy in combination with total or partial pharyngectomy and cervical esophagectomy via a cervical approach. Larynx-preserving procedures with resection of the cervical esophagus via median sternotomy or trans-tracheal approach have been described.[56] The major risk of esophagectomy without laryngectomy is uncontrollable aspiration. Trans-hiatal esophagectomy can be performed in combination with laryngopharyngoesophagectomy when there is tumor extension below the cervical esophagus or second esophageal primary malignancy.[57] Frozen-section evaluation should be obtained due to submucosal tumor extension. Bilateral neck dissections should be performed at resection because of the high risk of regional lymph node metastases.[58] A selective neck dissection of levels II, III, and IV is appropriate in the clinically negative

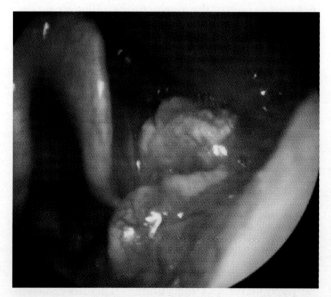

Figure 10–6.   Fiberoptic endoscopic appearance of a patient with a carcinoma of the right pyriform sinus suitable for a partial laryngopharyngectomy.

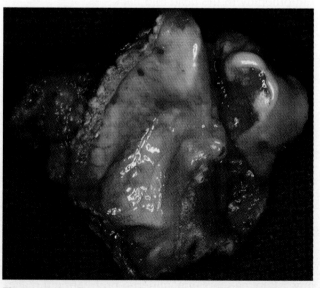

Figure 10–7.   Operative specimen of the patient in Figure 10-6 shows the extent of resection at partial laryngopharyngectomy.

neck because of the low risk of metastatic disease in the submandibular triangle (level I) and posterior triangle (level V).[59] Primary tracheoesophageal puncture can be performed regardless of reconstruction technique for speech restoration.[60]

Reconstruction

The selection of technique to reconstruct the pharynx and cervical esophagus following ablative surgery is largely determined by the size of the defect, presence or absence of laryngeal structures, and the availability of microvascular expertise. Small defects following endoscopic resection will heal by secondary intention. External partial pharyngectomy can be repaired by primary closure, tongue flap, local rotation flap, and skin, dermal, or mucosal grafts.[61] The Wookey procedure has historical significance, and may be employed in salvaging multiple failures of other procedures.[62] Although cervical skin, platysma, latissimus dorsi, and deltopectoral flaps have been used, pectoralis major myocutaneous (Figure 10–8) or revascularized radial forearm flaps are the most common choices for reconstruction of larger pharyngeal defects, following total laryngectomy with partial pharyngectomy.

Reconstruction becomes more challenging following partial resection of the larynx for hypopharynx and cervical esophagus carcinoma. Primary closure or local rotation flaps using residual laryngeal/hypopharyngeal mucosa, cervical skin, and sternohyoid myofascia have been described.[63] Many techniques use remaining laryngeal structures in combination with regional myocutaneous flaps or gastric pull-up to preserve laryngeal function. A single layer closure does not have higher fistula rates and speech restoration and swallowing are improved compared to multiple layer closure.[64] Cricopharyngeal myotomy is often performed to improve swallowing and acquisition of tracheoesophageal speech.[65] Although reported complication rates are low, patients should be prepared for the possibility of a permanent tracheostomy.

Circumferential defects of the upper aerodigestive tract require circumferential tissue replacement

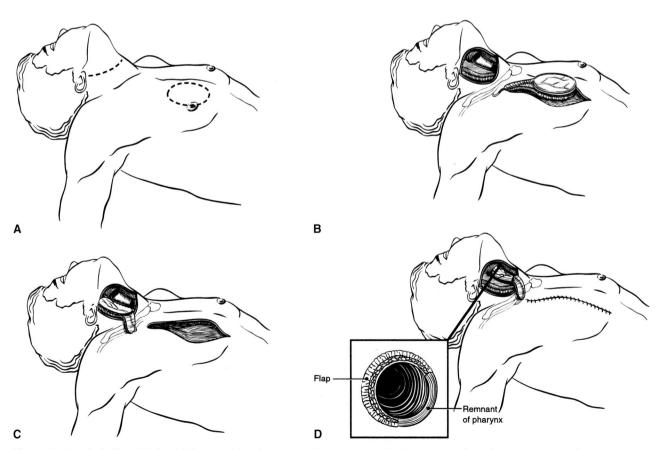

Figure 10–8. *A, B, C* and *D*, Partial defects of the pharynx can be reconstructed using a pectoralis major myocutaneous flap.

to reestablish continuity between the residual pharynx and esophagus. Both regional and free fasciocutaneous and musculocutaneous flaps can be tubed, but the preferred methods are free radial forearm, free jejunal interposition, or pharyngogastrostomy after pull-through esophagectomy (gastric pull-up).[66] Each of these techniques has their proponents, and the choice of technique is based on the preferred method of the operating surgeons and the size of the defect.

The advantages of radial forearm flaps include ease of harvest and avoidance of intra-abdominal surgery. Free jejunal transplantation (Figure 10–9) has the advantage of fewer mucosal sutures and can be harvested endoscopically. In addition, longer segments of jejunum can be harvested for defects which extend into the nasopharynx. Gastric pull-up is indicated for lesions extending into the thoracic esophagus or when total esophagectomy is indicated (Figure 10–10). A combination of techniques is occasionally required when additional structures, such as anterior neck skin, oropharynx, and oral cavity are included in the ablation. Among the three methods of recon-struction, free jejunal transplantation is recommended for primary reconstruction following laryngopharyngoesophagectomy.

NONSURGICAL TREATMENT

Chemotherapy

As stated previously, chemotherapy for patients with head and neck cancer has evolved from palliation to primary combined-modality treatment in the last decade. Prospective, randomized studies comparing induction chemotherapy plus definitive radiation therapy with conventional treatment (total laryngectomy, pharyngectomy, neck dissection, and postoperative irradiation) have shown that larynx preservation without decreased survival is possible in patients with cancer of the hypopharynx.[35] These protocols require frequent endoscopic evaluation, and those patients with limited or no response to treatment proceed to salvage surgery with postoperative radiation. Salvage surgery is also performed when patients relapse after chemotherapy and irradiation.

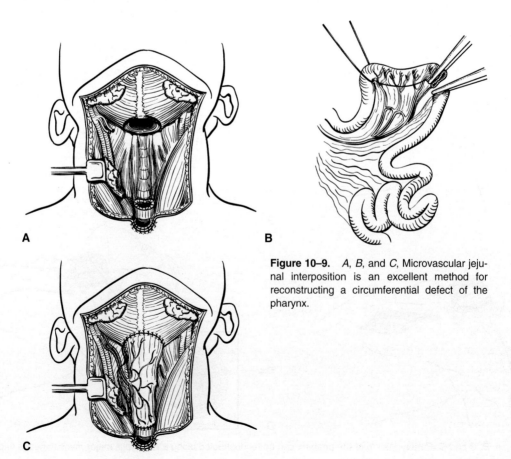

A

B

C

Figure 10–9. *A*, *B*, and *C*, Microvascular jejunal interposition is an excellent method for reconstructing a circumferential defect of the pharynx.

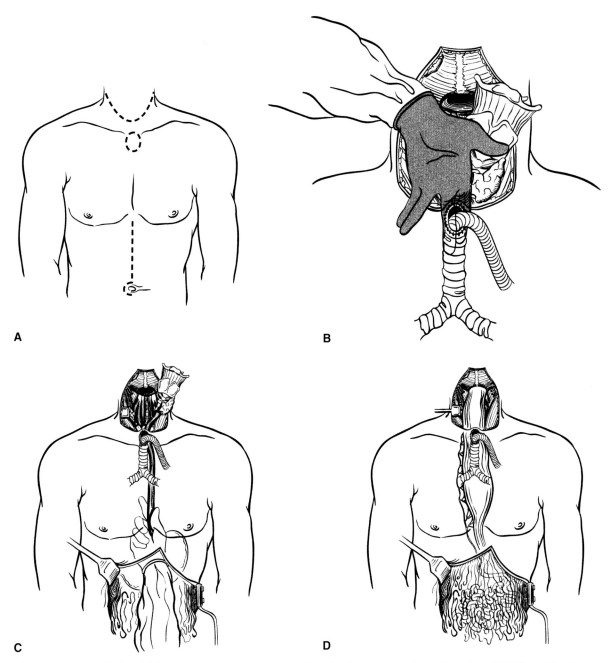

Figure 10–10. *A, B, C* and *D,* Pharyngogastrostomy after gastric pull-up for reconstructing a circumferential defect of the pharynx.

Survival is comparable in surgical and nonsurgical groups for the following reasons: chemotherapy appears to decrease the rate of distant failure, and patients who undergo successful surgical salvage following chemoradiation are included in the nonsurgical group with respect to survival.[67] The 5-year estimate of retaining a functional larynx is about 35 percent.[35] Intra-arterial chemotherapy has been employed to increase the intra-tumor dose and limit systemic exposure.[68] Several arteries, including lingual, ascending

pharyngeal, facial and superior thyroidal arteries are available for drug delivery. Selective arterial infusion combined with external radiation therapy is a feasible alternative to standard chemoradiation protocols and offers comparable rates of disease control and survival. For many institutions and clinicians, induction chemotherapy followed by radiation with surgical salvage is offered as standard treatment for patients with advanced carcinoma of the hypopharynx.[35] Because there are no prospective randomized trials comparing treatment options for carcinoma of the cervical esophagus, the approach to these lesions is more varied.

Radiotherapy

Radiation therapy can be used as single modality treatment for early stage hypopharyngeal carcinoma with acceptable results.[69] Neck dissection alone followed by radiation to both the primary site and necks is a reasonable treatment plan for early T stage lesions with bulky neck disease. Postoperative radiation therapy offers improved locoregional control rates when compared to preoperative RT.[70] Newer chemoradiation protocols offer larynx preservation with similar survival rates when compared to surgical resection. Hyperfractionation (twice daily) schedules have shown improved control rates in many studies.[71] A variety of schedule modifications and radiosensitizers have been reported in the literature with varying degrees of success.

There is wide variation in the indications, treatment regimens, and dosimetry for brachytherapy in the definitive and palliative treatment of cancer of the esophagus.[72] According to the American Brachytherapy Society (ABS), candidates for brachytherapy include patients with unifocal thoracic adenocarcinomas and squamous cell carcinomas less than 10 cm in length with no evidence of intra-abdominal or metastatic disease.[72] Contraindications include tracheal or bronchial involvement, cervical esophagus location, or stenosis that cannot be bypassed.[72] ABS guidelines will likely evolve as clinical data and treatment techniques are refined.

Stents

Significant dysphagia and an inability to manage normal secretions often accompany hypopharynx and cervical esophagus malignancies. Temporary relief can be achieved with the use of a nasopharyngeal airway or silicone salivary bypass tube from the nasopharynx or oropharynx to the cervical esophagus.[73] Self-expanding metal stents represent a major advancement in the palliative treatment of dysphagia caused by neoplasms of the esophagus.[74] Most patients report a significant improvement of dysphagia and some return to a normal diet. Problems with these devices include foreign body sensation,

chronic pain, proximal or distal prosthesis migration, insufficient expansion and neoplastic obstruction.[74] Other options include repeat or multiple stent placement, balloon dilation and percutaneous endoscopic gastrostomy (PEG).[74]

Laser Ablation

Palliative therapy for obstructing cervical esophageal carcinoma is possible with neodymium:yttrium-aluminum-garnet (Nd:YAG) laser. Vaporization of obstructing esophageal carcinoma followed by stent placement is effective for patients who are not candidates for curative therapy.[75] Photodynamic therapy (PDT) has reportedly been effective in a variety of head and neck malignancies that fail conventional therapy.[76] The technique involves intravenous or oral administration of a chemosensitizing drug selectively retained by neoplastic and reticuloendothelial tissues. When exposed to a 630-nm argon laser, the laser energy catalyzes a photochemical reaction which releases free oxygen radicals and results in cell death and tumor necrosis. There are only anecdotal reports in the literature in cases of hypopharynx and cervical esophagus cancer; therefore, no definitive statements can be made regarding clinical efficacy of this technique.

Sequelae, Complications, and their Management

Surgery

Fistula, stenosis, flap loss, and persistent dysphagia can complicate surgical resection of the hypopharynx and cervical esophagus.[77] Other complications include wound infection, wound necrosis, cervical skin necrosis, hemorrhage, and carotid artery rupture.[78] Positive histologic margins by frozen section indicate significantly increased risk of complications, including local recurrence and death from disease. Reported rates of perioperative mortality range from 5 to 18 percent. The use of microvascular jejunal flaps can result in anastomotic leak, flap loss, and intra-abdominal complications including hemorrhage. However, successful microvascular tissue transfer can be achieved in greater than 95 percent of patients.[79] Patients who undergo gastric pull-up reconstruction often complain of postprandial regurgitation due to impaired gastric peristalsis. Gastric emptying after gastric interposition is dependent on upright posture after meals and patients should be counseled accordingly. The morbidity rate of tracheoesophageal puncture is low and should be considered for patients requiring laryngectomy. Significant endocrine dysfunction (hypothyroidism, hypoparathyroidism) occurs with regularity following the treatment of hypopharyngeal and cervical esophageal carcinoma.[80] Clinicians should maintain a high index of suspicion for postsurgical endocrine dysfunction.

Approximately 20 percent of total laryngectomies require treatment for pharyngeal stenosis, and the highest incidence is found in patients treated for hypopharyngeal lesions.[81] Neck disease and inclusion of radical neck dissection are both significant factors in the development of hypopharyngeal stenosis. The best treatment of hypopharyngeal stenosis is its prevention through the use of regional or microvascular flaps to augment residual mucosa. Persistent fistulae or strictures can be corrected with local or regional flaps. Secondary jejunal interposition and radial forearm reconstruction are also effective surgical options. Tracheoesophageal puncture (TEP) may be complicated by poor speech because of hypertonicity or spasm of the pharyngoesophageal segment (PES). Treatment options include speech therapy, PES dilation, pharyngeal neurectomy, botulinum toxin injection into the PES, and myotomy.[82]

Radiotherapy

Complications of radiotherapy include mucositis, stenosis, complete stricture, persistent dysphagia, tissue necrosis, recurrence, and Lhermitte's syndrome.[83] Careful treatment planning is necessary to avoid damage to the spinal cord. Hypoparathyroidism and hypothyroidism can occur in patients treated with radiotherapy as well.

Chemotherapy

Patients who receive platinum-based chemotherapy should be informed of the potential risks of myelotoxicity, stomatitis, sepsis, dysphagia, hearing loss,

peripheral neuropathy, recurrence, weight loss and death. Neutropenia ($< 1{,}000$ cells/mm^3) and anemia are common hematologic side effects of chemotherapy.[84] Mucositis and stomatitis are compounded when concurrent radiotherapy is administered.

Rehabilitation and Quality of Life

Health-related quality of life (QOL) measurements provide an assessment of a patient's perception of his or her illness, and a variety of questionnaires specific for head and neck cancer have been developed.[85,86] For many head and neck cancer patients, quality of life, speech and swallowing are compromised before, during, and after treatment. Depression, anxiety, disability, and psychological distress are common. As one might expect, quality of life measurements vary based on patient personality, treatment type, and time elapsed from therapy.[87] The patient's attitude about their disease and their physical and social abilities following treatment plays a major role in quality of life measurements. Surprisingly, clinical stage of disease or degree of malnutrition does not seem to correlate with the patient's self-rated QOL.[88]

It is clear that total laryngectomy results in a major alteration in function of the upper aerodigestive tract. However, post-laryngectomy QOL scores are not significantly different from pre-laryngectomy scores in patients with advanced larynx cancer.[86] Though loss of voice is disabling, the functional limitations caused by a laryngectomy do not necessarily translate into a worse overall QOL.[86] Approximately 30 percent of patients develop esophageal speech and many others are rehabilitated by an electro-larynx or tracheoesophageal puncture.

Laryngeal radiotherapy results in significant but temporary deterioration of physical functioning and an exacerbation of many head and neck symptoms.[85] The frequency of oral side effects correlate with radiation treatment fields and dose as well as clinical stage.[85] Oral complaints include difficulty chewing/eating, pain, dry mouth, altered taste, dysphagia, altered speech, difficulty with dentures, and increased tooth decay in dentate patients. There is also a high level of depressive symptomatology followed by an improvement after treatment.[85] Despite physical deterioration, there is an improvement of emotional functioning and quality of life after treatment, and often these measurements return to their pre-treatment level.

When comparing total laryngectomy, hemilaryngectomy and radiotherapy for laryngeal cancer, the total laryngectomy group recovers most slowly, without achieving normal functioning by 6 months. Most hemilaryngectomees return to normal functioning by 3 months and radiotherapy-only patients show little overall dysfunction at 6 months.[89] However, there is no significant difference in overall QOL between groups or over time.[89] Ability to eat and/or speak is not associated with overall QOL or with any other specific QOL measurement.[89] Similarly, pre- and post-treatment QOL scores are similar for advanced oropharyngeal cancer patients treated surgically and nonsurgically.[86] The surgical group tends to complain of poorer appearance and speech, and the nonsurgical group reports higher pain scores.[86] Surgery results in greater measurable dysfunction, but psychological functioning and general well-being are similar between patients treated surgically and those receiving radiotherapy.[90] The data regarding QOL in patients enrolled in organ preservation protocols for hypopharynx and cervical esophagus cancers is evolving, and future studies will provide greater insight into this aspect of head and neck cancer care.

Outcomes and Results of Treatment

Recent reviews of the data collected by the United States National Cancer Database reveals that carcinoma of the hypopharynx continues to have the worst prognosis of any head and neck site.[91] Overall, 5-year survival is approximately 30 percent.[91]

Surgery

The 5-year survival rates following surgical resection for carcinoma of the hypopharynx are related to TNM stage at presentation (clinical: stage I, 74%; stage II, 45 to 63%; stage III, 32%; and stage IV, 0 to 14%) (neck: N0, 57%; N1, 28 to 30%; N2, 6 to 16%; and N3, 0 to 10%).[18,92] Local control rates are 57 to 80 percent and recurrences occur at the upper resection margin.[18,92] Five-year overall and disease-free survival rates are 30 percent and 41 percent, respectively, with surgical resection and postoperative radiotherapy.[92] Prognosis is better in patients with limited disease: local disease permitting larynx-sparing surgery, N0/N1 clinical neck, and stage I/II/III disease.[92] Supracricoid hemilaryngopharyngectomy (SCHLP) for selected T2 pyriform sinus carcinoma offers a 5-year disease-specific survival rate of 55 percent and excellent local control rates.[53] Voice preservation is possible in many patients following partial laryngopharyngectomy and neck dissection. Extent of surgery is associated with a higher risk of complications but does not affect local recurrence rates. The majority of neck dissection specimens will contain pathologically positive lymph nodes. Modified neck dissections sparing level I appear to offer similar control rates and less morbidity in the clinically negative neck when compared to classic radical neck dissections.[93]

Carcinoma of the cervical esophagus extends into the hypopharynx in the majority of patients. Less than half of patients are surgically resectable following preoperative or intraoperative evaluation. Perioperative mortality rates average 10 percent with gastric pull-up reconstruction, and are lower with free flap reconstruction. Total laryngopharyngoesophagectomy offers the lowest rate of local recurrence.[39] Almost half of the patients who undergo resection without laryngectomy will either aspirate or recur locally.[39] The cumulative 5-year survival rate for carcinoma of the cervical esophagus is between 9 and 16 percent.[39] Attempts at palliative resection should be carefully considered due to the extremely low probability of survival and durable symptom relief.[39]

Reconstruction-associated complications such as wound infection and anastomotic leakage occur less often after gastric pull-up reconstruction when compared to myocutaneous flaps, but are associated with more serious outcome.[92] Overall complication rates in the range of 25 to 30 percent have been reported.[92] Surgical mortality ranges from 0 to 12 percent and is often due to sepsis or cardiac problems.[39,92] Higher morbidity and mortality rates are associated with gastric pull-up when compared to free flap reconstruction.[94] Free jejunal grafts and radial forearm flaps are successful in excess of 90 to 95 percent of cases.[79] When compared to other forms of reconstruction, free jejunal transfer offers higher rates of oral nutrition, lower morbidity and shorter length of hospital stay.[95] Most patients resume oral intake following resection, and the duration of their hospitalization is approximately 2 weeks.[79,94] Despite wide excision, surgical margins are microscopically positive in a significant number of patients. Fluency in tracheoesophageal speech can be achieved in 75 percent of patients within 4 to 5 months following total laryngectomy.[60]

Recurrence in the neck is about 30 to 40 percent overall and is related to clinical neck stage at presentation (N0, 20%; N1, 37%; N2, 48%; and N3, 83%).[92] Failure in the contralateral unoperated neck occurs in 14 percent of patients with medial pyriform sinus lesions and bilateral neck dissections should be performed.[96] Second primary malignancy remains a significant cause of death in these patients.

Radiotherapy

Excellent local control rates (70 to 85%) can be achieved for early stage (T1 to T2) lesions using both standard and hyperfractionated radiotherapy.[97] As with patients treated surgically, treatment success is correlated with stage at presentation. The 5-year survival rates for T3 to T4 disease treated with definitive radiation are approximately 18 percent.[97] Radiotherapy as primary treatment usually reserves surgical resection for salvage. Locoregional recurrence rates of 45 to 50 percent over 5 years following primary radiotherapy for cure have been reported for advanced disease.[98]

Higher total dose increases the risk of both early and late complications.[97] At 5 years, 40 to 50 percent of patients will be alive and with a larynx following radiotherapy for early stage hypopharynx cancer.[97] Successful surgical salvage is infrequent and approaches 20 percent at 5 years.[98] Complication rates are higher when surgery is performed for salvage following radiation therapy.[98] Regional or free flaps offer the advantage of non-irradiated tissue for reconstruction. Intraoperative brachytherapy in combination with surgical salvage has been reported, but the experience is limited at the present time. Survivorship is extremely poor if disease recurs after salvage surgery.

Planned postoperative radiotherapy improves locoregional control and survival and decreases the risk of peristomal recurrence.[18,50,92] Postoperative radiation should be started within 6 weeks after surgery for the best results.[99]

Organ Preservation/Chemoradiation

Neoadjuvant chemotherapy in combination with radiotherapy has shown an overall response rate of 87 percent and a complete remission (CR) rate of 67 percent in patients with carcinoma of the hypopharynx.[100] Similarly, high rates of local control have been reported in cervical esophageal carcinoma.[101] Concurrent delivery of chemoradiation is considerably more toxic but may improve locoregional control and overall survival.[101] Significant complications include grade 3 to 4 granulocytopenia, severe mucositis, dysphagia, and death due to sepsis.[101] Half of the patients will require gastrostomy.[100] Incomplete response after chemotherapy has a high likelihood of treatment failure, even with no clinical evidence of tumor following subsequent radiotherapy.[100] Reported larynx preservation rates range from 30 to 67 percent of patients without compromising survival.[100,102] The range of preservation rates represents differences in protocol reporting and follow-up duration. Overall survival rates range from 20 to 40 percent at 3 years.[103] Local recurrences are more frequent in the laryngeal preservation group, and distant metastases are more frequent with standard therapy.[102] Although local control is decreased among organ preservation patients, there is no compromise in overall survival when combined with prompt surgical salvage.[102]

Thirty to thirty-five percent of patients require total laryngectomy for salvage as a consequence of poor response to induction chemotherapy or recurrent disease after completion of chemotherapy and radiation.[104] Surgical salvage may not be possible due to unresectable local disease or distant metastases. Postoperative pharyngocutaneous fistulae occur in almost 40 percent of patients, resulting in prolonged hospitalization.[104] Long-term survivorship is extremely poor in this situation, with some authors reporting no patients alive at 5 years.[104]

Table 10–1. CARCINOMA OF THE HYPOPHARYNX

Summary of Chemoradiation versus Surgery+RT Protocols

Author	Type	Patients	CR Primary	CR Neck	Mean Survival CRT (months)	Mean Survival SRT (months)	Preservation of Larynx (5-yr)	Local Failure CRT/SRT (%)	Regional Failure CRT/SRT (%)	Distant Failure CRT/SRT (%)	2 yr % CRT/SRT Survival (disease)	2 yr % CRT/SRT Survival (overall)	5 yr % CRT/SRT Survival (disease)	5 yr % CRT/SRT Survival (overall)
Lefebrve	P, R	194	52(54%)	31/61(51%)	44	25	35%	17/12	23/19	25/36	–/–	41/39	–/–	30/35
Zelefsky	RE, NR	56	12(46%)	–/–				42/30	38/30	23/40	–/–	–/–	30/42	15/22
Kraus	RE, NR	25	17(68%)	11(61%)	–	–	32%	48/–	24/–	24/–	–/–	–/–	44/–	–/–
Lavertu	RE, NR	20	20(100%)	–/–	–	–	85%*	15/–	–	–	–/–	–/–	62/–	–/–
Samant	RE, NR	25	(92%)	16(76%)	–	–	–	–	–	–	–/–	–/–	50/–	23/–
Robbins	RE, NR	8	–	–	–	–	–	–	–	–	–			
Shiinian	P, NR	29	15(52%)	–	–	–	28%	20/–	–/–	13/–	–/–	38/–	–/–	–/–
Clayman	RE, NR	87	24(83%)	–	–	–		31/–	–/–	–/–		55/67	–/–	–/–

*4 year data

Summary of Surgery and Radiation Therapy**

Author	Type	Patients	Surgery +RT Failure	Surgery	RT	Surgery Alone				RT Alone			Surgery & RT		
						5 yr Survival (overall) (%)	Local Failure (%)	Regional Failure (%)	Distant Failure (%)	Local Failure (%)	Regional Failure (%)	Distant Failure (%)	Local Failure (%)	Regional Failure (%)	Distant Failure (%)
Carpenter[13]	RE, NR	162	50	22	22	47	18	24	–	23	14	–	17	27	–
Shah[58]	RE, NR	301	39	234	28	25	–	–	–	–	–	–	–	–	–
Fein[71]	RE, NR	75	–	–	75	–	–	–	–	45	30	17	–	–	–
Kraus[92]	RE, NR	132	106	26	70	30	–	–	–	–	–	–	18	17	12
Garden[97]	RE, NR	70	–	–	70	–	–	–	–	19	–	–	–	–	–
Alcock[98]	RE, NR	189	–	–	189	–	–	–	–	45	–	–	–	–	–

**RT alone survival data includes surgical salvage. P = prospective; R = randomized; NR = non-randomized; RE = retrospective; CR = complete response; CRT = chemoradiation; SRT = surgery + radiation.

SUMMARY

The survival of patients with carcinoma of the hypopharynx and cervical esophagus remains poor in spite of multimodality treatment. The mean survival following diagnosis is usually less than 20 months and cumulative 5-year survival is less than 20 percent for advanced disease. Failure to control local disease remains a major cause of death in these patients. Locoregional control affects the risk of distant metastases, and tumors of the hypopharynx have a higher probability of micrometastatic dissemination at the time of initial diagnosis.[105] For all head and neck tumor sites, except for the hypopharynx and nasopharynx, improvements in locoregional control are likely to improve survival. Until effective methods to treat disseminated disease and second primary malignancies are developed, improvements in locoregional control will have little effect on ultimate survival for patients with hypopharynx and cervical esophagus malignancies.[105]

REFERENCES

1. Crafts RC. A textbook of human anatomy. New York: Churchill Livingstone; 1985.
2. American Joint Committee for Cancer. AJCC cancer staging manual. 5th ed. Chicago: Lippincott-Raven Publishers; 1997.
3. Horwitz SD, Caldarelli DD, Hendrickson FR. Treatment of carcinoma of the hypopharynx. Head Neck Surg 1979; 2(2):107–11.
4. Schwartz SI, Shires GT, Spencer FC. Principles of surgery. New York: McGraw-Hill; 1989.
5. Meyer GW, Austin RM, Brady CE III, Castell DO. Muscle anatomy of the human esophagus. J Clin Gastroenterol 1986;8(2):131–4.
6. Mu L, Sanders I. Neuromuscular organization of the human upper esophageal sphincter. Ann Otol Rhinol Laryngol 1998;107(5 Pt 1):370–7.
7. Liebermann-Meffert DM, Walbrun B, Hiebert CA, Siewert JR. Recurrent and superior laryngeal nerves: a new look with implications for the esophageal surgeon. Ann Thorac Surg 1999;67(1):217–23.
8. Goyal RK, Martin SB, Shapiro J, Spechler SJ. The role of cricopharyngeus muscle in pharyngoesophageal disorders. Dysphagia 1993;8(3):252–8.
9. Lang IM, Shaker R. Anatomy and physiology of the upper esophageal sphincter. Am J Med 1997;103(5A):S50–5.
10. Ribeiro U Jr, Posner MC, Safatle-Ribeiro AV, Reynolds JC. Risk factors for squamous cell carcinoma of the oesophagus. Br J Surg 1996;83(9):1174–85.
11. Gustavsson P, Jakobsson R, Johansson H, et al. Occupational exposures and squamous cell carcinoma of the oral cavity, pharynx, larynx, and oesophagus: a case-control study in Sweden. Occup Environ Med 1998;55(6):393–400.
12. Hoffman RM, Jaffe PE. Plummer-Vinson syndrome. A case report and literature review. Arch Intern Med 1995; 155(18):2008–11.
13. Carpenter RJ III, DeSanto LW, Devine KD, Taylor WF. Cancer of the hypopharynx. Analysis of treatment and results in 162 patients. Arch Otolaryngol 1976;102(12):716–21.
14. Jung TT, Adams GL. Dysphagia in laryngectomized patients. Otolaryngol Head Neck Surg 1980;88(1):25–33.
15. Lefebvre JL, Castelain B, De la Torre JC, et al. Lymph node invasion in hypopharynx and lateral epilarynx carcinoma: a prognostic factor. Head Neck Surg 1987;10(1):14–8.
16. Lawson W, Som HL, Biller HF. Papillary adenocarcinoma of the thyroid invading the upper air passages. Ann Otol Rhinol Laryngol 1977;86(6 Pt 1):751–5.
17. Deleyiannis FW, Weymuller EA Jr, Garcia I, Potosky AL. Geographic variation in the utilization of esophagoscopy and bronchoscopy in head and neck cancer. Arch Otolaryngol Head Neck Surg 1997;123(11):1203–10.
18. Haughey BH, Gates GA, Arfken CL, Harvey J. Meta-analysis of second malignant tumors in head and neck cancer: the case for an endoscopic screening protocol. Ann Otol Rhinol Laryngol 1992;101(2 Pt 1):105–12.
19. Parker JT, Hill JH. Panendoscopy in screening for synchronous primary malignancies. Laryngoscope 1988;98(2):147–9.
20. Thabet HM, Sessions DG, Gado MH, et al. Comparison of clinical evaluation and computed tomographic diagnostic accuracy for tumors of the larynx and hypopharynx. Laryngoscope 1996;106(5 Pt 1):589–94.
21. Righi PD, Kelley DJ, Ernst R, et al. Evaluation of prevertebral muscle invasion by squamous cell carcinoma. Can computed tomography replace open neck exploration? Arch Otolaryngol Head Neck Surg 1996;122(6):660–3.
22. Becker M, Zbaren P, Delavelle J, et al. Neoplastic invasion of the laryngeal cartilage: reassessment of criteria for diagnosis at CT. Radiology 1997;203(2):521–32.
23. Curtin HD, Ishwaran H, Mancuso AA, et al. Comparison of CT and MR imaging in staging of neck metastases. Radiology 1998;207(1):123–30.
24. Wenig BL, Ziffra KL, Mafee MF, Schild JA. MR imaging of squamous cell carcinoma of the larynx and hypopharynx. Otolaryngol Clin N Am 1995;28(3):609–19.
25. Mukherji SK, Mancuso AA, Kotzur IM, et al. Radiologic appearance of the irradiated larynx. Part II. Primary site response. Radiology 1994;193(1):149–54.
26. Kotwall C, Sako K, Razack MS, et al. Metastatic patterns in squamous cell cancer of the head and neck. Am J Surg 1987;154(4):439–42.
27. Troell RJ, Terris DJ. Detection of metastases from head and neck cancers. Laryngoscope 1995;105(3 Pt 1):247–50.
28. Korver KD, Graham SM, Hoffman HT, et al. Liver function studies in the assessment of head and neck cancer patients. Head Neck 1995;17(6):531–4.
29. Chaiken L, Rege S, Hoh C, et al. Positron emission tomography with fluorodeoxyglucose to evaluate tumor response and control after radiation therapy. Int J Radiat Oncol Biol Phys 1993;27(2):455–64.
30. Fagan JJ, Collins B, Barnes L, et al. Perineural invasion in squamous cell carcinoma of the head and neck. Arch Otolaryngol Head Neck Surg 1998;124(6):637–40.
31. Collin CF, Spiro RH. Carcinoma of the cervical esophagus: changing therapeutic trends. Am J Surg 1984;148(4):460–6.
32. Persky MS, Daly JF. Combined therapy vs. curative radiation in the treatment of pyriform sinus carcinoma. Otolaryngol Head Neck Surg 1981;89(1):87–91.

33. Arriagada R, Eschwege F, Cachin Y, Richard JM. The value of combining radiotherapy with surgery in the treatment of hypopharyngeal and laryngeal cancers. Cancer 1983; 51(10):1819–25.

34. Pfister DG, Shaha AR, Harrison LB. The role of chemotherapy in the curative treatment of head and neck cancer. Surg Oncol Clin N Am 1997;6(4):749–68.

35. Lefebvre JL, Chevalier D, Luboinski B, et al. Larynx preservation in pyriform sinus cancer: preliminary results of a European Organization for Research and Treatment of Cancer phase III trial. EORTC Head and Neck Cancer Cooperative Group. J Natl Cancer Inst 1996;88(13):890–9.

36. Pfister DG, Strong E, Harrison L, et al. Larynx preservation with combined chemotherapy and radiation therapy in advanced but resectable head and neck cancer. J Clin Oncol 1991;9(5):850–9.

37. Lavertu P, Adelstein DJ, Saxton JP, et al. Aggressive concurrent chemoradiotherapy for squamous cell head and neck cancer: an 8-year single-institution experience. Arch Otolaryngol Head Neck Surg 1999;125(2):142–8.

38. Zelefsky MJ, Kraus DH, Pfister DG, et al. Combined chemotherapy and radiotherapy versus surgery and postoperative radiotherapy for advanced hypopharyngeal cancer. Head Neck 1996;18(5):405–11.

39. Kelley DJ, Wolf R, Shaha AR, et al. Impact of clinicopathologic parameters on patient survival in carcinoma of the cervical esophagus. Am J Surg 1995;170(5):427–31.

40. Thompson AC, Quraishi SM, Morgan DA, Bradley PJ. Carcinoma of the larynx and hypopharynx in the elderly. Eur J Surg Oncol 1996;22(1):65–8.

41. Jones AS, Beasley N, Houghton D, Husband DJ. The effects of age on survival and other parameters in squamous cell carcinoma of the oral cavity, pharynx and larynx. Clin Otolaryngol 1998;23(1):51–6.

42. van Bokhorst-de van der Schueren MA, van Leeuwen PA, Sauerwein HP, et al. Assessment of malnutrition parameters in head and neck cancer and their relation to postoperative complications. Head Neck 1997;19(5):419–25.

43. Dubray B, Mosseri V, Brunin F, et al. Anemia is associated with lower local-regional control and survival after radiation therapy for head and neck cancer: a prospective study. Radiology 1996;201(2):553–8.

44. Kamei S, Takeichi Y, Oyama S, Baba S. Reconstruction using a free jejunal graft for surgery of the hypopharynx and the cervical esophagus in patients with a history of previous upper gastro-intestinal surgery. Acta Otolaryngol Suppl (Stockh) 1996;525:35–9.

45. Jones AS, Roland NJ, Hamilton J, et al. Malignant tumours of the cervical oesophagus. Clin Otolaryngol 1996;21(1): 49–53.

46. Leon X, Quer M, Burgues J, et al. Prevention of stomal recurrence. Head Neck 1996;18(1):54–9.

47. McLaughlin MP, Mendenhall WM, Mancuso AA, et al. Retropharyngeal adenopathy as a predictor of outcome in squamous cell carcinoma of the head and neck. Head Neck 1995;17(3):190–8.

48. Alvi A, Johnson JT. Development of distant metastasis after treatment of advanced-stage head and neck cancer. Head Neck 1997;19(6):500–5.

49. Candela FC, Kothari K, Shah JP. Patterns of cervical node metastases from squamous carcinoma of the oropharynx and hypopharynx. Head Neck 1990;12(3):197–203.

50. Hirano M, Kurita S, Tanaka H. Histopathologic study of carcinoma of the hypopharynx: implications for conservation surgery. Ann Otol Rhinol Laryngol 1987;96(6):625–9.

51. Nakatsuka T, Harii K, Ueda K, et al. Preservation of the larynx after resection of a carcinoma of the posterior wall of the hypopharynx: versatility of a free flap patch graft. Head Neck 1997;19(2):137–42.

52. Stern SJ. Anatomy of the lateral pharyngotomy approach. Head Neck 1992;14(2):153–6.

53. Laccourreye O, Merite-Drancy A, Brasnu D, et al. Supracricoid hemilaryngopharyngectomy in selected pyriform sinus carcinoma staged as T2. Laryngoscope 1993;103(12):1373–9.

54. Shenoy AM, Plinkert PK, Nanjundappa N, et al. Functional utility and oncologic safety of near-total laryngectomy with tracheopharyngeal speech shunt in a Third World oncologic center. Eur Arch Otorhinolaryngol 1997;254(3):128–32.

55. Urken ML, Blackwell K, Biller HF. Reconstruction of the laryngopharynx after hemicricoid/hemithyroid cartilage resection. Preliminary functional results. Arch Otolaryngol Head Neck Surg 1997;123(11):1213–22.

56. Omura K, Urayama H, Kanehira E, et al. Larynx-preserving resection of the cervical esophagus for cervical esophageal carcinoma limited to the submucosal layer. J Surg Oncol 1998;69(2):113–6.

57. Morton KA, Karwande SV, Davis RK, et al. Gastric emptying after gastric interposition for cancer of the esophagus or hypopharynx. Ann Thorac Surg 1991;51(5):759–63.

58. Shah JP, Shaha AR, Spiro RH, Strong EW. Carcinoma of the hypopharynx. Am J Surg 1976;132(4):439–43.

59. Wenig BL, Applebaum EL. The submandibular triangle in squamous cell carcinoma of the larynx and hypopharynx. Laryngoscope 1991;101(5):516–8.

60. Medina JE, Nance A, Burns L, Overton R. Voice restoration after total laryngopharyngectomy and cervical esophagectomy using the duckbill prosthesis. Am J Surg 1987; 154(4):407–10.

61. Lore JM Jr, Klotch DW, Lee KY. One-stage reconstruction of the hypopharynx using myomucosal tongue flap and dermal graft. Am J Surg 1982;144(4):473–6.

62. Silver CE. Reconstruction after pharyngolaryngectomy-esophagectomy. Am J Surg 1976;132(4):428–34.

63. Cook DW, Canepa C, Winek T, Sasaki TM. Laryngeal flap for hypopharynx reconstruction. Head Neck 1991;13(4): 318–20.

64. Olson NR, Callaway E. Nonclosure of pharyngeal muscle after laryngectomy. Ann Otol Rhinol Laryngol 1990;99 (7 Pt 1):507–8.

65. Blom ED, Pauloski BR, Hamaker RC. Functional outcome after surgery for prevention of pharyngospasms in tracheoesophageal speakers. Part I: Speech characteristics. Laryngoscope 1995;105(10):1093–103.

66. Kato H, Watanabe H, Iizuka T, et al. Primary esophageal reconstruction after resection of the cancer in the hypopharynx or cervical esophagus: comparison of free forearm skin tube flap, free jejunal transplantation and pull-through esophagectomy. Jpn J Clin Oncol 1987;17(3):255–61.

67. Paccagnella A, Orlando A, Marchiori C, et al. Phase III trial of initial chemotherapy in stage III or IV head and neck cancers: a study by the Gruppo di Studio sui Tumori della Testa e del Collo. J Natl Cancer Inst 1994;86(4):265–72.

68. Robbins KT, Fontanesi J, Wong FS, et al. A novel organ preservation protocol for advanced carcinoma of the larynx and pharynx. Arch Otolaryngol Head Neck Surg 1996;122(8):853–7.

69. Garden AS, Morrison WH, Clayman GL, et al. Early squamous cell carcinoma of the hypopharynx: outcomes of

treatment with radiation alone to the primary disease. Head Neck 1996;18(4):317–22.

70. Wennerberg J. Pre- versus post-operative radiotherapy of resectable squamous cell carcinoma of the head and neck. Acta Otolaryngol (Stockh) 1995;115(4):465–74.

71. Fein DA, Mendenhall WM, Parsons JT, et al. Pharyngeal wall carcinoma treated with radiotherapy: impact of treatment technique and fractionation. Int J Radiat Oncol Biol Phys 1993;26(5):751–7.

72. Gaspar LE, Nag S, Herskovic A, et al. American Brachytherapy Society (ABS) consensus guidelines for brachytherapy of esophageal cancer. Clinical Research Committee, American Brachytherapy Society, Philadelphia, (PA). Int J Radiat Oncol Biol Phys 1997;38(1):127–32.

73. Montgomery WW. Salivary bypass tube. Ann Otol Rhinol Laryngol 1978;87(2 Pt 1):159-62.

74. Conio M, Caroli-Bosc F, Demarquay JF, et al. Self-expanding metal stents in the palliation of neoplasms of the cervical esophagus. Hepatogastroenterology 1999;46(25):272–7.

75. Moon BC, Woolfson IK, Mercer CD. Neodymium: yttrium-aluminum-garnet laser vaporization for palliation of obstructing esophageal carcinoma. J Thorac Cardiovasc Surg 1989;98(1):11–4; [discussion 14–5].

76. Schweitzer VG. Photodynamic therapy for treatment of head and neck cancer. Otolaryngol Head Neck Surg 1990; 102(3):225–32.

77. de Vries EJ, Myers EN, Johnson JT, et al. Jejunal interposition for repair of stricture or fistula after laryngectomy. Ann Otol Rhinol Laryngol 1990;99(6 Pt 1):496–8.

78. Gall AM, Sessions DG, Ogura JH. Complications following surgery for cancer of the larynx and hypopharynx. Cancer 1977;39(2):624–31.

79. Bradford CR, Esclamado RM, Carroll WR, Sullivan MJ. Analysis of recurrence, complications, and functional results with free jejunal flaps. Head Neck 1994;16(2): 149–54.

80. Thorp MA, Levitt NS, Mortimore S, Isaacs S. Parathyroid and thyroid function five years after treatment of laryngeal and hypopharyngeal carcinoma. Clin Otolaryngol 1999;24(2):104–8.

81. Kaplan JN, Dobie RA, Cummings CW. The incidence of hypopharyngeal stenosis after surgery for laryngeal cancer. Otolaryngol Head Neck Surg 1981;89(6):956–9.

82. Singer MI, Blom ED, Hamaker RC. Pharyngeal plexus neurectomy for alaryngeal speech rehabilitation. Laryngoscope 1986;96(1):50–4.

83. Mendenhall WM, Million RR, Bova FJ. Carcinoma of the cervical esophagus treated with radiation therapy using a four-field box technique. Int J Radiat Oncol Biol Phys 1982;8(8):1435–9.

84. Shirinian MH, Weber RS, Lippman SM, et al. Laryngeal preservation by induction chemotherapy plus radiotherapy in locally advanced head and neck cancer: the M. D. Anderson Cancer Center experience. Head Neck 1994; 16(1):39–44.

85. De Graeff A, de Leeuw RJ, Ros WJ, et al. A prospective study on quality of life of laryngeal cancer patients treated with radiotherapy. Head Neck 1999;21(4):291–6.

86. Deleyiannis FW, Weymuller EA Jr, Coltrera MD, Futran N. Quality of life after laryngectomy: are functional disabilities important? Head Neck 1999;21(4):319–24.

87. McDonough EM, Boyd JH, Varvares MA, Maves MD. Relationship between psychological status and compliance in a sample of patients treated for cancer of the head and neck. Head Neck 1996;18(3):269–76.

88. Hammerlid E, Wirblad B, Sandin C, et al. Malnutrition and food intake in relation to quality of life in head and neck cancer patients. Head Neck 1998;20(6):540–8.

89. List MA, Ritter-Sterr CA, Baker TM, et al. Longitudinal assessment of quality of life in laryngeal cancer patients. Head Neck 1996;18(1):1–10.

90. Morton RP. Laryngeal cancer: quality-of-life and cost-effectiveness. Head Neck 1997;19(4):243–50.

91. Hoffman HT, Karnell LH, Funk GF, et al. The National Cancer Data Base report on cancer of the head and neck. Arch Otolaryngol Head Neck Surg 1998;124(9):951–62.

92. Kraus DH, Zelefsky MJ, Brock HA, et al. Combined surgery and radiation therapy for squamous cell carcinoma of the hypopharynx. Otolaryngol Head Neck Surg 1997;116(6 Pt 1):637–41.

93. Spiro RH, Gallo O, Shah JP. Selective jugular node dissection in patients with squamous carcinoma of the larynx or pharynx. Am J Surg 1993;166(4):399–402.

94. Cahow CE, Sasaki CT. Gastric pull-up reconstruction for pharyngo-laryngo-esophagectomy. Arch Surg 1994 Apr;129(4):425–9; [discussion 429–30].

95. Carlson GW, Schusterman MA, Guillamondegui OM. Total reconstruction of the hypopharynx and cervical esophagus: a 20-year experience. Ann Plast Surg 1992;29(5):408–12.

96. Johnson JT, Bacon GW, Myers EN, Wagner RL. Medial vs. lateral wall pyriform sinus carcinoma: implications for management of regional lymphatics. Head Neck 1994;16(5):401–5.

97. Garden AS, Morrison WH, Ang KK, Peters LJ. Hyperfractionated radiation in the treatment of squamous cell carcinomas of the head and neck: a comparison of two fractionation schedules. Int J Radiat Oncol Biol Phys 1995;31(3):493–502.

98. Alcock CJ, Fowler JF, Haybittle JL, et al. Salvage surgery following irradiation with different fractionation regimes in the treatment of carcinoma of the laryngopharynx: experience gained from a British Institute of Radiology study. J Laryngol Otol 1992;106(2):147–53.

99. Vikram B, Strong EW, Shah JP, Spiro R. Failure in the neck following multimodality treatment for advanced head and neck cancer. Head Neck Surg 1984;6(3):724–9.

100. Koch WM, Lee DJ, Eisele DW, et al. Chemoradiotherapy for organ preservation in oral and pharyngeal carcinoma. Arch Otolaryngol Head Neck Surg 1995;121(9):974–80.

101. Yu L, Vikram B, Malamud S, et al. Chemotherapy rapidly alternating with twice-a-day accelerated radiation therapy in carcinomas involving the hypopharynx or esophagus: an update. Cancer Invest 1995;13(6):567–72.

102. Clayman GL, Weber RS, Guillamondegui O, et al. Laryngeal preservation for advanced laryngeal and hypopharyngeal cancers. Arch Otolaryngol Head Neck Surg 1995;121(2): 219–23.

103. Kraus DH, Pfister DG, Harrison LB, et al. Larynx preservation with combined chemotherapy and radiation therapy in advanced hypopharynx cancer. Otolaryngol Head Neck Surg 1994;111(1):31–7.

104. Kraus DH, Pfister DG, Harrison LB, et al. Salvage laryngectomy for unsuccessful larynx preservation therapy. Ann Otol Rhinol Laryngol 1995;104(12):936–41.

105. Leibel SA, Scott CB, Mohiuddin M, et al. The effect of local-regional control on distant metastatic dissemination in carcinoma of the head and neck: results of an analysis from the RTOG head and neck database. Int J Radiat Oncol Biol Phys 1991;21(3):549–56.

11

Cancer of the Nasal Cavity and Paranasal Sinuses

RICHARD J. WONG, MD

DENNIS H. KRAUS, MD, FACS

Cancers of the nasal cavity and paranasal sinuses are rare, comprising less than 1 percent of all human malignancies and only 3 percent of those arising in the head and neck.[1] Sinonasal malignancies occur twice as often in males as in females, and are most often diagnosed in patients 50 to 70 years of age.[2] The majority of these tumors are squamous cell carcinoma, although a wide variety of other malignancies including sarcoma, adenoid cystic carcinoma, lymphoma, melanoma, and olfactory neuroblastoma may occur at this site.[3–4]

Sinonasal malignancies are very difficult tumors to treat and traditionally have been associated with a poor prognosis. One reason for these poor outcomes is the close anatomic proximity of the nasal cavity and paranasal sinuses to vital structures such as the skull base, brain, orbit, and carotid artery. This complex location makes complete surgical resection of sinonasal tumors a challenging and sometimes impossible task. In addition, tumors of the paranasal sinuses and nasal cavity tend to be asymptomatic at early stages, presenting more frequently at late stages once extensive local invasion has occurred. The unfortunate combination of complex surrounding anatomy with late, advanced stage presentation therefore leads to the frequent local recurrence and subsequent poor outcome associated with sinonasal maligancies.

ANATOMY

The nasal cavity represents the most superior aspect of the upper airway and is lined by a combination of cuboidal and pseudostratified ciliated columnar epithelium. The nasal mucosa contains mucous glands, minor salivary glands, and melanocytes as well as olfactory neuroepithelial cells superiorly. The nasal cavity is divided in the midline by the nasal septum, a partition of cartilage and bone lined by mucosa. The superior boundary of the nasal cavity is the ethmoid sinus, while the inferior boundary or floor of the nasal cavity is the hard palate. The lateral nasal cavity wall is also the medial wall of the maxillary sinus which includes the inferior turbinate and meatus, middle turbinate and meatus, and the nasolacrimal duct. The sphenoid sinus lies posterior and superior to the nasal cavity, while the nasopharynx is directly posterior to the nasal cavity. The blood supply to the nasal cavity comes posteriorly from the sphenopalatine branch of the internal maxillary artery, superiorly from the anterior and posterior ethmoid arteries, and anteriorly from the facial artery. The autonomic innervation of the nasal cavity is supplied by the greater superficial petrosal nerve, a branch of the facial nerve.[5]

The maxillary sinus is an air-containing bony chamber that lies lateral to either side of the nasal cavity. Each sinus is interposed between orbit and oral cavity; the roof of the sinus composes the orbital floor, and the floor of the sinus composes the hard palate. Lateral to the maxillary sinus lie the pterygoid musculature, mandibular ramus, and infratemporal fossa. The pterygopalatine fossa and pterygoid plates are posterior to the maxillary sinus.

The pterygopalatine fossa contains terminal branches of the internal maxillary artery, the vidian nerve, divisions of the trigeminal nerve, and the sphenopalatine ganglion. The pterygopalatine fossa serves as an important portal between several adjacent regions, including the paranasal sinuses, nasopharynx, infratemporal fossa, orbit, sphenoid, oral cavity, and middle cranial fossa.[5] Malignant invasion of the pterygopalatine fossa is therefore a particularly ominous feature.[6]

The orbit is a pyramid-shaped structure with its apex oriented posteromedially in close approximation with the paranasal sinuses and anterior cranial fossa. The orbital floor is the roof of the maxillary sinus; the medial orbital wall or lamina papyracea is the lateral wall of the ethmoid sinus; the superomedial wall forms the floor of the frontal sinus, and the orbital roof composes part of the anterior cranial base. The center of the anterior cranial base is formed by the cribriform plate and fovea ethmoidalis, or roof of the ethmoid sinus. The cribriform plate transmits olfactory nerve fibers from the central nervous system into the nasal cavity.

Deep to the zygoma and lateral to the maxillary sinus lies the infratemporal fossa. The infratemporal crest and the maxillary alveolus delineate the superior and inferior medial boundaries of this space, respectively. The mandibular ramus forms the lateral aspect of the infratemporal fossa, the lateral pterygoid plate lies medially, and the lateral wall of the maxillary sinus forms the anteromedial boundary. The roof of the infratemporal fossa is formed by both the greater sphenoid wing, the floor of the middle cranial fossa and an opening into the temporal fossa.[6] Also in communication with the infratemporal fossa are the inferior orbital fissure anteriorly and superiorly, and pterygopalatine fossa inferomedially.

The paranasal sinuses and nasal cavity therefore lie in a complex and intimate association with each other and with the orbits, infratemporal fossa, pterygopalatine fossa, and skull base. Sinonasal malignancies may extend through direct extension to these adjacent structures. A thorough understanding of the tumor's surrounding anatomical relationships is essential in determining the feasibility of surgical resection for a sinonasal tumor.

Staging

Öhngren described a difference in the prognosis of maxillary sinus malignancies depending on their anatomic location within the sinus.[7] He divided the maxillary sinus into 2 halves by an oblique, imaginary plane passing through the medial canthus of the eye and the angle of the mandible (Figure 11–1). Öhngren observed that this plane separates the topographically more favorable tumors which are anterior and inferior to the plane, from those of more unfavorable character which are superior and posterior to the plane. Öhngren's early insight into the topographical importance of maxillary sinus carcinoma proved to be highly significant. Cancers of the maxillary sinus originating anterior and inferior to this plane (in the "infrastructure"), present earlier with symptoms and are more amenable to surgical resection with a better overall prognosis. In contrast, malignancies originating posterior and superior to this plane, (in the "suprastructure"), tend to develop symptoms later in the course of the disease and are challenging to resect surgically due to the anatomic proximity of the pterygopalatine fossa, infratemporal fossa, orbit, and skull base. These principles of maxillary sinus carcinoma behavior continue to be reflected in the American Joint Committee for Cancer (AJCC) staging system for maxillary sinus carcinoma.[8]

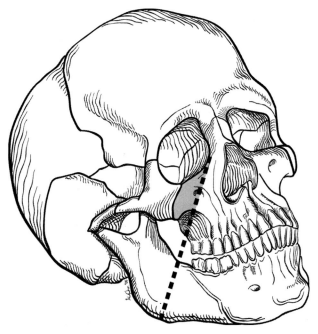

Figure 11–1. Anatomical diagram illustrating Öhngren's line.

Diagnosis

Symptoms

Nasal cavity and paranasal sinus malignancies often do not cause symptoms until they have expanded to a significant size or have extended through the bony confines of the sinus cavity. These tumors therefore tend to present at a more advanced stage. Symptoms may initially include nasal obstruction, epistaxis, pain, and episodes of sinusitis. Tumor expansion inferiorly towards the oral cavity may be associated with swelling of the gingiva or palate with loose teeth, while orbital invasion may lead to ocular symptoms such as proptosis, diplopia, decreased acuity, and restriction of ocular motion. Extension laterally into the pterygoid musculature may cause trismus and deeper invasion into the infratemporal fossa. Anterior extension through the anterior maxillary wall may cause visible cheek swelling and numbness from involvement of the infraorbital nerve. In rare cases, posterior and superior extension into the skull base, dura and brain may lead to headache, cerebrospinal fluid leak, and central nervous system deficits.

Physical Exam

A complete head and neck physical exam should always be performed, beginning with an assessment of overall facial symmetry and any areas of swelling or fullness. An eye examination should be performed with attention to the range of extraocular motion, visual acuity, pupillary response, and signs of globe displacement. Proptosis may be evident from the anterior displacement of the globe from a mass impinging on the orbit. An ear examination should inspect the tympanic membrane to assess middle ear aeration and to evaluate possible eustachian tube dysfunction or obstruction. Intraoral inspection of the hard palate, gingiva, and anterior maxillary wall should assess for fullness, signifying an expanding mass within the maxillary sinus or nasal cavity (Figure 11–2). Mandibular excursion should be assessed for trismus, a possible sign of pterygoid musculature invasion. Cranial nerves should be tested with particular attention to nerves I through VI along with a

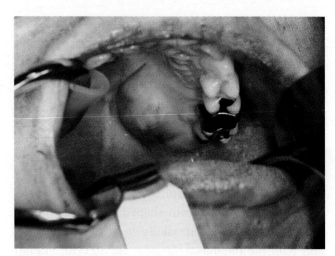

Figure 11-2. A hard palate and gingival bulge results from the inferior extension of a left maxillary sinus mass into the oral cavity.

general neurologic evaluation. A thorough intranasal exam is essential, using a flexible or rigid endoscope for optimal visualization of the nasal cavity and nasopharynx. Although gross tumor may be obvious, subtle irregularities in the nasal mucosal lining or fullness in the lateral or superior nasal cavity wall should also be carefully assessed. A thorough neck examination should be performed to evaluate for palpable lymph node metastases.

Imaging

Imaging studies are an essential component in the diagnosis, staging, and follow-up of sinonasal malignancies. Computed tomography (CT) scans give a good initial overview of the tumor's location with excellent bone detail (Figure 11–3). Because the paranasal sinuses and nasal cavity are mucosal-lined bony chambers, CT is helpful in determining whether a tumor remains confined within these natural boundaries or has eroded through the surrounding bone. CT provides details of the extent of local bone invasion, and is particularly useful in assessing the lamina papyracea, orbital floor, fovea ethmoidalis, cribriform plate, pterygoid plates, hard palate, and skull base.[9] The signal of the tumor is of soft-tissue density and may be either homogeneous or heterogeneous if focal areas of necrosis or hemorrhage exist. Intravenous contrast causes tumor enhancement, although inflamed mucosa may enhance similarly. Radiodensities within a mass may

mit intraluminal carotid assessment without the associated risks of conventional angiography. Inflamed mucosa, retained secretions, and benign polyps generally have a high signal on T2-weighted images. In contrast, tumors which are more cellular, with less

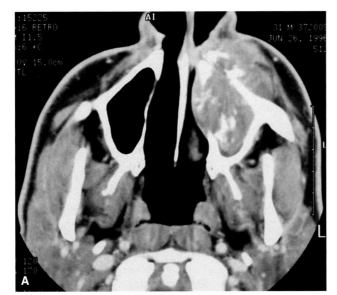

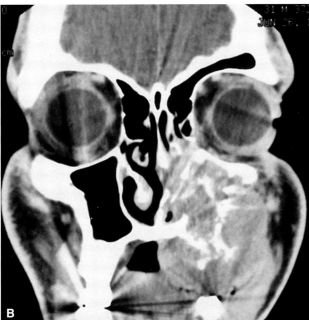

Figure 11–3. *A* and *B*, Axial and coronal CT scans accurately demonstrate the extent of bone destruction from a left-sided maxillary sinus tumor.

have particular characteristics suggestive of tumoral mineral deposition, residual destroyed bone from tumor invasion, or chronic fungal sinusitis.[10]

In comparison to CT, magnetic resonance imaging (MRI) allows a better distinction of tumor from adjacent soft tissue (Figure 11–4). MRI is particularly useful for determining invasion of the orbital contents, dura, brain, and cavernous sinus.[9] MRI may also be better for assessing carotid artery invasion, and newer techniques such as MR angiography per-

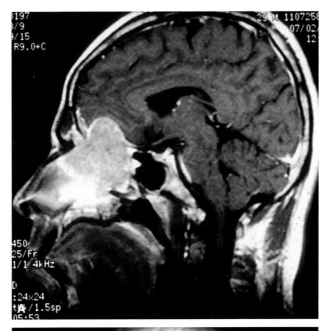

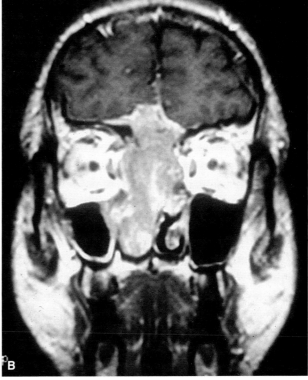

Figure 11–4. *A* and *B*, A saggital and coronal MRI scan with gadolinium contrast shows a large ethmoid malignancy completely filling both ethmoid sinuses and the right nasal cavity, with extensive intracranial extension.

amounts of extracellular water, exhibit an intermediate signal on T2-weighted images.[11] The exceptions to this characteristic are some schwannomas, minor salivary gland tumors, and a subgroup of inverted papillomas. Benign tumors extending intracranially tend to be more heterogeneous on MRI than malignant tumors.[12] With gadolinium injection on T1-weighted images, tumors enhance less intensely than inflamed mucosa, while secretions do not enhance. Mucoceles may be distinguished from tumors by peripheral enhancement.[13] CT and MRI therefore complement one another in the assessment of sinonasal tumors. CT provides excellent bone detail, while MRI offers better soft tissue imaging.

Biopsy

Once the site of the tumor has been identified, tissue diagnosis is required. A fundamental principle should be to obtain representative tissue by the least invasive method possible. Avoiding an open procedure is advantageous in preventing (1) the disturbance of intact anatomical structures and boundaries, (2) the possible tumor contamination of normal tissues, and (3) the disturbance of the tumor's location and obfuscation of its margins, making future localization and surgical treatment significantly more difficult.

An optimal procedure for biopsy of sinonasal malignancies is an endoscopic approach through the nares. This approach offers several advantages, including excellent visualization, low morbidity, and minimal alteration of the tumor and its surrounding structures. Even small, lateral tumors within the maxillary sinus may be accessible with the creation of a middle meatal antrostomy, visualization with a 30° or 70° endoscope, and biopsy using a long, curved giraffe instrument. An endoscopic approach should not, however, be used for either debulking or an attempted resection of the tumor. If the tumor presents itself at the nasal vestibule, punch biopsy in the office may be considered. However, it is important to insure by clinical examination that the mass is neither contiguous with the cerebrospinal fluid space nor highly vascular. If the mass compresses easily or appears vascular, further imaging should be obtained prior to biopsy.

In cases where a maxillary sinus tumor is not accessible transnasally with the endoscope, a canine fossa puncture can be combined with endoscopic visualization and biopsy. Open biopsy may rarely be necessary for poorly accessible tumors, through either a Caldwell-Luc approach or an external ethmoidectomy (Lynch) incision. However, if an open approach is used, minimal dissection and disruption of surrounding normal tissues should be sought for the reasons described above. Alternatively, the definitive surgical resection may be planned at the time of the open biopsy with frozen-section analysis if preoperative consent for this possibility has been obtained.

Pathology

Squamous Cell Carcinoma

Squamous cell carcinoma is the most common malignancy of the sinonasal tract. These tumors are more common in men than in women with a peak incidence between 60 to 70 years of age. There is an association between sinonasal squamous cell carcinoma and nickel exposure. Workers at a nickel refinery in Norway developed squamous cell carcinoma at 250 times the expected rate, with a latent period varying from 18 to 36 years.[14] Although tobacco and alcohol are major risk factors for squamous cell carcinoma of the

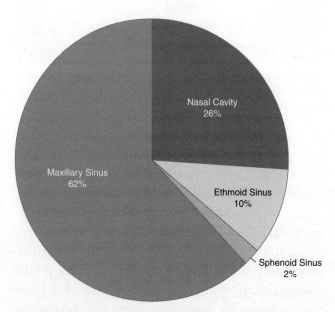

Figure 11–5. Site distribution of sinonasal squamous cell carcinoma. Data from Spiro et al.[70]

upper aerodigestive tract, they do not appear to be associated with sinonasal carcinogenesis.

The most frequent site of origin for squamous cell carcinoma is the maxillary sinus followed by the nasal cavity, ethmoid sinus, and sphenoid sinus (Figure 11-5). Within the nasal cavity, squamous cell carcinoma most commonly arises from the turbinates, followed by the nasal septum, floor, and vestibule.[15] Approximately 80 percent of these tumors are keratinizing carcinomas, with the remaining 20 percent the non-keratinizing subtype.[16] These lesions have a slight tendency to be of moderate histologic differentiation. Although less-differentiated lesions may exhibit a more rapid course of growth, the degree of differentiation does not carry as much prognostic significance as the extent of the disease.[15]

Adenocarcinoma

Adenocarcinomas exhibit a male predominance with a peak age incidence between 55 and 60 years.[5] Adenocarcinomas tend to arise superiorly in the sinonasal region and commonly involve the ethmoid sinuses. There is a significantly higher incidence of adenocarcinomas in workers exposed to wood dust particles. Acheson estimated that woodworkers in the furniture industry in southern England had an approximately 875-fold increased incidence in sinonasal adenocarcinoma when compared to the normal population.[17] Sinonasal adenocarcinomas may assume three basic histologic forms: papillary, sessile, and alveolar-mucoid.[15] Although one pattern may dominate a particular tumor, a combination of all three types also may coexist. The papillary form is the type associated with woodworkers and tends to be more localized with a better prognosis. In contrast, the sessile and alveolar-mucoid forms are locally more aggressive with a greater metastatic potential and carry a poorer prognosis.

Adenoid Cystic Carcinoma

Minor salivary glands lining the sinonasal tract may give rise to malignancies of salivary origin. Adenoid cystic carcinomas account for 5 to 15 percent of sinonasal malignancies and occur equally in both sexes with a peak age incidence between 40 and 60 years. Clinically, adenoid cystic carcinoma is marked by locally aggressive disease with a slow, relentless progression. Although regional lymphatic spread of adenoid cystic carcinoma is uncommon, both local recurrence and distant metastases may become evident in a delayed fashion, and in some cases even up to 20 years after treatment of the primary lesion. Perineural spread is the hallmark of adenoid cystic carcinoma. Cranial nerve invasion often provides an avenue of spread to the cranial base making local disease control particularly difficult.[5]

Mucosal Melanoma

Melanomas constitute about 3.5 percent of all neoplasms in the sinonasal tract, and orignate from neural crest-derived melanocytes present in the mucosa and submucosa. The nasal cavity is more commonly affected than the paranasal sinuses. Although some melanomas may appear heavily pigmented, others may be non-pigmented and appear pink or tan in color; melanin may or may not be present in these tumors. Histologically, sinonasal melanomas are quite varied, with both epithelioid and spindle cell features. As with all mucosal melanomas, the prognosis is quite poor with local recurrence and distant metastases ocurring in up to two-thirds of patients within 1 year.[12]

Olfactory Neuroblastoma

Olfactory neuroblastoma, also known as esthesioneuroblastoma, is a tumor of neural crest origin derived from olfactory epithelium. These tumors arise from the superior nasal cavity and typically form a mucosa-covered, soft mass with a congested appearance. These tumors occur with equal frequency in males and females with a bimodal age distribution; one peak occurs in a younger population aged 11 to 20 years, and the second peak in an older group aged 51 to 60 years.[15] The histologic appearance is marked by a characteristic rosette pattern of round cells with fibrillary material. Electron microscopy and special stains for neurofibrils are required to make the final diagnosis.[5] A staging system proposed by Kadish categorizes stage A as tumor confined to the nasal cavity, stage B as extension to the paranasal sinuses, and stage C as extension beyond, including cranial cavity, orbit, or with distant metastases.[18] The majority of these tumors are locally aggressive and tend to invade adjacent structures such as the orbit and cranial cavity. Regional lymph node metastases may occur in 20 to 40 percent of cases.[16] Prognosis is dependent on disease extent at presentation.

Sinonasal Undifferentiated Carcinoma

Sinonasal undifferentiated carcinoma is a highly aggressive, rapidly growing malignancy that frequently involves multiple sinuses and the nasal cavity. Histologically, sinonasal undifferentiated carcinoma is marked by pleomorphic cells arranged in sheets, nests, and trabeculae with a high nuclear to cytoplasmic ratio. There is an absence of any histologic differentiating features.[16] These tumors may be histologically confused with olfactory neuroblastoma, although the distinction is important because of their different clinical behaviors. The poor prognosis of sinonasal undifferentiated carcinoma is related to its propensity for extensive local invasion.

Other

Other malignancies which may arise in the sinonasal tract include a variety of lymphomas and sarcomas. Kraus reviewed non-squamous cell malignancies of the paranasal sinuses and identified the most common histologic sarcoma types as fibrosarcoma, rhabdomyosarcoma, and osteogenic sarcoma.[3] The lymphoma type most commonly involved was histiocytic, large cell lymphoma. Minor salivary gland carcinomas other than adenoid cystic carcinoma and adenocarcinoma may also arise in the sinonasal tract, such as mucoepidermoid carcinoma.

TREATMENT GOALS AND ALTERNATIVE FACTORS AFFECTING CHOICE OF TREATMENT

The treatment goals should be assessed individually for each patient prior to embarking on any course of therapy. These decisions should include careful consideration of many factors including (1) histology of the tumor, (2) tumor stage, (3) feasibility of a complete surgical resection, (4) the patient's underlying medical condition, (5) associated treatment risks and morbidity, (6) reconstructive options for the restoration of form and function, (7) socioeconomic issues, (8) the surgeon's technical ability, and (9) each patient's personal wishes.

A curative attempt is feasible for lesions that appear to be surgically resectable. Early maxillary sinus lesions or nasal cavity lesions are infrequent. These tumors may be removed surgically without any additional therapy if the resection completely encompasses the limited tumor. However, the overwhelming majority of sinonasal malignancies require multimodality therapy. The mainstay of treatment for resectable lesions is surgery combined with postoperative radiation therapy. Limited studies have suggested that the use of chemotherapy and radiation therapy may also be beneficial for more advanced tumors. Palliation may be the primary treatment goal for patients with extensive, unresectable local disease, distant metastatic disease, or poor physical constitution. Palliative treatment is most often applied as radiation therapy and/or chemotherapy in an attempt to reduce local morbidity.

The optimal management of sinonasal malignancies is not standardized, and many issues remain controversial. The difficulties in assessing treatment strategies derive from the relative rarity of these lesions, combined with a multitude of different histologic types and sites of involvement. Because squamous cell carcinoma is most common, most studies have focused their observations on this histologic type. The following recommendations reflect our approach to the treatment of sinonasal squamous cell carcinoma.

Surgery or Radiation Therapy Alone

Early squamous cell carcinoma of the maxillary sinus (T1) and small, contained, anterior nasal cavity malignancies may be amenable to surgical resection alone as definitive therapy. If the surgical margins from the specimen are widely negative with no evidence of perineural invasion and the tumor is of a low-grade histology, then no postoperative radiation therapy is required. The addition of any of these features, however, identifies a tumor that should be treated more aggressively with bimodal therapy, given its increased likelihood for local recurrence.

Radiation therapy alone for localized (T1) squamous cell carcinoma of the maxillary sinus and nasal cavity may also be effective. However, surgery is generally preferred because radiation therapy has a higher local morbidity in this anatomic location from close proximity to the orbit, brain, and salivary glands. Radiation therapy alone for larger (T2 to T4) squamous cell carcinoma gives significantly inferior results in comparision to combination therapy. Several series have shown that radiation therapy alone used for all T stage lesions yields 5-year survival rates of only 0 to 16 percent.[19–22]

Squamous cell carcinomas of the nasal vestibule behave more similarly to cutaneous squamous cell carcinoma than sinonasal malignancies, and are staged by the AJCC according to the cutaneous classification system.[8] Vestibular carcinomas have a more favorable prognosis than sinonasal malignancies. Primary radiation alone as external beam therapy and/or brachytherapy has been shown to be effective for T1 and T2 lesions, with a 94 percent 5-year local control rate and a 94 percent 5-year cause-specific survival rate.[23] Surgery alone is also effective for these early lesions, particularly for medial lesions that may be resected with low morbidity. Lateral or inferior lesions present a more difficult reconstructive challenge, and therefore radiation therapy is preferred.[24] T4 lesions are best treated with a combination of surgery and radiation therapy.

Surgery with Postoperative Radiation Therapy

Surgery combined with postoperative radiation therapy is the standard treatment for most sinonasal malignancies. Several series have shown that combination therapy of surgery with radiation is superior to surgery alone.[5] Most squamous cell carcinoma of the maxillary sinus (T2, T3, and most T4), nasal cavity, and ethmoid sinus may be treated by surgical resection followed by radiation therapy if the tumor is confined to an anatomic region that makes it removable in its entirety. Massive parenchymal brain invasion, extensive skull base invasion, massive tumor volume with trismus, and carotid artery inva-

sion are contraindications to surgical resection. Gross tumor invasion through the periorbita with infiltration of orbital fat or muscle requires orbital exenteration. Localized anterior skull base invasion does not necessarily preclude consideration of surgery, as these tumors may still be removed with craniofacial resection. Most 5-year survival figures for combination surgery and radiation treatment range from 35 to 50 percent for a variety of histologic lesions across all stages (Table 11–1).

Preoperative radiation therapy has been proposed as an alternative to postoperative radiation therapy. Yu-Hua reported an improved 5-year survival rate for patients treated with preoperative radiation when compared to postoperative treatment, although these findings have not been reproduced.[25] Sisson supported the use of preoperative radiation therapy, stating that the radiation treatment may change an inoperable lesion to an operable one, and may make orbital preservation possible.[26] However, shrinkage of the primary tumor in response to preoperative radiation should not influence the extent of surgical resection. Tumors do not shrink concentrically and may leave islands of viable cells behind in normal-appearing tissue. The surgical resection should therefore include the same area involved with tumor as prior to any radiation therapy.[27] In addition, postoperative wound complications increase with increasing doses of preoperative radiation therapy.

The advantages of postoperative radiation therapy include no delay in tumor resection, dissection through normal tissue planes during the surgery, improved postoperative wound healing, and less dose restriction. In addition, radiation therapy may be more effective as a postoperative treatment of microscopic disease, rather than as an initial treatment for massive, bulky disease.

Surgical Management of the Orbit

The specific indications for orbital preservation and exenteration have evolved over the past 40 years and remain a controversial subject. Although in the 1950s the orbit was almost routinely exenterated for any extension of maxillary sinus carcinoma toward the orbital floor, the emerging consensus is that the

Study	No. of Patients	Treatment Options	Site	Tumor Type	T stage, maxillary	5-Year Survival	Local Control
Yu-Hua[25] 1982	50	RT + surgery Surgery + RT	Maxillary	SCC	T1: 0 T2: 4 T3: 31 T4: 14	54% (preop RT 64%, postop RT 29%)	
Spiro[70] 1989	105	Surgery + RT RT + surgery RT alone Surgery alone	Maxillary Nasal cavity Ethmoid	SCC	T1: 2 T2: 8 T3: 32 T4: 13	37% (nasal 45%, maxillary 38%, ethmoid 13%)	49.2% for maxillary tumors (33/65)
Zaharia[71] 1989	149	Surgery + RT	Maxillary	Multiple	T1: 2 T2: 12 T3: 117 T4: 18	36.2%	67.1%
Lavertu[72] 1989	54	Surgery Surgery + RT RT + surgery	Maxillary Ethmoid	SCC	T1: 3 T2: 9 T3: 20 T4: 16	38.2% for maxillary tumors	37.5% for maxillary tumors
Sisson[26] 1989	60	RT + surgery Surgery + RT Surgery alone Chemo alone	Maxillary Ethmoid	Multiple	T1: 2 T2: 13 T3: 16 T4: 15	49% (preop RT 65%, postop RT 63%, maxillary sinus only 42.8%)	56% for surgery + RT 41% for RT + surgery
Jiang[47] 1991	73	Postop RT	Maxillary	Multiple	T1: 3 T2: 16 T3: 32 T4: 22	51%	78%
Paulino[73] 1998	48	Surgery + RT RT alone	Maxillary	Multiple	T1: 1 T2: 6 T3: 17 T4: 24	46.9% (surgery + RT 51.5%, RT alone 0%)	50.5% (surgery + RT 59.2%, RT alone 22.7%)

Table 11–1. SURGERY AND RADIATION THERAPY

RT = radiation therapy; SCC = squamous cell carcinoma.

orbit can often be preserved without compromising overall survival or local control of disease. This approach has been complicated, however, by differing criteria that have been used to determine the indications for orbital preservation.

Carrau examined 58 patients with bony orbital invasion by squamous cell carcinoma of the sinonasal tract and found that 3-year survival was not affected by orbital preservation in the absence of orbital soft tissue invasion. The authors concluded that the orbit may be spared if the full thickness of the periorbita is not breached by tumor.[28] McCary and Perry concluded from their review of 36 patients that periorbital invasion does not necessarily indicate a need for orbital exenteration. They found that preoperative radiation therapy followed by intraoperative frozen section and selected resection of the involved periorbita may save the eye without a compromised outcome.[29–30] Tumor exten-

sion through the periorbita does not necessarily condemn the eye to exenteration. Tiwari has noted that a thin fascial layer exists around the periorbital fat that is distinct from the periorbita and believes that invasion of this layer should determine the need for exenteration.[31] Quatela has taken an even more aggressive approach by resecting intraorbital tumor with involved orbital fat and extraocular muscles off of Tenon's fascia surrounding the globe, and then preserving or "banking" the residual, nonfunctional globe in vivo.[32]

Care must be taken to avoid attempting orbital preservation at the potential cost of decreased local disease control and survival. Our approach is to resect involved periorbita and preserve the orbital contents in cases where there is no invasion of orbital fat, orbital musculature, or involvement of the orbital apex. The invasion of any of these structures is an indication for orbital exenteration.

Chemotherapy for Advanced Tumors

In attempts to improve the survival rates and local control of advanced sinonasal tumors, chemotherapy has been administered as an adjuvant treatment in a wide variety of methods. Chemotherapy has been given (1) with radiation and daily tumor debridement,[33–36] (2) by topical application,[35] (3) selectively to the head and neck through intra-arterial infusion,[33,37–39] (4) as a neoadjuvant treatment prior to further local treatment,[40–42] and (5) concomitantly with hyperfractionated radiation therapy[43–45] (Tables 11–2 and 11–3). Unfortunately, many studies have been published with a wide variety of different chemotherapy agents and treatment regimens, small numbers of patients, short follow-up periods, varying tumor histologies, and varying outcomes, all of which make a universal interpretation of these results difficult. The preliminary data from these studies suggest that advanced stage sinonasal tumors derive a significant benefit from combination chemotherapy regimens and are appropriate for locally extensive tumors not amenable to surgical resection. However, larger reviews with longer follow-up and randomized trials are needed for a more thorough assessment of the role of chemotherapy in the management of sinonasal malignacies.

Treatment of the Neck

Clinically positive metastatic disease in the neck is generally managed with neck dissection, the type depending on the extent and location of the nodal metastases. The spinal accessory nerve may be preserved if it is not grossly involved with disease. Postoperative radiation therapy to the neck is indicated for multiple positive nodes, any single node > 3 cm in size, or extracapsular spread.

The management of the clinically negative neck remains controversial. Some studies have supported the use of elective neck irradiation for maxillary squamous cell carcinoma.[46–47] Paulino noted a 28.9 percent rate of neck recurrence in 38 patients with maxillary squamous cell carcinoma and initially untreated N0 necks.[46] However, traditional guidelines have not indicated a need for prophylactic neck treatment unless the sinonasal tumor encroaches upon areas of increased risk for lymphatic spread such as the nasopharynx or soft palate.[48] Penzer argued against elective neck irradiation, reporting that although elective neck irradiation resulted in improved regional control, no survival benefit was noted.[49] Our approach is to not treat the N0 neck electively in cases of sinonasal squamous cell carcinoma.

Radiation Therapy for Palliation

Radiation therapy alone as a treatment modality is primarily reserved for palliative care. Palliation is an appropriate treatment goal for patients with massive unresectable tumors, distant metastatic disease, extensive medical co-morbidities, and poor physical constitution precluding more aggressive therapy.

Table 11–2. CHEMOTHERAPY AND ROUTINE TUMOR DÉBRIDEMENT					
Study	No.	Treatment Regimen	Site	Tumor Type	Results
Sato[33] 1970	57	Surgery + RT + intra-arterial 5-FU (superficial temporal artery) + antral cleaning	All sinuses	Multiple	Complete response: 38/57 22/57 needed no further Rx
Sakai[34] 1983	134	RT + 5-FU + cryosurgery + immunotherapy + antrostomy + antral cleaning	Maxillary	Multiple	4-yr survival: 54% 4-yr local control: 45.2%
Knegt[35] 1985	60	Surgery + low dose RT + topical 5-FU + antral cleaning	All sinuses	Multiple	5-yr survival: 65% 5-yr survival for SCC and Undifferentiated carcinoma: 52%
Sakata[36] 1993	33	Low dose RT + intra-arterial 5-FU/BUdR + antral cleaning	Maxillary	SCC	5-yr survival: 46%
	45	Low dose RT + antral cleaning	Maxillary	SCC	5-yr survival: 24%
	14	Single tumor debulking + pre- and postop RT	Maxillary	SCC	5-yr survival: 7.2%
	15	intra-arterial 5FU/cisplatin + surgery + pre- and postop RT	Maxillary	SCC	5-yr survival: 53%

BUdR = 5-bromodeoxyuridine; 5-FU = 5-fluorouracil; RT = radiation therapy; SCC = squamous cell carcinoma..

Table 11–3. CHEMOTHERAPY AND RADIATION THERAPY					
Study	No.	Treatment Regimen	Site	Tumor Type	Results
Lee[37] 1989	24	Intra-arterial cisplatin, bleomycin (internal maxillary artery) + subsequent IV 5-FU + surgery and/or RT	All sinuses	Multiple	2 pts died, 1 tech failure; CR: 9/21 (43%), PR: 10 (48%), MR: 2 (9%); (SCC: CR 5, PR 7, MR 1)
LoRusso[40] 1989	24	Neoadjuvant cisplatin, vincristine, bleomycin, or 5-FU, cisplatin, or 5-FU, MTX + surgery and/or RT	All sinuses	Multiple	CR: 44%, PR 38%; survival of previously untreated pts—CR: 21+ mo, PR 13.5 mo, NR 3mo
Choi[43] 1991	14	Hyperfractionated RT + concomitant cisplatin	All sinuses Nasopharynx	Multiple	CR: 11/12 7/12 (58%) alive at 47 mo 5 NED, 2 local recurrences
Rosen[42] 1993	12	Neoadjuvant 5-FU, cisplatin + surgery and RT ± concomitant chemo	All sinuses	Multiple	CR: 11/12 11/12 (92%) alive at 55 mo One death from disease
Harrison[44] 1998	52	Delayed accelerated RT + concomitant cisplatin (± mitomycin) + postRT cisplatin and vinblastine	All H&N (12 with paranasal sinus sites)	Multiple	CR: 60% for all sites; paranasal sinus local control: 78% 3-yr survival: 42%

H&N = head and neck; 5-FU = 5-fluorouracil; MTX = methotrexate ; RT = radiation therapy; SCC = squamous cell carcinoma; CR = complete response; MR = minimal response; NR = no response; PR = partial response; NED = no evidence of disease.

Radiation therapy alone may be of benefit in decreasing local morbidity from advanced sinonasal tumors, but is unlikely to provide a significant survival advantage except for early lesions. Surgical salvage reserved for primary radiation failures does not offer a survival advantage over conventional surgery with postoperative radiation therapy.[50] In addition, 26 percent of these primary radiation failures were subsequently considered unresectable due to extensive disease, further arguing against the use of radiation alone as initial therapy.

Surgical Treatment

The type of surgical resection required for tumors of the nasal cavity and paranasal sinuses is dictated by each lesion's anatomic location and sites of extension. Tumors originating in the maxillary sinus are removed by some form of maxillectomy. Several different subtypes of maxillectomy have been described, each characterized by the extent of the maxilla resected with tumor. Although terms such as limited, partial, medial, subtotal, total, radical, and extended have been used to differentiate these types of maxillectomy, there is still a lack of a standard nomenclature and some confusion exists between terms. To clarify these discrepancies, a classification system was recently described which categorized maxillectomies into limited, subtotal, and total max-

illectomies.[51] The limited maxillectomy removes primarily one wall of the maxilla, while the subtotal maxillectomy removes at least two walls, including the palate. Total maxillectomy is a term reserved for procedures resecting the entire maxilla. This system of classification requires that the soft-tissue approach to the maxilla, as well as the specific portion of bone removed, be described for limited and subtotal maxillectomies. Any extension of the resection to include adjacent structures such as the orbit should also be clarified.

The limited maxillectomy is most frequently performed with either resection of the medial wall or the floor of the maxillary sinus. Medial maxillectomy is appropriate for limited, low-grade tumors of the medial wall of the maxillary sinus, nasal cavity, and ethmoid sinus, such as inverted papilloma. The entire medial maxillary wall, lamina papyracea and ethmoid sinus are removed in this procedure (Figures 11–6 and 11–7). The infraorbital nerve is preserved, along with the majority of the anterior maxillary wall, orbital floor, and entire lateral maxillary wall and floor. The fragile nature of the ethmoid air cells, lamina papyracea, and lateral nasal wall makes the en bloc removal of an entire medial maxillectomy specimen challenging.[52]

Malignancies of the floor and lower half of the maxillary sinus may extend inferiorly into the hard palate or alveolar ridge. If such tumors are limited in extent and anteriorly located, they may be resected by a limited maxillectomy of the maxillary floor by an approach through the open mouth (Figures 11–8 and 11–9). Intraoral mucosal incisions are made on the hard palate and extended into the gingival-buccal sulcus, allowing elevation of the cheek soft tissues off the anterior maxillary wall. Osteotomies along the inferior maxilla are then made with a high-speed power saw and osteotome.

Larger tumors of the maxillary sinus may be resected by subtotal maxillectomy, a procedure that removes at least two walls of the sinus including a portion of the hard palate. The tumor location determines the particular subtotal variant that is appropriate. Total maxillectomy is the least common maxillary resection, and is defined as the complete removal of the maxilla (Figures 11–10 and 11–11). Orbital exenteration may be included, and has been performed in up to 71 percent of cases requiring total maxillectomy.[51] Extensions of total maxillectomy are more common and may involve any number of adjacent sites.

The choice of soft-tissue approach depends on the type of maxillectomy being performed. Limited maxillectomy for small lesions of the hard palate or floor of the maxillary sinus may occasionally be approached transorally without the need for any facial incisions. A midface degloving or Denker's approach offers better inferior maxillary exposure while also avoiding any external skin incisions. Medial maxillectomy requires a lateral rhinotomy incision with a Lynch extension for improved ethmoid exposure superiorly. Larger nasal cavity and maxillary lesions require a Weber-Ferguson incision. Total maxillectomy requires a much wider lateral exposure with a full elevation of the cheek flap and division of the infraorbital nerve. This exposure may be achieved by a Weber-Ferguson incision with a subciliary or transconjunctival extension. An alternate approach for total maxillectomy is a Weber-Ferguson incision with an extended Lynch extension curving superiorly and laterally across the brow. This incision, when combined with gentle orbital retraction laterally, permits adequate lateral exposure for total maxillectomy without requiring either a subciliary or transconjunctival extension. A combination subciliary and supraciliary extension of the Weber-Ferguson incision is indicated for total maxillectomy with orbital exenteration.[52]

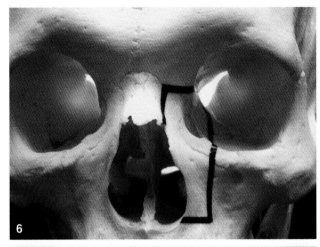

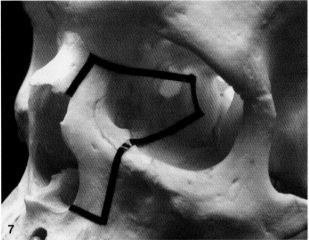

Figures 11–6 and 11–7. Anteroposterior and oblique views of a skull delineating the osteotomies required for a medial maxillectomy.

Nonsurgical Treatment

Chemotherapy with Maxillary Debridement

Chemotherapy has been incorporated into numerous different treatment regimens with varying agents, methods of delivery, and combinations with radiation and/or surgery. In the 1970s several groups in Japan began trying a combination of chemotherapy, radiation therapy and routine tumor débridement or cryosurgery within the maxillary sinus. The regimens included 5-fluorouracil (5-FU) or cisplatin with delivery through intravenous,[34,36] selective intra-arterial,[33] and topical methods.[35] Responses to these treatments were encouraging. Four- to 5-year survival rates for squamous cell carcinoma were in the 46 to 65 percent range for all histologic types combined (see Table 11–2). Sakata initially tried a

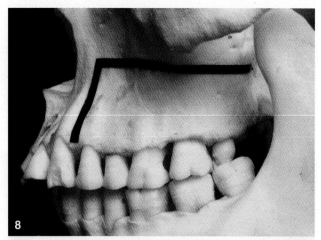

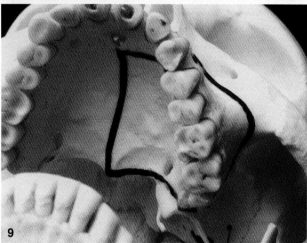

Figures 11–8 and 11–9.   Lateral and palatal views of a skull delineating the osteotomies required for an "infastructure" maxillectomy.

regmen of 5-FU, bromodeoxyuridine, low-dose radiation therapy, and daily tumor débridement and reported a 5-year survival of 46 percent. Modifications of this regimen without chemotherapy or without daily débridement led to significantly worse survival. However, the additions of (1) cisplatin to the 5-FU, (2) a more aggressive surgical maxillectomy, and (3) higher dose radiation therapy both pre- and post-operatively ultimately yielded the best survival results.[36] Difficulties of these routine débridements included significant pain as well as risk of injury to adjacent structures such as the orbit and brain.

Selective Intra-arterial Chemotherapy

The selective administration of chemotherapy through intra-arterial infusion offers the advantage of a more direct drug delivery to the tumor site at a

higher local concentration than can be achieved with systemic therapy. This technique was initially attempted with modest results similar to those obtained by surgery and postoperative radiation therapy.[53] Shibuya suggested that one problem was the multiplicity of feeding arteries supplying the maxillary sinus causing an irregular, lower distribution of intra-arterially infused chemotherapy.[54] A study by Lee reviewed 24 patients treated with selective intra-arterial cisplatin and bleomycin through the internal maxillary artery, combined with intravenous 5-fluorouracil, and followed by radiation therapy and/or surgery. Although long-term follow-up was not available, 43 percent achieved a complete response, 48 percent a partial response, and only 9 percent a minimal response.[37] Two patients died from complications related to the selective chemotherapy. Robbins has treated a variety of advanced head and neck cancers using selective intra-arterial cisplatin with con-

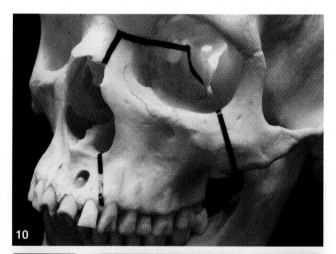

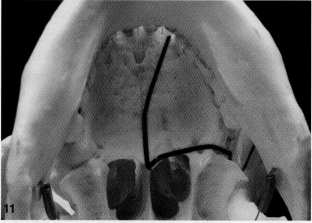

Figures 11–10 and 11–11.   Oblique and palatal views of a skull delineating the osteotomies required for a total maxillectomy.

comitant radiation therapy and intravenous sodium thiosulfate neutralization. Sodium thiosulfate binds covalently to cisplatin and forms a product that is nontoxic and devoid of antitumor activity, thereby reducing side effects and permitting a high cisplatin concentration to be delivered to the tumor site. In a group of 24 patients with all types of stage IV head and neck carcinoma, Robbins reported an impressive complete response rate of 96 percent, and an overall and disease-free 3-year survival of 88 percent and 53 percent respectively.[38–39]

Neoadjuvant or Concurrent Chemotherapy

Despite the encouraging results described above, both routine tumor débridement and intra-arterial cannulation present technical demands and may not be available for widespread use. Chemotherapy may be administered intravenously as a neoadjuvant agent prior to treatment with other modalities. LoRusso gave 24 patients with stage III or IV disease various chemotherapy combinations, including 5-FU and cisplatin, and followed this with surgery and/or radiation therapy. Overall 5-year survival was only 9.5 percent, but 29 percent of patients remained disease free at a median of 15 months.[40] Bjork-Eriksson treated 12 patients with 5-FU and cisplatin followed by radiation therapy and then limited surgery. Local control was achieved in 11 patients and 10 remained alive without disease at a mean follow up of 27 months.[41] Rosen treated 12 patients with 5-FU and cisplatin followed by surgery and radiation with or without concomittant chemotherapy. Of these 12 patients, 11 had complete responses and had no evidence of disease at a mean follow up of 55 months with a range of 13 to 105 months.[42] The latter 2 studies showed particularly impressive initial response rates for neoadjuvant 5-FU and cisplatin, although they contained only small numbers of patients with limited follow-up.

Both cisplatin and 5-FU act as radiosensitizers by enhancing the effect of radiation therapy on tumor cells, and concomitant chemo-radiation delivery may take advantage of this effect. In addition, radiation may be more effective when delivered twice a day as either accelerated fractionation reducing overall treatment time, or as hyperfractionation increasing total dose delivery.[55] Choi gave cisplatin alone with concomitant hyperfractionated radiation therapy for T4 paranasal sinus and nasopharyngeal tumors. He found initial complete responses in 11 of 12 patients, with an overall 58 percent survival at a mean follow-up period of 47 months.[43] Harrison treated 52 patients with a variety of unresectable head and neck cancers, all T4 or N3, 12 of whom had paranasal sinus carcinoma. Many of these patients had brain and/or dural invasion, as well as orbital invasion. Treatment included delayed accelerated radiation therapy with concomitant cisplatin (+/- mitomycin), with or without adjuvant post-radiation cisplatin and vinblastine. Of all patients in the study, 60 percent had an initial complete response. The subgroup of patients with paranasal sinus carcinomas had a 3-year local control rate of 78 percent with an overall 3-year survival of 42 percent.[44,45]

In summary, cisplatin and 5-FU are currently the most effective chemotherapy agents in the treatment of sinonasal malignancy (see Table 11–3). Their adminstration may be most effective as neoadjuvant agents prior to other treatment modalities, or concurrently with hyperfractionated radiation therapy. Although initial responses seem encouraging, longer follow-up from these retrospective reviews and prospective randomized studies are required for a more thorough assessment. The use of chemotherapy in a multimodality regimen should be considered for all advanced sinonasal tumors not amenable to complete surgical resection in a non-palliative setting.

Sequelae, Complications and their Management

Surgery

The most common perioperative complications which may accompany surgical resection of sinonasal malignancies include intraoperative or postoperative bleeding, wound infection, cerebrospinal fluid leak, and visual or orbital injury if orbital preservation was planned. Visual complications including diplopia, lacrimal duct dysfunction, ectropion, and exposure keratopathy may occur in cases of maxillectomy with orbital preservation. Local morbidity from a maxillectomy defect depends on the extent of resection. Although historically maxillectomy defects have not always been reconstructed, the significant functional and cosmetic deficits from this procedure coupled with a larger selection of surgical and prosthetic reconstructive options now available make the reconstuction of maxillectomy defects a desired goal.

Hard palate defects from limited and subtotal maxillectomy may be fitted with a palatal obturator to separate the oral cavity from the sinus and nasal cavities. This closure is essential for swallowing and speech. The obturator is fabricated preoperatively with dental impressions taken by the prosthodontist and then fitted intraoperatively according to the extent of the surgical resection. A split-thickness skin graft is used to cover the undersurface of the cheek flap as well as the remaining bare bony interior of the maxillary sinus. Xeroform gauze packing is placed in the cavity and supported by fixation of the palatal obturator to remaining teeth or alveolus. The obturator allows for immediate swallowing function. One week postoperatively the initial obturator is removed with the packing, and an interim obturator is fashioned and fitted by the prosthodontist. The final permanent palatal obturator is placed in another 6 to 8 weeks.[52] A significant correlation has been established between the degree of obturator function and measurements of the patient's quality of life.[56]

Microvascular free tissue transfer may be used in selected cases for palatal reconstruction, obviating the need for a dental obturator. The radial forearm free flap may be used to reconstruct the hard or soft palate by folding it over and using one skin layer to line the nasal side, and the other the oral side of the defect[57–58] (Figures 11–12 and 11–13). The scapular free flap offers the additional option of vascularized bone with soft tissue for hard palate reconstruction.[59] Bone reconstruction may be particularly desirable in patients requiring osseointegrated dental implants. The latissimus dorsi may be transferred in conjunction with a bony scapular free flap as an additional soft tissue source.[60]

Surgical reconstruction of the lacrimal duct system and medial canthal ligament should always be addressed to avoid postoperative epiphora and pseudo-telecanthis, respectively. During elevation of the cheek flap at the time of maxillectomy, the lacrimal sac and duct are elevated out of the lacrimal fossa and transected flush with the orbital rim. The medial canthal ligament is detached from the nasal bone and retracted laterally with the orbital periosteum with a silk suture left long for identification. The interrupted lacrimal system is later restored during closure with the creation of a dacryocystorhinostomy. The medial canthal ligament is later sutured back to a drill hole in the nasal bone at the same level as the contralateral medial canthus.[52] During this reattachment, McCary has recommended a slight overcorrection in the superior direction to compensate for later inferior globe displacement.[61]

In cases of maxillectomy with orbital floor resection, reconstruction of the floor is critical to retaining the function of a preserved globe. Stern reviewed 18 patients treated with maxillectomy and orbital floor resection without reconstruction, 9 of whom also received radiation therapy. Only 3 patients (17%) retained any useful function within the preserved eye.[62] A globe that has been preserved without the support of the orbital floor is unlikely to retain significant function, especially if radiation therapy is used. Stern concluded that orbital exenteration should be considered in this setting. However, another interpretation is that there is a need to perform a reconstructive procedure restoring the support of the orbital floor for cases with orbital preservation.

Cordeiro successfully reconstructed maxillectomy and orbital floor defects in 14 patients who had orbital preservation. The orbital floor was restored using a nonvascularized bone graft such as split rib, split calvaria, or iliac crest (Figures 11–14 and 11–15). A rectus free flap was used in 12 patients and temporalis transposition in 2 elderly patients for soft-tissue reconstruction. There were no flap failures but there was one postoperative death. All 13 remaining patients were left with adequate functional vision. All of the orbital floor bone grafts were covered with well vascularized tissue and remained intact without evidence of resorption or infection, even in cases with postoperative radiation therapy. As Stern's findings had suggested, Cordeiro found that attention to orbital floor reconstruction assists in preserving ocular function.[63]

Total maxillectomy defects, particularly in cases with orbital exenteration or skin and soft-tissue defects, may be reconstructed in a single stage with

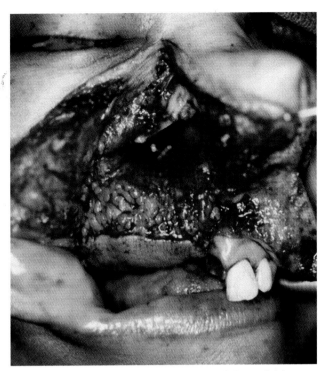

Figures 11–12. Intraoperative photograph of the radial forearm free flap placed in a right partial maxillectomy defect.

microvascular free tissue transfer. One of the most effective sources for maxillectomy and orbital defect reconstruction is the rectus abdominis free flap, a reliable source of tissue which provides both tissue bulk and skin[64] (Figure 11–16). The rectus flap may be folded on itself within the surgical defect such that the cutaneous flap restores the palate. To restore the volume defects and recontour the malar eminence, the maxillary cavity should be overcorrected initially and maximally filled with the flap; atrophy will later reduce its volume by up to one-third. Sus-

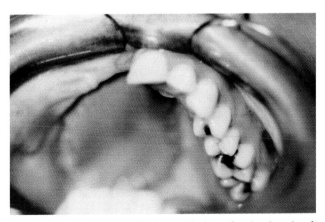

Figure 11–13. Postoperative intraoral view of a hard and soft palate reconstruction using a radial forearm free flap.

pension sutures around the flap prevent prolapse of the flap into the oral cavity.[65]

Radiation Therapy

The complications that may arise from radiation treatment of the paranasal sinuses can be quite significant and are related to the anatomic proximity of adjacent structures. Jiang reviewed the ocular complications that developed in 219 patients treated with radiation therapy for various sinonasal cancers. Sixty patients developed ipsilateral visual impairment, 8 patients developed ipsilateral blindness from optic neuropathy, and 11 developed bilateral visual impairment from optic chiasm injury. Corneal injury was highly significant (> 80%) with corneal and lacrimal gland irradiation > 55 Gy, but was preventable with corneal and lacrimal shielding. Radiation-induced retinopathy occurred in 20 percent of patients with doses of 50 to 60 Gy. Optic neuropathy was rare (< 5%) at doses $\leq$ 60 Gy, although the risk rapidly increased at higher doses. Bilateral blindness from optic chiasm injury was low (< 10%) at doses $\leq$ 60 Gy, although doses of 61 to 76 Gy caused a significantly higher rate (24%).[66]

Soft-tissue complications may include septal perforation, nasal cartilage necrosis, fistula, epiphora, nasal synechiae, nasal stenosis, trismus, pituitary insufficiency, and brain necrosis. Osteoradionecrosis, bone exposure, hearing loss, and loss of dentition may also occur. The risk of injury to these structures is related to both daily fraction size and total dose.[67]

Chemotherapy

The 2 most common chemotherapy agents used for sinonasal malignancies are cisplatin and 5-fluorouracil. Systemic cisplatin toxicity most commonly includes nausea and vomiting, renal failure, myelosuppression—with repeated treatment cycles, alopecia, and ototoxicity and neurotoxicity as a cumulative effect. 5-Fluorouracil may cause myelosuppression, mucositis, gastritis and diarrhea.[68]

The impressive results achieved with aggressive chemoradiotherapy regimens for advanced disease are associated with an increased toxicity. Harrison's regimen of cisplatin (+/–mitomycin) and concomi-

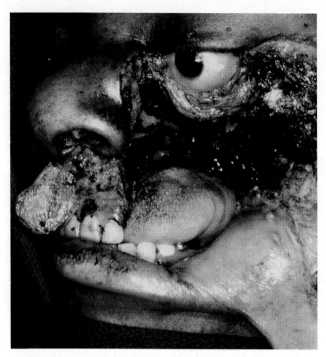

Figure 11–14.   Intraoperative photograph of a left total maxillectomy defect with resection of the orbital floor but preservation of the orbital contents.

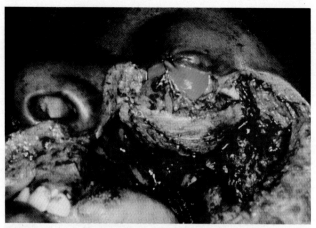

Figure 11–15.   Reconstruction of the orbital floor, with a split rib graft, in the same patient shown in Figure 11–14.

tant hyperfractionated radiation therapy followed by additional cisplatin and vinblastine caused significant mucositis in all 52 patients during the radiation phase. Of the 27 patients treated with both cisplatin and mitomycin, 2 (7.4%) died from sepsis resulting in the removal of mitomycin from the protocol. Treatment breaks were required in 38 percent of the patients, and only 44 percent of patients were able to tolerate two cycles of the post-radiation adjuvant treatment. There were *severe* acute complications in 34 percent of patients, including severe mucositis, granulocytopenia and sepsis, lung toxicity, blindness, frontal lobe necrosis, and osteoradionecrosis.[44]

The selective intra-arterial administration of high dose chemotherapy may lead to different complications. Lee's series of 24 patients treated with intra-arterial cisplatin and bleomycin through the internal maxillary artery followed by 5-fluorouracil had 2 deaths: the first 2 days after infusion following a generalized seizure, and the second 6 days after infusion without apparent cause. One additional patient suffered a cerebrovascular accident.[37] Robbins has noted that the administration of sodium thiosulfate following intra-arterial cisplatin decreases systemic toxicity by forming a

nontoxic product and permitting higher regional doses of cisplatin to be delivered to the tumor site.[38,39] The added morbidity of selective arterial cannulation with the still unclear effects of high-dose regional chemotherapy must be weighed together when considering the use of selective intra-arterial chemotherapy.

Outcomes and Results of Treatment

The prognosis for sinonasal malignancies has remained poor for the past several decades despite refinements in both surgical technique and radiation therapy. Stern reviewed the M.D. Anderson experi-

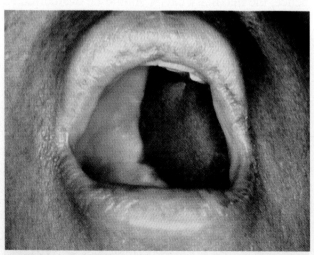

Figure 11–16.   An intraoral view of a rectus abdominus free flap filling a left total maxillectomy defect. Facial contour following total maxillectomy is improved by the soft-tissue bulk of a rectus abdominus free flap reconstruction.

ence for maxillary squamous cell carcinoma and found no significant improvement in survival when compared to a similar study there 20 years earlier.[69] However, another study from M.D. Anderson has shown an improved survival with surgery and postoperative radiation therapy when reviewing all types of malignancies.[47]

The various chemotherapy and radiation therapy regimens described above have shown survival improvements for advanced stage disease, although some of these reports have been for small numbers of patients with relatively short follow-up periods. Surgery with postoperative radiation therapy remains the standard treatment for resectable sinonasal carcinoma. A brief review of the larger series reporting outcomes for surgery with postoperative radiation therapy is shown in Table 11–1.

Spiro reviewed 105 patients at Memorial Sloan-Kettering Cancer Center with nasal cavity, maxillary, and ethmoid squamous cell carcinoma treated with combination surgery and radiation therapy, radiation therapy alone, or surgery alone. The majority of these patients presented with extensive disease with 82 percent of newly treated patients having stage III or stage IV disease. Survival is correlated to stage at presentation (Figure 11–17), and the overall 5-year survival was 37 percent. The survival rates for nasal, maxillary, and ethmoid tumors were 45 percent, 38 percent, and 13 percent respectively (Figure 11–18). The local control for maxillary sinus

tumors was 49 percent, and local recurrence was the most common site of failure.[70]

Zaharia reported the outcome of 149 patients treated with surgery and postoperative radiation therapy for a variety of malignant histologies. The 5-year actuarial survival was 36.2 percent overall, while for squamous cell carcinoma alone it was 35 percent.[71] Sisson reported a 49 percent 5-year survival after treating 60 patients with sinonasal malignancies with a variety of regimens.[26] Jiang reviewed the M.D. Anderson experience of 73 patients with maxillary sinus malignancies of varying histologies treated with surgery and postoperative radiation therapy. Overall 5-year relapse free survival was 51 percent, with a local control rate of 78 percent.[47] Lavertu treated 54 patients with squamous cell carcinoma of the sinuses: all received surgery and/or radiation therapy with an overall survival of 38.2 percent for the maxillary sinus group.[72]

SUMMARY

The overall treatment of sinonasal maligancies has resulted in 5-year survival rates in the 30 to 50 percent range, with most of the larger series near the lower end of this spectrum. Local control is a particularly difficult problem, with the majority of failures occurring at the primary site. These difficulties with sinonasal cancer treatment are linked to the complex anatomy of the paranasal sinus region, and a propen-

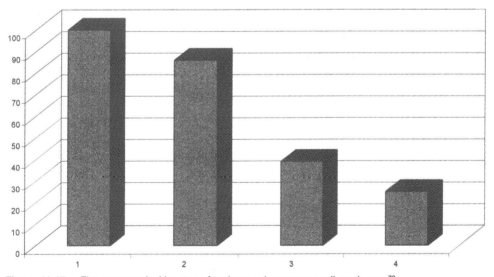

Figure 11-17. Five-year survival by stage for sinonasal squamous cell carcinoma.[70]

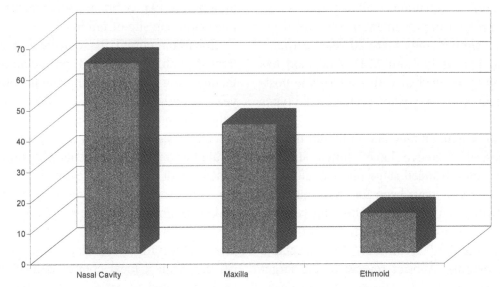

Figure 11–18.   Five-year survival by site for sinonasal squamous cell carcinoma.[70]

sity for late presentation due to the absence of symptoms in early stage disease. Complete surgical removal of the tumor with postoperative radiation therapy remains the standard of care for resectable lesions. Improved reconstructive techniques including microvascular free flaps and prosthetic obturators have significantly decreased the functional and cosmetic morbidity from aggressive surgical resection. The orbital contents may be preserved in cases where the orbital fat, musculature, and apex are free of disease. If the orbital floor is resected with orbital preservation, then reconstruction of the orbital floor is essential to maintaining good postoperative ocular function, particularly in the setting of additional planned radiation therapy. The use of chemotherapy and accelerated radiation therapy preliminarily appear to offer a substantial benefit for advanced stage tumors. The addition of these modalities may ultimately improve the long-prevailing poor prognosis of these challenging tumors.

REFERENCES

1. Grant RN, Silverberg E. Cancer Statistics 1970. New York: American Cancer Society; 1970.
2. Carrau RL, Myers EN, Johnson JT. Paranasal sinus carcinoma—diagnosis, treatment, and prognosis. Oncology 1992;6:43–50.
3. Kraus DH, Roberts JK, Medendorp SV, et al. Non squamous cell malignancies of the paranasal sinuses. Ann Otol Rhinol Laryngol 1990;99:5–11.
4. Spiro JD, Soo KC, Spiro RH. Non squamous cell malignant neoplasms of the nasal cavities and paranasal sinuses. Head Neck 1995;17:114–8.
5. Stern SJ, Hanna E. Cancer of the nasal cavity and paranasal sinuses. In: Myers EN, Suen JY, editors. Cancer of the Head and Neck. Philadelphia (PA): W.B. Saunders Co.; 1996. p.205–33.
6. Pearson BW. Surgical anatomy of the nasal cavity and paranasal sinuses. In: Thawley SE, Panje WR, Batsakis JG, Lindberg RD, editors. Comprehensive Management of Head and Neck Tumors. Philadelphia (PA): W.B. Saunders Co.; 1999. p.540–57.
7. Öhngren LG. Malignant tumors of the maxillo-ethmoidal region. Acta Otolaryngol Suppl 1933;19:101–6.
8. American Joint Committee on Cancer. AJCC Cancer Staging Manual. New York: Lippincott-Raven; 1997.
9. Kraus DH, Lanzieri CF, Wanamaker JR, et al. Complementary use of computed tomography and magnetic resonance imaging in assessing skull base lesions. Laryngoscope 1992;102:623–9.
10. Mosesson RE, Som PM. The radiographic evaluation of sinonasal tumors. Otolaryngol Clin N Am 1995;28:1097–115.
11. Som PM, Shapiro MD, Biller HF, et al. Sinonasal tumors and inflammatory tissues: differentiation with MR imaging. Radiology 1988;167:803–8.
12. Som PM, Dillon WP, Sze G, et al. Benign and malignant sinonasal lesions with intracranial extension: differentiation with MR imaging. Radiology 1989;172:763–6.
13. Lanzieri CF, Shah M, Kraus D, Lavertu P. Use of gadolinium-enhanced MR imaging for differentiating mucoceles from neoplasms in the paranasal sinuses. Radiology 1991;178:425–8.
14. Pedersen E, Hogetveit AC, Andersen A. Cancer of respiratory organs among workers at a nickel refinery in Norway. Int J Cancer 1973;12:32–41.
15. Batsakis JG. Pathology of tumors of the nasal cavity and

paranasal sinuses. In: Thawley SE, Panje WR, Batsakis JG, Lindberg RD, editors. Comprehensive Management of Head and Neck Tumors. Philadelphia (PA): W.B. Saunders Co.; 1999. p.522–39.

16. Wenig BM. Atlas of Head and Neck Pathology. Philadelpia (PA): W.B. Saunders Co.; 1993.

17. Acheson ED. Nasal cancer in the furniture and boot and shoe manufacturing industries. Prev Med 1976;5:295–315.

18. Kadish S, Goodman M, Wang CC. Olfactory neuroblastoma: a clinical analysis of 17 cases. Cancer 1976;37:1571–6.

19. Parsons JT, Stringer SP, Mancuso AA, Million RR. Nasal vestibule, nasal cavity, and paranasal sinuses. In: Million RR, Cassisi NJ, editors. Management of Head and Neck Cancer. Philadelphia (PA): J.B. Lippincott Co.; 1994. p.551–98.

20. Kurohara SS, Webster JH, Ellis F, et al. Role of radiation therapy and surgery in the management of localized epidermoid carcinoma of the maxillary sinus. Am J Roentgenol 1972;114:35–42.

21. Lee F, Ogura JH. Maxillary sinus carcinoma. Laryngoscope 1981;91:133–9.

22. St. Pierre S, Baker SR. Squamous cell carcinoma of the maxillary sinus: analysis of 66 cases. Head Neck Surg 1983;5:508–13.

23. Mendenhall WM, Stringer SP, Cassisi NJ, Mendenhall NP. Squamous cell carcinoma of the nasal vestibule. Head Neck 1999;21:385–93.

24. Goepfert H. Editorial comment: the vex and fuss about nasal vestibular cancer. Head Neck 1999;21:383–4.

25. Yu-Hua H, Gui-Yi T, Yu-Qin Q, et al. Comparison of pre- and postoperative radiation in the combined treatment of carcinoma of the maxillary sinus. Int J Radiat Oncol Biol Phys 1982;8:1045–9.

26. Sisson GA, Toriumi DM, Atiyah RA. Paranasal sinus malignancy: a comprehensive update. Laryngoscope 1989;99:143–50.

27. Shah JP, Zelefsky MJ, O'Malley BB. Squamous cell carcinoma of the oral cavity. In: Harrison LB, editor. Head and Neck Cancer: A Multidisciplinary Approach. New York: Lippincott-Raven;1999. p.421.

28. Carrau RL, Segas J, Nuss DW, et al. Squamous cell carcinoma of the sinonasal tract invading the orbit. Laryngoscope 1999;109:230–5.

29. McCary WS, Levine PA, Cantrell RW. Preservation of the eye in the treatment of sinonasal malignant neoplasms with orbital involvement. Arch Otolaryngol Head Neck Surg 1996;122;657–9.

30. Perry C, Levine PA, Williamson BR, Cantrell RW. Preservation of the eye in paranasal sinus cancer surgery. Arch Otolaryngol Head Neck Surg 1988;114:632–4.

31. Tiwari R, van der Wal J, van der Wal I, Snow G. Studies of the anatomy and pathology of the orbit in carcinoma of the maxillary sinus and their impact on preservation of the eye in maxillectomy. Head Neck 1998;20:193–6.

32. Quatela VC, Futran ND, Boynton JR. Eye banking: techniques for eye preservation in selected neoplasms encroaching on the globe. Otolaryngol Head Neck Surg 1993;108:662–70.

33. Sato Y, Morita M, Takahashi H, et al. Combined surgery, radiotherapy, and regional chemotherapy in carcinoma of the paranasal sinuses. Cancer 1970;25:571–9.

34. Sakai S, Hohki A, Fuchihata H, Tanaka Y. Multidisciplinary treatment of maxillary sinus carcinoma. Cancer 1983;52:1360–4.

35. Knegt PP, de Jong PC, van Andel JG, et al. Carcinoma of the paranasal sinuses: results of a prospective pilot study. Cancer 1985;56:57–62.

36. Sakata K, Aoki Y, Karasawa K, et al. Analysis of the results of combined therapy for maxillary carcinoma. Cancer 1993;71:2715–22.

37. Lee Y, Dimery I, Van Tassel P, et al. Superselective intra-arterial chemotherapy of advanced paranasal sinus tumors. Arch Otolaryngol Head Neck Surg 1989;115:503–11.

38. Robbins KT, Vicario D, Seagren S, et al. A targeted supradose cisplatin chemoradiation protocol for advanced head and neck cancer. Am J Surg 1994;168:419–22.

39. Robbins KT, Storniolo AM, Kerber C, et al. Rapid superselective high-dose cisplatin infusion for advanced head and neck malignancies. Head Neck 1992;14:364–71.

40. LoRusso P, Tapazoglou E, Kish JA, et al. Chemotherapy for paranasal sinus carcinoma: a 10 year experience at Wayne State University. Cancer 1988;62:1–5.

41. Bjork-Eriksson T, Mercke C, Petruson B, Ekholm S. Potential impact on tumor control and organ preservation with cisplatin and 5-fluorouracil for patients with advanced tumors of the paranasal sinuses and nasal fossa. Cancer 1992;70:2615–20.

42. Rosen A, Vokes EE, Scher N, et al. Locoregionally advanced paranasal sinus carcinoma: favorable survival with multimodality therapy. Arch Otolaryngol Head Neck Surg 1993;119:743–6.

43. Choi KN, Rotman M, Aziz H, et al. Locally advanced paranasal sinus and nasopharynx tumors treated with hyperfractionated radiation and concomitant infusion cisplatin. Cancer 1991;67:2748–52.

44. Harrison LB, Raben A, Pfister DG, et al. A prospective phase II trial of concomitant chemotherapy and radiotherapy with delayed accelerated fractionation in unresectable tumors of the head and neck. Head Neck 1998;20:497–503.

45. Harrison LB, Pfister DG, Fass DE, et al. Concomitant chemotherapy-radiation therapy followed by hyperfractionated radiation therapy for advanced unresectable head and neck cancer. Int J Radiat Oncol Biol Phys 1991;21:703–8.

46. Paulino AC, Fisher SG, Marks JE. Is prophylactic neck irradiation indicated in patients with squamous cell carcinoma of the maxillary sinus? Int J Radiat Oncol Biol Phys 1997;39:283–9.

47. Jiang GL, Ang KK, Peters LJ, et al. Maxillary sinus carcinomas: natural history and results of postoperative radiotherapy. Radiother Oncol 1991;21:193–200.

48. The American Society for Head and Neck Surgery and the Society of Head and Neck Surgeons. Clinical Practice Guidelines for the Diagnosis and Management of Cancer of the Head and Neck, 1996.

49. Penzer RD, Moss WT, Tong D, et al. Cervical lymph node metastasis in patients with squamous cell carcinoma of the maxillary antrum: the role of elective irradiation of the clinically negative neck. Int J Radiat Biol 1979;5:1977–80.

50. Curran AJ, Gullane PJ, Waldron J, et al. Surgical salvage after failed radiation for paranasal sinus malignancy. Laryngoscope 1998;108:1618–22.

51. Spiro RH, Strong EW, Shah JP. Maxillectomy and its classi-fication. Head Neck 1997;19:309–14.

52. Shah JP. Head and Neck Surgery. New York: Mosby-Wolfe; 1996. p. 49–83.

53. Goepfert H, Jesse RH, Lindberg RD. Arterial infusion and radiation therapy in the treatment of advanced cancer of the nasal cavity and paranasal sinuses. Am J Surg 1973;126:464–8.

54. Shibuya H, Suzuki S, Horiuchi J, et al. Reappraisal of tri-modal combination therapy for maxillary sinus carci-noma. Cancer 1982;50:2790–4.

55. Milas L, Peters LJ. Biology of radiation therapy. In: Thawley SE, Panje WR, Batsakis JG, Lindberg RD, editors. Com-prehensive Management of Head and Neck Tumors. Philadelphia (PA): W.B. Saunders Co.; 1999. p. 99–123.

56. Kornblith AB, Zlotolow IM, Gooen J, et al. Quality of life of maxillectomy patients using an obturator prosthesis. Head Neck 1996;18:323–34.

57. Hatoko M, Harashina T, Inoue T, et al. Reconstruction of palate with radial forearm flap: a report of 3 cases. Br J Plastic Surg 1990;43:350–4.

58. MacLeod AM, Morrison WA, McCann JJ, et al. The free radial forearm flap with and without bone for closure of large palatal fistulae. Br J Plastic Surg 1987;40:391–5.

59. Urken ML, Sullivan MJ. Scapular and parascapular fasciocu-taneous and osteocutaneous free flaps. In: Urken ML, Cheney ML, Sullivan MJ, Biller HF, editors. Atlas of Regional and Free Flaps for Head and Neck Reconstruc-tion. New York: Raven Press; 1995. p.217–36.

60. Aviv JE, Urken ML, Vickery C, et al. The combined latissimus dorsi-scapular free flap in head and neck reconstruction. Arch Otolaryngol Head Neck Surg 1991;117:1242–50.

61. McCary WS, Levine PA. Management of the eye in the treat-ment of sinonasal cancers. Otolaryngol Clin N Am 1995;28:1231–8.

62. Stern SJ, Goepfert H, Clayman G, et al. Orbital preservation in maxillectomy. Otolaryngol Head Neck Surg 1993;109:111–5.

63. Cordeiro PG, Santamaria E, Kraus DH, et al. Reconstruction of total maxillectomy defects with preservation of the orbital contents. Plast Reconstr Surg 1998;102:1874–84.

64. Olsen KD, Meland B, Ebersold MJ, et al. Extensive defects of the sino-orbital regions: results with microvascular reconstruction. Arch Otolaryngol Head Neck Surg 1992; 118:828–33.

65. Browne JD, Burke AJ. Benefits of routine maxillectomy and orbital reconstruction with the rectus abdominis free flap. Otolaryngol Head Neck Surg 1999;121:203–9.

66. Jiang GL, Tucker SL, Guttenberger R, et al. Radiation-induced injury to the visual pathway. Radiother Oncol 1994;30:17–25.

67. Rabin A, Pfister DG, O'Malley BB. Nonsurgical manage-ment of carcinoma of the nasal vestibule, nasal cavity, and paranasal sinuses. In: Harrison LB, editor. Head and Neck Cancer: A Multidisciplinary Approach. New York: Lip-pincott-Raven; 1999. p.595–638.

68. Stupp R, Vokes EE. Chemotherapy of head and neck tumors. In: Thawley SE, Panje WR, Batsakis JG, Lindberg RD, editors. Comprehensive management of Head and Neck Tumors. Philadelphia (PA): W.B. Saunders Co.; 1999. p.141–56.

69. Stern SJ, Goepfert H, Clayman G, et al. Squamous cell car-cinoma of the maxillary sinus. Arch Otolaryngol Head Neck Surg 1993;119:964–9.

70. Spiro JD, Soo KC, Spiro RH. Squamous cell carcinoma of the nasal cavity and paranasal sinuses. Am J Surg 1989;158:310–4.

71. Zaharia, M, Salem LE, Travezan R, et al. Postoperative radiotherapy in the management of cancer of the maxil-lary sinus. Int J Radiat Oncol Biol Phys 1989;17:967–71.

72. Lavertu P, Roberts JK, Kraus DH, et al. Squamous cell carci-noma of the paranasal sinuses: the Cleveland Clinic expe-rience 1977–1986. Laryngoscope 1989;99:1130–6.

73. Paulino AC, Marks JE, Bricker P, et al. Results of treatment of patients with maxillary sinus carcinoma. Cancer 1998; 83:457–65.

12

Skull Base: Anterior and Middle Cranial Fossa

PAUL A. KEDESHIAN, MD
DENNIS H. KRAUS, MD, FACS
JATIN P. SHAH, MD, FACS

Tumors that arise from or extend to the base of the skull pose a significant management challenge secondary to the proximity of critical neurovascular structures. Until very recently, the accurate assessment of the extent of these lesions met with imprecision, while their treatment involved significant morbidity, and the overall results were dismal. However, the advent of modern radiographic imaging (computed tomography [CT] and magnetic resonance imaging [MRI]), advancements in microsurgical reconstruction and rigid fixation, and most significantly, the pioneering efforts of a handful of surgeons, essentially defined a new surgical sub-discipline which we now recognize as skull base surgery.

In 1941, Dandy[1] described his experience with a transcranial approach for orbital tumors. This approach, via the anterior cranial fossa, allowed for adequate tumor visualization through the orbital roof and thereby permitted gross total tumor removal. Over a decade later, Smith and colleagues[2] first described a combined intracranial/extracranial (facial) approach for tumors that occupied the frontal, sphenoid, ethmoid, and maxillary sinuses as well as the orbit and nasal cavity. This combined approach was the first to permit the operating surgeon to apply the basic oncologic principle of en bloc tumor resection with grossly negative margins to tumors in this area, thus achieving an accurate intraoperative assessment of tumor extent. Soon after this initial description, Ketcham and colleagues[3] applied a craniofacial approach to a series of patients with tumors involving the sinonasal tract

and anterior skull base and reported good success in safely achieving gross tumor clearance. At approximately the same period of time, Parsons and colleagues[4] first described the en bloc resection of tumors of the temporal bone, demonstrating that lesions of the lateral skull base could also be removed through a combined surgical approach, rather than in a piecemeal fashion. These early forays into surgery for tumors of the skull base are all-the-more astounding when one considers that they were all accomplished prior to the availability of either CT or MR imaging.

With the development and application of computed tomography (CT) in the 1970s and the later introduction of magnetic resonance imaging (MRI), skull base surgery was revolutionized. Clinicians were now able to make precise determinations of a skull base tumor's pretreatment extent, allowing for improved treatment planning, patient selection, risk assessment, and post-treatment follow-up. To supplement the information regarding a tumor's radiographic extent, angiography, magnetic resonance angiography (MRA), and functional assessments of cerebral circulation such as balloon occlusion studies, xenon and single photon emission computed tomography (SPECT) scans became available, providing important information—particularly in the case of tumors of the middle cranial fossa. In addition, the ability to embolize vascular tumors such as glomus jugulare tumors has also contributed greatly to the precision and success of skull base surgery. Moreover, the availability of microsurgical instrumentation, the widespread use of neuroanesthetic measures to prevent brain edema (intravenous mannitol, controlled hyperventilation, lumbar subarachnoid drain placement), and the ability to intraoperatively monitor cranial nerve and brain function have all been important features in the evolution of cranial base surgery. All of these developments, combined with improvements in microvascular free tissue transfer and the consequent assembly of a management team with a spirit of cooperation, have made surgical resection the optimal treatment modality for most tumors of the skull base.

As the details of tumor diagnosis, treatment, and prognosis intimately depend upon the specific area of the cranial base in question, this review will be accordingly subdivided into lesions of the anterior and middle skull base, separately discussing the particular features of these two distinct regions. While many laterally-arising lesions around the temporal bone and surrounding skin will be addressed in the middle fossa section, lesions such as acoustic neuromas and other lesions of the cerebellopontine angle and the posterior fossa will not be included and the reader is referred to neurotology texts for the specific consideration of these lesions.

ANTERIOR CRANIAL FOSSA

Anatomy

The anterior skull base is the bony partition between the frontal lobes in the anterior cranial fossa and the upper midline and paramedian facial structures including the nasal cavity and the eyes. In particular, this bony partition is defined by the superior-most portion of the nasal cavity and the interorbital paranasal sinuses (ethmoid/sphenoid), the cribriform plate of the ethmoid bone, the planum sphenoidale, and the orbital roof (Figure 12–1). The clivus serves as the defining osseous component of the central skull base. It extends from the dorsum sellae to the foramen magnum and can be anatomically separated into an upper, middle and lower segment. The upper clivus extends from the dorsum sellae to the petrous apex. Immediately anterior to this upper clival segment lies the sphenoid sinus; the intracavernous carotid artery and the optic nerve are

lateral, and the midbrain and basilar artery posterior. The middle clival segment extends from the petrous apex down to the pars nervosa of the jugular foramen. The nasopharynx and retropharyngeal soft tissues are situated anterior to this segment, while the inferior petrosal sinus, and seventh and eighth cranial nerves are lateral. The lower clivus extends from the pars nervosa of the jugular foramen to the foramen magnum. The retropharyngeal soft tissues are situated anteriorly while the sigmoid sinus, jugular bulb and hypoglossal nerves are situated laterally.

Diagnosis

The majority of lesions that involve the anterior cranial base are tumors arising in the sinonasal cavity and which cause symptoms associated with their site of origin, although the signs may be quite nonspecific or subtle and therefore not appreciated until significant

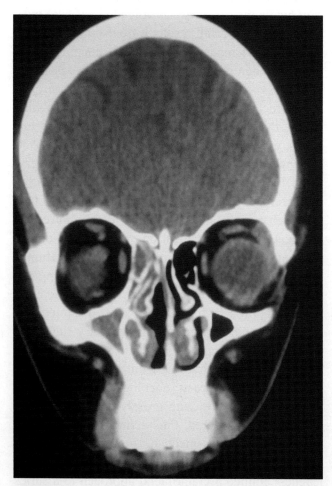

FIGURE 12–1. Coronal CT scan demonstrating anatomy of anterior base of skull as well as a right ethmoid sinus squamous cell carcinoma.

tumor growth and extension have occurred. In particular, a careful medical history is often able to elicit nasal obstruction, epistaxis, anosmia/hyposmia, facial pain, or minor visual changes.[5] A head and neck physical examination that includes anterior rhinoscopy and nasal endoscopy may demonstrate a lesion in the sinonasal cavity. CT and MR radiographs are critical in the diagnostic evaluation of anterior skull base lesions as well. In most cases, these studies are complementary in accurately defining a tumor's extent and its relationship to bony and soft tissue structures.

The pathologic diagnosis of lesions of the anterior skull base can be obtained, particularly when a significant intranasal tumor mass is present, via an office biopsy under local anesthesia. However, prudence must be exercised when performing a biopsy if a lesion appears vascular or if it is located in the superior nasal vault and its potential connection with the anterior cranial fossa could precipitate a cerebrospinal fluid (CSF) leak.

Lesions that involve or extend to the anterior skull base include a range of both benign and malignant histologies. While benign tumors including inverting papilloma (schneiderian papilloma), and juvenile nasopharyngeal angiofibroma (JNA) can require craniofacial approaches for surgical resection, the majority of tumors of the anterior skull base are malignant and include: adenocarcinomas and adenoid cystic carcinomas arising from the minor salivary glands of the sinonasal tract, squamous carcinomas arising from either the sinonasal cavity or the nasopharynx, chondrosarcomas or osteogenic sarcomas arising from the various bony and cartilaginous elements of the sinonasal cavity, soft tissue sarcomas, mucosal melanomas, esthesioneuroblastomas, and extensive skin cancers of the midface with deep penetration and skull base extension. Additionally, lymphomas (particularly in patients with human immunodeficiency virus [HIV]) and small cell neuroendocrine carcinomas may involve the anterior skull base although their treatment is generally nonsurgical. While there are significant differences in the prognoses associated with these tumor types (as well as the need for adjuvant therapy), their surgical treatments do not significantly differ and they will therefore be discussed as a group. The differences in the biologic behavior of these various malignant histologies will become more apparent when treatment results are discussed.

Treatment—Surgery

The varied histologies as well as the relative rarity of the tumors of the anterior skull base make objective comparisons of treatments impossible. However, as safe surgical resection with low morbidity is now feasible with the craniofacial approach, most anterior skull base lesions are treated with surgical resection.[6] In cases in which surgery is contraindicated, nonsurgical treatment protocols may offer an equivalent likelihood of benefit with less morbidity.[7] While it is difficult to enumerate absolute contraindications to anterior skull base surgery, and a tumor's histology and biologic behavior are exceedingly important considerations (particularly in the case of esthesioneuroblastoma),[8] some important issues to address prior to embarking upon a craniofacial resection include:

1. whether gross total tumor removal is achievable—unlikely for tumors in which distant metastases are present, tumors with extensive dural and/or brain parenchymal invasion, or tumors with extensive cavernous sinus invasion;
2. whether surgical resection would cause an unacceptable degree of morbidity—such as tumors involving the only seeing eye, tumors involving the optic chiasm, or tumors encasing the internal carotid artery.[9, 10]

Surgical Preparation

Prior to craniofacial resection, all patients receive intravenous steroids and antibiotics whose spectrums include broad coverage for skin flora, upper aerodigestive tract flora, and a cephalosporin with good CSF penetration. At our institution, we employ vancomycin, metronidazole, and ceftazidime based on the local and known pathogens. Following the introduction of general endotracheal anesthesia, a lumbar spinal drain is placed and, depending upon the posterosuperior tumor extent, controlled CSF drainage, hyperventilation and/or mannitol diuresis are used to minimize the need for frontal lobe retraction.[9,11–13]

Operative Procedure

The surgical procedure commences with a bifrontal craniotomy. The bicoronal skin incision in the scalp is deepened to a level just superficial to the pericranium which is then incised approximately 5 cm posterior to the scalp incision. The galea and pericranium are elevated to the level of the supraorbital rims and the nasofrontal suture line, preserving the neurovascular (supraorbital) pedicle as it emerges from the supraorbital notch (Figure 12–2). Once this flap has been successfully elevated, a frontal craniotomy is performed. We utilize a single burr hole on either side of the saggital sinus and a side-cutting craniotome for the bone flap with the inferior osteotomy located subfrontally at approximately the level of the nasion. The dura overlying the frontal lobe is then carefully explored and, based upon the tumor's extent, the decision whether to proceed by an extradural or intradural route is made. Upon dissection of the anterior cranial fossa floor, the olfactory bulbs are sharply divided and their dural sleeves

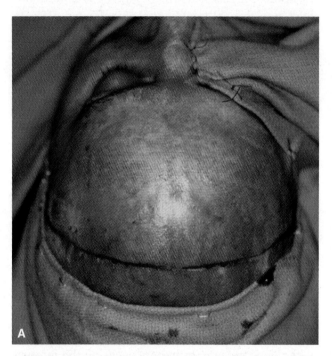
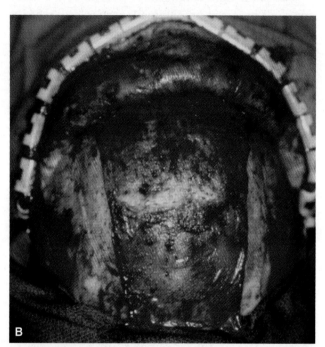
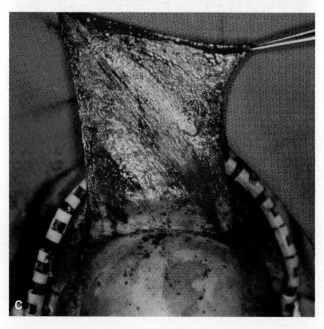

Figure 12–2. *A*, Incision for bifrontal craniotomy. *B* and *C*, Galeal-pericranial flap.

are oversewn to prevent a CSF leak. Once an adequate degree of frontal lobe relaxation is achieved, the bony anterior fossa floor can be fully visualized and the superior bone cuts made (Figure 12–3). These cuts frequently involve a posterior cut at approximately the level of the anterior sphenoid wall, variable portions of the superior orbital roof, and the entire cribriform plate and superior ethmoid complex. This frontal bone flap is later cranialized by removing the posterior bony sinus wall and stripping the mucosa from the anterior sinus wall to prevent the formation of a frontal sinus mucocele.

We have found this bifrontal cranial approach to offer outstanding access with minimal morbidity and good cosmesis.[13,14] In an effort to minimize the morbidity associated with this bifrontal craniotomy, the use of less extensive subcranial exposures have been described.[15–17] While some of these approaches may, in selected circumstances, offer adequate access and permit visualization of the full superior extent of a tumor, their potential for inadequate exposure outweighs any perceived cosmetic benefit.

Once the tumor has been adequately encompassed from above, and all bone cuts at the anterior cranial base performed, facial exposure of the tumor is obtained. Depending upon the extent of the tumor, this is accomplished via either an isolated lateral rhinotomy or a Weber-Ferguson approach (Figure 12–4). If significant lateral extension of the tumor is present, the Weber-Ferguson approach can be modified through a lateral extension which we prefer to

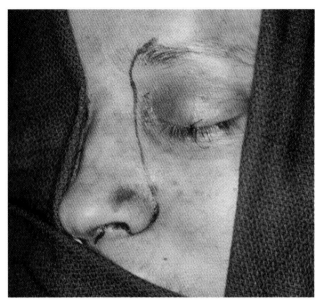

Figure 12–4. Incision for lateral rhinotomy.

carry out through a transconjunctival incision into the ipsilateral fornix of the conjunctiva (rather than through a subciliary incision). With this exposure, tumor can be successfully mobilized encompassing complete anatomic units (maxilla/orbit/sinus) en bloc with the bony skull base. Once the tumor has been resected with tumor-free margins, reconstruction of the anterior skull base defect can proceed. When orbital exenteration and/or total maxillectomy are performed and a significant soft tissue defect is present, free tissue transfer offers the best option for satisfactory reconstruction. However, if a significant soft tissue defect has not been created, reconstruction focuses on establishing a water-tight seal around the intracranial contents and isolating the sinonasal tract. In order to achieve this, the scalp flap that includes both galea and pericranium is now dissected in a plane superficial to the galea, leaving galea on each side of the incision to allow for closure. This well-vascularized galeal-pericranial flap is then sutured to the basal dura and the perimeter of the bony defect (Figure 12–5).[12,14,18]

We have recently adopted additional reconstructive nuances in an effort to minimize the postoperative morbidity and sequelae of craniofacial resection. While many descriptions of craniofacial surgical techniques indicate that the nasofrontal duct can be transsected and marsupialized to the surrounding soft tissue,[6] our experience with postoper-

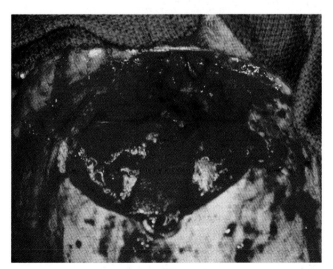

Figure 12–3. Exposure of cribriform plate/anterior base of skull.

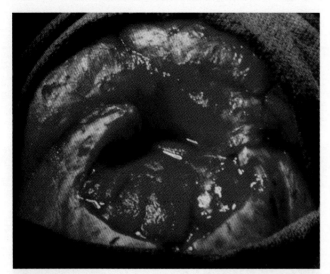

Figure 12–5. Repair of anterior base of skull defect with galeal-pericranial flap.

cially when postoperative radiotherapy was employed. The authors used this data to make the case that orbital exenteration should be more strongly considered at the time of the initial surgical resection if major loss of eye support and postoper-

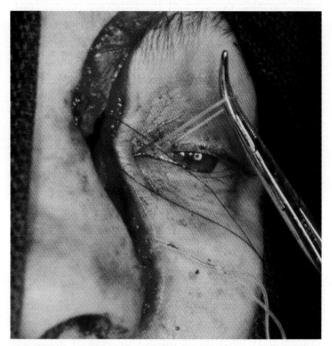

Figure 12–6. Placement of nasolacrimal duct stent.

ative nasolacrimal duct stenosis and epiphora would argue otherwise.[14] We currently stent the naso-lacrimal duct after it has been transsected (Figure 12–6), and remove this stent after the completion of radiotherapy. In addition to nasolacrimal duct stenting, we have also focused attention on the accurate repositioning of the medial canthus. A permanent suture is placed in the divided medial canthal tendon and it is overcorrected in both the superior and posterior planes in anticipation of postoperative laxity of the tendon (Figure 12–7). If this overcorrection is not performed, variable degrees of orbital dystopia and telecanthus can occur and occasionally result in visual disturbances. These two technical aspects of craniofacial reconstruction are critical, as Andersen and colleagues[19] noted that nearly 50 percent of patients undergoing craniofacial resection for tumors of the anterior skull base develop ocular sequelae from their treatment.

Tumors of the anterior skull base can extend laterally and closely approach (if not directly invade) the orbital periosteum and orbital soft tissues. In these cases, resection of the majority of the bony and fascial support of orbit may be required, although the globe is preserved. The loss of support for an otherwise normal eye (especially when most/all of the orbital floor is resected) was recently addressed by Stern and colleagues,[20] who noted a decrease in the likelihood of eventual eye function when the orbital floor was resected for sinonasal cancer, espe-

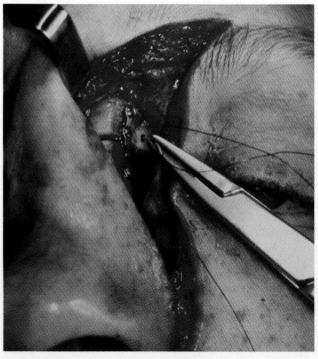

Figure 12–7. Repair of medial canthal tendon.

ative radiotherapy were anticipated. However, most would not resect an eye unless gross invasion of the orbital contents (fat, muscle, or globe) and/or significantly decreased ocular function were present. This conservative approach is supported by a recent meta-analysis by Carrau and colleagues[21] that could not document any increase in local recurrences with such an approach. An alternative solution to the issue of eye function following the loss of the orbit's physical support was recently offered by Cordeiro and colleagues.[22] These authors noted improved eye function (as well as cosmesis) when the resected orbital floor was reconstructed using a combination of a bone graft (either split calvarium or rib) and a vascularized flap (either pedicled or free) regardless of whether postoperative radiotherapy was administered.

Nonsurgical Treatment

As previously noted, most malignant tumors that arise from or involve the anterior skull base are considered primary surgical lesions unless: a tumor possess features that make its resection too risky, if surgery is unlikely to achieve total tumor removal, or if a patient's medical condition precludes surgery. It is primarily in these situations that nonsurgical modalities are considered for tumors of the anterior skull base. In light of the relative rarity of anterior skull base tumors, their varied histologies and biologic behavior, and the fact that the majority of these tumors are treated with primary surgery, there are no studies that specifically address the use of nonsurgical treatment when compared to surgery. External beam radiotherapy has been employed as the primary treatment modality for tumors of the paranasal sinuses with extension to the anterior skull base. These treatments use a combination of both anterior and lateral portals with every effort made to minimize the dose received by the eye, optic nerve/chiasm, spinal cord, and lacrimal ducts.[23] At the Memorial Hospital we have, over the past decade, employed a regimen of concomitant chemotherapy/radiotherapy for patients with tumors of the head and neck deemed to be surgically unresectable.[7] Within this cohort of patients, a subset presented with tumors of the nasopharynx and paranasal sinuses—many of whom had involvement of the anterior skull base.

This protocol consists of an initial 4-week course of conventionally-delivered external beam radiotherapy (1.8 Gy/day) to both the sites of gross and potential microscopic disease during which concomitant cisplatin (100 mg/m^2) is delivered on days 1 and 22. During the subsequent 2 weeks, hyperfractionated radiotherapy (1.8 Gy in the morning and 1.6 Gy in the afternoon) is delivered with the evening dose directed exclusively to the site(s) of gross disease. The total radiotherapy dose therefore approximates 70 Gy. The 3-year local control rate for patients treated with this protocol was 58 percent while their overall survival was 36 percent.

In addition to these experiences with the use of radiotherapy either with or without chemotherapy for tumors of the anterior skull base, the use of chemotherapy specifically for esthesioneuroblastomas is well described and was first reported by Wade and colleagues.[24] Although chemotherapy is still employed as part of a combined treatment protocol in selected centers,[25] we have found esthesioneuroblastomas to have the most favorable prognosis of all malignant anterior skull base histologies.[13] Consequently, although esthesioneuroblastomas are chemotherapy-sensitive tumors,[26] we consider systemic chemotherapy for only those esthesioneuroblastomas that have locally unresectable disease or distant metastases.

Complications

As alluded to earlier, the potential complications of anterior craniofacial resection have always been at the forefront when considering the treatment options available for tumors of the anterior base of skull. Although the morbidity and mortality associated with anterior craniofacial resection have declined significantly from Ketcham's initial description in which 23 major/minor complications and 2 deaths occurred in a series of 31 operative procedures,[27] the reported complication rate for patients undergoing craniofacial resections for malignant tumors is still close to 40 percent.[9] While the incidence of complications can be difficult to compare between different centers secondary to differences in reporting and the definition of major and minor complications, the morbidity and mortality associated with anterior craniofacial resection for malignant tumors from a number of skull base centers is summarized in Table 12–1. These include a variety of infectious complications (abscesses, meningitis, bone and scalp flap infections), CSF leaks, pneumocephalus, diabetes insipidus, retro-orbital hematoma, blindness, transient impairment in neurologic function, coma, stroke and death.[13,24,27–37] While anterior craniofacial resection is unavoidably associated with a variable degree of operative morbidity, if careful patient selection, adequate perioperative preparation, and meticulous surgical technique are employed, the complication rate and morbidity of craniofacial resection can be maintained at an acceptable rate.

Results of Treatment

When all of the malignant tumors involving the anterior skull base are considered, the 5-year survival for patients who undergo anterior craniofacial resection is approximately 50 to 60 percent (see Table 12–1). While these series do demonstrate some consistency, if one further analyzes these results by histology, some striking differences emerge. Within our series of 115 consecutive anterior craniofacial resections, the 5-year disease-specific survival for patients with esthesioneuroblastomas is 100 percent, as compared to 67 percent for patients with squamous carcinoma arising from the skin, 50 to 60 percent for sinonasal carcinomas/sarcomas/minor salivary tumors, and only 33 percent for patients with mucosal melanomas.[13] More specifically, local tumor control was obtained in 65 percent of patients and the disease-specific survival was 58 percent at 5 years and 48 percent at 10 years. Moreover, a statistically significant improvement in survival was seen for patients whose tumors could be encompassed with a limited craniofacial resection as compared to those that required a more extensive resection including palate, orbit, dura or brain. These results, which are consistent with those reported by other smaller series, emphasize the critical importance of tumor histology and biology in the prognosis of anterior skull base lesions. In addition to the importance of tumor histology, several other studies have demonstrated the significance of dural invasion by tumor (irrespective of histology) as well as positive tumor margins as prognostic factors associated with both local recurrence and survival.[38–40] These studies serve to reiterate the vital importance of preoperative tumor assessment and tumor biology when formulating a treatment plan and confirm the role of postoperative radiotherapy.

The reported 5-year survival for patients with extensive tumors that involve the anterior skull base treated with primary radiotherapy is 10 to 15 percent.[23] In contrast, when the results of concurrent chemotherapy and radiotherapy (unresectable treatment protocol) in the subgroup of patients with paranasal sinus tumors is examined, there was a 42 percent overall survival at 3 years of follow-up.[7] All patients in this cohort had stage IV tumors with the predominant histologies being squamous carcinoma, adenocarcinoma, mucoepidermoid carcinoma, adenoid cystic carcinoma, and undifferentiated carcinoma. Local control was successfully achieved in 78 percent of patients while regional control was obtained in 57 percent. While all of these patients did not have tumors that involved the anterior skull base, these very advanced-staged lesions were all judged to be surgically unresectable by a multidisci-

Table 12–1. ANTERIOR CRANIOFACIAL RESECTION FOR MALIGNANT TUMORS (50 OR MORE PATIENTS)								
Author	Year	No. of Patients	Malignant (%)	Primary/ Secondary (%)	Survival (%)	Follow-up	Mortality (%)	Comp (%)
Shah et al.[13]	1997	115	100	61/39	58 (5-yr)	4.7 yrs	3.5	35
Cantu et al.[32]	1999	91	100	46/54	47 (5-yr)	47 mos	7.7	N/A
McCaffrey et al.[33]	1994	54	100	N/A	49 (5-yr)	31 mos	0	30
Catalano et al.[34]	1994	73	85	60/40	N/A	3 yrs	3	36
Ketcham et al.[35]	1985	89	100	24/76	44 (4 yrs minimum)	10 yrs	3	N/A
Jackson et al.[36]	1991	68	100	16/84	69 (1 yr minimum)	6.5 yrs	1	N/A
Janecka et al.[37]	1995	50	100	46/54	74 (N/A)	40 mos	0	6

N/A = Not available.

plinary disease management team, and therefore, this nonsurgical treatment protocol merits consideration in patients with advanced tumors of the anterior skull base. Additionally, the results of this treatment protocol suggest that consideration must be given to its use in less advanced lesions as well.

MIDDLE CRANIAL FOSSA

Anatomy

The middle cranial fossa is that portion of the skull base that lies between the orbit anteriorly and the temporal bone posteriorly. The temporal lobes rest upon the bony middle fossa plate and numerous critical neurovascular structures pass through various foramina within this area. These nerves and blood vessels are some of the structures from which tumors can develop and either invade or abut the middle fossa. Within the area referred to as the middle cranial fossa, one can identify 2 fairly distinct regions. These include the anterior middle cranial fossa (Figure 12–8) which is comprised of: the infratemporal fossa, the pterygopalatine fossa, the foramen ovale which transmits V-3, the foramen rotundum which transmits V-2, the foramen lacerum into which the carotid artery passes, the cavernous sinus, and the middle fossa dura. The posterior middle cranial fossa contains structures both in and around the temporal bone and includes the tegmen of the middle cranial fossa, sigmoid sinus, petrous apex and petrous portion of the carotid artery, middle ear, cochlea, vestibular apparatus and the facial nerve.

Diagnosis

A careful history and head and neck physical examination (including a detailed neurologic examination) may reveal a variety of signs and symptoms associated with a lesion arising in the middle fossa, or lesions that occupy both the anterior and middle fossa such as tumors of the lacrimal gland. These signs and symptoms include facial numbness and pain secondary to involvement of any of the three divisions of the trigeminal nerve, trismus from involvement of the muscles of mastication, paralysis or paresis of cranial nerves IX to XII, Horner's syn-

drome from involvement of the sympathetic chain, facial swelling from masses within the infratemporal fossa, serous otitis media from obstruction of the eustachian tube orifice, or even facial paralysis from facial nerve invasion.[5]

Since many of the lesions that extend to the middle cranial fossa are not easily accessible, in many instances, pretreatment tissue biopsies are not feasible. Particularly in these circumstances, radiographic imaging by CT and MRI are essential. The imaging characteristics of a lesion and the pattern of displacement or destruction of the surrounding bony and soft tissue structures can suggest particular diagnostic entities and/or sites of tumor origin.

Unlike tumors of the anterior skull base that are primarily malignant, tumors at the middle cranial base include a mix of both benign and malignant pathologies. In particular, some of the lesions that are present at the middle cranial base can vary from T4 tumors of the maxillary sinus that extend into the pterygopalatine fossa with involvement of V-2 at the foramen rotundum, to neurilemmomas of the lower cranial nerves (IX to XII) or the sympathetic chain,

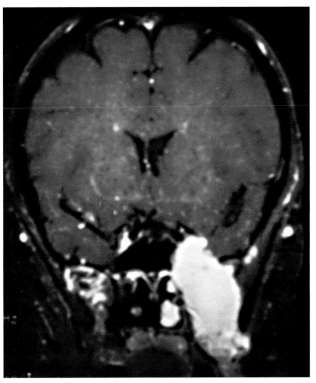

Figure 12–8. Coronal MRI scan demonstrating a sarcoma involving anterior, and middle cranial fossa as well as infratemporal fossa sarcoma.

glomus tumors of either the jugular bulb (jugulare) or the vagus nerve (intravagale), deep lobe parotid tumors with significant retromandibular extension, soft tissue sarcomas of the masticatory muscles, carcinomas (squamous, basal, or minor salivary) of the external ear canal and temporal bone, and carcinomas of the nasopharynx.

Factors Affecting Choice of Treatment

Because of the varied benign and malignant histologies that can involve the middle cranial fossa, the choice of a particular treatment for tumors in this area needs to be individualized. Treatment selection must consider factors such as the biology of the tumor (if its histology is known), the tumor's location and radiographic appearance, and the morbidity that is likely to be associated with a particular treatment modality. While general recommendations for treating tumors of the middle cranial fossa are difficult to make, a reasonable rule of thumb is that patients with malignant tumors of the middle fossa are best treated by primary surgical resection when gross tumor removal can be accomplished with acceptable morbidity; while patients with benign tumors, particularly those whose removal might require sacrifice of a major neurovascular structure, may need to balance the morbidity of surgical resection with either external radiotherapy (in an attempt to arrest tumor growth) or, less commonly, clinical observation.

Surgery

Prior to proceeding with surgery for a tumor in the area of the middle cranial fossa, it is important to determine a patient's pulmonary reserve since sacrifice of one or more of the lower cranial nerves (IX to XII) can result in aspiration. Additionally, the circulatory pattern of the carotid arterial system should be preoperatively assessed by either conventional or MR angiography while the potential functional effect of carotid sacrifice should be determined by balloon occlusion and subsequent SPECT or xenon scanning. If the ipsilateral carotid artery is found to be dominant and there is the likelihood of interruption of carotid arterial flow, the potential neurologic consequences of a surgical approach may be deemed

unacceptable. Moreover, with respect to cavernous sinus resection, a recent series by Saito and colleagues separates the types of cavernous sinus dissections into types 1 to 3, with the type 3 resections requiring carotid artery sacrifice and demonstrating poor 2-year survival.[41]

Approaches

The surgical approach for tumors at the middle cranial base was first systematically described in 1979 by Fisch and colleagues.[42] In this landmark publication, tumors of the temporal bone, clivus, and parasellar/para-sphenoid region were accessed via progressively more anterior approaches labeled Type A, B, and C respectively. More recently, Janecka and colleagues[43] described an approach to the middle cranial base in which the facial skeleton is extensively osteotomized and translocated, permitting access to the critical skull base regions. While each of these approaches can be used to approach lesions that are at the middle cranial base, they can also be used in combination with some of the approaches previously described for anterior fossa lesions. Such a combination of surgical approaches (anterolateral approach) is particularly useful when a lesion arises from an anterior or paramedian structure (such as the sphenoid sinus, pterygoid region, lateral orbit, or lacrimal gland), with significant lateral extension.[5]

Infratemporal Fossa

This surgical approach has been extensively employed for tumors that involve the nasopharynx, including squamous carcinoma and juvenile nasopharyngeal angiofibroma.[44] It begins with a retroauricular incision extending from the frontal area down into the neck. The extra-temporal facial nerve is then identified and the temporalis muscle inferiorly reflected. A segment of the zygomatic arch, and/or the lateral orbital wall, is then osteotomized and also displaced inferiorly with the masseter muscle remaining attached to it, or it is resected as a unit and replaced to its correct position at the end of the operative procedure. Additional exposure of the carotid artery is obtained through either disarticulation or resection of the mandibular condyle. Radical mastoidectomy for the identification of the vertical segment of the facial nerve as well as the intrapetrous internal carotid artery are completed, and the facial nerve is anteriorly displaced—facilitating a lateral approach to the tumor. If necessary, particularly with the more anterior Type B and C approaches, concomitant pterional craniotomy can be performed ensuring that the superior-most extent of the tumor in the region of the foramen ovale and spinosum is adequately visualized and surgically encompassed.

Facial Translocation

This surgical approach begins with a hemi-coronal incision posterior to the hairline and is carried inferiorly into the preauricular region around the lobule of the ear, and then extended to the upper neck if exposure of the carotid sheath structures is planned (Figure 12–9). A horizontal incision is then carried from the pre-auricular incision medially. This incision passes over the superior edge of the zygomatic arch to the level of the lateral canthus and sometimes severs the upper branches of the facial nerve. If they are to be divided, these branches should be identified, isolated, and labeled prior to their division in order to facilitate nerve re-anastomosis at the end of the operative procedure. An ipsilateral Weber-Ferguson approach is then completed with a trans-conjunctival incision in the inferior fornix of the conjunctiva joining the horizontal incision previously made over the zygomatic arch. Soft tissue overlying the anterior maxillary face is then elevated, and both the lacrimal duct and infraorbital nerves are divided. The facial skin flap is inferiorly reflected while the frontotemporal scalp flap is medially reflected, providing access to the zygomatic arch, lateral orbit and maxilla. Frontozygomatic, zygomaticomaxillary, and orbitomaxillary osteotomies permit translocation of segments of the facial skeleton. Finally, the temporalis muscle can be released from its insertion into the temporal line of the scalp and, if its blood supply from the internal maxillary artery is preserved, it can be transposed and used for reconstruction of the post-resection defect if necessary. In addition to the aforementioned osteotomies, the coronoid process of the mandible can be either retracted or osteotomized to facilitate greater exposure. Modifications and extensions of the

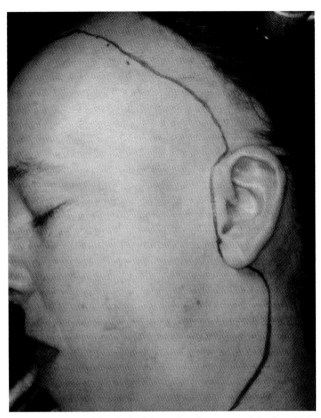

Figure 12–9. Incision for facial translocation approach to the middle cranial fossa.

facial translocation approach can additionally permit bilateral surgical exposure when necessary.[45]

At the conclusion of the tumor resection, the mobilized temporalis muscle may be used to partially reconstruct or seal off the surgical defect. The segments of the facial skeleton are then repositioned and rigidly fixated to the cranium utilizing reconstruction plates. Large soft-tissue defects are reconstructed using free tissue transfer (rectus abdominis or radial forearm) in an attempt to prevent a CSF leak, with reestablishment of orbital support as described previously.

Nonsurgical Therapy

If one excludes carcinoma of the nasopharynx for which radiotherapy and chemotherapy are extremely effective (see chapter on "Cancer of the Nasopharynx"), there is a paucity of data on the use of nonsurgical modalities specifically for the treatment of malignant tumors involving the middle cranial base. However, if one considers tumors of specific histologies such as glomus tumors, neurilemmomas, and juvenile nasopharyngeal angiofibromas (JNAs), whose resection occasionally requires access to the middle cranial fossa, some data can be extracted from the literature.

When external beam radiotherapy is employed for the treatment of glomus jugulare tumors, growth arrest ensues, although a clinically and radiographically detectable mass may persist. This growth arrest is thought to be due to fibrosis of the tumor's vasculature.[46,47] If surgical resection of glomus jugulare tumors is compared to external radiotherapy, a review of multiple series indicates that the rates of disease recurrence and persistence are equivalent.[48] These findings suggest that treatment morbidity may be the critical factor in choosing the appropriate therapy for this tumor. With respect to treatment of schwannomas using external beam radiotherapy (for tumors of the eighth cranial nerve), although there is a great deal of controversy regarding its appropriateness in this setting, recent reports appear to demonstrate that it provides excellent tumor control without significant morbidity.[49] External beam radiotherapy has also been employed, with good reported success, for the treatment of JNAs.[50,51] However, secondary to the effectiveness of surgical resection, and the potential effects of radiation on the growth of the facial skeleton in adolescents, most radiotherapy use for primary JNA treatment has been limited to the setting of very extensive tumors whose surgical resection might entail significant morbidity.[50, 51]

Sequelae and Rehabilitation

The morbidity of surgical resection of tumors of the middle cranial fossa, irrespective of the surgical approach that is chosen, relate to paralysis or paresis of the lower cranial nerves as well as the facial mimetic musculature.[52] If vagus nerve injury or sacrifice occur, paralysis of the pharynx, palate, and the vocal cord will ensue. In many instances, the initial breathiness and aspiration of liquids that can occur will gradually resolve as there is compensatory movement of the contralateral vocal cord. However, if this compensation is inadequate, complete glottic closure can be reestablished by surgically medializing the paralyzed vocal cord (Figure 12–10).[52,53]

Additionally, velopharyngeal insufficiency may result from paralysis of the palatal branch of the vagus nerve. To decrease the degree of nasal regurgitation that occurs, Netterville[52] has successfully employed unilateral palatal adhesion in which the nasopharyngeal surface of the palate is sutured to the posterior pharyngeal wall.

When the spinal accessory nerve is injured and the sternomastoid and trapezius muscles subsequently paralyzed, shoulder pain and restricted range of motion may occur. In these situations, aggressive postoperative physical therapy can prevent the development of adhesive capsulitis and scapular "winging," although normal shoulder range of motion and strength are not possible.[54] Isolated glossopharyngeal or hypoglossal nerve paralysis is not usually associated with significant morbidity, although speech and swallowing therapy may assist with any resultant dysphagia or articulatory difficulties. However, combinations of nerve paralyses such as a simultaneous

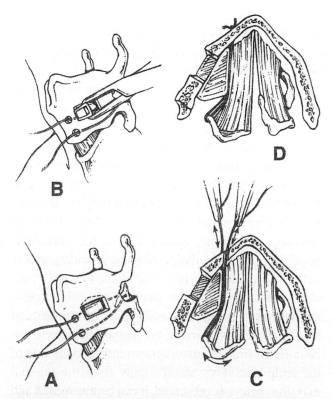

Figure 12–10. *A*, Arytenoid adduction sutures placed prior to placement of silastic implant. *B*, Placement of silastic implant. *C* and *D*, Gradual tightening of arytenoid adduction suture with medialization closure of the posterior commissure. Reprinted with permission from Arytenoid adduction as an adjunct to type I thyroplasty for unilateral vocal cord paralysis. Kraus DH, Orlikoff RF, Rizk SS, Rosenberg DB. Head Neck 1999;21:52–29. Copyright © 1999 John Wiley & Sons Inc.

hypoglossal and vagal injury may result in significant aspiration necessitating gastrostomy.

Surgical interruption of the facial nerve, such as during a middle cranial fossa approach, can result in either partial or total paralysis of the facial musculature. The resulting corneal exposure, oral incompetence, and cosmetic deformity are formidable rehabilitation challenges. While a variety of surgical procedures are available for providing either static or dynamic facial reanimation including nerve crossovers, muscle transfers, and skin tightening procedures (brow/face lifts), immediate attention should be focused on the reestablishment of complete eye closure and the prevention of exposure keratopathy. This can be effectively performed by the subcutaneous placement of a gold weight in the upper eye lid (Figure 12–11).[55] Such measures may be quite helpful as return of facial function, in instances where the anatomic integrity of the nerve has been maintained, may take 6 to 12 months.

Results

In light of the wide variety of benign and malignant histologies whose resection requires exposure of the middle cranial base, an objective assessment of the results of treatment is difficult to determine. However, data regarding the results of treatment for advanced parotid neoplasms is one area in which clinical series may be compared. Leonetti and colleagues described their experience in the surgical management of advanced (stage IV) parotid neoplasms.[56] In this series of 27 patients, they identified three categories of disease: tumors adjacent to either the bony or cartilaginous external auditory canal (EAC) and tumor extending into the EAC (both of which could be treated with the resection of the involved segment of the EAC), and tumor invading the middle ear and/or jugular bulb necessitating sacrifice of both the jugular foramen and the cochlea. With a mean follow-up period of 31.8 months, the resection of these advanced tumors resulted in 60 percent of the patients being alive without disease. A few, small series of extensive adenoid cystic carcinomas of the sinonasal cavity requiring anterior/middle fossa resections have also been published. Shotton and colleagues[57] reported 11 of 13 patients

tumor-free at 1 to 15 years after infratemporal fossa dissection for T2 to T4 adenoid cystic carcinoma. More recently, Pitman and colleagues[58] reported a 41 percent overall survival at 36 months and a 36 percent rate of local recurrence in a series of 35 patients whose sinonasal adenoid cystic carcinoma required either an anterior or anterolateral craniofacial resection. With respect to extensive adenoid cystic carcinoma involving the skull base, neutron radiotherapy has also been employed with a 53 percent reported locoregional control rate at 5 years.[59] Additionally a small series of middle cranial fossa resections reported by Fisch[60] demonstrated good success in achieving either subtotal or total tumor removal in patients with very extensive juvenile nasopharyngeal angiofibromas extending to or invading the cavernous sinus.

Another area in which some uniformity with respect to tumor histology allows for the critical assessment of the results of surgical therapy is in the case of temporal bone resection for squamous cell carcinoma of the external ear canal. Temporal bone resection for tumors arising from the ear/EAC or impinging upon it has evolved greatly, with improvements in radiographic imaging. Consequently, the bony erosion associated with a tumor, extension of the tumor into the middle ear, and an assessment of the ipsilateral parotid are all evaluable and highlight the critical importance of obtaining a deep resection

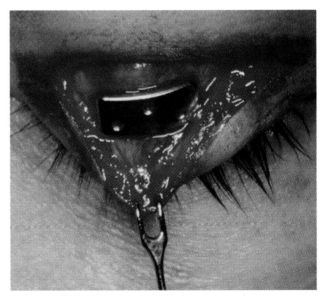

Figure 12–11. Placement of gold weight in upper eyelid for paralysis of the upper division of the facial nerve.

margin as well as the need to identify the facial nerve and carotid artery.[61] In a review of a series of 26 studies on this topic, Prasad and Janecka[61] determined that when a squamous carcinoma of the external auditory canal extends to the middle ear cleft, patients who undergo a subtotal temporal bone resection (whose medial margin is the internal carotid artery) had a 41.7 percent 5-year survival as compared to only a 28.7 percent 5-year survival for any less extensive resection. These results, as well as the fact that nearly 90 percent of those patients who died of their tumors in this series experienced local tumor recurrence, strongly suggest that when surgery is performed, an appropriately aggressive approach and resection of the middle cranial base is mandatory.

REFERENCES

1. Dandy WE. Orbital tumors: Results following the transcranial operative attack. New York: Oskar Priest; 1941.

2. Smith RR, Klopp CT, Williams JM. Surgical treatment of cancer of the frontal sinus and adjacent areas. Cancer 1954;7:991–4.

3. Ketcham AS, Wilkins RH, Van Buren JM, Smith RR. A combined intracranial facial approach to the paranasal sinuses. Am J Surg 1963;106:698–703.

4. Parsons H, Lewis JS. Subtotal resection of the temporal bone for cancer of the ear. Cancer 1954;7:995–1001.

5. Nuss DW, Janecka IP. Cranial base tumors. In: Myers EN, Suen JY, editors. Cancer of the head and neck, 3rd ed. Philadelphia (PA): W.B. Saunders Co.; 1996. p. 234–75

6. Schramm VL. Anterior craniofacial resection. In: Jackson CG, editor. Surgery of skull base tumors. New York: Churchill Livingstone. 1991.

7. Harrison LB, Raben A, Pfister DG, et al. A prospective phase II trial of concomitant chemotherapy and radiotherapy with delayed accelerated fractionation in unresectable tumors of the head and neck. Head Neck 1998;20:497–503.

8. Bilsky MH, Kraus DH, Strong EW, et al. Extended anterior craniofacial resection for intracranial extension of malignant tumors. Am J Surg 1997;174:565–8.

9. Boyle JO, Shah KC, Shah JP. Craniofacial resection for malignant neoplasms of the skull base: an overview. J Surg Oncol 1998;69:275–84.

10. O'Malley BW, Janecka IP. Evolution of outcomes in cranial base surgery. Semin Surg Oncol 1995;11:221–7.

11. Shah JP, Sundaresan N, Galicich J, Strong EW. Craniofacial resections for tumors involving the base of the skull. Am J Surg 1987;154:352–8.

12. Shah JP, Kraus DH, Arbit E, et al. Craniofacial resection for tumors involving the anterior skull base. Otolaryngol Head Neck Surg 1992;106:387–93.

13. Shah JP, Kraus DH, Bilsky MH, et al. Craniofacial resection for malignant tumors involving the anterior skull base. Arch Otolaryngol Head Neck Surg 1997;123:1312–17.

14. Kraus DH, Shah JP, Arbit E, et al. Complications of cranio-

15. Cheesman AD, Lund VJ, Howard DJ. Craniofacial resection for tumors of the nasal cavity and paranasal sinuses. Head Neck 1986;8:429–35.

16. Panje WR, Dohrmann GJ, Pitcock JK, et al. The transfacial approach for combined anterior craniofacial tumor ablation. Arch Otolaryngol Head Neck Surg 1989;115:301–7.

17. Raveh J, Laedrach K, Speiser M, et al. The subcranial approach for fronto-orbital and anteroposterior skull-base tumors. Arch Otolaryngol Head Neck Surg 1993;119:385–93.

18. Snyderman CH, Janecka IP, Sekhar LN, et al. Anterior cranial base reconstruction: Role of galeal and pericranial flaps. Laryngoscope 1990;100:607–14.

19. Andersen PE, Kraus DH, Arbit E, Shah JP. Management of the orbit during anterior fossa craniofacial resection. Arch Otolaryngol Head Neck Surg 1996;122: 1305–7.

20. Stern SJ, Goepfert H, Clayman G, et al. Orbital preservation in maxillectomy. Otolaryngol Head Neck Surg 1993;109:111–5.

21. Carrau RL, Segas J, Nuss DW, et al. Squamous cell carcinoma of the sinonasal tract invading the orbit. Laryngoscope 1999;109:230–5.

22. Cordeiro PG, Santamaria E, Kraus DH, et al. Reconstruction of total maxillectomy defects with preservation of the orbital contents. Plast Reconstr Surg 1998;102:1874–84.

23. Parsons JT, Stringer SP, Mancuso AA, Million RR. Nasal vestibule, nasal cavity, and paranasal sinus. In: Million RR, Cassisi NJ, editors. Management of head and neck cancer—A multidisciplinary approach. Philadelphia (PA): JB Lippincott Co.; 1994.

24. Wade PM, Smith RE, Johns ME. Response of esthesioneuroblastoma to chemotherapy. Cancer 1984;53:1036–41.

25. Levine PA, Debo RF, Meredith SD, et al. Craniofacial resection at the University of Virginia (1976–1992): survival analysis. Head Neck 1994;16:574–7.

26. McElroy EA Jr, Buckner JC, Lewis JE. Chemotherapy for advanced esthesioneuroblastoma: the Mayo Clinic experience. Neurosurgery 1998;42(5):1023–7.

27. Ketcham AS, Hoye RC, Van Buren JM, Johnson RH. Complications of intracranial facial resection for tumors of the paranasal sinuses. Am J Surg 1966;112:591–6.

28. Arbit E, Shah J, Bedford R, Carlon G. Tension pneumocephalus: treatment with controlled decompression via a closed water-seal drainage system. J Neurosurg 1991;74: 139–42.

29. Richtsmeier WJ, Briggs RJS, Koch WM, et al. Complications and early outcome of anterior craniofacial resection. Arch Otolaryngol Head Neck Surg 1992;118:913–7.

30. Terz JJ, Young HF, Lawrence W. Combined craniofacial resection for locally advanced carcinoma of the head and neck: tumors of the skin and soft tissues. Am J Surg 1980;140:613–7.

31. Terz JJ, Young HF, Lawrence W. Combined craniofacial resection for locally advanced carcinoma of the head and neck: carcinoma of the paranasal sinuses. Am J Surg 1980;140:618–24.

32. Cantu G, Solero CL, Mariani L, et al. Anterior craniofacial resection for malignant ethmoid tumors—a series of 91 patients. Head Neck 1999;21:185–91.

33. McCaffrey TV, Olsen KD, Yohanan JM, et al. Factors affect-

facial resection for tumors involving the anterior skull base. Head Neck 1994;16:307–12.

ing survival of patients with tumors of the anterior skull base. Laryngoscope 1994;104:940–5.

34. Catalano PJ, Hecht CS, Biller HF, et al. Craniofacial resection: an analysis of 73 cases. Arch Otolaryngol Head Neck Surg 1994;120:1203–8.

35. Ketcham AS, Van Buren JM. Tumors of the paranasal sinuses: a therapeutic challenge. Am J Surg 1985;150:406–13.

36. Jackson IT, Bailey H, Marsh WR, Juhasz P. Results and prognosis following surgery for malignant tumors of the skull base. Head Neck 1991;13:89–96.

37. Janecka IP, Sen C, Sekhar L, Curtin H. Treatment of paranasal sinus cancer with cranial base surgery: results. Laryngoscope 1994;104:553–5.

38. Van Tuyl R, Gussak GS. Prognostic factors in craniofacial surgery. Laryngoscope 1991;101:240–4.

39. Kraus DH, Sterman BM, Levine HL, et al. Factors influencing survival in ethmoid sinus cancer. Arch Otolaryngol Head Neck Surg 1992;118:367–72.

40. Clayman GL, DeMonte F, Jaffe DM, et al. Outcome and complications of extended cranial-base resections requiring microvascular free-tissue transfer. Arch Otolaryngol Head Neck Surg 1995;121:1253–7.

41. Saito K, Fukata K, Takahashi M, et al. Management of the cavernous sinus in en bloc resections of malignant skull base tumors. Head Neck 1999;21:734–42.

42. Fisch U, Pillsbury HC. Infratemporal fossa approach to lesions in the temporal bone and base of the skull. Arch Otolaryngol Head Neck Surg 1979;105:99–107.

43. Janecka IP, Sen CN, Sekhar LN, Arriaga M.. Facial translocation: a new approach to the cranial base. Otolaryngol Head Neck Surg 1990;103:413–9.

44. Fisch U. The infratemporal fossa approach for nasopharyngeal tumors. Laryngoscope 1983;93:36–44.

45. Janecka IP. Classification of facial translocation approach to the skull base. Otolaryngol Head Neck Surg 1995;112:579–85.

46. Guedea F, Mendenhall WM, Parsons JT, Million RR. Radiotherapy for chemodectoma of the carotid body and ganglion nodosum. Head Neck 1991;13:509–13.

47. Cole JM, Beiler D. Long-term results of treatment for glomus jugulare and glomus vagale tumors with radiotherapy. Laryngoscope 1994;104:1461–5.

48. Carrasco V, Rosenman J. Radiation therapy of glomus jugulare tumors. Laryngoscope 1993;103 Suppl 60:23–7.

49. Kondziolka D, Lunsford LD, McLaughlin MR, Flickinger JC. Long-term outcomes after radiosurgery for acoustic neuromas. N Engl J Med 1998;339:1426–33.

50. Kasper ME, Parsons JT, Mancuso AA, et al. Radiation therapy for juvenile angiofibroma: evaluation by CT and MRI, analysis of tumor regression, and selection of patients. Int J Radiat Oncol Biol Phys 1993;25:689–94.

51. Cummings BJ, Blend R, Keane T, et al. Primary radiation therapy for juvenile nasopharyngeal angiofibroma. Laryngoscope 1984;94(12 Pt 1):1599–605.

52. Netterville JL, Civantos FJ. Rehabilitation of cranial nerve deficits after neurotologic skull base surgery. Laryngoscope 1993;103 Suppl 60:45–54.

53. Kraus DH, Orlikoff RF, Rizk SS, Rosenberg DB. Arytenoid adduction as an adjunct to type I thyroplasty for unilateral vocal cord paralysis. Head Neck 1999;21(1):52–9.

54. Roberts WL. Rehabilitation of the head and neck cancer patient. In: McGarvey CL, editor. Physical therapy for the cancer patient. New York: Churchill Livingstone; 1990. p. 47–65.

55. Tucker HM. Postoperative management and rehabilitation of cranial nerve deficits. In: Jackson CG, editor. Surgery of skull base tumors. New York: Churchill Livingstone; 1991. p. 273–86.

56. Leonetti JP, Smith PG, Anand VK, et al. Subtotal petrosectomy in the management of advanced parotid neoplasms. Otolaryngol Head Neck Surg 1993;108:270–6.

57. Shotton JC, Schmid S, Fisch U. The infratemporal fossa approach for adenoid cystic carcinoma of the skull base and nasopharynx. Otolaryngol Clin North Am 1991;24:1445–64.

58. Pitman KT, Prokopakis EP, Aydogan B, et al. The role of skull base surgery for the treatment of adenoid cystic carcinoma of the sinonasal tract. Head Neck 1999;21:402–7.

59. Douglas JG, Lee S, Laramore GE, et al. Neutron radiotherapy for the treatment of locally advanced major salivary gland tumors. Head Neck 1999;21:255–63.

60. Andrews JC, Fisch U, Valavanis A, et al. The surgical management of extensive nasopharyngeal angiofibromas with the infratemporal fossa approach. Laryngoscope 1989;99:429–37.

61. Prasad S, Janecka IP. Efficacy of surgical treatment for squamous cell carcinoma of the temporal bone: a literature review. Otolaryngol Head Neck Surg 1994;110:270–80.

13

Salivary Tumors

JEFFREY D. SPIRO, MD, FACS
RONALD H. SPIRO, MD, FACS

The salivary glands are an uncommon site for cancer arising in the upper aerodigestive tract. Tumors arising in these glands comprise only about 7 percent of epithelial malignant neoplasms encountered in the head and neck, with an incidence of 1 per 100,000 population per year.[1-3] Considering the variety of anatomic sites and the number of different histologic subtypes encountered, it is easy to understand how oncologists may accumulate only limited experience with specific types of salivary gland cancer. Many of these tumors behave in an indolent fashion and the need for prolonged follow-up complicates the ability of the clinician to draw conclusions about the efficacy of treatment. For these reasons, most of the data about results are based on the experience reported from major referral centers.

ANATOMY

Salivary glands encountered in the head and neck consist of the "major" salivary glands and the "minor" salivary glands. The term "major" refers to the paired parotid, submandibular, and sublingual glands (Figure 13–1). The minor glands are small, predominantly mucus-secreting glands located beneath the mucosa of the upper aerodigestive tract. These glands are found in highest concentration in the palate, nasal cavity and oral cavity.

The parotid gland overlies the angle of the mandible and is closely related to the cartilage of the ear canal posteriorly, the zygoma superiorly, the parapharyngeal space medially, and the sternomastoid and posterior digastric muscles inferiorly. The facial nerve

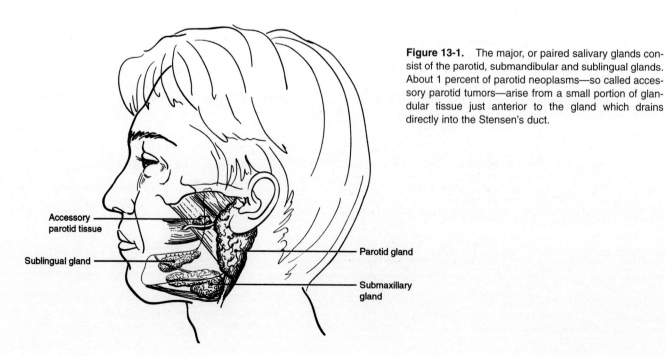

Figure 13-1. The major, or paired salivary glands consist of the parotid, submandibular and sublingual glands. About 1 percent of parotid neoplasms—so called accessory parotid tumors—arise from a small portion of glandular tissue just anterior to the gland which drains directly into the Stensen's duct.

Accessory
parotid tissue

Sublingual gland

Parotid gland

Submaxillary
gland

exits the stylomastoid foramen and runs through the substance of the parotid gland, splitting into its 5 main branches in the process. The exact pattern of arborization of the nerve is quite variable.[4] The plane of the facial nerve is used to divide the gland into its "superficial" and "deep" lobes, with about 20 percent of the substance of the gland lying beneath the nerve.

The submandibular gland abuts the body of the mandible superolaterally, the lingual and hypoglossal nerves medially, the mylohyoid muscle anteriorly and the tail of the parotid gland posteriorly (Figure 13–2). The marginal branch of the facial nerve runs along the lateral surface of the gland, just deep to the platysma.

DIAGNOSIS

As summarized in Figure 13–3, the parotid gland is the most common site of origin of salivary neoplasms, almost 80 percent of which are benign.[5–7] Submandibular gland neoplasms are far less common, and about half will be malignant. According to

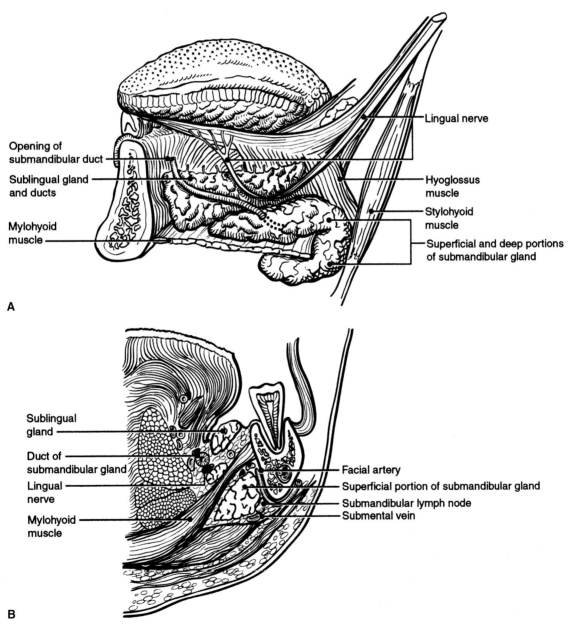

Figure 13–2. *A*, The relation of the submandibular gland to its muscular "bed" (digastric, mylohyoid and hyoglossus muscles) and major nerves is illustrated. *B*, Coronal view showing the location of the gland between the lingual cortex of the mandible and the floor of the mouth.

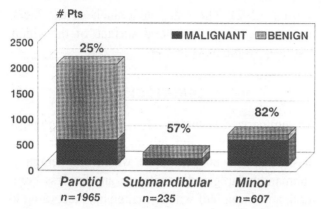

Figure 13–3. This bar graph shows the relative incidence of parotid, submandibular and minor salivary gland tumors in the Memorial Hospital experience. Percentages represent the proportion malignant at each site. The incidence of malignant minor salivary gland tumors is probably much lower in community practice.

reports from referral centers, minor salivary glands most often give rise to malignant tumors. The proportion of malignant minor salivary tumors arising in the oral cavity is lower in series from the community setting. It is uncommon to find a benign minor salivary neoplasm outside of the oral cavity or oropharynx.[5,8]

For cancer arising in major salivary glands, the most common presentation is a painless swelling of the affected gland. When small, malignant tumors of the major salivary glands are indistinguishable clinically from benign tumors. The duration of the swelling may be brief in patients with cancer, but it is not uncommon for patients with low-grade salivary cancers to present with a swelling that has been evident for years. Intermittent swelling of the submandibular gland related to salivary stimuli most likely represents inflammatory disease, and may be associated with pain. Because obstruction of the parotid gland is far less common, the presence of pain in association with a mass in the parotid may be suggestive of malignant disease.

Findings in patients with major salivary gland tumors that are highly indicative of malignancy include paralysis of all or part of the facial nerve, and the presence of associated lymphadenopathy. In patients with parotid cancer, these findings are noted at presentation in 9 to 25 percent and 13 to 25 percent, respectively.[2,3,9–13] Fixation of the tumor to overlying skin or adjacent deep structures is also suggestive of a malignant neoplasm.

The presenting complaint of patients with minor salivary cancer obviously will vary depending on the

site of the lesion, as will the findings on physical examination (Figure 13–4). Most often, these lesions present as a submucosal swelling (Figure 13–5), but they may be ulcerated when the overlying mucosa has been traumatized. As such, they may be clinically indistinguishable from squamous cell carcinomas.

Diagnostic imaging of major salivary cancers is not routinely indicated, but may be useful in various situations.[14] For lesions fixed to adjacent bony structures, such as the mandible or temporal bone, radiographs can delineate the extent of bone involvement (Figure 13–6). In cases where a lesion appears to involve the parapharyngeal space, MRI can distinguish deep-lobe parotid or minor salivary tumors from other parapharyngeal neoplasms. Imaging studies are important in patients with minor salivary cancers arising in the palate, nasal cavity, nasopharynx and paranasal sinuses where the full extent of the tumor usually cannot be defined by clinical exam alone.

Tumors arising in major salivary glands are easily accessible to fine needle aspiration biopsy (FNAB). Experienced cytopathologists can reliably distinguish salivary from non-salivary pathology and benign from malignant,[15–16] but precise histologic classification based only on an aspirate is an unrealistic goal. While some advocate routine FNAB of all major salivary neoplasms, it is our belief that such a practice adds little to the management of small, obvious parotid tumors. On the other hand, FNAB of submandibular masses is important because only a minority will prove to be primary tumors arising in

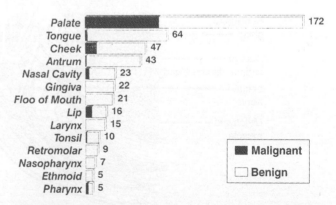

Figure 13–4. Sites of origin of minor salivary gland tumors as seen at Memorial Hospital. The palate was involved in almost 40 percent of patients, reflecting the high density of minor salivary glands in this site. Black shading indicates malignant tumors, almost all of which arose in the oral cavity.

the submandibular gland. Most minor salivary tumors are accessible for direct open biopsy in the office or the operating room. Care must be taken to insure that representative material is obtained for pathologic

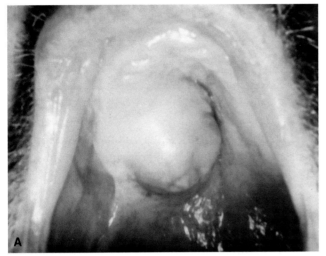

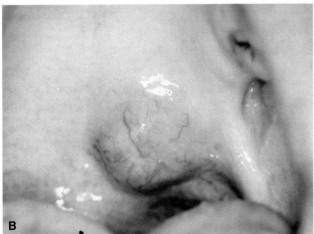

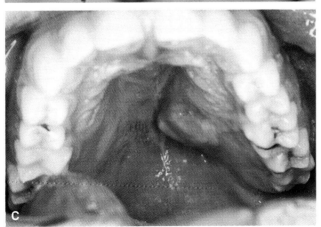

Figure 13–5. *A*, Pleomorphic adenoma of right hard palate, and *B*, adenoid cystic carcinoma at junction of left hard and soft palate. Benign minor salivary tumors are clinically indistinguishable from their malignant counterparts. *C*, Mucoepidermoid carcinoma of the hard palate.

analysis, particularly if the lesion is located in the nasal cavity or paranasal sinuses where confusion with many other types of cancer is possible.

The classification of malignant salivary gland tumors is complex and challenging to pathologists (Tables 13–1 and 13–2). Specific histologic types of salivary cancer vary in incidence, depending on their site of origin. Mucoepidermoid carcinoma is the most common cancer of the parotid gland, and adenoid cystic carcinoma is the most common malignant tumor arising in the submandibular gland.[2,3,5–7,17–28] In minor salivary sites, adenoid cystic carcinoma and adenocarcinoma are most prevalent.[8,29,30]

TREATMENT GOALS AND ALTERNATIVES

Role of Multidisciplinary Treatment

As with head and neck cancer in general, the goals of treatment for salivary cancer are cure of the disease while minimizing the morbidity of treatment. Surgical resection has long been the mainstay of treatment of salivary cancer, but has the potential to create significant functional deficits. For cancers arising in the parotid gland, loss of the facial nerve is the greatest functional concern, while the hypoglossal nerve, lingual nerve and marginal mandibular branch of the facial nerve are at risk when carcinomas of the submandibular salivary

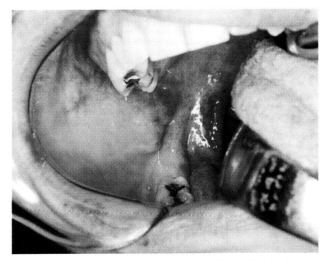

Figure 13–6. Adenoid cystic carcinoma arising in the left retromolar trigone extending into the adjacent cheek mucosa. Tumors of this histologic type are always more extensive than can be appreciated either clinically or radiographically.

Table 13–1. MEMORIAL HOSPITAL CLASSIFICATION AND INCIDENCE OF MALIGNANT SALIVARY TUMORS

	1939 through 1973		1988 through 1993	
	Number of Patients	Incidence (%)	Number of patients	Incidence (%)
Mucoepidermoid carcinoma	439	34	119	34
Adenoid cystic carcinoma	281	22	72	21
Adenocarcinoma	225	17	73	21
Malignant mixed tumor	161	13	22	6
Acinic cell carcinoma	84	7	25	7
Epidermoid carcinoma	53	4	19	6
Anaplastic and other	35	3	16	5
Total	1278	100.0	346	100.0

gland are resected. Excision of malignant salivary gland neoplasms arising at minor salivary sites may jeopardize structures such as the larynx or the orbital contents. Unfortunately, more extensive surgery does not necessarily yield better salvage in patients with locally advanced salivary cancer.

In an effort to reduce the morbidity associated with "radical" surgical resection while maintaining or even improving chances for cure, there has been increasing use of combinations of surgery and radiotherapy during the past 2 decades. This strategy, which will be discussed later in this chapter, has proven to be effective in advancing these treatment goals.

Factors Affecting Choice of Treatment

The single most important factor affecting the choice of treatment for salivary gland cancer is the extent of the lesion at diagnosis (ie, the clinical stage). In general, smaller lesions arising in major or minor salivary glands are amenable to surgical resection with minimal morbidity and good control of disease. Larger tumors that have invaded adjacent structures not only will require more extensive resection, but also the addition of adjuvant radiotherapy to increase the chances of cure. In some cases, disease may be so extensive as to be unresectable. Finally, patients with disseminated disease usually will not benefit from aggressive local or regional therapy. The exception may be patients with adenoid cystic carcinoma, who can live for many years despite pulmonary metastases.

Location is also an important factor in treatment selection. Borderline resectable lesions in inaccessi-

ble locations, such as sinus tumors involving the base of the skull, may be better suited for nonsurgical therapy such as chemoradiotherapy or neutron beam irradiation. When resection margins are close because of tumor proximity to vital structures, the evidence suggests that adjunctive radiotherapy can improve results.

Histology may influence treatment planning as well. Adenoid cystic carcinoma, for example, with its propensity for perineural spread and insidious local extension, is often very difficult to adequately encompass with surgical resection alone. Other lesions that are high grade histologically more often present with locally extensive disease, and also have a higher incidence of distant metastases than their low grade counterparts, which suggests the need for effective systemic therapy in this subset of patients.

Table 13–2. WORLD HEALTH ORGANIZATION (WHO) CLASSIFICATION OF MALIGNANT SALIVARY GLAND TUMORS

Acinic cell carcinoma
Mucoepidermoid carcinoma
Adenoid cystic carcinoma
Polymorphous low-grade adenocarcinoma
Epithelial-myoepithelial carcinoma
Basal cell adenocarcinoma
Sebaceous carcinoma
Papillary cystadenocarcinoma
Mucinous adenocarcinoma
Oncocytic carcinoma
Salivary duct carcinoma
Adenocarcinoma
Malignant myoepithelioma
Carcinoma in pleomorphic adenoma
Squamous cell carcinoma
Small cell carcinoma
Undifferentiated carcinoma

Surgical Treatment

Surgical resection remains the mainstay of treatment for salivary tumors. Specific considerations pertaining to various sites are discussed below.

Parotid Gland

In most cases, the minimum surgical procedure recommended for tumors arising in the parotid gland is excision of the superficial "lobe" of the parotid gland with dissection and preservation of the facial nerve. In carefully selected patients with small lesions arising in the tail of the gland, a more limited local excision without formal nerve dissection may be feasible. When surgery is performed for parotid cancer, every effort should be made to preserve the facial nerve unless it is imbedded in, or adherent to, the tumor. Piecemeal excision of a malignant parotid tumor in order to spare the nerve violates basic oncologic principles, and is mentioned only to be condemned. Sacrifice of all or part of the facial nerve has been required in 29 to 40 percent of reported patients with carcinoma of the parotid gland.[10,12,17] As discussed below, immediate cable grafting using branches of the cervical plexus or the sural nerve is indicated when feasible after facial nerve resection.

When a tumor arises deep to the facial nerve, several surgical approaches are possible. For small lesions that do not extend significantly into the parapharyngeal space, the facial nerve is initially exposed by superficial parotidectomy and then the branches can be displaced to allow for tumor removal (Figure 13–7). When there is significant extension into the parapharyngeal space (Figure 13–8), the submandibular gland can be removed to facilitate transcervical access. A paramedian mandibulotomy will occasionally be required for adequate access to the parapharyngeal space in patients with large lesions.

Submandibular Gland

Excision of this gland will occasionally be adequate treatment when a carcinoma is small and surrounded by normal parenchyma. More often, the tumor extends to or through the gland capsule to involve adjacent structures. In this setting, the resection may have to include the "bed" of the gland (ie, digastric,

mylohyoid and hyoglossal muscles), adjacent nerves (lingual, hypoglossal, ramus marginalis), the mandible or the floor of the mouth and/or sublingual gland. This is probably best acccomplished in conjunction with removal of levels 1, 2 and 3 lymph nodes as an "extended" supraomohyoid neck dissection. Tumor extent will obviously determine which additional structures to resect. Patients with high-stage tumors may actually require a composite resection. Given the difficulty in obtaining adequate microscopic margins of resection in adenoid cystic carcinoma, there has been a trend toward combining less radical surgery with postoperative radiotherapy.

Minor Salivary Sites

The surgical approach to tumors arising in minor salivary sites will obviously vary depending on the site of origin, but is generally similar to that utilized for squamous cell carcinoma arising at the same site. Lesions arising in the larynx may be amenable to either conservation laryngeal surgery or total laryngectomy. A tumor arising in the tongue base can be approached utilizing a paramedian mandibulotomy, and palatal salivary cancer may require a peroral partial or conventional subtotal maxillectomy. For those

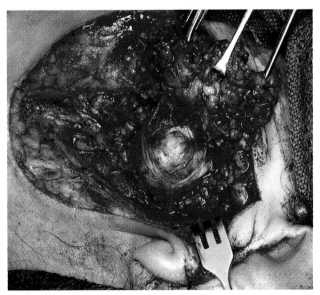

Figure 13–7. Tumors situated lateral to the mandible but medial to the facial nerve are seldom diagnosed preoperatively as deep-lobe tumors. Only during the course of superficial parotidectomy was it appreciated that this pleomorphic adenoma was deep to the bifurcation of the nerve. With careful dissection, it is almost always possible to remove these tumors and preserve the facial nerve.

lesions arising in the nasal cavity or paranasal sinuses, adequate resection must include these structures, and occasionally a combined craniofacial resection or orbital exenteration is necessary in cases of more extensive disease.

Neck Treatment

Those few patients who initially present with obvious nodal involvement require therapeutic neck dissection. In carefully selected patients who have limited disease in the first echelon of nodal drainage, selective neck dissection may be adequate. Those with more extensive neck disease should undergo comprehensive neck dissection with preservation of the accessory nerve when feasible.

Because the incidence of occult neck disease in salivary cancer is low overall, elective dissection of the neck is not routinely indicated. It may be appropriate, however, in patients with sizeable N0 squamous cell or high-grade mucoepidermoid carcinoma, which have a higher incidence of cervical lymph node metastases. In these cases, a selective neck dissection encompassing the nodal levels at greatest risk should be adequate to identify those patients with occult disease.

Nonsurgical Treatment

For many years, salivary cancer was believed to be resistant to radiation therapy. In recent years, radiotherapy has assumed an important role in the treatment of salivary cancer, particularly in combination with surgical resection. When malignant salivary neoplasms arise in locations that are relatively inaccessible, such as the nasopharynx or the base of the skull, primary radiotherapy becomes a more attractive option. The use of neutron beam irradiation has been advocated in recent years as a primary therapy for salivary cancer in this setting, particularly in patients with adenoid cystic carcinoma.[31,32] Encouraging locoregional control rates are reported, but the significant associated morbidity raises the question of whether neutrons might best be reserved for patients with recurrent or unresectable tumors.

The indications for postoperative radiotherapy include: advanced stage disease, concern over ade-

quacy of surgical margins, and adverse findings in the surgical pathology report.[13,33,34] Unilateral therapy is usually adequate for lesions arising in major salivary glands, and at least the first echelon lymphatic drainage basin is often included in the treatment field. When disease involves the nasal cavity or paranasal sinuses, careful treatment planning is obviously needed to minimize dose to the adjacent central nervous system or to orbital contents.

As noted previously, distant metastases are a frequent occurrence in certain types of salivary cancer,

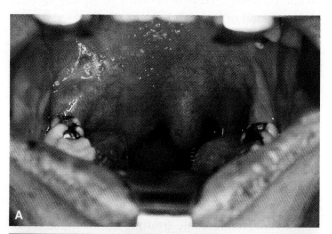

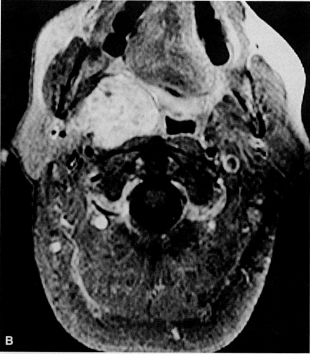

Figure 13–8.   *A,* Typical parapharyngeal presentation of a retromandibular, pleomorphic adenoma arising in the deep lobe of the left parotid gland. *B,* MRI scan showing the paraphyaryngeal tumor, contiguous with the parotid gland and extending through the stylomandibular window.

such as adenoid cystic carcinoma and high-grade lesions of any histology. This suggests the need for effective systemic therapy, but effective drug regimens are not presently available.

Sequelae, Complications and their Management

When salivary neoplasms are limited to the major glands, the aftereffects of treatment are usually limited. Unintentional injury to the facial nerve during parotidectomy, or disruption of the lingual or hypoglossal nerves during excision of the submandibular gland, are quite uncommon. If the resection is extended beyond the parotid or submandibular gland to include adjacent structures such as the mandible or the temporal bone, the risk of complications increases.

When "salivary-type" tumors arise in locations other than the major salivary glands, potential treatment sequelae and complications will obviously vary according to the site of disease. These problems will be similar to those encountered when treating squamous cell carcinoma at similar sites, and are described elsewhere in this volume.

Rehabilitation and Quality of Life

As noted above, all or part of the facial nerve may be paralyzed at presentation in patients with parotid gland cancer. In addition, resection of the facial nerve may be required at the time of surgical resection. Loss of the mimetic function of the face has a significant negative impact on the quality of life, and inability to close the eye may result in problems from corneal exposure.

As mentioned above, primary cable grafting of the facial nerve at the time of ablative surgery is desirable, providing that proximal and distal disease-free nerve branches are available. Sensory nerve branches harvested from the cervical plexus provide the most convenient source of nerve grafts, but the sural nerves provide a good substitute when these are unavailable. Although the results of grafting often leave much to be desired, there is usually improvement in muscle tone, particularly in younger patients, regardless of postoperative radiotherapy.[35,36]

When the proximal stump of the facial nerve is not available, the hypoglossal nerve can be anastamosed to the distal portion of the facial nerve. Gold weight eyelid implants and fascial slings have proved useful when nerve grafting is not possible, or is unsuccessful.

Outcomes and Results of Treatment

General Considerations

Several issues must be considered when assessing treatment results. Reported series are often small, and outcomes can vary widely depending on the anatomic sites of origin and the histologic subtypes included in the study population. More importantly, the indolent course of many salivary neoplasms mandates clinical follow-up of at least 10 years in order to draw valid conclusions. Finally, the inclusion of patients over an extended time period may mean that considerable variation exists in diagnostic and therapeutic capabilities over the study period.

In the Memorial Hospital experience with previously untreated major salivary gland carcinoma, the reported 5-, 10- and 15-year cumulative survival rates were 82 percent, 67 percent and 55 percent, respectively. Similarly, survival rates for those with previously untreated malignant minor salivary gland tumors were 73 percent, 56 percent, and 46 percent, respectively.[37,38]

Results by Histology

Differences in treatment outcome have been noted depending on the specific histology of salivary cancer. For those tumor types where histologic grading is possible, such as mucoepidermoid carcinoma or adenocarcinoma, high-grade lesions carry a worse prognosis (Figure 13–9).[37] High-grade cancers tend to be locally advanced at presentation, and are more often associated with regional and distant metastases.[39,40]

Results by Treatment

While surgery has historically been the mainstay of therapy for salivary cancer, considerable experience with adjuvant radiotherapy has accumulated over the past 2 decades. Results indicate that combining radiotherapy and surgery has resulted in improved

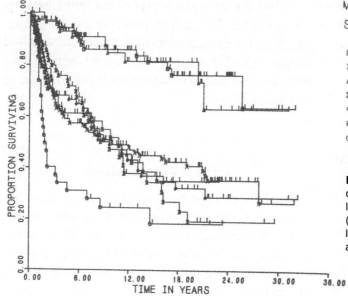

MAJOR SALIVARY CA: 1939-1982
SURVIVAL BY HISTOLOGY

⊡	MUCOEP GR1	(72 PTS..	58 CENSORED)
X	MUCOEP OTHER	(132 PTS..	57 CENSORED)
△	ACINIC	(56 PTS..	48 CENSORED)
⊠	ADENOIDCYSTIC	(53 PTS..	20 CENSORED)
◇	MMT	(67 PTS..	25 CENSORED)
✳	ADENO CA	(47 PTS..	21 CENSORED)
○	S& CA OR ANAPL CA	(34 PTS..	8 CENSORED)

TICK MARK (!) INDICATES LAST FOLLOW-UP

Figure 13–9. Cumulative survival rates according to histologic diagnosis fall into 3 groups. The best prognosis was seen with low-grade mucoepidermoid carcinoma and acinic cell carcinoma (upper 2 curves). Epidermoid and anaplastic carcinoma had the lowest survival rates (lowest curve). Results were intermediate and similar for all other histologic tumor types.

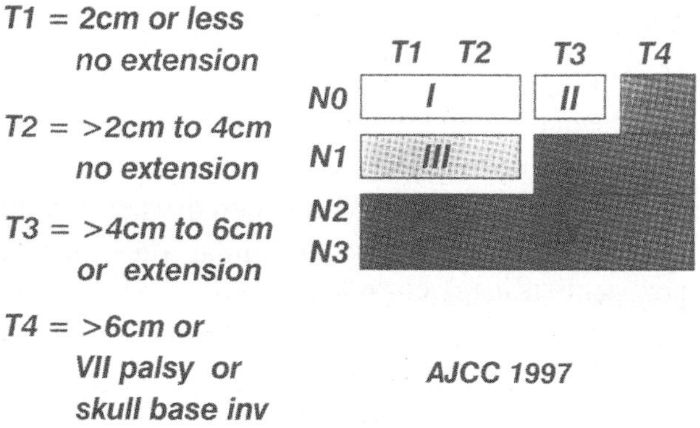

Figure 13–10.   T staging and stage groupings according to the 1997 edition of the AJCC Cancer Staging Manual. The N staging is identical to that used for squamous cell carcinoma.

T1 = 2cm or less
   no extension

T2 = >2cm to 4cm
   no extension

T3 = >4cm to 6cm
   or extension

T4 = >6cm or
   VII palsy or
   skull base inv

AJCC 1997

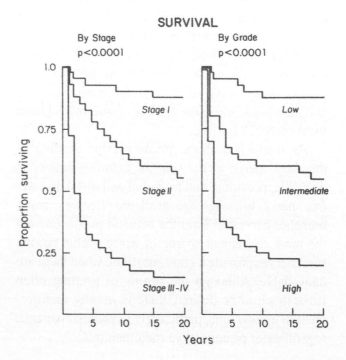

Figure 13–11.   Significant differences in survival were noted when tumors arising in all sites, regardless of histology, were analyzed according to the clinical stage. For those tumors that could be graded (mucoepidermoid, adenocarcinoma, squamous cell carcinoma) similar survival differences were noted.

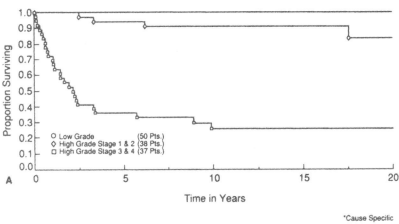

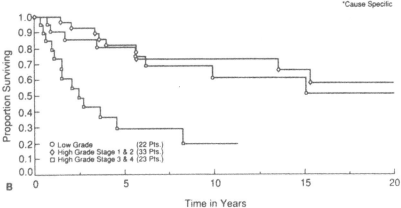

Figure 13–12. Cumulative survival curves for *A*, mucoepidermoid carcinoma and *B*, adenocarcinoma of minor salivary gland origin. For both tumor types, there was no difference in survival when low-grade tumors were compared to high-grade but low-stage lesions, confirming that clinical stage is more important than grade as a prognostic factor.

local and regional control of disease.[33,34] Unfortunately, this has not always translated into improved survival, because of distant metastases, which again suggests the need for effective systemic therapy in salivary cancer.

Results by Stage of Disease

The stage of disease at presentation is the most reliable predictor of treatment outcome in salivary cancer (Figure 13–10).[41] Cumulative survival according to clinical stage and histology is shown in Figure 13–11.[5] This includes patients with minor salivary gland cancers, which were staged using the criteria for squamous carcinomas in similar sites (Figure 13–12).[37] Aside from the fact that not all salivary gland carcinomas are gradeable, the data clearly indicate that clinical stage is a more important predictor of survival.

REFERENCES

1. National Cancer Institute, Biometry Branch. The Third National Cancer Survey: Advanced three year report 1969–1971 Incidence. National Cancer Institute, Bethesda MD, 1974.
2. Pedersen D, Overgaard J, Sogaard H, et al. Malignant parotid tumors in 110 consecutive patients: Treatment results and prognosis. Laryngoscope 1992;102:1064–9.
3. Renehan A, Gleave EN, Hancock BD, et al. Long-term follow-up of over 1000 patients with salivary gland tumours treated in a single center. Br J Surg 1986;83:1750–4.
4. Katz AD, Catalano P. The clinical significance of the various anastamotic branches of the facial nerve: report of 100 patients. Arch Otolaryngol 1987;113:959–62.
5. Spiro RH. Salivary neoplasms: overview of a 35 year experience with 2,807 patients. Head Neck Surg 1986;8:77–84.
6. Eneroth CM. Salivary gland tumors in the parotid gland, submandibular gland, and the palate region. Cancer 1971; 27:1415–8.
7. Eveson JW, Cawson RA. Salivary gland tumours: a review of 2,410 cases with particular reference to histological types, site, age and sex distribution. J Pathol 1985;146:51–8.
8. Waldron CA, El-Mofty SK, Gnepp DR. Tumors of the intraoral minor salivary glands: A demographic and histologic study of 426 cases. Oral Surg Oral Med Oral Pathol 1988;66:323–33.
9. Woods JE, Cheng GC, Beahrs OH. Experience with 1,360 primary parotid tumors. Am J Surg 1975;130:460–2.
10. Spiro RH, Huvos AW, Strong EW. Cancer of the parotid gland: a clinicopathologic study of 288 primary cases. Am J Surg 1975;130:452–9.
11. Borthune A, Kjellevold, Kaalhus O, Vermund H. Salivary gland malignant neoplasms: treatment and prognosis. Int J Radiat Oncol Biol Phys 1986;12:747–54.

12. Frankenthaler RA, Luna MA, Lee SS, et al. Prognostic variables in parotid cancer. Arch Otolaryngol Head Neck Surg 1991;117:1251–6.

13. Tu G, Hu Y, Jiang P, Qin D. The superiority of combined therapy in parotid cancer. Arch Otolaryngol 1982;108:710–3.

14. Weissman JL. Imaging of the salivary glands. Semin Ultrasound CT MR 1995; 16:546–68.

15. Atula T, Greenman R, Laippala P, Klemi PJ. Fine-needle aspiration biopsy in the diagnosis of parotid gland lesions: evaluation of 438 biopsies. Diagn Cytopathol 1996;15:185–90.

16. Al-Khafaji BM, Nestok BR, Katz RL. Fine-needle aspiration of 154 parotid masses with histologic correlation: Ten year experience at the University of Texas M.D. Anderson Cancer Center. Cancer (Cancer Cytopathology) 1998;84:153–9

17. Hodgkinson DJ. The influence of facial nerve sacrifice in surgery of malignant parotid tumors. J Surg Oncol 1976;8:425–32.

18. Friedman M, Levin B, Grybauskas V, et al. Malignant tumors of the major salivary glands. Otolaryngol Clin North Am 1986;19:625–36.

19. Guillamondegui OM, Byers RM, Luna MA, et al. Aggressive surgery in treatment for parotid cancer: the role of adjunctive postoperative radiotherapy. Am J Roentgenol 1975;1213:49–54.

20. Rafla S. Malignant parotid tumors: natural history and treatment. Cancer 1977;40:136–44.

21. Hollander L, Cunningham MP. Management of cancer of the parotid gland. Surg Clin North Am 1973;53:113–9.

22. Hugo NE, McKinney P, Griffith BH. Management of tumors of the parotid gland. Surg Clin North Am 1973;53:105–11.

23. Spiro RH, Hajdu SI, Strong EW. Tumors of the submaxillary gland. Am J Surg 1976;132:463–8.

24. Byers RM, Jesse RH, Guillamondegui OM, Luna MA. Malignant tumors of the submaxillary gland. Am J Surg 1973;126:458–63.

25. Lowe JT Jr, Farmer JC Jr. Submaxillary gland tumors. Laryngoscope 1974;84:542–52.

26. Trial ML, Lubritz J. Tumors of the submandibular gland. Laryngoscope 1974;84:1225–32.

27. Pyper PL, Beverland DE, Bell DM. Tumors of the submandibular gland. J Royal Coll Surg Edin 1987;32:233-5.

28. Rafla S. Submaxillary gland tumors. Cancer 1970;26:821–6.

29. Spiro RH, Koss LG, Hajdu SI, Strong EW. Tumors of minor salivary origin: A clinicopathologic study of 492 cases. Cancer 1973;31:117–29.

30. Chou C, Zhu G, Luo M, Xue G. Carcinoma of the minor salivary glands: results of surgery and combined treatment. J Oral Maxillofac Surg 1996;54:448–53.

31. Buchholz TA, Laramore GE, Griffen BR, et al. The role of fast neutron therapy in the management of advanced salivary gland malignant neoplasms. Cancer 1992;69:2779–88.

32. Krull A, Schwarz R, Brackrock S, et al. Neutron therapy in malignant salivary gland tumors: Results at European centers. Recent Results Cancer Res 1998;150:88–99.

33. Garden AS, El-Naggar AK, Morrison WH, et al. Postoperative radiotherapy for malignant tumors of the parotid gland. Int J Radiat Oncol Biol Phys 1997;37:79–85.

34. Armstrong JG, Harrison LB, Spiro RH, et al. Malignant tumors of major salivary origin: a matched pair analysis of the role of combined surgery and postoperative radiotherapy. Arch Otolaryngol Head Neck Surg 1990;116:290–3.

35. Reddy PG, Arden RL, Mathog RH. Facial nerve rehabilitation after radical parotidectomy. Laryngoscope 1999;109:894–9.

36. Kerrebijn JD, Freeman JL. Facial nerve reconstruction: Outcomes and failures. J Otolaryngol 1998;27:183–6.

37. Spiro RH, Thaler HT, Hicks WS, et al. The importance of clinical staging of minor salivary tumors. Am J Surg 1991;162:330–6.

38. Spiro RH, Armstrong J, Harrison LB, et al. Carcinoma of major salivary glands: recent trends. Arch Otolaryngol Head Neck Surg 1989;115:316–21.

39. Renehan AG, Gleave EN, Slevin NJ, McGurk M. Clinicopathological and treatment-related factors influencing survival in parotid cancer. Br J Surg 1999;80:1296–1300.

40. Gallo O, Franchi A, Bottai GV, et al. Risk factors for distant metastases from carcinoma of the parotid gland. Cancer 1997;80:844–51.

41. American Joint Commission for Cancer Staging and End Results Reporting. Manual for staging of cancer. Chicago (IL): American Joint Commission; 1997.

14

Thyroid and Parathyroid Tumors

ASHOK R. SHAHA, MD, FACS
SNEHAL G. PATEL, MD, MS, FRCS

THYROID TUMORS

Diseases of the thyroid gland represent a common medical and surgical problem. A variety of inflammatory lesions and neoplasms are noted by endocrinologists and surgeons interested in thyroid pathology. Various pathologic conditions include Hashimoto's thyroiditis, nodular goiter, solitary thyroid nodule, adenomas and thyroid cancer.

Although thyroid disease is extremely common, thyroid cancer is relatively uncommon and forms less than 2 percent of all human cancers. Approximately 19,500 new patients with thyroid cancer will be seen in the United States during the year 2001, while approximately 1,300 patients will die of thyroid cancer.[1] The prevalence of nodular goiter has decreased considerably in the United States due to the routine use of iodized salt. However, it is still quite prevalent in other parts of the world, particularly in certain European countries around the Alps, and in Asia near the Himalayas. The routine use of ultrasonography has shown a very high incidence of occult thyroid lesions in the general population, although the incidence of clinically palpable thyroid nodularity is only approximately 5 percent.[2,3] The prevalence of malignancy in solitary thyroid nodules ranges between 5 and 20 percent, while the incidence of thyroid cancer in multi-nodular goiter is less than 5 percent.[2,3] Even though the incidence and mortality rate of thyroid cancer is not very high, this subject has generated considerable discussion and controversies. Major controversial issues are related to the diagnostic work-up and the extent of thyroidectomy.

Various groups of physicians are involved in the management of thyroid disease, including family practitioners, internists, endocrinologists, radiotherapists, nuclear medicine physicians, general surgeons, otolaryngologists, surgical oncologists, head and neck surgeons and endocrine surgeons. Even though thyroid surgery appears to be one of the safest surgical procedures, the morbidity and complications of thyroid surgery can be devastating to the patient in relation to voice dysfunction and permanent hypoparathyroidism.

It is interesting to note that Samuel Gross, in 1866, stated, "Thyroid surgery is horrid butchery. No honest and sensible surgeon would ever engage in thyroid surgery."[4] On the other hand, toward the turn of the twentieth century, the first surgeon ever to win the Nobel Prize was Theodore Kocher for his contributions to the understanding of thyroid physiology, as well as for perfecting the technique of thyroidectomy. In his hands, the mortality rate from thyroidectomy was less than 1 percent.[4]

Anatomy

The thyroid gland develops from the pharyngeal pouch, starting at the base of the tongue in the region of the foramen cecum, during the fourth week of gestation. As the thyroid gland descends to the lower neck, it brings with it a tract called the thyroglossal duct. An undescended thyroid gland, though rare, is occasionally seen as a lingual thyroid. A more common anomaly of the thyroglossal tract is the thyroglossal duct cyst, commonly presenting as a midline cervical mass in children. This is one of the most common midline neck masses in children, the treatment of which is generally complete surgical excision (Sistrunk operation), where the cyst is removed in its entirety, along with a central portion of the hyoid bone. The thyroglossal duct track is invaginated by the hyoid or is intimately adherent to the hyoid bone. In the latter instance, the central portion of the hyoid and the core of the tissue of the base of the tongue should be removed to secure complete removal of the thyroglossal duct tract to avoid recurrences. The lingual thyroid is a rare condition where a patient may present with an enlargement of thyroid tissue on the base of the tongue. It is important, whenever a lingual thyroid is suspected, to determine the presence or absence of normal thyroid in the neck, prior to any surgical undertaking, since surgical excision may precipitate hypothyroidism. Most patients with a lingual thyroid, however, can be treated conservatively.

The three important structures surrounding the thyroid gland are the recurrent laryngeal nerves, the superior laryngeal nerves, and the parathyroid glands (Figures 14–1 to 14–3). Any surgeon undertaking a surgical procedure on the thyroid must be quite familiar with the normal anatomy and variations of these important structures surrounding the thyroid gland to reduce complications and morbidity.

The superior laryngeal nerve runs parallel to the vagus nerve at the base of the skull, and then turns medially to divide into external and internal branches. The external branch supplies the cricoarytenoid muscle, which makes the vocal cord tight.[5] This nerve is popularly called the "singer's nerve," since injury to this nerve will lead to the lack of ability to raise the voice or sing at high pitch. The true incidence of injury to the superior laryngeal nerve is unclear in the literature, although this complication can be devastating, especially for a professional singer.

The recurrent laryngeal nerve supplies all the intrinsic muscles of the larynx—with the exception of the cricoarytenoid muscle. During thyroid surgery, the nerve may be injured near its entry into the larynx, close to the cricoid cartilage, or where the nerve crosses the inferior thyroid artery.[6] The nerve may be injured below the thyroid gland in the superior mediastinum near the trachea, but the most common site of injury is the area of Berry's ligament, or where the nerve crosses the inferior thyroid artery.[5] Berry's ligament is thickened, pre-tracheal fascia that suspends

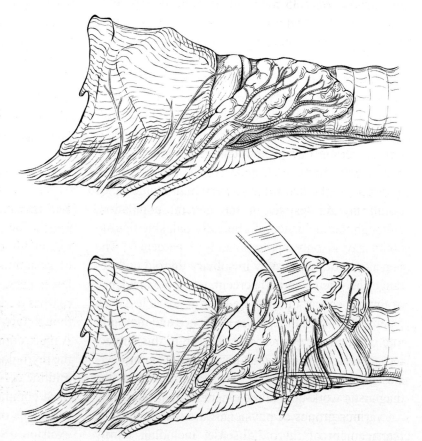

Figure 14–1. Schematic representation of the lateral and superior aspects of the thyroid gland, showing the superior laryngeal nerve running parallel to the vessels.

Figure 14–2. Exposure of the tracheoesophageal groove, depicting the recurrent laryngeal nerve and its relation to the branches of the inferior thyroid artery.

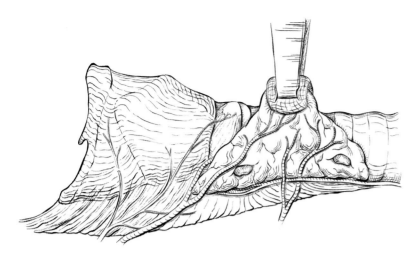

Figure 14–3. Anatomic relation of the parathyroid glands to the inferior thyroid artery.

the thyroid gland from the trachea and the cricoid cartilage. Several capsular veins course through this ligament, which makes surgical resection tedious and carries a high risk of injury to the recurrent laryngeal nerve. Occasionally the recurrent laryngeal nerve may divide into two or three branches external to the cricoid cartilage, and this should be kept in mind to avoid injury to any of these branches.

The parathyroid glands are generally located on the posterior surface of the thyroid gland, each weighing approximately 35 mg. Identification and preservation of the parathyroid glands and their blood supply is extremely critical in thyroid surgery—especially in patients undergoing total thyroidectomy. The blood supply to the parathyroids generally comes from the inferior thyroid artery, however in some instances there are small branches exclusively supplying the superior parathyroid gland from the superior thyroid artery.[7] Some of the anteriorly placed parathyroid glands may receive their blood supply directly from the thyroid gland and these glands are at high risk of injury during total thyroidectomy. An understanding of the anatomy of the parathyroid glands, as well as their blood supply, is essential for the surgeon contemplating thyroid surgery.

Diagnosis

When a patient presents with a solitary thyroid nodule or a diffuse enlargement of the thyroid, a variety of diagnostic studies can be employed.[8–12] Although an extensive work-up can be performed (including various imaging studies), probably the most cost-effective approach is a good history and physical examination followed by a fine-needle aspiration biopsy (Table 14–1).

The three main indications for surgery on the thyroid gland are suspicion of malignancy, compression symptoms, and cosmesis. There continues to be considerable controversy regarding the optimal work-up of a thyroid mass. The most appropriate, cost-effective, and accurate initial test available today is a fine-needle aspiration biopsy. The accuracy, sensitivity and positive-predictive value of this method exceeds 90 percent.[9]

Certain clinical features need to be carefully looked for in every patient with a thyroid mass as these masses are commonly associated with malignancy (Table 14–2). Age is an important factor, since benign thyroid disease is more common in middle-aged individuals and thyroid cancer is more prevalent among the young and the elderly. A young child presenting with a thyroid mass has a greater than 40 percent chance of having thyroid cancer. Every effort should be made to rule out thyroid cancer in young individuals. Similarly, in older patients, a thyroid mass is more likely to be neoplastic rather than a benign nodular goiter. Thyroid disease is more common in women, but thyroid cancer, per se, is more common in men

Table 14–1. INVESTIGATION OF A THYROID NODULE	
History/physical	Radiography of neck/chest
Thyroid function tests	Thyroid scan
CBC/SMAC/calcium	Ultrasound
Thyroid antibodies	CT scan
Indirect laryngoscopy	MRI
	PET scan
	Fine-needle aspiration cytology
	Core biopsy

Table 14–2. CLINICAL FEATURES INDICATIVE OF A MALIGNANT THYROID NODULE

Age (very young or old)
Sex (male)
Presence of distant (pulmonary) metastases
Neck node metastases
Vocal cord paralysis
History of irradiation to the neck
Clinical characteristics: hard, fixed nodule
Rapid growth
Sudden change in size of thyroid nodule
Residence of the individual
Pressure effects

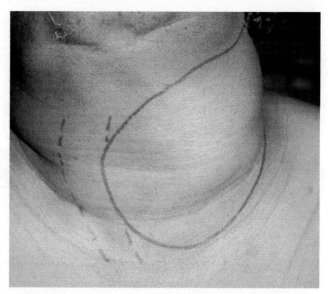

Figure 14–5. A large substernal goiter with tracheal deviation.

(Figure 14–4). The overall incidence of colloid goiter has decreased in the United States due to the routine use of iodized salt over the past half century.

A history of radiation to the neck is also an important factor in the genesis of thyroid cancer. Radiation was commonly used in years gone by for benign diseases such as acne, enlarged tonsil, adenoids, enlarged thymus, or skin infections. The common dose of external radiation used by the dermatologists was generally between 800 and 1,200 cGy. There is a very high incidence of thyroid cancer in individuals presenting with a thyroid mass in the setting of previous exposure to radiation. A majority of these tumors are multifocal and involve both lobes of the thyroid, and the most common histopathology is papillary carcinoma. The Chernobyl nuclear accident in 1986 exposed certain regions of Belarus, the Ukraine, and Russia to environmental radiation and since 1990 there has been an upsurge in the incidence of thyroid cancer (up to a 30-fold increase) in these areas.

Other clinical features such as vocal cord paralysis, the presence of lymph node metastasis, or a hard and fixed thyroid mass are highly suggestive of thyroid cancer (Figures 14–5 and 14–6). Other symptoms may be related to the presence of distant disease such as pulmonary metastases (Figure 14–7). A family history of medullary carcinoma of the thyroid or multiple endocrine neoplasia, type I or II, should prompt appropriate evaluation.

Most patients presenting with thyroid cancer or solitary thyroid nodule are euthyroid and blood tests

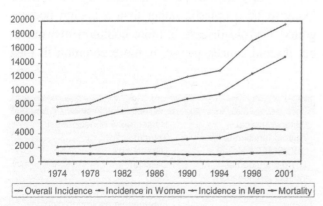

Figure 14–4. Incidence of thyroid cancer and mortality in the United States, 1974 to 1996.

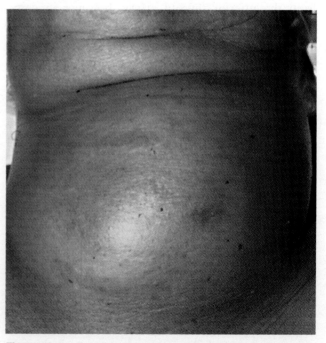

Figure 14–6. A patient with an anaplastic thyroid carcinoma.

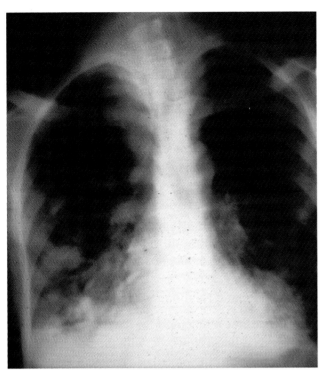

Figure 14–7. Multiple pulmonary metastases from differentiated thyroid carcinoma.

done as a routine do not aid the differential diagnosis of a solitary thyroid nodule. However, thyroid antibody estimation is helpful in young women with diffuse goiter or for the diagnosis of Hashimoto's thyroiditis.

Imaging Studies

Although various imaging studies have been used in the evaluation of a thyroid mass, none can routinely confirm the diagnosis of malignancy.

Thyroid Ultrasonography

A thyroid ultrasound examination is commonly performed as the initial evaluation of a thyroid mass to rule out a solid versus a cystic mass, and to confirm whether a clinically solitary nodule is indeed a single thyroid nodule as opposed to a dominant nodule within a multinodular goiter.[13,14] Between 15 and 20 percent of solitary thyroid nodules are malignant, while the corresponding rate is less than 5 percent in cystic thyroid nodules. The incidence of malignancy may be slightly higher in cysts that recur after initial aspiration or thyroid masses that are more than 3.0

cm in size. Ultrasonography is also helpful in the evaluation of incidentally-noted thyroid nodules, the so-called incidentalomas of the thyroid picked up on a CT or MRI scan of the neck done for other reasons. Since most of these incidentalomas are clinically non-palpable, ultrasound-guided fine-needle aspiration biopsy may be performed in an effort to get tissue diagnosis.[13] Another indication for thyroid ultrasonography is to monitor the size of the thyroid mass in patients who are managed conservatively, eg, pregnant women. For patients undergoing ipsilateral thyroid lobectomy it may be helpful to monitor the contralateral lobe and to rule out local recurrence in the thyroid bed during follow-up.

Thyroid Scintigraphy

Thyroid scintigraphy using technetium 99m or iodine-123 may be used to evaluate the hormonal secretory status of a thyroid nodule. A cold nodule represents nonfunctioning thyroid tissue (Figure 14–8) while a hot nodule is indicative of functioning or hyperfunctioning tissue. The incidence of malignancy in a cold thyroid nodule ranges between 15 and 20 percent, while the incidence of malignancy in a hot thyroid nodule is generally less than 5 percent.[10] A thyroid scan is also helpful in distinguishing a solitary thyroid nodule from a thyroid nodule that is part of a multinodular pathology.

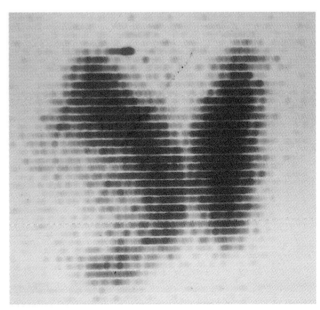

Figure 14–8. Thyroid scan showing a cold right thyroid nodule.

Not all patients with differentiated thyroid cancer have radioiodine avid tumors and it is not uncommon for a patient with elevated serum thyroglobulin (TG) to have a negative radioactive iodine (RAI) scan. In these patients, the residual or recurrent tumor may be too small to be resolved on the scan. Alternatively, the tumor cells may have lost their iodine-concentrating ability in spite of being able to secrete detectable levels of TG. When these patients are treated empirically with high-dose RAI, post-treatment scans often demonstrate uptake in micrometastatic deposits.

Another alternative for imaging differentiated thyroid cancer that has lost its iodine-trapping ability is to employ one of the newer imaging modalities such as thallium-201 total body scan or ^{18}FDG-PET scan. Thallium-201 has been in clinical use for evaluation of myocardial function and has been reported to be sensitive in imaging differentiated thyroid tumors. Less well-differentiated thyroid carcinomas that do not concentrate RAI may be better imaged with a ^{18}FDG-PET scan. The role of these modalities is currently under investigation and needs to be better defined before recommending their use in routine clinical practice.

Computed Tomography (CT) Scan

A CT scan is not routinely recommended in patients with thyroid masses, especially those with a clinically solitary thyroid nodule. However, it may be of great help in evaluating large tumors (Figure 14–9), especially those with substernal extension, or in patients with lymphoma or anaplastic thyroid can-

cer. In patients with recurrent thyroid masses or recurrent thyroid cancer, a CT scan may be indicated to evaluate the extent of the disease and its relation to the airway. In patients with anaplastic thyroid cancer and recurrent thyroid cancer who present with airway problems, it can define the presence and extent of endo-luminal pathology. Features such as the position of the trachea, involvement of either the tracheal wall or esophageal lumen, and the status of the tracheoesophageal grooves can be assessed quite reliably. Other issues such as minimal invasion of the laryngotracheal cartilage or pharyngoesophageal musculature are more difficult to interpret and are most often resolved only at surgical exploration.

Magnetic Resonance Imaging (MRI)

An MRI scan is rarely used for the routine evaluation of thyroid nodules. However, with the frequent use of MRI for investigating other head and neck conditions, including neurologic problems, an "incidentaloma of the thyroid" may be picked up (Figure 14–10). Further investigation of such incidentalomas may be performed by an ultrasound-guided needle biopsy. However, most of these incidentally discovered thyroid nodules are less than 1.0 cm in greatest dimension and, if non-palpable, they can be kept under observation with close follow-up (Figure 14–11).

Needle Biopsy

Fine-needle aspiration biopsy is probably the most important and cost-effective diagnostic study currently available for evaluation of a solitary thyroid

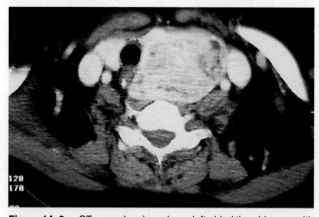

Figure 14–9.   CT scan showing a large left-sided thyroid mass with calcification.

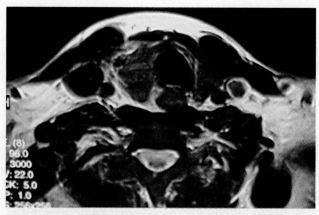

Figure 14–10.   MRI scan for evaluation of cervical trauma picked up an "incidentaloma" of the thyroid.

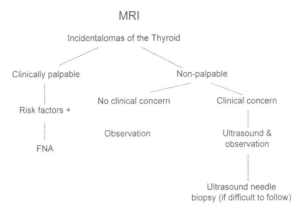

Figure 14–11. Suggested algorithm for the management of thyroid incidentalomas.

Table 14–4. INTERPRETATION OF FINE-NEEDLE ASPIRATION BIOPSY OF THE THYROID			
Malignant	Suspicious	Benign	Inadequate

Papillary
Medullary
Anaplastic
	Cellular smears
	Follicular
	  neoplasm
	Hürthle cell
	  lesion
	Lymphoma
		Colloid goiter
		Colloid cyst
		Thyroiditis
			Technical
			  problems
			Degenerative
			  nodule
			Hemorrhagic
			  cyst

nodule. The fear of needle-track implantation that was generated in the mid-1950s is no longer a consideration today. While the technique of fine-needle aspiration biopsy is familiar to most surgeons, endocrinologists and pathologists, one needs to be aware of certain pitfalls of the procedure (Table 14–3).

A number 22, 23, or 25 guage needle is generally used for thyroid mass aspiration and the smears are preserved in 95 percent alcohol. The results of fine-needle aspiration biopsy are usually interpreted as definite malignant pathology (such as papillary carcinoma, medullary carcinoma or anaplastic carcinoma) or clearly benign (such as thyroid cyst, colloid goiter, or Hashimoto's thyroiditis) (Table 14–4). The intermediate gray area of "suspicious" pathology includes findings that may be consistent with a follicular or Hürthle cell neoplasm. Most of these patients are recommended to undergo surgical intervention as the distinction between a benign follicular neoplasm and a malignant follicular tumor is generally possible only after removal of the entire thyroid mass and evaluating the tumor for capsular and vascular invasion. In the indeterminate group, where there may have been a technical problem or difficulties in interpretation, the investigation can be easily and safely repeated.

Patients who have an unequivocally benign needle aspiration result with no clinical suspicion of a malignant process could be observed. Whether or not suppressive therapy is indicated in these patients remains controversial. The likelihood that the thyroid nodule will disappear on suppressive therapy is small, but if the nodule exists in the background of a multinodular goiter, it may decrease in overall size. It is important to appreciate that while the diagnosis of malignancy is easy and reliable on fine-needle aspiration biopsy, a negative result cannot rule out malignancy. With the more widespread use of fine-needle aspiration biopsy, there has been a 50 percent reduction in the number of patients undergoing routine thyroidectomy, while the prevalence of malignancy has doubled in these specimens—most likely due to the selection associated with this approach.

Pathology

Although a variety of histologic types of tumors can occur in the thyroid (Table 14–5), an overwhelming majority of malignant thyroid tumors are well-differentiated tumors (Figure 14–12), and include papillary, follicular, mixed, and Hürthle cell tumors. The Hürthle cell tumors of the thyroid are an independent group consisting of oncocytic cells (also know as oxyphil or Askanazy cells). In the recent WHO classification, although Hürthle cell tumors are included as a variant of follicular tumors, the behavior of

Table 14–3. PITFALLS IN NEEDLE ASPIRATION BIOPSY OF THE THYROID
Adequacy of specimen—quantitative and qualitative
Accuracy of specimen—nonhomogeneity of needle placement
Accuracy of cytopathologic interpretation
Cysts—difficulties with degenerative nodules
Follicular lesions—benign versus malignant
Hürthle cell lesions—benign versus malignant
Lymphocytic lesions—lymphocytic thyroiditis versus lymphoma

Table 14–5. PATHOLOGIC TYPES OF THYROID CANCER	
Well-differentiated	Other Group
Papillary carcinoma	Medullary carcinoma
Follicular carcinoma	Anaplastic carcinoma
Mixed	Lymphoma
Hürthle cell carcinoma	Squamous cell carcinoma
	Sarcoma
	Metastatic tumors to the thyroid

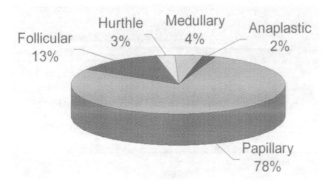

Figure 14–12. The histologic distribution of thyroid tumors.

Hürthle cell tumors is quite distinct and, overall, the prognosis of Hürthle cell cancer is much poorer than papillary or follicular thyroid cancers. Papillary carcinoma has a better outcome in comparison to follicular thyroid cancer.

Hundahl and colleagues have recently reported the data from the NCDB (National Cancer Data-Base) on thyroid cancer in the United States.[15] In their report of 53,865 cases, 78 percent were papillary thyroid cancer, 13 percent were follicular cancer while medullary and anaplastic thyroid cancer comprised 3 percent and 2 percent respectively. Papillary thyroid carcinoma is the most common histologic type, with a high incidence of multicentricity and lymph node metastasis. On the other hand, follicular thyroid cancer has a high likelihood of hematogenous spread with prevalence of distant metastasis of

approximately 30 percent. It is interesting to note that thyroid cancer represents a spectrum of diseases ranging from the most common and favorable papillary thyroid cancer to the highly lethal anaplastic or giant and spindle cell thyroid cancer.

In the group of differentiated thyroid cancers, Rosai and colleagues recently observed variants of differentiated thyroid cancer such as tall cell (Figure 14–13), scirrhous, trabecular, and insular varieties, which represent more aggressive forms of differentiated thyroid cancer commonly grouped as poorly-differentiated thyroid tumors.[16] These are more likely to present with extra-thyroidal extension of the disease and generally affect elderly male patients.

Medullary thyroid cancer (MTC) is a tumor of the thyroid originating from the parafollicular C cells, which produce calcitonin. MTC may present either as a sporadic or familial form. The familial variety is transmitted as an autosomal dominant inheritance and may occur as a part of multiple endocrine neoplasia, types I/II. Recently, molecular studies have revealed the presence of the RET proto-oncogene mutation in MTC. Screening of siblings and family members is now performed for RET mutation and if the family members are RET-positive they are considered candidates for prophylactic total thyroidectomy, which may be performed as early as age 5 or 6. Most of these young individuals are found to have C-cell hyperplasia or early medullary carcinoma.

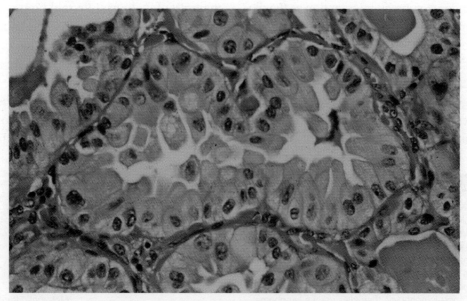

Figure 14–13.   Tall cell variant of papillary carcinoma of the thyroid (Hematoxylin-eosin stain; ×400).

Anaplastic thyroid cancer comes in different forms, the most common being giant and spindle cell anaplastic thyroid cancer. Most of these tumors grow rapidly and have a very high likelihood of lymph node and distant metastasis. Accurate pathologic diagnosis of anaplastic thyroid cancer is critical to rule out either small cell anaplastic thyroid cancer or a lymphoma of the thyroid, as these are managed very differently and have a more favorable clinical course.

Metastatic tumors to the thyroid are quite rare, but occasionally a primary tumor of the lung, breast or kidney, or a melanoma may metastasize to the thyroid, presenting a diagnostic dilemma in differentiation from a solitary thyroid nodule.

Treatment Goals and Treatment Alternatives—The Role of Multidisciplinary Treatment

The goals of treatment in the management of thyroid tumors are to cure the disease while minimizing the complications of thyroid surgery and side effects of adjuvant therapeutic modalities. The mainstay of treatment in thyroid cancers is complete surgical extirpation of the primary tumor. The extent of surgery should be tailored to the biologic aggressiveness of the disease.

Adjuvant therapeutic options available include radioactive iodine and external beam radiation therapy. In the low risk patient, surgical removal of all gross tumor is generally quite satisfactory. However, in the more aggressive forms of thyroid cancer or in the high risk group, a combined modality approach using surgery followed by radioactive iodine is indicated. After a total thyroidectomy, radioactive iodine dosimetry is used to document any evidence of residual thyroid tissue, and ablative treatment can then kill any residual normal or abnormal thyroid remnant tissue. Radioactive iodine scans also facilitate documentation of distant metastasis, most commonly pulmonary metastasis, which can be controlled satisfactorily in the early stages when the gross disease may not be evident on a routine chest radiograph.

The role of chemotherapy in the management of thyroid cancer is extremely limited, and is restricted to treatment of high-grade, poorly-differentiated or anaplastic cancers. External beam radiation therapy also has limited application in the management of thyroid cancer.[17] Experience in the United States with postoperative external radiation therapy is limited, but it has been routinely used in France, where improved local control of disease has been reported with this approach. External beam radiation therapy may be utilized when gross residual tumor remains or when an aggressive tumor exhibits extra-thyroidal extension at surgery. The most common indication for postoperative external radiation therapy is a high-grade tumor in a high risk patient, especially when the tumor is adherent to the esophageal or tracheal wall. Primary external beam radiation therapy, along with chemotherapy, is utilized in the management of anaplastic thyroid cancer.

Factors Affecting Choice of Treatment

The treatment plan for differentiated thyroid cancer can be rationally formulated by taking into account prognostic factors and assigning risk groups. Before considering any definitive treatment procedure in the management of thyroid cancer, it is extremely important to understand the factors that impact prognosis in this disease. Our understanding of thyroid cancer has improved considerably over the last 2 decades, with the definition of patient-related factors (eg, age and sex) and tumor-related factors (eg, size of the tumor, grade of the tumor, extra-thyroidal extension of the primary tumor, and the presence or absence of distant metastasis) as prognostic factors of importance. The Mayo Clinic[18,19] based their classification system (AGES) on prognostic factors of age, grade of the tumor, extra-thyroidal extension, and size of the tumor, while the Lahey Clinic used age, distant metastasis, extra-thyroidal extension, and size (AMES).[20,21] Both institutions divided their patients into low and high risk groups based on their respective prognosticators. Outcomes in the low risk group were uniformly excellent, with a long-term mortality of less than 2 percent. Conversely, mortality in the high risk group was as high as 46 percent. A similar experience was reported from the European Organization for Research and Treatment of Cancer (EORTC),[22] the University of Chicago, and Memorial Sloan-Kettering Cancer Center. Shaha and colleagues from Memorial Sloan-Kettering Cancer Center

Table 14–6. RISK GROUPS IN THYROID CANCER

Low Risk	Low risk patients/low risk tumors
Intermediate Risk	Low risk patient/high risk tumor High risk patient/low risk tumor
High Risk	High risk patient/high risk tumor
Patient Factors	Age, Gender
Tumor Factors	Grade, Size, Extrathyroidal extension, Distant metastasis

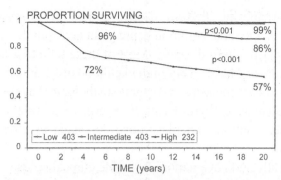

Figure 14–14. Survival in differentiated thyroid carcinoma stratified by low, intermediate and high risk-groups. Numbers in box indicate, number of patients in each risk group.

divided their patients into low, intermediate, and high risk groups[23] (Tables 14–6 and 14–7). The significant prognostic factors in their series were grade of the tumor, age, distant metastasis, extra-thyroidal extension, and size of the tumor (GAMES).[24] Their low risk group included low risk patients (below the age of 45) with low risk tumors, while the high risk group included high risk patients (above the age of 45) with high risk tumors. The intermediate risk group included two separate categories: young patients with more aggressive tumors and older patients with less aggressive tumors. The reported long-term survival in the low-risk group was 99 percent, while the intermediate risk group was 85 percent and the high risk group was 57 percent[24] (Figure 14–14).

Hay and colleagues, in a recent report from the Mayo Clinic, described the prognostic factors of importance as MACIS (distant metastasis, age, completeness of resection, extra-thyroidal tumor invasion, and size of the tumor).[25] They emphasize completeness of resection as a major prognostic factor. This is especially vital in patients who present with extra-thyroidal tumor extension. Thus, the experience of several different institutions based on a large number of patients followed for a long period of time essentially point to the fact that a relatively uniform set of prognostic factors can be used to reliably classify patients with differentiated thyroid cancer into well-defined risk groups.

Based on the excellent outcome in the low risk group, a lobectomy and isthmusectomy is quite satisfactory if the disease is confined to only one lobe. The decision to subject a patient to total thyroidectomy should be based on gross intraoperative findings, prognostic factors and risk-group analysis rather than

the fact that the patient has thyroid cancer (Table 14–8). The role of radioactive iodine dosimetry and ablation remains undefined in the low risk group, since the overall outcome is excellent and routine use of these modalities may represent overtreatment.

However, in patients with high risk tumors, appropriate surgical aggressiveness is crucial, as is consideration of adjuvant radioactive iodine therapy. If the patient is likely to require radioactive iodine therapy, it is important to proceed with total thyroidectomy to facilitate dosimetry and treatment at a later date. It is also vital to review the pathology to rule out areas of poorly-differentiated thyroid cancer within the specimen, a situation that is not uncommon in elderly patients or in patients who present with extra-thyroidal extension. These patients are at high risk for local recurrence and should be considered for adjuvant external beam radiation therapy. Table 14–9 presents the common indications for employing external beam radiation therapy in thyroid cancer.

Patients with certain histologic subtypes such as tall cell, insular, scirrhous, solid trabecular, and those

Table 14–7. RISK-GROUP DEFINITIONS IN DIFFERENTIATED CARCINOMA OF THE THYROID

	Low Risk	Intermediate Risk		High Risk
Age (years)	<45	<45	>45	>45
Distant metastasis	M0	M+	M0	M+
Tumor Size	T1, T2 (<4 cm)	T3, T4 (>4 cm)	T1, T2 (<4 cm)	T3, T4 (>4 cm)
Histology and grade	Papillary	Follicular and/or high-grade	Papillary	Follicular and/or high-grade
5-Year survival	100%	96%	96%	72%
20-year survival	99%	85%	85%	57%

Table 14–8. INDICATIONS FOR TOTAL THYROIDECTOMY

Multicentricity of thyroid cancer, varying between 30 and 70%
The incidence of local recurrence in the opposite thyroid lobe
  may be 5 to 15%
High incidence of mortality in patients with local recurrence
To facilitate the routine use of radioactive iodine dosimetry and
  ablation
Follow-up with thyroglobulin, which is difficult in presence of
  normal thyroid tissue
Theoretical consideration of anaplastic transformation of
  residual thyroid tissue
High incidence of complications in reoperative thyroid surgery
Minimal complications of total thyroidectomy in experienced
  hands

with undifferentiated areas respond relatively poorly and generally do not show avidity for radioactive iodine. The role of external radiation therapy, especially in this category, still remains to be defined.

Other prognostic factors including DNA ploidy, adenylate cyclase receptor, epidermal growth factor (EGF) receptor, vascular endothelial growth factor (VEGF), telomerase content, and cathepsin have been examined in various reports over the years. The role of the tumor suppressor gene p53 has also been studied extensively and a higher expression has been reported in poorly-differentiated or anaplastic thyroid cancers. Techniques such as comparative genomic hybridization have been used to screen for genomic aberrations, and a more detailed molecular and genetic understanding of the spectrum of thyroid tumors can be expected over the next few years.

Surgical Treatment

Considerable controversy exists regarding the extent of thyroidectomy in patients presenting with a differentiated thyroid cancer in a solitary nodule. There are strong proponents of routine total thyroidectomy, an approach that is mainly based on the premise of being able to treat multicentric microscopic disease in the opposite lobe. The incidence of microscopic thyroid cancer in the opposite lobe has been reported to range between 30 and 80 percent. However, the clinical significance of this "laboratory cancer" remains unclear, as the incidence of recurrence in the opposite lobe after ipsilateral lobectomy is only 5 to 7 percent. In the absence of level I evidence for the advantage of such an approach, as discussed above, a rational risk-group based approach should be used to

determine the extent of thyroidectomy. Another argument used to promote routine total thyroidectomy is that it allows for radioactive iodine dosimetry and ablation, as well as the use of serum thyroglobulin as a tumor marker in the follow-up of patients. However, in low risk-group patients these are of minimal value and are generally not necessary.

A detailed description of the technique of thyroidectomy is beyond the scope of this book, but a few technical considerations will be discussed. The most commonly used incision for thyroid operations is the low "collar" incision. An appropriate transverse skin crease is chosen and the incision should preferably be marked out with the patient sitting up before induction of anesthesia. This is especially important in women as anatomic orientation changes when the patient is supine with the neck hyperextended. The usual extent of the incision is from the anterior border of one sternocleidomastoid muscle to that of the other, and this provides adequate exposure for safe conduct of the operation. Smaller incisions may be adequate in patients with thin necks and a centrally situated nodule, but surgical exposure should never be compromised for the questionable benefit of better cosmesis associated with small incisions. Obviously, larger tumors may need more extensive exposure and the horizontal incision can be extended laterally if neck dissection becomes unexpectedly necessary. Superior and inferior flaps are developed in a subplatysmal plane and held apart with a self-retaining retractor. Certain maneuvers such as dividing the fascia over the sternocleidomastoid muscle and lateral to it, and dividing one or both strap muscles can provide extra exposure when required. Division of the sternothyroid muscle close to the thyroid cartilage facili-

Table 14–9. INDICATIONS FOR EXTERNAL RADIATION THERAPY

Anaplastic thyroid cancer
Medullary thyroid cancer with extensive nodal or mediastinal
  disease
Residual medullary thyroid cancer
High risk differentiated thyroid cancer patient with high risk
  tumor
Patient with extrathyroidal extension and microscopic residual
  tumor
Gross residual tumor
Poorly-differentiated thyroid cancer invading central
  compartment
Selected patients with distant metastasis, such as bone or brain

tates safe mobilization of the superior thyroid pole and allows accurate identification of the superior laryngeal nerve. Mobilization of the thyroid lobe generally proceeds from the lateral to medial direction after identification of the recurrent laryngeal nerve caudad to the inferior cornu of the thyroid cartilage in the tracheoesophageal groove. Once the middle and inferior thyroid veins and the superior thyroid pedicle have been divided, the lobe can be rotated medially to expose its posterolateral surface. If the parathyroid glands are identified, they are dissected off the thyroid to preserve their blood supply. Routine division of the inferior thyroid artery lateral to the recurrent nerve is not only unhelpful in mobilization of the thyroid lobe, but can also devascularize both parathyroid glands on that side. Instead, the branches of the inferior thyroid artery are divided medial to and between the parathyroid and thyroid glands. The areolar tissue containing the parathyroid gland can then be swept away laterally along with the inferior thyroid artery. It should be noted that the recurrent nerve is intimately related to the inferior parathyroid gland and great care is essential in this dissection. Obviously, the presence of gross tumor or abnormal lymph nodes in the tracheoesophageal groove may make it impossible to accomplish this part of the procedure without compromising complete tumor excision and placing the recurrent nerve at risk. If the parathyroid gland is devascularized, it should be autotransplanted into the sternocleidomastoid muscle. As described under the **Anatomy** section, it is well recognized that the recurrent laryngeal nerve is at highest risk of injury in the region of Berry's ligament. Meticulous and careful dissection using a fine microclamp is vital if complete excision of all thyroid tissue is to be safely accomplished without injuring the recurrent nerve. It is also crucial to recognize that the recurrent nerve may be at risk if the region of the Berry's ligament is dissected medial to the superior pole of a low-lying thyroid gland without demonstrating the entire course of the nerve.

Management of Locally Invasive Differentiated Thyroid Cancer

Unlike poorly-differentiated or anaplastic carcinoma, well-differentiated thyroid carcinoma is only rarely locally invasive. Although the presence of extra-thyroidal extension is a significant predictor of treatment failure and outcome, this finding should not be automatically construed as a sign of unresectability. Extended resections may be necessary to achieve palliation, but if complete excision of all gross tumor is achieved, the presence of extra-thyroidal extension has been shown to have no adverse impact on prognosis in younger patients.[26] The most commonly involved structures that need resection include the infrahyoid strap muscles, the recurrent laryngeal nerve, the cartilage of the laryngotracheal complex or the pharyngoesophageal musculature. The majority of tumors adherent to the larynx or trachea can be grossly resected by conservative measures such as "shaving" the cartilage. However, in the presence of obvious cartilage or endo-luminal invasion, partial or even circumferential sleeve resection of the trachea is justifiable. Tumors adherent to the pharyngoesophageal wall can be adequately resected by excising the involved muscle up to the submucosal layer. Other structures such as the strap muscles or the internal jugular vein can be sacrificed without much consequence if they are involved. Obviously, total thyroidectomy must be performed in these patients even if the opposite lobe is grossly normal to facilitate monitoring and treatment with radioactive iodine. As these tumors are more likely to be of poorer differentiation, they may not concentrate radioactive iodine and external beam radiation must be considered when appropriate.

Management of the Neck

Elective neck dissection is not recommended in the management of differentiated thyroid cancer, but clinically or radiologically demonstrable nodes must be appropriately addressed. Although the incidence of regional nodal metastases is highest in young patients, this finding is of no prognostic significance if the neck is managed appropriately.[27] Suspicious nodes encountered during thyroidectomy can be sampled and submitted for frozen-section evaluation, but there is no merit in the so-called berry picking procedure. Central compartment dissection including the tracheoesophageal groove lymph nodes is the preferred operation and is carried out taking precautions to preserve the recurrent laryngeal nerve and the parathyroids with their vascular supply. For lateral compartment nodal disease, a comprehensive neck dissection including levels II to V becomes necessary. Level I can be safely spared if there are no clinically abnormal nodes in the region. A type III modified neck dissection preserving the internal jugular vein, the sternocleidomastoid muscle and the spinal accessory nerve is preferred if there is no evidence of extra-thyroidal or extra-nodal extension of disease. Although not essential, we prefer to stage neck dissections for patients with bilateral lymphatic metastases a few days apart to increase the safety of an otherwise long and tedious operation. Every effort must be made to preserve the recurrent laryngeal nerve, even in patients with bulky disease in the tracheoesophageal groove. It is often possible to dissect the nerve free of the nodes without leaving gross residual disease; although tedious, this is a worthwhile endeavor as preservation of laryngeal function significantly impacts the patient's quality of life after surgery. In contrast, preservation of the parathyroid glands, especially their vascular supply, may be impossible under these circumstances and if a normal parathyroid gland is identified, autotransplantation must be considered. Patients with bulky nodal disease are at high risk for pulmonary micrometastases, and should be evaluated with a postoperative radioactive iodine scan followed by ablative therapy if indicated. In contrast to young patients, the presence of regional nodal metastases does predict a higher rate of neck failure in older patients in whom comprehensive neck dissection should be followed by adjuvant radioactive iodine therapy.

Complications

Even though thyroid surgery is considered to be one of the safest surgical procedures in modern practice, a variety of complications can occur. The most important complications directly related to the surgical procedure include injury to the recurrent laryngeal nerve, the superior laryngeal nerve, and the parathyroid glands.

The recurrent laryngeal nerve is a branch of the vagus; on the right side it loops around the subclavian artery, while on the left side it originates in the mediastinum and curves around the arch of the aorta, supplying all the intrinsic muscles of the larynx with the exception of the cricoarytenoid muscle. Injury to the recurrent laryngeal nerve may occur in the paratracheal area, in the region where it crosses the inferior thyroid artery, or in the vicinity of the ligament of Berry.[6] The recurrent laryngeal nerve may cross the inferior thyroid artery either superficial or deep to it, or it may indeed course between the branches of the artery. The inferior parathyroid gland is also commonly located in intimate relation to these two important structures. The recurrent laryngeal nerve then proceeds close to Berry's ligament to enter the larynx at the level of the cricoid cartilage. Most injuries to the recurrent laryngeal nerve probably occur in this area near Berry's ligament, where there are often tiny veins passing through. If one of these veins is injured during dissection of this region, the recurrent laryngeal nerve may be traumatized during efforts to attain hemostasis. It is also known that the recurrent laryngeal nerve can branch into tiny filaments before entering the larynx, and injury to any of these has the potential for altering laryngeal function. Generally, traction injury to the recurrent laryngeal nerve will improve over a period of 3 to 4 weeks. Transection of the recurrent laryngeal nerve, however, obviously leads to permanent paralysis of the vocal cord, but the final resting position of the paralyzed vocal cord may vary over a period of time. In a majority of young individuals, the paralyzed vocal cord may come to rest in the median or paramedian position where the opposite cord may be able to compensate for the ipsilateral paralyzed one. If adequate compensation occurs, the quality of voice may be acceptable under most circumstances, but never does return to normal. Laryngoplasty with vocal cord medialization may be undertaken in selected patients to improve the quality of the voice.

Injury to the superior laryngeal nerve leads to an inability to raise the voice to a high pitch, resulting in difficulty with yelling, screaming or singing. On routine examination of the larynx, the findings are often very subtle, but careful comparison of the vocal cords shows bowing on the affected side. Special investigations such as videostroboscopy or voice analysis may be better able to help define the problem. There is no effective treatment for injury to the superior laryngeal nerve except for voice training and speech therapy.

One of the most distressing complications of total thyroidectomy is permanent hypoparathyroidism which may result from total removal of all four parathyroid glands or from damage to their blood supply. During the surgery, if the parathyroid gland is identified and if the blood supply is thought to be compromised, a biopsy of a sliver of tissue should be sent for frozen-section analysis to confirm the presence of parathyroid tissue. The compromised gland can then be minced into small pieces and implanted into a pocket created within the strap muscles or the sternomastoid muscle.[7] The minced parathyroid will pick up blood supply from the surrounding musculature and, over a period of a few weeks, will regain its normal function. For thyroid surgery, it is not necessary to autotransplant the parathyroid into the forearm, which is the usual practice in patients undergoing parathyroidectomy for secondary hyperparathyroidism due to renal failure.

The vocal cord function should be evaluated after surgery, and the status of the vocal cords should be documented in the patient's chart. In patients undergoing total thyroidectomy and para-tracheal nodal dissection, it is important to check calcium levels 24 and 48 hours after surgery to be certain that normal levels are maintained. Routine postoperative supplementation of calcium has been advocated by some authors in all patients undergoing thyroidectomy. We prefer to observe the patient clinically and monitor the blood for serum calcium, reserving calcium supplementation for symptomatic patients and those with a significant downward trend in serum calcium levels. Asymptomatic patients are followed with serial calcium levels and close clinical observation. If the parathyroid glands have been preserved in situ, calcium supplements can generally be eliminated within 3 to 4 weeks after the surgical procedure.

Another dreaded complication of thyroid surgery is postoperative hematoma[28] which usually occurs between 6 to 24 hours after surgery, leading to increased central compartment pressure and airway distress. It has traditionally been a routine practice to keep a tracheostomy tray by the bedside in the event that the patient develops airway distress. An emergent tracheostomy is rarely indicated in modern practice, since the patient can easily be re-intubated if necessary, prior to exploration. If a wound hematoma is noted, it is generally best to bring the patient back to the operating room, explore the wound, achieve hemostasis, and place a drain. Most of these patients are then ready to be discharged from the hospital within 24 to 48 hours.

There appears to be recent interest in outpatient thyroidectomies, or else discharging the patient within 23 hours after the surgical procedure. There also seems to be some interest in thyroidectomy under local anesthesia. Obviously, the surgeon must be quite familiar with the technique of local anesthesia and the patient must be cooperative. We feel more comfortable performing these surgical procedures under general anesthesia. Drains are not commonly used in patients undergoing routine thyroidectomy. However, drains are indicated if there is excessive bleeding, or a subtotal thyroidectomy has been performed for Grave's disease (where there is an increased chance of bleeding from the cut surface of the thyroid), or in patients with a large dead space after removal of colloid goiter or substernal goiter. With judicious selection, the author has been able to avoid the use of drains in approximately 70 percent of patients undergoing thyroidectomy.

Clearly, safe and successful thyroidectomy requires meticulous and careful dissection, reinforcing Halsted's statement that the "technique of thyroidectomy reveals the triumph of surgical procedure."

Radioactive Iodine Therapy

The use of radioactive iodine (RAI) in the diagnosis and management of differentiated thyroid cancer (DTC) is based on the physiologic property of the thyroid follicular cell to trap and retain iodine. Undifferentiated tumors and medullary carcinomas therefore are not amenable to this form of treatment. DTC is reported to take up approximately 0.5 percent of the administered dose of RAI per gram of tissue with a biologic half-life of about 4 days.[29] In radiobiologic terms, this delivers approximately five times the absorbed dose of external beam radiation therapy. Also, because of this differential uptake in functioning cells, tumor tissue, including distant metastases, receives a several hundredfold higher dose compared to normal tissue.

Table 14–10 presents some common indications for considering RAI in the management of patients with thyroid cancer. A dose of 3 to 5 mCi of RAI is used for a diagnostic scan that is usually performed 4 to 6 weeks after total thyroidectomy. After a well-executed total thyroidectomy, less than 1 to 2 percent of the diagnostic dose of RAI is generally concentrated in the region of the thyroid bed. Older patients, those with Hürthle cell or poorly-differentiated tumors, and those with bone metastases generally do not benefit from RAI therapy because these tumors do not effectively concentrate RAI. If the RAI scan demonstrates a significant thyroid remnant, 75 to 150 mCi of RAI is administered to ablate this tissue before any further RAI imaging or treatment can proceed.

Patients scheduled for RAI scan, dosimetry or treatment are generally required to be off their supplemental thyroxine for at least 4 to 6 weeks to allow a hypothyroid state to develop. The resultant elevation of serum TSH to around 40 mU/ml creates optimal conditions for any functioning thyroid tissue to concentrate RAI. However, the symptoms of hypothyroidism can be debilitating, and until recently patients either had to endure them, or were switched over to exogenous T_3 from their usual dose of thyroxine for 2 to 4 weeks. Exogenous T_3 would then have to be discontinued and followed about 2 weeks later by RAI scan and/or therapy. A recent advance has been the use of recombinant human TSH which can be administered exogenously to elevate the patient's serum TSH level with the aim of increasing the RAI-concentrating ability of thyroid tissue. The experience with recombinant human TSH is, however, not mature and initial reports seem to suggest that the traditional hypothyroid approach may be more effective. Other precautions that are important in patients undergoing RAI evaluation or therapy include avoidance of iodine-containing food or medication and radiographic contrast.

If imaging does demonstrate the presence of RAI-avid tumor, the appropriate dose for safe and effective treatment needs to be calculated. The therapeutic dose of RAI has usually empirically varied between 100 to 200 mCi depending upon the extent of local and metastatic disease. Dosimetry studies based on the estimated tumor volume and the radiobiologic characteristics of RAI have been reported with some correlation of response rates. However, on a practical basis we prefer to use dosimetry to assess and deliver the maximum tolerable dose of RAI. RAI therapy can be repeated at intervals of 6 to 12 months until there is no longer any demonstrable evidence of functioning disease.

Complications of RAI include thyroiditis that usually resolves within 2 to 3 weeks. Parotitis may also occur but is self-limiting. More serious side effects like bone marrow depression and pulmonary fibrosis are generally associated only with high cumulative doses of RAI.

Following total thyroidectomy and RAI therapy, serial measurements of serum thyroglobulin (TG) can be used to monitor patients for development of recurrent disease. While elevated serum Tg levels in patients receiving thyroxine-suppressive therapy are a relatively reliable indicator of recurrent disease, low or borderline levels do not necessarily exclude recurrence. Skeletal and pulmonary metastases are associated with the highest Tg levels while patients with lymphatic metastases generally have lower levels. Borderline patients should be investigated by taking the patient off exogenous thyroxine to induce hypothyroidism as discussed above. It should be noted that serum Tg estimation is reliable only in the absence of thyroglobulin antibodies.

PARATHYROID TUMORS

The parathyroid glands are the smallest of the endocrine glands and yet their proper function in controlling calcium and phosphorus metabolism is vital in normal calcium homeostasis and is avoiding osteoporosis.[30] The routine use of serum multi-channel chemistry has made it possible to document hypercalcemia in an increasing number of otherwise totally

---

Table 14–10. INDICATIONS FOR RADIOACTIVE IODINE THERAPY

Ablation of remnant thyroid tissue following total thyroidectomy
Gross or microscopic residual disease after surgical resection
Adjuvant therapy of bulky cervical nodal metastases to evaluate for pulmonary micrometastases
Management of the patient presenting with clinically apparent distant metastases
Treatment of distant metastases, especially pulmonary disease

asymptomatic patients—individuals who require further endocrinologic evaluation to rule out primary hyperparathyroidism. The incidence of primary hyperparathyroidism is 1 out of 700 individuals and occurs most commonly in women above the age of 45.

There is considerable interest in hyperparathyroidism related to the multiple endocrine neoplasia (MEN) syndromes type I and II. MEN, type I, known as Wermer's syndrome, includes pancreatic, parathyroid and pituitary adenomas; MEN, type II, known as Sipple's syndrome, includes medullary carcinoma of the thyroid, pheochromocytoma, and hyperparathyroidism. MEN, type II is divided into MEN, type IIA and IIB, the latter of which includes mucosal neuromas.[30] Most parathyroid tumors associated with the MEN syndromes are functional and only 1 percent are malignant.

Recent advances in management of hyperparathyroidism relate to the development of more accurate localization studies and investigations such as the quick parathormone assay.[31,32] Other advances include minimally invasive parathyroidectomy, minimal access surgery, the use of intraoperative gamma probes for localization, and endoscopic parathyroidectomy.[33,34,35]

Anatomy

The parathyroid glands develop during the sixth week of gestation, with the superior parathyroids originating from the fourth pharyngeal pouch along with the thyroid gland. They may come to rest behind the upper pole of the thyroid or may descend into the posterior mediastinum. The inferior parathyroid glands develop from the third pharyngeal pouch along with the thymus, and may remain buried under the thymic capsule. Likewise, the superior parathyroid glands may also be buried under the thyroid capsule.

Approximately 10 percent of individuals have supernumerary parathyroid glands (ranging from five to eight), and approximately 2 to 3 percent of individuals have less than four parathyroid glands. The most common location of the superior parathyroid is on the posterior capsule of the superior pole of the thyroid. Anatomically, the superior parathyroid glands are generally superior and lateral to the

Table 14–11. ANATOMIC LOCATION OF PARATHYROID GLANDS	
Superior Parathyroid Glands	**Inferior Parathyroid Glands**
Superior thyroid pole	Submanubrial space
Tracheoesophageal groove	Thymic fat pad
Behind the esophagus	In the thyroid crypt or capsule
In the carotid sheath	
Within the thyroid gland	

recurrent laryngeal nerve while the inferior parathyroid glands are inferior and medial to the nerve. Due to the more tortuous course of their embryologic descent, the inferior parathyroids are more variable in their location as compared with the superior glands (Table 14–11).

The parathyroids are generally oval or irregularly-shaped, tan-colored, small glands that measure between 4.0 to 5.0 mm x 1.0 to 3.0 mm in size. Each parathyroid gland weighs approximately 35 mg. The blood supply to the inferior parathyroid glands generally comes from the branches of the inferior thyroid artery. The superior parathyroid may receive its blood supply either from a branch of the inferior thyroid artery or, occasionally, from the posterior branch of the superior thyroid artery. The inferior thyroid artery branches to the parathyroid glands before dividing into multiple branches and supplying the thyroid gland (Table 14–12).

Diagnosis

Although most patients with hyperparathyroidism present with hypercalcemia,[36] a variety of disorders may cause hypercalcemia and should be ruled out in the differential diagnosis (Table 14–13). The most common symptoms include vague fatigue, weight loss, discomfort, forgetfulness, and renal stones. The classic symptoms of "bones, moans, groans and psychic overtones" are rarely encountered in modern

Table 14–12. BLOOD SUPPLY TO THE PARATHYROID GLANDS	
Superior Parathyroid Glands	**Inferior Parathyroid Glands**
Branch of inferior thyroid artery	Branch of the inferior thyroid artery
Superior thyroid artery	From thyroid gland
Branches from the anastomotic loop between superior and inferior thyroid artery	

Table 14–13. CAUSES OF HYPERCALCEMIA

Metastatic cancer from lungs, kidneys, prostate, breast, etc.
Primary hyperparathyroidism
Milk alkali syndrome
Thiazide diuretic therapy
Multiple myeloma
Paget's disease
Sarcoidosis
Pseudohyperparathyroidism
Benign familial hypocalciuric hypercalcemia
Immobilization
Hypervitaminosis D
Hyperproteinemia
Acute Addison's disease
Chronic or acute leukemia
Hyperthyroidism

practice. The hallmarks of primary hyperparathyroidism are high calcium, low phosphorus, and high parathormone serum levels.

Hyperparathyroidism is classified into three groups: primary hyperparathyroidism (which represents intrinsic derangement of the parathyroid gland), secondary hyperparathyroidism, (which refers to a reaction to hypocalcemia generally resulting from renal failure), and tertiary hyperparathyroidism (which is the autonomous development of parathyroid hyperfunction generally subsequent to secondary hyperparathyroidism in patients with renal failure who may be on long-term dialysis). Evaluation of the intact parathyroid hormone level is extremely important in the diagnosis of primary hyperparathyroidism. Other diagnostic studies such as 24-hour urinary calcium, chloride-to-phosphorus ratio, and urinary cyclic AMP are rarely utilized since the advent of bone densitometry, which is used for assessing the need for surgery in patients with asymptomatic hyperparathyroidism so as to prevent future osteoporosis (Table 14–14).

Bone densitometry is typically performed on the lumbar spine and neck of the femur or distal radius.

Pathology

The most common pathologic finding in patients presenting with suspected primary hyperparathyroidism is a single gland adenoma (found in 85% of individuals). Approximately 14 percent present with multiglandular disease or hyperplastic parathyroid glands, whereas only 1 percent present with parathyroid carcinoma. In spite of its rarity, parathyroid carcinoma generates considerable interest because of its uncertain clinical behavior, a problem compounded by the lack of long-term prospective data. Recently, Hundahl and colleagues reported a collected series from the National Cancer Data Base of 286 patients with parathyroid carcinoma, which is the largest series in the literature.[37]

The pathologic diagnosis of parathyroid cancer may be difficult based on histopathologic features alone. The final diagnosis of parathyroid cancer is based on its clinical behavior, and tumors that develop local recurrence, lymph node metastasis, or distant metastasis are classified as malignant.[38] Approximately 4 to 5 percent of patients present with multiple adenomas, which is one of the prime reasons for persistent or recurrent hyperparathyroidism after initial exploration and removal of single enlarged glands.

Localization Studies

There is considerable interest and controversy related to the role of preoperative localization studies in primary hyperparathyroidism. Generally, the success of surgical exploration in correctly diagnosed primary hyperparathyroidism exceeds 95 percent. There are several specific indications for relying on localization studies in patients with primary hyperparathyroidism[39] (Table 14–15). Parathyroid localization may also be very helpful in documenting ectopically located parathyroid glands.

Table 14–14. DIAGNOSTIC EVALUATION OF PRIMARY HYPERPARATHYROIDISM

Laboratory tests
  Blood
  Calcium
  Phosphorus
  Parathormone
  Chloride—P ratio
  Urinary cAMP
  Ionized calcium
  Tubular reabsorption of phosphorus

Bone Analysis
  Photon beam bone densitometry
  Metacarpal bone thickness
  Quantitative bone histomorphometry

PTH—chemimmunoluminometric assay, N terminal, C terminal, intact

Table 14–15. INDICATIONS FOR PARATHYROID LOCALIZATION PRIOR TO PRIMARY EXPLORATION

Diagnostic Problems—Associated Malignancies	Technical Problems	Patient Factors
Mild asymptomatic hypercalcemia	Patients with previous neck or thyroid surgery	Poor risk patients where unilateral exploration is crucial
Hypercalcemia crisis for urgent diagnosis	Obese individuals with short neck Associated palpable thyroid abnormality	Poor risk patients where surgery under local anesthesia is considered For better patient counseling prior to surgery

Localization studies can be classified as noninvasive and invasive tests[40] (Table 14–16). The latter are generally used for patients with a previous failed exploration. The experience with invasive tests (such as angiogram or selected venous parathormone assay) is very limited and very few centers have such expertise. Noninvasive studies are most commonly utilized and the experience frequently depends on institutional practice. The most common tests include ultrasonography, CT, MRI and the recently-popularized sestamibi scan.

Sestamibi (99^m-technetium isobutyl isonitrile radionuclide) has a selective affinity for parathyroid glands and is one of the most sensitive localization studies currently available (Table 14–17). Sestamibi scan has been utilized for intraoperative gamma probe-assisted localization of enlarged parathyroid glands (Figure 14–15). This is a physiologic approach to parathyroid localization, as opposed to the older, anatomic approach. It has also been described as a minimally-invasive radio-guided parathyroidectomy and has been popularized by Norman and colleagues.[34] This procedure is based on the same principle as lymphoscintigraphy and sentinel node biopsy for melanoma and breast carcinoma. Using this technique, Norman and colleagues have reported a significant decrease in the operative time and expense, because of the ability to perform these surgical procedures under local anesthesia through a small incision.[33,34]

Ultrasonography of the neck (Figure 14–16) is also a good test, but it is highly dependent upon the experience of the ultrasonographer involved in the parathyroid evaluation. Its advantage is its ability to guide an ultrasonographic needle biopsy, and the aspirate can be evaluated by cytology or by PTH assay.

CT scan is of limited value, since there may be artifacts which are difficult to interpret. However, an MRI scan may document a glowing enlarged parathyroid gland on a T2-weighted image (Figure 14–17). The addition of sestamibi SPECT (single photon emission computed tomography) imaging assists the operating surgeon to locate the exact position of the parathyroid gland and can facilitate minimal access surgery. The SPECT scan is also helpful to the operating surgeon as it can locate and localize the parathyroid gland in three dimensions.

Surgical Treatment

Once the diagnosis of primary hyperparathyroidism is made, the typically recommended treatment is surgical exploration of the neck and appropriate parathyroidectomy. However, in elderly, feeble patients, conservative medical treatment may be

Table 14–16. PARATHYROID LOCALIZATION STUDIES

Noninvasive Studies	Invasive Studies
Esophagogram	Arteriography
Ultrasonography—US-guided needle biopsy	Selective venous catheterization
	Digital subtraction angiography
Thallium technetium scan	
CT scan	
MRI	
Sestamibi scan	
PET scan	
Monoclonal antibodies (experimental)	

Table 14–17. REPORTED SENSITIVITIES OF VARIOUS PARATHYROID LOCALIZATION STUDIES

Localization Study	Sensitivity (%)
High-resolution ultrasonography	80
CT scan	63
MRI	74
Technetium thallium subtraction scan	55–82
Venous sampling	65–80
Technetium—99m sestamibi scan	80–100

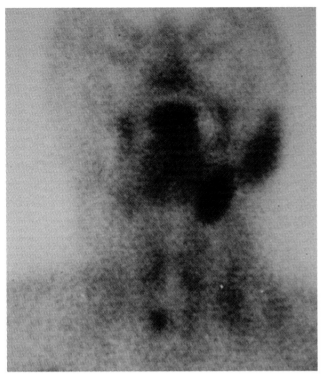

Figure 14–15. Sestamibi scan obtained prior to radio-guided parathyroidectomy.

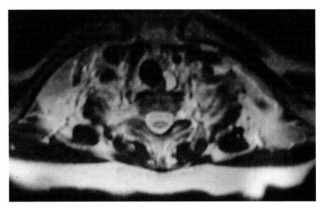

Figure 14–17. MRI scan showing a large, left-sided parathyroid gland.

entertained with a close follow-up. Even in this group, if indicated, the surgical procedure could be performed under local anesthesia.

In selected patients, a preoperative localization study is performed as discussed above. A transverse skin incision is usually made for bilateral exploration. Despite the fact that unilateral exploration is proposed by some authors (especially with the use of

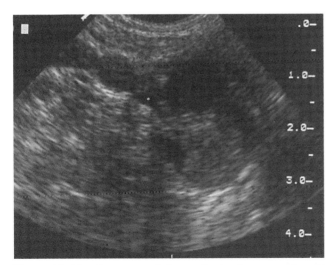

Figure 14–16. Sonogram of the neck showing a parathyroid adenoma.

preoperative sestamibi scan and quick-PTH), the usual approach is to explore both sides of the neck even when a large parathyroid gland is noted on the ipsilateral side (Table 14–18). The reasons for exploration of both sides include the fact that 5 to 15 percent of patients may have multiglandular disease and multiple adenomas, and it may be difficult to distinguish between uniglandular versus multiglandular disease based on examining only one side.[41] Exploration of the other side adds to the operative time, but it does give the surgeon the security of having excluded gross parathyroid or thyroid abnormality on the other side. During surgery, the parathyroid glands may be anatomically confused with thyroid tissue, lymph node, thymic remnant or a fat pad. The usual practice is to remove the enlarged parathyroid gland, along with a biopsy of one normal-appearing parathyroid gland for the pathologist to use as comparison. However, it is not absolutely necessary to biopsy the normal parathyroid glands in every case.

In patients presenting with multiglandular disease, subtotal parathyroidectomy leaving behind

Table 14–18. APPROACHES TO PARATHYROID EXPLORATION	
Unilateral	**Bilateral**
Scan-directed exploration	Uniglandular versus multiglandular disease
Look for second normal gland on same side	Multiple adenomas
Less operating time	Look on other side for abnormal glands
Reduced complications	Does not take too much extra time in the OR
	It is easy to explore both sides in primary exploration

normal-appearing parathyroid tissue, equivalent in amount to one-third or one-quarter of a normal parathyroid gland, is recommended. If subtotal parathyroidectomy is undertaken, it is vitally important to preserve adequate blood supply to the remnant parathyroid gland.

The surgical results and the outcome in patients undergoing exploration for a single adenoma are excellent. However, for patients presenting with hyperplasia, a small percentage of patients may return with persistent hypercalcemia or mild hyperparathyroidism. In patients with multiglandular disease, some may return after subtotal parathyroidectomy for a reoperative procedure due to persistent hyperparathyroidism. Occasionally, an enlarged parathyroid gland may not easily be located at cervical exploration. Under these circumstances, it is extremely important to carefully look for certain areas where parathyroid glands are known to lie hidden: deep to the thyroid capsule, behind the carotid artery, within the carotid sheath, behind the esophagus, high up to the hyoid or low down in the posterior mediastinum.[42–44] The parathyroid gland may sometimes be intra-thyroidal, but the true intra-thyroidal parathyroid adenoma within the substance of the thyroid gland is very rare. Most parathyroid glands are situated on the surface of the thyroid gland, deep to the thyroid capsule or within a crypt of the thyroid. A thyroid lobectomy may be necessary to check if a parathyroid adenoma lies within the substance of the thyroid gland.

Various advances have played an important role in the surgery of hyperparathyroidism over the past decade (Table 14–19).[31,32] The use of quick-PTH (chemi-immuno-luminescent PTH) is of great assistance during parathyroid surgery since the assay can be completed within 15 minutes. A preoperative quick-PTH is measured and after the adenoma is removed, the test is repeated within 5 and 15 minutes to check for a fall in the PTH level. A decrease of more than 50 percent over the preoperative value is a reliable indicator of successful parathyroidectomy. Another major advance is radio-guided parathyroid surgery in which sestamibi is injected approximately 2 hours prior to surgery. A parathyroid scan is performed and combined with scan-directed surgical exploration using an intraoperative gamma probe. Once the enlarged parathyroid is removed, the background activity and the activity of the parathyroid gland are compared. Radionuclide activity of more than 20 percent is indicative of a parathyroid adenoma.

There is considerable recent interest in endoscopic parathyroid surgery, but it has not yet become standard practice in the United States.

Reoperative Parathyroid Surgery

The success of parathyroid surgery ranges between 90 and 95 percent in most series. However, primary exploration may be unsuccessful in certain select circumstances such as multiglandular disease, an enlarged parathyroid gland located in the mediastinum, parathyroid carcinoma, or multiple adenomas. In the patient with failed parathyroid surgery, the most important initial issue is to confirm the diagnosis to make sure that one is not dealing with familial hypocalciuric hypercalcemia or other causes of hypercalcemia. After the diagnosis of primary hyperparathyroidism is confirmed by repeating the appropriate blood studies (including serum calcium, phosphorus, and PTH), it is important to obtain more information from the previous operating surgeon, analyze the operative findings, and to re-review the pathology from the primary surgery. Noninvasive localization studies (including sestamibi scan and ultrasonography) are extremely important under these circumstances. Occasionally, ultrasound-guided needle aspiration is needed to confirm the diagnosis of an enlarged parathyroid gland. In very rare circumstances, invasive studies (such as angiogram, selective PTH, or venous assay) may be necessary. Figure 14–18 depicts an algorithmic schema for parathyroid reexploration.

During reoperative surgery, it is extremely important to preserve any normal-appearing parathyroid tissue specifically so as to avoid perma-

Table 14–19. ADVANCES IN PARATHYROID SURGERY

Sestamibi-guided unilateral exploration
Scan-guided surgery with quick-PTH
Outpatient parathyroidectomy
Scan-directed parathyroidectomy with intraoperative gamma probe (physiologic approach to parathyroid disease)
Endoscopic parathyroidectomy
Endoscopy-assisted parathyroidectomy—sestamibi-assisted minimal incision approach

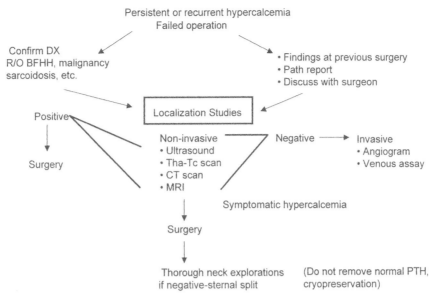

Persistent or recurrent hypercalcemia
Failed operation

Confirm DX
R/O BFHH, malignancy
sarcoidosis, etc.

• Findings at previous surgery
• Path report
• Discuss with surgeon

Positive

Localization Studies

Surgery

Non-invasive
• Ultrasound
• Tha-Tc scan
• CT scan
• MRI

Negative ⟶ Invasive
• Angiogram
• Venous assay

Symptomatic hypercalcemia

Surgery

Thorough neck explorations
if negative-sternal split

(Do not remove normal PTH,
cryopreservation)

Figure 14–18.   Algorithm for parathyroid reexploration.

nent hypoparathyroidism.[42,43] The surgeon should be familiar with cryopreservation of the parathyroid, which can be preserved in the patient's own serum or in a specially formulated medium.

Parathyroid Cancer

Approximately 1 percent of cases of primary hyperparathyroidism are due to parathyroid carcinoma.[37] Criteria for diagnosis of parathyroid carcinoma are generally not well defined, but the presence of capsular invasion is an indicator of malignancy (Figure 14–19). As discussed above, the absolute diagnosis of parathyroid carcinoma is based on its clinical behavior with lymph node metastasis, recurrent parathyroid disease or distant metastasis being taken as indicators of malignancy.

A preoperative suspicion of parathyroid carcinoma is based mainly on a palpable parathyroid gland or markedly elevated calcium levels with intra-

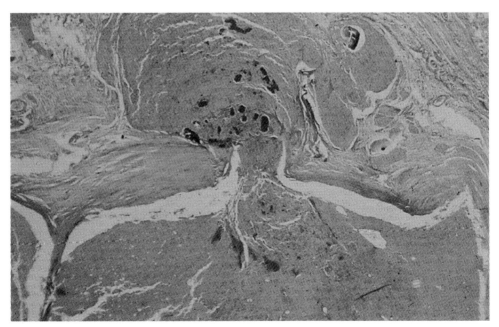

Figure 14–19.   Parathyroid carcinoma showing major capsular invasion (Hematoxylin-eosin stain; ×100).

operative findings of a firm parathyroid mass adherent to the surrounding structures and thyroid gland. If the parathyroid gland is intimately adherent to the thyroid capsule and the dissection between the two is difficult, it is generally appropriate to remove the enlarged parathyroid along with the thyroid gland. It is important not to dissect into the parathyroid capsule so as to avoid spillage of the parathyroid tumor. If the suspicion of malignancy exists, wide local excision of the parathyroid gland, adjacent thyroid tissue, and adherent muscles, etc. should be performed. A modified neck dissection should be considered for abnormal and enlarged lymph nodes.

Parathyroid carcinoma is a rare disease and the efficacy of one treatment regimen over another cannot be established, as only approximately 500 patients with parathyroid carcinoma have been described in the literature. Approximately one-third of patients develop local recurrence, about 17 percent develop regional nodal metastasis and approximately 25 percent have recurrence at distant sites such as the lungs, bones or liver. The experience with chemotherapy (using a drug such as dacarbazine) and radiation therapy is extremely limited. The National Cancer Database review of 286 patients with parathyroid carcinoma reported a 5-year survival of 86 percent and a 10-year survival of 49 percent.[37]

Complications and Postoperative Follow-up

The proof of success in parathyroid surgery is a normal postoperative calcium level, which usually occurs within 24 to 48 hours after surgery. In patients who present initially with severe hyperparathyroidism and long-standing hypercalcemia, there may be persistent hypocalcemia due to severe bone hunger and/or requirements of large doses of calcium supplementation prior to stabilization of the calcium to normal levels. During the postoperative period, intravenous calcium supplementation may be instituted if necessary, but most patients can subsequently be stabilized on oral calcium supplementation. The occasional patient may require vitamin D supplementation.

Secondary Hyperparathyroidism

Secondary hyperparathyroidism is usually noted in patients with renal failure and in those on dialysis.

The most common indication for surgery in these patients is osteoporosis, bone weakness, and severe pruritus. Identification of the parathyroid glands in these cases in general is quite easy during surgery, where all four parathyroid glands are markedly enlarged. The surgical treatment usually consists of total parathyroidectomy with autotransplantation of a portion of the parathyroid gland into the forearm muscles. The parathyroid gland may occasionally be autotransplanted into the abdominal fat or rectus muscle. Another surgical approach in these patients is subtotal parathyroidectomy, but the former method is generally preferred. Infrequently, patients with parathyroid autotransplantation may regrow their parathyroid gland in the transplanted site, requiring re-excision of the hypertrophic parathyroid gland. Most of these patients benefit from surgical intervention and the symptoms such as pruritus improve almost instantaneously.

REFERENCES

1. Greenlee RT, Hill-Harmon MB, Murray T, Thun M. Cancer statistics, 2001. CA Cancer J Clin 2001;51:15–37.
2. Mazzaferri EL. Management of the solitary thyroid nodule. N Engl J Med 1993;328:553–9.
3. Jossart GH, Clark OH. Well-differentiated thyroid cancer. Curr Prob Surg 1994;31:935–1011.
4. Shaha AR. Controversies in the management of thyroid nodule. Laryngoscope 2000;110:183–93.
5. Cernea CR, Ferray AR, Nishio S, et al. Surgical anatomy of the external branch of the superior laryngeal nerve. Head Neck 1992;14:380–3.
6. Lore JM Jr. Practical anatomical considerations in thyroid tumor surgery. Arch Otolaryngol 1983;109:568–74.
7. Shaha AR, Jaffe BM. Parathyroid preservation during thyroid surgery. Am J Otolaryngol 1998;19:113–7.
8. Rojeski MT, Gharib H. Nodular thyroid goiter, evaluation and management. N Engl J Med 1985;313:428–36.
9. Gharib H, Goellner JR. Fine-needle aspiration biopsy of the thyroid: an appraisal. Ann Int Med 1993;118:282–9.
10. Ashcraft MW, Van Herle AJ. Management of thyroid nodules-II: Scanning techniques, thyroid suppression therapy, and fine-needle aspiration biopsy. Head Neck Surg 1981;3:297–322.
11. Blum M, Yee J. Advances in thyroid imaging: thyroid sonography—when and how should it be used. Thyroid Today 1997;20:1–13.
12. Rosen IB, Azadian A, Walfish PG, et al. Ultrasound-guided fine-needle aspiration biopsy in the management of thyroid disease. Am J Surg 1993;166:346–9.
13. Ezzat S, Sarti DA, Cain DR, et al. Thyroid incidentalomas—prevalence by palpation and ultrasonography. Arch Int Med 1994;154:1838–40.

14. Bumstead RM. Thyroid disease: a guide for the head and neck surgeon. Ann Otol Rhinol Laryngol 1980;89 Suppl:72.

15. Hundahl SA, Fleming ID, Fremgen AM, Menck HR. A National Cancer Data Base report on 53,856 cases of thyroid carcinoma treated in the United States, 1985–1995. Cancer 1998;83:2638–48.

16. Rosai J, Carcangiu ML, DeLellis RA. Tumors of the thyroid gland. Atlas of tumor pathology. 3rd series. Washington (DC): Armed Forces Institute of Pathology; 1992.

17. Brierley JD, Tsang RW. External-beam radiation therapy in the treatment of differentiated thyroid cancer. Semin Surg Oncol 1999;16:42–9.

18. Hay ID, Grant CS, Taylor WF, et al. Ipsilateral lobectomy versus bilateral lobar resection in papillary thyroid carcinoma: a retrospective analysis of surgical outcome using a novel prognostic scoring system. Surgery 1987;102:1088–95.

19. Hay ID, Taylor WF, McConahey WM. A prognostic score for predicting outcome in papillary thyroid carcinoma. Endocrinology 1986;119 Suppl:1–15.

20. Cady B, Ross R, Silverman M, Wool M. Further evidence of the validity of risk-group definition in differentiated thyroid gland. Surgery 1985;98:1171–8.

21. Cady B, Ross RL. An expanded view of risk group definition in differentiated thyroid carcinoma. Surgery 1988;104: 947–53.

22. Byar DP, Green SB, Dor P, et al. A prognostic index for thyroid carcinoma. A study of the E.O.R.T.C. Thyroid Cancer Cooperative Group. Eur J Cancer 1979;15:1033–41.

23. Shaha AR, Loree TR, Shah JP. Intermediate risk group for differentiated carcinoma of the thyroid. Surgery 1994;116:1036–41.

24. Shah JP, Loree TR, Dharker D, et al. Prognostic factors in differentiated carcinoma of the thyroid gland. Am J Surg 1992;164:658–61.

25. Hay ID, Bergstralh EJ, Goellner JR, et al. Predicting outcome in papillary thyroid carcinoma: development of a reliable prognostic scoring system in a cohort of 1779 patients surgically treated at one institution during 1940 through 1989. Surgery 1993;114:1050–8.

26. Anderson PE, Kinsella J, Loree TR, et al. Differentiated carcinoma of the thyroid with extrathyroidal extension. Am J Surg 1995;170:467–70.

27. Hughes CJ, Shaha AR, Shah JP, et al. Impact of lymph node metastasis in differentiated carcinoma of the thyroid: a matched-pair analysis. Head Neck 1996;18:127–32.

28. Shaha AR, Jaffe BM. Practical management of post-thyroidectomy hematoma. J Surg Oncol 1994;57:235–8.

29. Pochin EE. Radioiodine therapy of thyroid cancer. Semin Nucl Med 1971;1:503.

30. Wells SA, Leight GF, Ross A. Primary hyperparathyroidism. Curr Prob Surg 1980;170:398.

31. Irvin GL, Prudhomme DL, Periso GT, et al. A new approach to parathyroidectomy. Ann Surg 1994;219:574–81.

32. Irvin GL, Dembrow VD, Prudhomme DL. Operative monitoring of parathyroid gland hyperfunction. Am J Surg 1991;162:299–302.

33. Greene AK, Mowschenson P, Hodin RA. Is sestamibi-guided parathyroidectomy really cost-effective? Surgery 1999; 126:1036–41.

34. Norman J, Denham D. Minimally invasive radioguided parathyroidectomy in the reoperative neck. Surgery 1998;124:1088–93.

35. Murphy C, Norman J. The 20% rule: A simple, instantaneous radioactivity measurement defines cure and allows elimination of frozen sections and hormone assays during parathyroidectomy. Surgery 1999;126:1023–9.

36. National Institute of Health, California. Diagnosis and management of asymptomatic primary hyperparathyroidism: Consensus development conference statement. Ann Intern Med 1991;114:593.

37. Hundahl SA, Fleming ID, Fremgen AM, et al. Two hundred eighty-six cases of parathyroid carcinoma treated in the United States 1985–1995: A National Cancer Data Base Report. The American College of Surgeons Commission on Cancer and the American Cancer Society. Cancer 1999; 86:538–44.

38. Shaha AR, Shah JP. Parathyroid carcinoma—a diagnostic and therapeutic challenge. Cancer 1999;86:378–80.

39. Norton JA, Shawker TH, Jones BL, et al. Intraoperative ultrasound and reoperative parathyroid surgery: an initial evaluation. World J Surg 1986;10:631–9.

40. Shaha AR, La Rosa CA, Jaffe BM. Parathyroid localization prior to primary exploration. Am J Surg 1993;166:289–94.

41. Shaha AR, Sarkar S, Strashun A, Yeh S. Sestamibi scan for preoperative localization in primary hyperparathyroidism. Head Neck 1997;19:87–91.

42. Duh QY, Uden P, Clark OH. Unilateral neck exploration for primary hyperparathyroidism-analysis of a controversy using a mathematical model. World J Surg 1992;16: 654–62.

43. Brennan AF, Norton JA. Reoperation for persistent and recurrent hyperparathyroidism. Ann Surg 1985;201:40.

44. Saxe AW, Brennan MF. Strategy and technique of reoperative parathyroid surgery. Surgery 1981;89:417.

15

Management of Cervical Metastasis

PETER E. ANDERSEN, MD, FACS
SCOTT SAFFOLD, MD

Head and neck cancer represents less than 5 percent of all cancers in the United States and will be responsible for approximately 11,800 deaths in 2001.[1] However, worldwide it ranks as the sixth most common cancer,[2] thus making head and neck cancer a major health problem. While the term "head and neck cancer" refers to tumors of myriad sites of origin and histologic types, over 90 percent of these are squamous carcinomas arising from the epithelium of the upper aerodigestive tract (oral cavity, oropharynx, hypopharynx and larynx) and for the purposes of this discussion the term shall refer exclusively to these tumors.

The status of the regional lymphatics is one of the most important prognostic indicators in patients with head and neck cancer. Head and neck cancers that are localized to the primary site without regional lymph node metastasis have excellent cure rates with either surgery or radiation therapy. The presence of regional metastases results in cure rates that are approximately half of those obtainable if metastasis to the regional lymphatics is not present. Thus the treatment of the neck has become one of the most actively debated topics in the field of head and neck oncology. Treatment of the neck in patients with clinical evidence of nodal metastasis has traditionally been surgical. In recent decades this has been extended to include a combination of surgery and radiation therapy. The role of chemotherapy in the management of neck disease remains controversial and is currently being actively investigated.

Butlin[3] was the first surgeon to systematically address the cervical lymph nodes by excising the nodal tissue of the submandibular triangle in continuity with the primary lesion in patients with cancer of the tongue. This did not remove all of the lymphatic tissue in the neck that was at risk for metastasis and it was not until the radical neck dissection (RND) described by Crile[4] and later popularized by Martin[5,6] that systematic removal of all of the lymphatic tissue in the lateral neck became routine.

Radical neck dissection, however, is cosmetically deforming and produces a characteristic shoulder disability that has been termed the "shoulder syndrome."[7] In an effort to lessen the morbidity of classic RND, various modifications have been proposed that preserve non-lymphatic structures that are normally sacrificed during this procedure but still remove all of the nodal tissue excised in RND. These modifications in general include preservation of the spinal accessory nerve (SAN) and can also involve preservation of the internal jugular vein (IJV) and/or the sternocleidomastoid muscle (SCM). More recently, further modifications of neck dissection have been proposed which preserve all of the non-lymphatic structures removed in "then-RND" but do not remove all of the lymphatic tissue on the involved side of the neck. These operations, which have been termed selective neck dissections, are based on observations that cancers of the head and neck tend to metastasize in predictable patterns based on the location of the primary tumor. Whether these modifications avoid all of the morbidity of RND is ambiguous, however there is evidence that shoulder function is retained when the spiral accessory nerve is preserved.[8,9,10]

Anatomy of Cervical Lymphatics

The lymphatics of the head and neck are a rich plexus of vessels whose anatomy was described by Rouviere and others.[11,12] There are many methods of clinically describing locations of lymph nodes; however the method that is in widest use and most reproducible is the system described by the Head and Neck Service at Memorial Sloan-Kettering Cancer Center. This system divides the neck into 5 nodal groups or levels, which are described in Figure 15–1.[13]

Classification of Neck Dissections

With the development of the many modifications of the classic RND there has been a proliferation of terms to describe these various procedures. This has resulted in a nomenclature that is non-uniform and confusing. To facilitate communication and to ensure standardization, the American Academy of Otolaryngology, Head and Neck Surgery has proposed a classification scheme for neck dissection.[13] In this scheme, RND, which is defined as the removal of nodal groups I to V with the SCM, IJV, and SAN, is considered to be the standard basic neck dissection, while all other procedures are considered to be modifications of RND. Modified radical neck dissection (MRND) consists of preservation of one or more of the non-lymphatic structures normally removed in RND. Selective neck dissection consists of removal of one or more regional lymph node groups with preservation of the SAN, SCM, and IJV. This nomenclature is described in greater detail in Table 15–1 and Figure 15–2. The typical postoperative appearance of patients after various neck dissections are shown in Figure 15–3, Figure 15–4, Figure 15–5, and Figure 15–6. The routine use of a standardized system will greatly reduce the confusing nomenclature currently used in describing neck dissections.

Patterns of Lymphatic Flow

The entire concept of selective or limited neck dissection is based on the clinical observation that

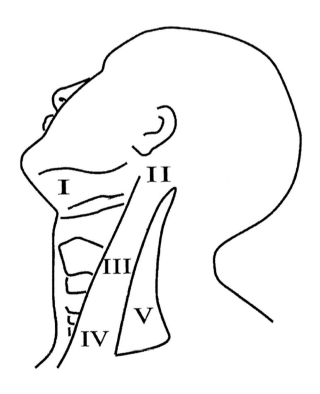

Group	Description
I	**Submental group**-The nodal tissue lying between the anterior belly of the digastric muscles and above the hyoid bone.
	Submandibular group-Nodal tissue lying in the triangle bounded by the anterior and posterior bellies of the digastric muscle and the inferior border of the mandible.
II	**Upper jugular group**-Nodal tissue lying around the upper portion of the IJV and the upper SAN. Extending from the skull base to the bifurcation of the carotid artery or the hyoid bone (clinical landmark), the posterior limit is the posterior border of the SCM and the anterior border is the lateral border of the sternohyoid muscle.
III	**Middle jugular group**-Nodal tissue lying around the middle third of the IJV from the inferior border of level 2 to the omohyoid muscle or the cricothyroid membrane (clinical landmark). The anterior and posterior borders are the same as those for level 2.
IV	**Lower jugular group**-Nodal tissue lying around the inferior third of the IJV from the inferior border of level 3 to the clavicle. The anterior and posterior borders are the same as those for level 2 and 3.
V	**Posterior triangle group**-Nodal tissue around the lower portion

Figure 15–1.   System for describing location of cervical lymphatic metastases. IJV = internal jugular vein; SAN = spinal accessory nerve; SCM = sternocleidomastoid.

Table 15–1. Classification of Neck Dissections		
Type of Neck Dissection	Nodal Levels Dissected	Structures Preserved
Radical neck dissection (RND)	I–V	None
Type I modified radical neck dissection (MRND I)	I–V	SAN
Type II modified radical neck dissection (MRND II)	I–V	SAN SCM
Type III modified radical neck dissection (MRND III)	I–V	SCM IJV SAN
Supraomohyoid neck dissection (SOHND)	I–III	SCM IJV SAN
Lateral (jugular) neck dissection (LND)	II–IV	SCM IJV SAN
Anterolateral neck dissection (ALND)	I–IV	SCM IJV SAN
Posterolateral neck dissection (PLND)	II–V	SCM IJV SAN

SAN = spinal accessory nerve; SCM = sternocleidomastoid; IJV = internal jugular vein.

squamous cell carcinomas of the upper aerodigestive tract metastasize to the cervical lymph nodes in a predictable pattern. Strong experimental evidence of this concept's validity is provided by Fisch,[14] who performed lymphography using oil-based contrast media injected into postauricular lymphatics. Twenty-four hours after injection the patients underwent complete neck dissection and filling of the lymph nodes was verified in almost every one of his 100 cases. The flow of the contrast material was observed with radiography. From observations obtained from 8 cases that were free of lymph node metastases, Fisch was able to document the normal pattern of flow in the cervical lymphatics.

After injection in the postauricular lymphatics, contrast first flowed into a group of nodes just below and behind the angle of the mandible. These nodes were called the junctional nodes by Fisch and probably represent either high level V or high level II nodes. From the junctional nodes, contrast

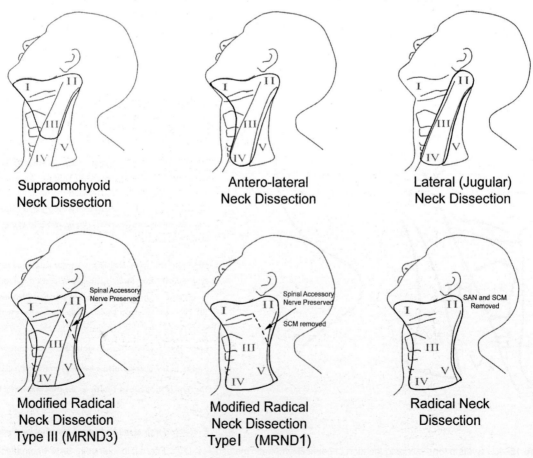

Supraomohyoid Neck Dissection

Antero-lateral Neck Dissection

Lateral (Jugular) Neck Dissection

Modified Radical Neck Dissection Type III (MRND3)

Modified Radical Neck Dissection Type I (MRND1)

Radical Neck Dissection

Figure 15–2. Cervical lymph node groups removed in various types of neck dissection.

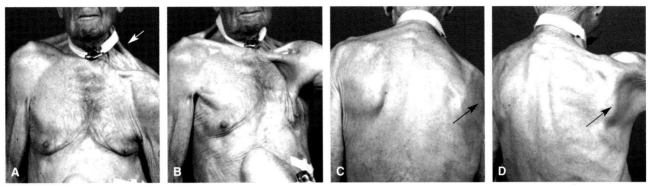

Figure 15–3. Cosmetic and functional deformity resulting from radical neck dissection. *A,* Anterior view demonstrating anterior and inferior displacement of shoulder and trapezius muscle (*arrow*). *B,* Anterior view demonstrating decreased shoulder abduction. *C and D,* Posterior view demonstrating winging of scapula. (Photos courtesy of James I. Cohen, MD, PhD.)

flowed first into both the lymphatics along the spinal accessory nerve and the internal jugular vein. Contrast in the lymphatics along the spinal accessory nerve then flowed into the transverse cervical chain, and through this medially into the low jugular chain. Of particular interest is the observation that contrast contained within the lymphatics of the spinal accessory chain could reach the jugular chain lymphatics by connecting vessels which occurred at many places along the spinal accessory chain. Contrast contained within the jugular chain could not, however, reach the spinal accessory chain by retrograde flow along the same route. Flow to contralateral lymphatics or retrograde lymphatic flow was not observed. These patterns are shown in Figure 15–7. A critical question

left unanswered by the studies of Fisch is the precise location of the junctional nodes he described. If these nodes are commonly involved by head and neck cancer metastasis, it is possible virtually anywhere in the neck, and the concept of selective neck dissection would seem to be unsound. However, as will be shown in the section on patterns of nodal metastasis from squamous carcinomas of the upper aerodigestive tract, these junctional nodes are probably uninvolved in most cases of head and neck cancer since metastasis to level V is uncommon, except in nasopharyngeal carcinoma.

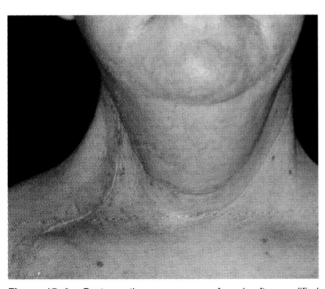

Figure 15–4. Postoperative appearance of neck after modified radical neck dissection, type I.

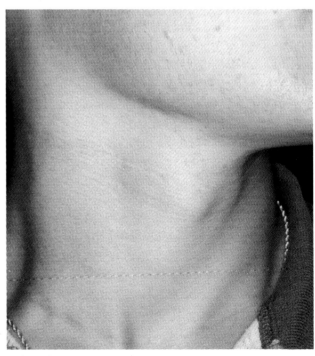

Figure 15–5. Postoperative appearance of neck after supraomohyoid neck dissection.

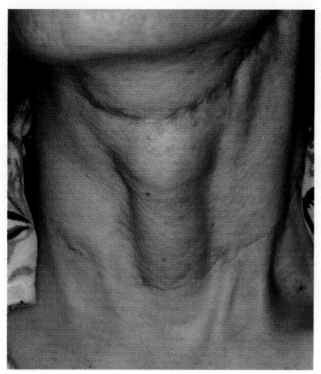

Figure 15–6. Postoperative appearance of neck after bilateral modified radical neck dissections, type III.

Incidence and Pattern of Nodal Metastasis

The rational use of modifications of RND, especially selective neck dissection, is based upon work describing the patterns of lymphatic metastasis. These studies have shown that patterns of metastasis can be predicted based upon knowledge of the primary tumor location. Without such validation the concept of selective neck dissection would be invalid, since by definition nodal tissue at risk for metastasis would be left behind in the neck.

Lindberg published the location of nodal metastases in patients with squamous carcinoma of the upper aerodigestive tract as determined by clinical examination[15] in 1972. This review consisted of 2,044 previously untreated patients with squamous carcinoma of the head and neck. The presence of nodal metastasis and their location was assessed and correlated with the location and stage of the primary site. Primary sites were divided into oral tongue, floor of mouth, retromolar trigone/anterior faucial pillar, soft palate, tonsillar fossa, base of tongue, oropharyngeal walls, supraglottic larynx, hypopharynx and nasopharynx. Fifty-seven percent

of patients presented with clinical evidence of metastasis in the cervical nodes. Lindberg showed that for lesions of the oral tongue, floor of mouth, retromolar trigone/anterior faucial arch and soft palate, the incidence of cervical nodal metastasis increased with the size of the primary tumor. However, the incidence of nodal metastasis did not correlate with the size of the primary in tumors of the tonsillar fossa, base of tongue, supraglottic larynx, and hypopharynx.

Lindberg demonstrated that squamous cell carcinomas of the upper aerodigestive tract tend to metastasize to the neck in a predictable pattern. By far the most common site of metastasis by all tumors is to the ipsilateral level II nodes. Tumors that lie within the oral cavity anterior to the circumvallate papillae have a propensity to metastasize to levels I through III, with levels IV and V seldom involved. Tumors of the oropharynx have a low propensity to metastasize to level I; metastasis is most common to level II with decreasing incidence of metastasis in levels III and IV. These tumors have a higher rate of metastases to level V than oral cavity tumors but the rate is still low. Tumors of the supraglottic larynx and hypopharynx rarely metastasize to level I, again metastases were most com-

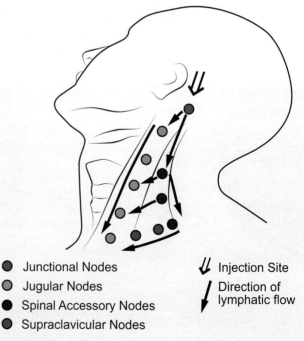

● Junctional Nodes
○ Jugular Nodes
● Spinal Accessory Nodes
● Supraclavicular Nodes

⇓ Injection Site
↓ Direction of lymphatic flow

Figure 15–7. Pattern of lymphatic flow as demonstrated by Fisch. Data from Fisch UP, et al. Cervical lymphatic system as visualized by lymphography. Ann Otol Rhinol Laryngol 1964;73:869-82.

mon to level II with a decreasing incidence in levels III and IV and metastases to level V were infrequent. Tumors of the nasopharynx are unique among squamous cell carcinomas of the upper aerodigestive tract in that they metastasize widely to levels II through V. Contralateral metastases were uncommon in cancers of the floor of mouth, oral tongue, hypopharynx, and retromolar trigone/anterior faucial arch. In contrast, tumors of the nasopharnyx, base of tongue, oropharyngeal walls, soft palate, supraglottic larynx, and tonsil have substantial rates of contralateral metastases.

Lindberg's data clearly showed that in cases of squamous cell carcinoma of the upper aerodigestive tract, with the exception of nasopharyngeal carcinoma, nodal metastasis occurs in a predictable pattern and it may, in certain instances, be sound to exclude dissection of the level V lymph nodes. However, this study provides only information on clinically positive nodal metastasis—it provides no information on the incidence and location of occult nodal metastasis. Such information on microscopic metastasis can only be obtained from a surgical specimen. Byers and colleagues published one such study[16] in 1988. They examined the specimens of 428 patients undergoing 648 modified neck dissections and correlated the location of the pathologically positive lymph nodes with the primary site. The majority of these neck dissections were selective neck dissections and therefore not all of the lymph node levels at risk were examined in each patient. This study essentially confirms the clinical data of Lindberg,[15] that lesions anterior to the circumvallate papillae are most likely to metastasize to lymph nodes levels I through III and lesions within the hypopharynx and larynx to levels II through IV. It must be pointed out, however, that the majority of these dissections were less than comprehensive and therefore the low incidence of metastasis to certain nodal levels may simply reflect the lack of sampling of those levels.

In order to fully assess all the lymph node levels at risk for a particular primary site, surgical specimens should include all lymph node levels (comprehensive neck dissection). Just such information is provided in a series of studies by Shah and colleagues,[17,18,19] which involved 1,081 previously untreated patients who underwent 1,119 classic RNDs for squamous carcinoma of the upper aerodigestive tract. The operations consisted of 343 elective RND in the clinically N0 setting and 776 therapeutic RND in the clinically N+ setting.

The results of Shah's studies are shown in Figure 15–8. Each lymph node level shows the percentage of patients with pathologically N+ neck dissections who had metastasis at that level. In patients with primary tumors of the oral cavity undergoing therapeutic RND, the majority of metastatic nodes were located in levels I to III; level IV was involved in 20 percent of specimens and level V in only 4 percent. In those with primary oropharyngeal tumors, the majority of metastases were located in levels II to IV; levels I and V were involved in 17 percent and 11 percent of the specimens respectively. Therapeutic neck dissection in hypopharyngeal tumors showed that the majority of metastases were located in levels II to IV, while levels I and V were involved in 10 percent and 11 percent of the specimens respectively. Primary tumors of the larynx metastasized to levels II through IV with levels I and V being involved in 8 percent and 5 percent of the specimens respectively.

In the setting of elective RND in patients with primary tumors of the oral cavity, the majority of metastases were located in levels I to III; levels IV and V were involved in 9 percent and 2 percent of the specimens respectively. In patients with primary tumors located in the oropharynx, the majority of metastases were located in levels II to IV; levels I and V were involved in 7 percent of the specimens each. Patients with tumors of the hypopharynx undergoing elective RND had the majority of metastases in levels II to IV, while levels I and V were not involved in any of the specimens. Primary tumors of the larynx metastasized primarily to levels II through IV, while levels I and V were involved in 14 percent and 7 percent of the specimens respectively.

The question of metastasis to level V was addressed by another study from Memorial Hospital by Davidson and colleagues.[20] They examined the specimens of 1,123 patients undergoing 1,277 RNDs and found metastases to level V in only 3 percent of patients. Level V metastases were highest in patients with hypopharyngeal and oropharyngeal primary sites (7% and 6% respectively). Only 3 of the 40 patients with level V metastases had these in the face

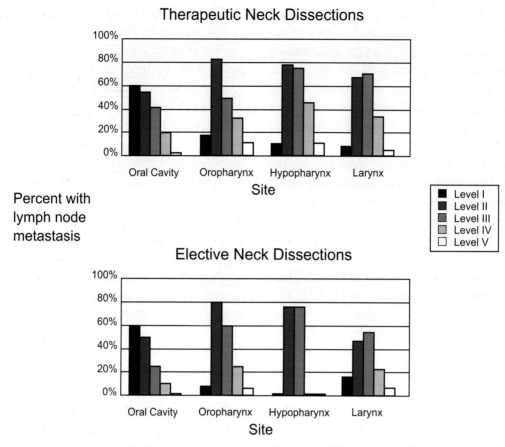

Figure 15–8.   Incidence of metastasis to lymph node levels by primary site in N+ and N0 patients. (Data from Shah JP, et al. The patterns of cervical lymph node metastases from squamous carcinoma of the oral cavity. Cancer 1990;66:109–13, and Shah JP. Patterns of cervical lymph node metastasis from squamous carcinomas of the upper aerodigestive tract. Am J Surg 1990;160:405–9.)

of a clinical N0 stage. They concluded that the incidence of metastases to level V was small in general, and extremely unlikely in the clinically N0 patient.

Evaluation of the Neck

Pre-surgical staging of the neck has become more complex over the years. Clinical assessment of the neck by palpation, while providing critical information, is inadequate in its sensitivity for detecting metastatic disease to the cervical nodes. Error rates as high as 40 percent have been reported when physical examination alone is used to evaluate the neck.[21] Patient factors such as a short, obese neck, as well as prior irradiation play a role in decreasing the accuracy of this technique. Clearly, radiologic assessment of the neck adds to the sensitivity and specificity of preoperative neck evaluation.

Computerized tomography (CT) and magnetic resonance imaging (MRI) have become the workhorses of imaging modalities in head and neck squamous cell carcinoma (HNSCC). Size criteria are frequently used as indicators of metastatic involvement. Other features such as central necrosis or ring-enhancement aid in specificity but are relatively infrequent findings. Generally, a subdigastric node measuring > 15 mm, a submandibular node > 12 mm, and other nodes > 10 mm are suspicious for involvement. Using criteria such as these, the accuracy of detecting neck disease approaches 90 percent.[22,23] Size, however, is certainly not pathognomonic for cancerous involvement of lymph nodes. Even in the patient with an identified squamous cell carcinoma of the upper aerodigestive tract, a myriad of alternative causes of enlarged lymph nodes exist. Further, microscopic foci of disease may exist in nodes of normal size. As CT or MRI is often employed to evaluate the primary lesion, inclusion of the neck in the area of study incurs nominal additional expense and no morbidity. Although CT and MRI provide excellent anatomic detail and are the current modalities of choice, they provide little information on the biology of the lymph node.

Due to its non-invasiveness and affordability, ultrasound (US) has been investigated as a potential tool in evaluating neck disease. Factors such as size, irregular margins, and echo characteristics of lymph nodes have been shown to have predictive value in assessing involved nodes. The overall sensitivity of this approach, however, is limited due to the operator-dependent nature of ultrasound.[24] Some authors have proposed ultrasound in combination with ultrasound-guided fine needle aspiration as an approach to diagnosis. Takes and colleagues[25] examined, with ultrasonography, 64 necks staged N0 based on physical examination. Those with nodes greater than 5 mm in size underwent ultrasound-guided needle biopsy. Results were further verified with histopathologic examination and the findings compared with CT of the neck for detection of involved nodes. They found a 48 percent sensitivity, 100 percent specificity, and 79 percent accuracy for ultrasound versus 54, 92, and 77 percent respectively for CT. These results demonstrate that, in experienced hands, ultrasound can be a useful tool. Its widespread application, however, is limited by the technical expertise required for accurate interpretation.

Positron emission tomography (PET) has been employed to assess metabolic changes in a variety of tissues including those of the head and neck. PET localizes regions of increased glucose metabolism by using the radionuclide 2-[^{18}F]-fluoro-2-deoxy-D-glucose. Hanasono[26] and colleagues demonstrated a potential role of this technique in evaluating unknown primaries, distant metastases, and for tumor surveillance. They suggest that it may be effective as an adjuvant to CT and MRI in selected cases. Another study, however, found sensitivity of 78 percent and specificity of 100 percent when PET was used to evaluate patients clinically staged N0.[27] Although their numbers were small, the results compare favorably to other imaging modalities. Another interesting approach attempts to combine the sensitivity of PET with the anatomic detail of CT and MRI. Wong and colleagues[28] used computer-combined imaging to evaluate primary lesions in the head and neck. They found enhanced detail and accuracy as compared to clinical exam or single modality imaging alone. Whether this approach can be extended to evaluation of nodal disease is unclear, and cost-benefit issues may preclude its widespread utilization.

Selection of Surgical Therapy

The proliferation of different types of modified neck dissection has the potential to lead to confusion regarding what type of neck dissection is appropriate for a particular clinical situation. This is complicated by the lack of data from randomized studies comparing the effectiveness of the variations of neck dissection. The goal of any neck dissection, however, should be: to remove all clinically obvious metastatic disease, to sample the lymph node levels at highest risk for metastasis in order to detect the presence of occult metastasis, and to perform this in such a way as to minimize the morbidity of the procedure without compromising the 2 previous goals. With this in mind, 2 dominant clinical scenarios emerge: the clinically N0 and the clinically N+ neck. A general algorithm is presented in Figure 15–9.

In the clinically N0 setting, the first decision to be made is whether to perform a neck dissection at all or to simply observe the neck for the development of metastasis. There is no firm data to suggest that elective neck dissection improves survival; in fact the only randomized trial addressing this question failed to find any survival advantage to elective neck dissection.[29] However, some authors have reported improved survival in patients treated during a time period when elective neck dissection is frequently performed as compared to earlier periods where observation of the neck was more common.[30] It seems likely, however, that if elective neck treatment is to improve survival, that it will be of most benefit to those patients with a high risk of occult metastasis—thus some authors have recommended elective neck treatment in patients with a greater than 20 to 25 percent risk of occult metastasis.[31] In addition it is often assumed that if the neck is observed closely, any metastatic disease that occurs will be detected at an early stage. This assumption is, in fact, erroneous, as Andersen and colleagues[32] reported on a series of 47 patients who recurred in the neck during observation. In these patients, 60 percent were pathologically N2 or greater and extracapsular spread was present in half when the failure was detected.

Due to the high rates of occult metastasis in patients with primary tumors located in the hypopharynx, oropharynx, and supraglottic larynx, elective treatment of the neck (with neck dissection if surgical resection of the primary tumor is planned, or with radiotherapy if the primary tumor is to be irradiated for cure) is indicated.[15] Occult metastasis from tumors of the oral cavity (specifically tongue and floor of mouth) has been correlated with tumor stage[15] and tumor thickness[33] (Figure 15–10). Therefore, elective treatment of the neck is indicated in patients with tumor greater than 2 mm thick or in T3 or T4 primaries. Other indications for elective neck dissection include the need to enter the neck, either to resect the primary tumor (eg, mandibulotomy, lateral pharyngotomy, supraglottic laryngectomy), or for reconstruction (eg, free tissue transfer). In these situations it is convenient to electively dissect the neck. Another factor, which may lead the surgeon to electively dissect the neck, is the case of the patient is believed unlikely to return for the close follow-up that is necessary if observation of the neck is to be employed.

When deciding the type of neck dissection to perform in the elective setting, 2 factors must be considered: the likelihood of occult metastasis, and the most likely location of the metastases based on the location of the primary tumor. Since in the clinically N0 patient the majority of neck dissections are likely to be negative for occult metastasis,[21,34,35] the neck dissection chosen must be the least morbid possible. Selective neck dissections are ideally suited for the elective setting. On examining Figure 15–8, the operations that remove the nodal levels most at risk are

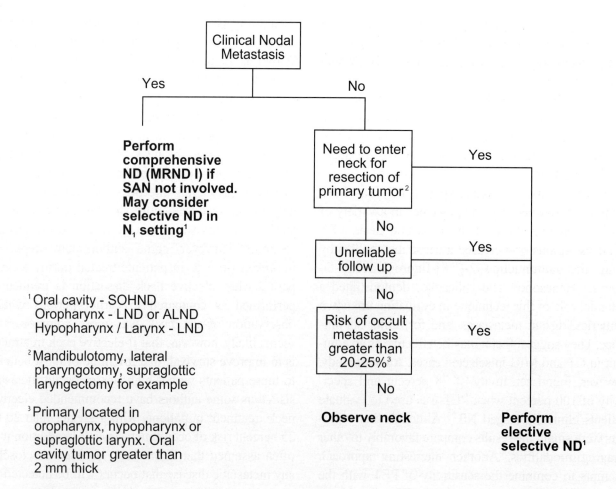

Figure 15–9.   General algorithm for selection of neck dissection.

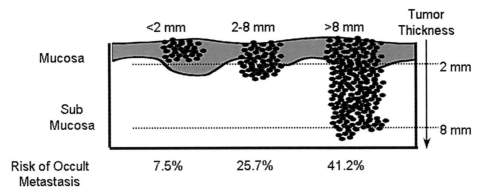

Figure 15–10. Risk of occult nodal metastasis with increasing thickness of oral cavity cancers (tongue and floor of mouth). Data from Spiro RH, et al. Predictive value of tumor thickness in squamous carcinoma confined to the tongue and floor of the mouth.[33]

obvious. Primary tumors in the oral cavity should undergo supraomohyoid neck dissection (SOHND); oropharyngeal tumors would best be treated with lateral neck dissection (LND). However, since surgical resection of the primary often involves an approach through level I, anterolateral neck dissection (ALND) may be a better choice, while tumors located in the hypopharynx or larynx should undergo LND. If the surgeon desires only one operation that is appropriate in all situations (for proficiency or for instruction of residents) then ALND is an excellent operation for the elective treatment of the neck in patients with head and neck cancer.

In the clinically N+ patient, the existence of lymphatic metastasis is established and therefore it is acceptable to perform a neck dissection with a greater potential for morbidity. It has been shown that preservation of the spinal accessory nerve in the N+ neck is not associated with increased risk of recurrence in the neck as long as the nerve is not involved by the tumor,[36] therefore even in this setting it is possible to potentially ameliorate some of the morbidity of RND. As Figure 15–8 demonstrates, the incidence of metastasis at all levels in the neck increases in the setting of clinically obvious neck metastasis. Therefore in the N+ patient, an acceptable and safe neck dissection to perform is a comprehensive neck dissection that spares the spinal accessory nerve if it is not involved with tumor (MRND I).

The use of selective neck dissections in the N+ patient is controversial. While Shah's study[17] shows that the rate of metastasis to all levels increases in the N+ neck, it also shows that the pattern of metastasis

still follows the general pattern seen in the N0 neck. There is in fact some evidence that selective neck dissection in the N+ neck yields control rates similar to more comprehensive neck dissections.[37,38] The efficacy of selective neck dissection in the N+ neck is still a matter of debate; however, its use in low-stage neck disease such as the N1 neck is not unreasonable. The type of selective neck dissection employed should be based on the patterns of nodal metastasis shown in Figure 15–8. Given the low risk of metastasis to level V reported by Davidson[20] and the increased risk of involvement of level IV in the N+ neck, the ALND might be the selective neck dissection of choice if one is to perform this type of operation in the N+ setting.

Radiation Therapy

The ability of radiotherapy to improve outcomes in squamous cell carcinoma of the head and neck is well demonstrated. Its efficacy in early T1 and T2 lesions of the upper aerodigestive tract approaches that of surgical management. Treatment of disease metastatic to the neck with radiation has also shown benefit. Studies have shown that, in the N0 neck, radiotherapy is as effective as elective neck dissection (END) in reducing locoregional recurrence.[39] Surgery combined with radiation has been shown to reduce local failure rates to 18 percent in N1 necks.[40] The timing of neck irradiation, however, has been a subject of debate. Preoperative radiation had been favored in the past due to the theoretical advantage of treating while the vascular supply of the tumor was undisturbed. Preoperative therapy may also help to reduce bulky disease and thus facilitate surgical extirpation. However, the increased incidence of radiation-related surgical complications following high-dose preoperative radiotherapy has led to the currently accepted practice of administering radiotherapy in the postoperative period. Typically, surgeons prefer postoperative radiation to avoid the wound healing difficulties encountered in operating on previously irradiated tissue. Further, Leemans et al has shown that histopathologic evaluation of the neck specimen can be used to select those patients who are more likely to benefit from combined therapy.[41] Patients with neck disease found to be metastatic to multiple nodes or extending beyond the lymph node capsule have been shown to have better locoregional control and survival with the addition of postoperative radiotherapy.[42] Delaying radiation allows the surgeon to select patients with these risk factors for further treatment. In fact, an RTOG study with long-term follow-up showed that patients treated with postoperative radiation had lower locoregional failure rates than those treated preoperatively. Due to a higher incidence of distant disease, however, they demonstrated no difference in survivals.[43]

More recently, neoadjuvant chemotherapy has shown some promise in management of advanced head and neck squamous cell carcinoma. Various organ preservation protocols have been proposed in which combined chemotherapy and radiation have been used as initial therapy of the primary lesion and neck metastases. These approaches reserve surgery for salvage in patients failing to develop a complete response. Their proponents suggest that for partial responders, following neoadjuvant multi-modality therapy, an oncologically sound surgical procedure can be performed that has a greater chance of preserving speech or swallowing. This potential benefit must be weighed against the increased risk of surgical complications that has been associated with preoperative therapy. Chemoradiotherapy protocols designed at preserving function at the primary site often fail to eradicate disease in the neck. This necessitates post-treatment surgical management of the neck even for those achieving a dramatic response at the primary site. Lavertu[44] and colleagues demonstrated a 46 percent complication rate in patients treated with neoadjuvant chemotherapy. Only 12 percent of these, however, were major complications, and they found no increased risk in those patients undergoing chemoradiotherapy. Other studies have shown similarly low wound-related complication rates; this is consistent with historically reported rates of neck wound complications following neck dissection alone.[45]

Controversies

A key controversy in management of the neck in head and neck squamous cell carcinoma relates to which and how much therapy is appropriate. In management of the N0 neck, it is generally accepted that a metastatic risk in excess of 20 percent warrants elective therapy. Although some advocates of a watchful waiting policy exist, current data supports liberal use of prophylactic therapy. Though little information in regard to impact on survival exists, a study from Memorial Sloan-Kettering Cancer Center demonstrated that, despite close follow-up, patients who were observed rather than electively treated presented with advanced neck disease. Sixty percent of patients who recurred in the neck presented with N2 or greater disease and 77 percent had evidence of extracapsular spread.[32] Such patients required more extensive therapy than if they had undergone elective treatment.

What therapy is indicated for treatment of the N0 neck is an issue of some debate. Advocates of elective radiotherapy suggest that its ability to control microscopic foci of disease render it comparable to neck dissection in control of neck disease. Its sequelae, including often-debilitating xerostomia, however, make it a more morbid treatment option, as compared to selective neck dissection. Certainly, selective lateral or supraomohyoid neck dissection can be performed quickly, safely and with minimal postoperative morbidity. The oncologic efficacy of selective neck dissection has been discussed earlier, and those factors make it the treatment of choice for the clinically uninvolved neck, unless radiotherapy is to be employed for the treatment of the primary site.

Management of the N1 neck is more controversial. Conventionally, radical neck dissection (RND) has been the treatment of choice for patients presenting with disease in the neck. Modifications of RND, including those sparing the eleventh nerve, in the past were criticized for their violation of traditional surgical oncologic principles. An *en bloc* resection is not possible and lymphatic channels must be cut to preserve such structures. It is now accepted that tumor metastasizes in an embolic fashion and therefore, effective treatment can still be rendered. This has been borne out by the work of Bocca.[46] An extensive review of functional neck dissection, preserving the eleventh nerve, sternocleidomastoid muscle, and internal jugular vein routinely showed a recurrence rate comparable to RND even in N1 disease in 171 patients. So long as nodes are not adherent to the structures of concern and a connective tissue plane of dissection can be established, it may be possible to preserve these structures. That the important structures traversing the neck are maintained within their own aponeurotic sheaths is validated by the work of Byers.[47] In an extensive review of functional and selective neck dissection, he found a 4.7 percent local recurrence rate for patients with pathologically positive jugulodigastric nodes despite preservation of the eleventh nerve, so long as postoperative radiotherapy was used.

As it has become more accepted to preserve important structures in the neck, the concept of removing only at-risk nodal groups even in the N+ neck has been considered. Spiro and colleagues[48] reviewed the Memorial Sloan-Kettering Cancer Center experience with supraomohyoid neck dissection and found that in 31 patients undergoing therapeutic dissection and radiotherapy, there was a 6 percent local failure rate. Traynor and colleagues[49] examined 29 patients with N1-N2C neck disease treated with various forms of selective neck dissection (SND) and found local recurrence rates of only 4 percent. Their group emphasized the importance of careful selection of patients. Shah demonstrated that, even in patients with clinically evident neck disease, of 776 pathologically evaluated RNDs only 3.7 percent had involvement of the level V nodes.[36] This data, in addition to early studies of patterns of lymphatic spread of head and neck squamous cell carcinoma, have led to broader application of selective neck dissection (SND) in management of the N1 neck, particularly if postoperative radiotherapy is utilized. Those with massive adenopathy, fixed nodes or gross extracapsular spread should be treated with classic radical neck dissection. They suggest, however, that the type of neck dissection can be individualized: nodal groups resected as well as structures of the neck to be preserved are based on known patterns of lymphatic spread as well as findings at the time of surgery.

FUTURE DIRECTIONS

As with many neoplastic diseases, the future of head and neck squamous cell carcinoma management likely will include emerging treatments such as immunotherapy. Novel approaches such as gene therapy, T cell manipulation, and cytokine therapy have been employed in experimental treatment of other solid tumors with limited success. While the application of such strategies is based on a limited understanding of tumor immunology at the primary site, even less is known about the immunoregulatory role of the draining lymphatics. Current treatment protocols focus on the goal of complete extirpation of the tumor. As Collins points out, however, HNSCC is more likely a systemic disease with a predilection for sites in the head and neck.[50] The role of lymph nodes in this process is unclear. Extrapolating conventional immunology to tumor biology, tumor antigens are transported from the primary site either by antigen-presenting cells (macrophages, dendritic cells, B cells) or by tumor cells themselves to the regional lymph node where an immunologic response is initiated. The propagation of this response is systemic rather than local. It follows, then, that lymph nodes are biologic rather than mechanical barriers to tumor advancement. Several investigators have found evidence of increased antitumor activity in lymph nodes draining HNSCC. Vetto and colleagues[51] found higher expression of the T cell activation marker OX40 on cells from draining lymph nodes than in the peripheral blood. Other studies have also shown that the draining lymph nodes have been exposed to tumor antigens.[52,53] Clearly, through tolerance or immunosuppression, this systemic immune response is ineffective in controlling disease. One study demonstrated a tumor-induced inhibitory effect on lymph node cells that was more pronounced in first echelon nodes than in nodes outside the primary drainage basin.[54] As our understanding of the immunologic interactions between the tumor and the host progresses, therapy guided at manipulating and enhancing the immune response may be developed. It is possible that the key to understanding this relationship lies within the draining lymph nodes.

REFERENCES

1. Greenlee RT, Hill-Harman MB, Murray T, Thun M. Cancer Statistics, 2001. CA Cancer J Clin 2001;51:15–36.

2. Parkin DM, Muir CS, Laara E. Global burden of cancer. Biennial report 1986–7. Lyon: IARC, World Health Organization and International Agency for Research on Cancer; 1987

3. Butlin HI, Spencer WG, Disease of the tongue, 2nd ed. London: Cassell, 1900.

4. Crile G. Excision of cancer of the head and neck with special reference to the plan of dissection based on one hundred and thirty-two operations. JAMA 1906;47:1780–6.

5. Martin H. The treatment of cervical metastatic cancer. Ann Surg 1944;114:972–86.

6. Martin H, DelValle B, Enrlich H, Cahan EG. Neck dissection. Cancer 1951;4:441–99.

7. Nahum AM, Mullally W, Marmor L. A syndrome resulting from radical neck dissection. Arch Otolaryngol 1961;74:82–6.

8. Ballantyne AJ, Guinn GA. Reduction of shoulder disability after neck dissection. Am J Surg 1966;112:662–7.

9. Short SO, Kaplan JN, Laramore GE, Cummings CW. Shoulder pain and function after neck dissection with or without preservation of the spinal accessory nerve. Am J Surg 1984;148:478–82.

10. Schuller DE, Reiches NA, Hamaker RC, et al. Analysis of disability resulting from treatment including radical neck dissection or modified neck dissection. Head Neck Surg 1983;6:551–8.

11. Rouviere H. Anatomy of the human lymphatic system. Ann Arbor (MI): Edwards Brothers; 1938.

12. Haagensen CD, Feind CR, Merter FP, et al, editors. The lymphatics in cancer. Philadelphia (PA): WB Saunders; 1972.

13. Robbins KT, Medina JE, Wolfe GT, et al. Standardizing neck dissection terminology. Arch Otolaryngol Head Neck Surg 1991;117:601–5.

14. Fisch UP, Sigel ME. Cervical lymphatic system as visualized by lymphography. Ann Otol Rhinol Laryngol 1964;73:869–82.

15. Lindberg R. Distribution of cervical lymph node metastases from squamous cell carcinoma of the upper respiratory and digestive tracts. Cancer 1972;29:1446–8.

16. Byers RM, Wolf PF, Ballantyne AJ. Rationale for modified neck dissection. Head Neck Surg 1988;10:160–7.

17. Shah JP, Candela FC, Poddar AK. The patterns of cervical lymph node metastases from squamous carcinoma of the oral cavity. Cancer 1990;66:109–13.

18. Candela FC, Kothari K, Shah JP. Patterns of cervical node metastases from squamous carcinoma of the oropharynx and hypopharynx. Head Neck 1990;12:197–203.

19. Candela FC, Shah J, Jaques DP, Shah JP. Patterns of cervical node metastases from squamous carcinoma of the larynx. Arch Otolaryngol Head Neck Surg 1990;116:432–5.

20. Davidson BJ, Kulkarny V, Delacure MD, Shah JP. Posterior triangle metastases of squamous cell carcinoma of the upper aerodigestive tract. Am J Surg 1993;166:395–8.

21. Teichgraeber JF, Clairmont AA. Incidence of occult metastases for cancer of the oral tongue and floor of mouth: Treatment rationale. Head Neck Surg 1984;7:15–21.

22. Som PM. Detection of metastasis in cervical lymph nodes: CT and MR criteria and differential diagnosis. Am J Roentgenol 1992;158:9619,

23. Friedman K, Shelton VK, Mafee K, et al. Metastatic neck disease. Arch Otolaryngol Head Neck Surg 1984;110:443–7.

24. John DJ, Williams SR, Ahuja A, et al. Palpation compared with ultrasound in the assessment of malignant cervical lymph nodes. J Otol Laryngol 1993;107:821–3.

25. Takes RP, Righi P, Meeuwis CA, et al. The value of ultrasound with ultrasound-guided fine needle aspiration biopsy compared to computed tomography in the detection of regional metastases in the clinically negative neck. Int J Radiat Oncol Biol Phys 1998;40:1027–32.

26. Hanasono W, Kunda LD, Segall GK, et al. Uses and limitations of FDG positron emission tomography in patients with head and neck cancer. Laryngoscope 1999;109:880–5.

27. Myers LL, Wax MK, Nabi H, et al. Positron emission tomography in the evaluation of the N0 neck. Laryngoscope 1998;108:232–6.

28. Wong WL, Hussain K, Chevretton E, et al. Validation and clinical application of computer-combined computed tomography and positron emission tomography with 2-[18F]fluoro-2-deoxy-D-glucose head and neck images. Am J Surg 1996 Dec;172(6):628–32.

29. Vandenbrouck C, Sancho-Garnier H, Chassagne D, et al. Elective versus therapeutic radical neck dissection in epidermoid carcinoma of the oral cavity. Cancer 1980;46:386–90.

30. Franceschi D, Gupta R, Spiro R, Shah J. Improved survival in the treatment of squamous carcinoma of the oral tongue. Am J Surg 1993;166:360–5.

31. Weiss MH, Harrison LB, Isaacs RS. Use of decision analysis in planning a management strategy for the stage N0 neck. Arch Otolaryngol Head Neck Surg 1994;120:699–702.

32. Andersen P, Cambronero E, Shaha AR, Shah JP. The extent of neck disease after regional failure during observation of the N0 neck. Am J Surg 1996 Dec;172(6):689–91.

33. Spiro RH, Huvos AG, Wong GY, et al. Predictive value of tumor thickness in squamous carcinoma confined to the tongue and floor of the mouth. Am J Surg 1986;152:345–50.

34. Spiro JD, Spiro RH, Shah JP, et al. Critical assessment of supraomohyoid neck dissection. Am J Surg 1988;156:286–9.

35. Shah JP. Patterns of cervical lymph node metastasis from squamous carcinomas of the upper aerodigestive tract. Am J Surg 1990;160:405–9.

36. Andersen P, Cambronero E, Spiro R, Shah J. The role of comprehensive neck dissection with preservation of the spinal accessory nerve in the clinically positive neck. Am J Surg 1994;168:499–502.

37. Byers RM. Modified neck dissection: A study of 967 cases from 1970 to 1980. Am J Surg 1985;150:414–21.

38. Traynor S. Cohen J, Andersen P, Everts F. Results of selective neck dissection in the clinically positive neck. Am J Surg 1996;172:654–7.

39. Fletcher GH. Elective irradiation of subclinical disease in cancers of the head and neck. Cancer 1972;29:1450.

40. Goffinet DR, Willard EF, Goode RL. Combined surgery and postoperative irradiation in the treatment of cervical lymph nodes. Arch Otolaryngol Head Neck Surg 1994;110:736–8.

41. Leemans CR, Tiwari R, Van der Waal I, et al. The efficacy of comprehensive neck dissection with or without postoperative radiotherapy in nodal metastases of squamous cell carcinoma of the upper respiratory and digestive tracts. Laryngoscope 1990;100:1194–8.

42. Huang DT, Johnson CR, Schmidt-Uhlrich R, Grimes M. Postoperative radiotherapy in head and neck carcinoma with extracapsular lymph node extension and/or positive margins: a comparative study. Int J Radiat Oncol Biol Phys 1992;23:737–42.

43. Tupchong L, Scott CB, Blitzer PH, et al. Randomized study of preoperative versus postoperative radiation therapy in advanced head and neck carcinoma: Long-term follow-up of RTOG Study 73-03. Int J Radiat Oncol Biol Phys 1991;20:21–8.

44. Lavertu P, Bonafede JP, Adelstein DJ, et al. Comparison of surgical complications after organ preservation therapy in patients with stage III or IV squamous cell head and neck cancer. Arch Otolaryngol Head Neck Surg 1998;124:401–6.

45. Davidson BJ, Newkirk KA, Harter KW, et al. Complications from planned posttreatment neck dissections. Arch Otolaryngol Head Neck Surg 1999;125:401–5.

46. Bocca E, Pignataro O, Oldini C, Cappa C. Functional neck dissection: an evaluation and review of 843 cases. Laryngoscope 1984;94:942–5.

47. Byers RM. Modified neck dissection. Am J Surg 1985;150:414–21.

48. Spiro RK, Morgan GJ, Strong EW, Shah JP. Supraomohyoid neck dissection. Am J Surg 1996;172:650–3.

49. Traynor SJ, Cohen JI, Gray J, et al. Selective neck dissection and the management of the node-positive neck. Am J Surg 1996;172:654–7.

50. Collins SL. Controversies in management of cancer of the neck. In: Thawley, Panje, Batsakis, et al. editors. Comprehensive management of head and neck tumors. New York: WB Saunders; 1999. p. 1479–1563.

51. Vetto JT, Lum S, Morris A, et al. Presence of the T-cell activation marker OX-40 on tumor infiltrating lymphocytes and draining lymph node cells from patients with melanoma and head and neck cancers. Am J Surg 1997;174:258–65.

52. Vitolo D, Letessier EM, Johnson JT, Whiteside TL. Immunologic effector cells in head and neck cancer. J Natl Cancer Inst Monogr 1992;16:203–8.

53. Romero P, Dunbar R, Valmori D, et al. Ex vivo staining of metastatic lymph nodes by class I major histocompatibility complex tetramers reveals high numbers of antigen-experienced tumor-specific cytolytic T lymphocytes. J Exp Med 1998;188:1641–50.

54. Wang MB, Lichtenstein A, Mickel RA. Hierarchical immunosuppression of regional lymph nodes in patients with head and neck squamous cell carcinoma. Otolaryngol Head Neck Surg 1991;105:517–27.

16

Neurogenic and Vascular Tumors of the Head and Neck

PAUL A. KEDESHIAN, MD

JATIN P. SHAH, MD, FACS

Neurovascular tumors of the head and neck are a varied group of neoplasms that can present clinically as isolated masses or in association with various familial syndromes. The majority of neurovascular tumors are benign lesions that can potentially exhibit local destruction from expansile growth, while some are overtly malignant, with aggressive growth capabilities and obvious metastatic potential. While the treatment for these lesions is overwhelmingly surgical, the selected treatment must carefully balance the functional and cosmetic sequelae of surgery against the indolent behavior of most of these tumors. This review will separately consider some of the more frequently encountered types of neurovascular tumors, emphasizing general principles of anatomy, diagnosis, treatment, and rehabilitation where applicable.

VASCULAR TUMORS

Hemangiomas

Hemangiomas are the most common tumor of the neonate/infant, occurring most often in the head and neck.[1] The terminology used to categorize these predominantly pediatric vasoformative tumors can be quite confusing and cumbersome. While capillary, cavernous, and mixed types of hemangiomas differ from one another with respect to their depth of penetration, a great deal of overlap within a particular tumor can be present.[2,3] For the purposes of this discussion, all hemangiomas will be considered together, and the biologic classification proposed by Mulliken and Glowacki will serve as the basis for distinguishing hemangiomas from other types of vascular malformations.[4] In this schema, hemangiomas are defined as vascular lesions: (1) that present in the neonatal period, (2) that demonstrate proliferative and then involutional growth patterns, and (3) whose endothelial cells exhibit increased mitotic activity during proliferation. The other major category of vasoformative growths to differentiate from hemangiomas are the vascular malformations, described as neonatal growths that: (1) fail to involute, (2) grow proportionately with the infant, and (3) demonstrate no endothelial cell proliferation.[4]

Anatomy

Head and neck hemangiomas, comprising as many as 0.5 percent of all head and neck neoplasms, commonly present at cutaneous sites (scalp, neck, face, ear, lip, nose), although they may arise within the musculature or deep soft tissues of the head and neck, as well as within the mucosa of the upper aerodigestive tract (subglottic larynx).[5] Vascular malformations on the other hand, usually are restricted to specific dermatomes, frequently presenting within the cutaneous territories innervated by one of the branches of the trigeminal nerve. The discussion that follows concentrates exclusively on hemangiomas of the head and neck.

Diagnosis

Hemangiomas usually present as erythematous, raised, mobile, cutaneous masses that appear at or

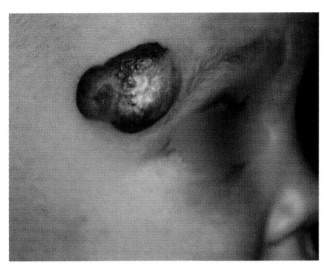

Figure 16–1. Cutaneous hemangioma.

soon after birth (Figure 16–1). This characteristic appearance, occasionally coupled with the reported history of rapid proliferation during early childhood (with or without subsequent involution), is usually adequate for diagnosis. Accordingly, biopsy of these lesions is rarely if ever performed or indicated unless a malignant neoplasm is suggested by aggressive invasion of local structures.

In those hemangiomas that arise deep within the substance of either the parotid gland or neck musculature (masseter, sternocleidomastoid, scalene or trapezius muscles), a mobile, ill-defined, deep neck mass without any overlying skin changes is the usual presentation (Figure 16–2).[5] The diagnosis of these hemangiomas may be confirmed by radiographic imaging with intravenous contrast (CT/MRI) that will demonstrate varying degrees of contrast enhancement.[5,6]

In the case of hemangiomas of the upper aerodigestive tract, the medical history and physical findings may include intermittent stridor (especially with crying or exertion), the concurrent presence of a cutaneous hemangioma (present in approximately 50% of children), or rarely, hemoptysis.[7] Endoscopically, the presence of an erythematous mass in the posterior subglottic region is frequently appreciated.[8]

Treatment

Prior to considering the treatment options available for hemangiomas, the natural history of these lesions needs to be appreciated. The vast majority of cutaneous hemangiomas will spontaneously undergo involution with approximately half having regressed by age 5, 70 percent by age 7, and as many as 90 percent by the onset of puberty.[9] However, it must be recognized that, even after complete regression, residual masses of fibrofatty tissue may remain. These masses can cause significant cosmetic and functional sequelae, particularly if a hemangioma arises from the nose, ear or lip.[1,9] Thus, determining which hemangiomas require treatment and the type and extent of treatment can be quite complicated.

The objectives of any proposed treatment beyond careful initial evaluation, parental reassurance, and monitoring for the development of complications (ulceration) must be very carefully defined. Exceptions to such a conservative approach to the treatment of hemangiomas are in the case of either a cutaneous hemangioma that arises from the periocular region that may require early treatment in order to prevent the development of disastrous functional consequences (deprivational amblyopia)[3] or a subglottic hemangioma that may require early treatment for airway compromise.[3]

In most cases, the surgical excision of all but the most pedunculated, cutaneous hemangiomas that are in a location that permits excision with camouflage of the surgical scar is questionable. The exception to this is that of periorbital hemangioma previously alluded to whose excision is considered a surgical emergency.[3] In the case of subglottic hemangiomas requiring treatment for airway compromise, the initial role for surgery may be in the establishment of an airway via a tracheostomy, with laser excision only considered for small, well-circumscribed lesions secondary to the risk of subglottic stenosis.[8,10] In the rare situation where an intramuscular hemangioma is suspected of causing functional compromise secondary to the compression of adjacent structures, surgical excision can be accomplished, keeping in mind the higher rate of recurrence of these tumors secondary to their more infiltrative pattern of growth.[6]

More commonly, nonsurgical modalities are employed for the treatment of hemangiomas. As the physics of lasers have become better understood and the technology for their precise delivery has

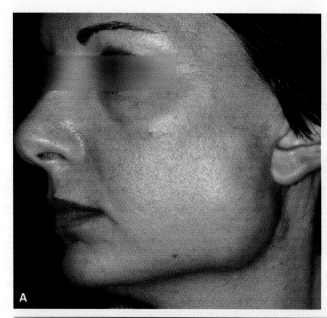

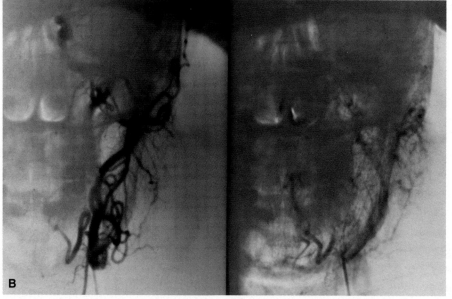

Figure 16–2. *A*, Parotid hemangio-lymphangioma. *B*, Angiogram.

advanced, this mode of treatment for cutaneous hemangiomas has gained popularity. Yellow light lasers (λ 578 to 985 nm) allow for their light to be preferentially absorbed by hemoglobin with only melanin acting as a mild competing chromophore. These yellow light lasers (which take the form of either a copper vapor laser or a flashlamp pulsed dye laser) allow for selective photo-thermolysis and have been used to treat hemangiomas. However, some of the original enthusiasm for the use of lasers to treat hemangiomas has dissipated as it has become apparent that due to the very superficial depth of penetration of these lasers (approximately

1.2 mm), they are only effective for the most superficial, plaque-like hemangiomas and, if used to treat lesions that have a deeper component, may leave these areas entirely untreated.[3]

In addition to the use of lasers for the treatment of hemangiomas, intra-tumoral and systemic steroid treatment for massive and life-threatening hemangiomas have long been employed, with approximately one-third of tumors showing a dramatic response within 1 week of treatment.[11] Corticosteroids in the range of 2 to 4 mg/kg/day appear to be tolerated quite well with acceptably low levels of toxicity (growth retardation, immunocompromise, hypertension),[3] however, steroids are generally regarded as a temporizing measure to effectively control the sequelae of a hemangioma's proliferative growth phase. More recently, the anti-angiogenic properties of interferon alfa-2a have been used for the treatment of massive and life-threatening hemangiomas,[12,13] while the anti-angiogenic properties of TNP-470, an agent initially developed to treat malignant tumors, has been found to demonstrate effectiveness in preclinical hemangioma model systems.[14] However, these treatments are not without significant risk as interferon alfa-2a can cause spastic diplegia.[11]

Cystic Hygroma

Cystic hygromas are rare malformations of the lymphatic system that usually present in infancy or in the neonatal period. While 90 percent of cystic hygromas present by 2 years of age, initial presentation in adulthood can occur.[2,5] Unlike hemangiomas, these lesions do not demonstrate spontaneous regression and therefore nearly always require treatment.[15]

Anatomy and Diagnosis

Although cystic hygromas can occur anywhere in the body, greater than 90 percent of these lesions are encountered in the head and neck, with the vast majority in the lateral neck and very few within the substance of the tongue.[15,16] These lesions usually present as soft, easily compressible, fluctuant, ill-defined posterior neck masses that may come to clinical attention following a recent upper respiratory infection (Figure 16–3). Other neck masses that should be considered in the differential diagnosis of cystic hygromas include lipomas, branchial cleft cysts, lymphomas, and thyroglossal duct cysts, however the clinical presentation and history, supplemented by radiographic imaging of the neck (CT with intravenous contrast), will usually make the diagnosis quite apparent.[17]

Treatment

Cystic hygromas are most successfully treated by complete surgical excision, preserving adjacent neurovascular structures, although multiple needle aspirations, the injection of sclerosing agents, and even radiation therapy have previously been employed.[18] The growth pattern of many cystic hygromas, with multiple superficial and deep extensions that insinuate between surrounding structures, can make complete removal a formidable challenge and likely accounts for the recurrences not infrequently encountered.[15,17] Moreover, multiple potential complications of surgery for cystic hygroma have been described including cranial nerve injury, chyle fistula formation, and wound infection, emphasizing

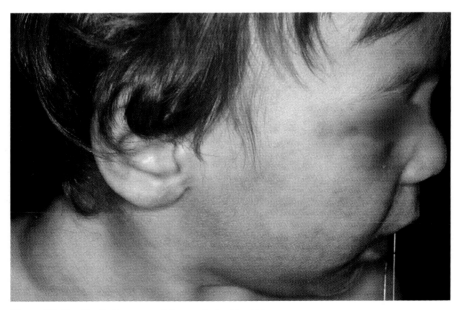

Figure 16–3.　Cystic hygroma of the posterior triangle.

the need for a conservative and meticulous surgical approach to these lesions.[15,16,18]

Hemangiopericytoma

Anatomy

Hemangiopericytomas are malignant tumors that arise from the capillary pericytes (pericytes of Zimmermann), structures within the outer capillary wall that are responsible for regulating the size of the capillary lumen.[19] These mesenchymal tumors can arise in any age group and from anywhere in the body that capillaries are present, with the extremities, pelvis, and retroperitoneum as the most common locations.[5] Approximately one-quarter of all hemangiopericytomas arise in head and neck sites with half of these originating in the sinonasal cavity, and the remainder arising from the neck, orbit, parotid, and oral cavity.[20,21] For reasons that are not entirely clear, hemangiopericytomas that arise from capillaries in the head and neck behave in a much less malignant fashion than their non-head and neck counterparts.[22]

Diagnosis

When it presents in the sinonasal cavity, a hemangiopericytoma frequently causes nasal obstruction and epistaxis. Clinically, an erythematous hemorrhagic mass is visible (Figure 16–4).[23] Radiographic imaging will frequently demonstrate a mass causing bone erosion that manifests enhancement with intravenous contrast administration. The other entities that must be considered in the differential diagnosis of sinonasal hemangiopericytoma include juvenile nasopharyngeal angiofibroma, pyogenic granuloma, and any benign or malignant spindle cell lesion of the sinonasal cavity.[23] When it arises from other sites in the head and neck, a hemangiopericytoma often presents as a painless, slowly enlarging vascular-appearing mass that can occasionally invade local structures through relentless growth.[24–26]

Whether it arises from the sinonasal area or elsewhere in the head and neck, the cytologic diagnosis of hemangiopericytoma, as with other spindle cell neoplasms, can be quite challenging, due to the absence of tissue architecture.[19] Therefore, the definitive diagnosis of a hemangiopericytoma usually relies upon suggestive clinical findings coupled with a tissue biopsy that demonstrates a well-vascularized submucosal or subcutaneous tumor containing irregular vascular spaces.[19]

Treatment

The treatment of choice for head and neck hemangiopericytomas is surgical resection. When these tumors arise from the sinonasal region, such a resection frequently involves an anterior craniofacial approach in order to ensure complete tumor exposure and *en bloc* excision. During such resections, neck dissection is not electively performed as the lungs are the overwhelming site of metastasis rather than the regional lymphatics.[5] At other head and neck sites, the surgical approach selected must afford the opportunity to completely encompass the tumor mass.

The results of treatment for head and neck hemangiopericytomas seem to favor a less aggressive biology as compared to the same histology at other body sites, although local recurrence of tumor in as many as 50 percent of patients may occur.[22] While the rarity of this tumor's occurrence in the head and neck precludes the existence of large series upon which to directly assess treatment results, if one extrapolates from the results of the treatment of other low-grade sarcomas of the head and neck, small primary tumor size and surgery that can achieve negative surgical margins are important prognostic features.[27]

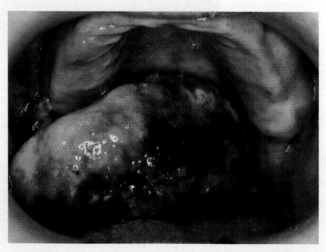

Figure 16–4. Hemangiopericytoma of the palate and maxilla.

While the literature includes many case descriptions of the use of radiotherapy for the treatment of hemangiopericytomas, particularly in the case of microscopically positive or close surgical margins or surgically inoperable lesions, the benefit of such therapy is unproven.[24,27,28] Finally, isolated descriptions of the use of a variety of chemotherapeutic regimens for distant metastases have not revealed any significant or durable clinical responses.[29]

Juvenile Nasopharyngeal Angiofibroma

Anatomy

Juvenile nasopharyngeal angiofibroma (JNA) is a rare, benign, vascular neoplasm that arises almost exclusively in adolescent males. JNAs arise in the area of the sphenopalatine foramen, at the junction of the palatine bone, the vomer, and the pterygoid root.[30] These tumors receive their predominant blood supply from branches of the external carotid artery (internal maxillary), although an internal carotid arterial supply can also be present.[31] With the introduction of computerized tomography (CT), assessment of the true anatomic extent of these tumors became possible, prompting the description of multiple staging systems, all of which attempt to assess the degree to which the tumor has extended out of the nasopharynx.[30,32,33] The simplest of these staging systems, first described by Chandler, identifies tumors that are confined to the nasopharynx (stage I), those that have extended anteriorly or superiorly into either the nasal cavity or sphenoid sinus (stage II), those that have extended into the paranasal sinuses or more laterally into the cheek and infratemporal fossa (stage III), and those tumors that extend intracranially (stage IV).[32]

Diagnosis

JNAs typically present with nasal obstruction and intermittent epistaxis in an adolescent male with nasal endoscopy revealing a vascular nasopharyngeal or nasal cavity mass (Figure 16–5).[34,35] Radiographically, the presence of a contrast-enhancing lesion in the nasopharynx with variable degrees of extension into contiguous structures may be appar-

ent (Figure 16–6). Moreover, magnetic resonance angiography (MRA) or conventional angiography can strikingly delineate the vascular nature of these tumors, identify the arteries that constitute their vascular supply, and permit subsequent embolization (Figure 16–7).[31,36–38] The differential diagnosis of these nasopharyngeal tumors includes hemangiopericytomas and antro-choanal polyps.

Biopsy of these tumors is rarely, if ever, indicated and can result in life-threatening epistaxis due to their extensive vascularity.

Treatment

The presumed endocrine-responsive nature of these tumors has long been appreciated, stimulating a trial of androgen-blocking agents as a potential treatment adjunct.[39] Despite these and other nonsurgical therapies, the preferred treatment for JNAs is complete surgical excision, often preceded by angiography and embolization to minimize the risk of intraoperative blood loss.[31,36,38] Although some regard intracranial extension and/or internal carotid artery vascular supply as contraindications to surgical resection,[31] the use of intracranial and skull base approaches for these extensive tumors has been described.[37,40] Recently, endoscopic intranasal surgical resection of

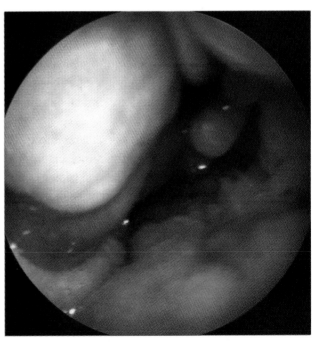

Figure 16–5. Juvenile nasopharyngeal angiofibroma (JNA).

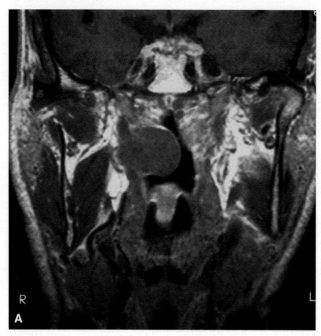 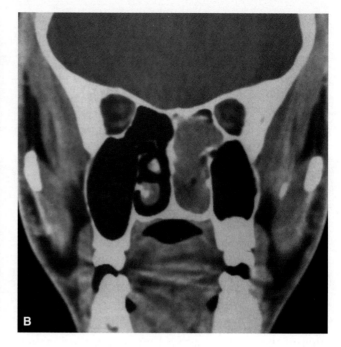

Figure 16–6.   *A,* MRI of JNA. *B,* CT of JNA.

JNAs has also been described and proposed for selected small lesions.[40,41]

Radiation therapy has been proposed as a treatment alternative to surgical resection for extensive tumors,[42,43] as well as postsurgical recurrences.[44] Total radiation doses of 20 to 30 Gy (approximately 150 cGy/fraction) have been reported to yield nearly 100 percent tumor growth arrest with minimal observable morbidity.[42,43] However, the long-term effects of radiation on facial development in this adolescent patient population are not known,[40] nor are the potential risks of radiation-induced malignant transformation.[45,46] Chemotherapy has even been suggested as a potential treatment option for extensive recurrent JNAs.[47]

The surgical approach that is used for the treatment of JNA will depend upon the tumor extent that is apparent on preoperative clinical and radiographic examination.[40] Surgical approaches include a transpalatal approach for small lesions confined to the midline, a medial maxillectomy approach for lesions with a greater degree of lateral extension, and craniofacial, infratemporal fossa, and facial translocation approaches for more extensive tumors. While no sufficiently large clinical series of various tumor stages exists in order to assess the efficacy of surgery as a single treatment modality, results taken

from a variety of small series seem to suggest that surgical resection is associated with a less than 10 percent rate of recurrence in smaller tumors and as much as a 40 percent risk of recurrence in more extensive tumors.[31,40]

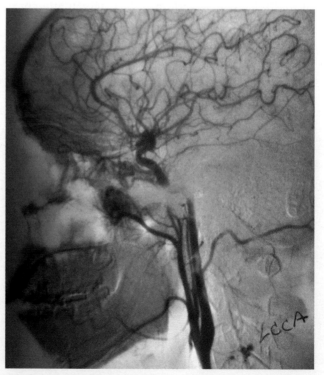

Figure 16–7.   Angiogram of JNA.

Paragangliomas

Introduction

The extra-adrenal paraganglia are neural crest-derived rests of tissue that migrate to sites in the body in close association with cranial nerves, the aorta and its branches.[48] These paraganglia are composed of two predominant cell types: the sustentacular cells and the chief cells. The sustentacular cells are modified Schwann cells whereas the chief cells produce and can release catecholamines and other neurotransmitter substances.[19,48] The tumors that arise from these cell rests, the paragangliomas, can occasionally release neurotransmitter substances or demonstrate malignant behavior.[49,50]

While paragangliomas produce symptoms of neurotransmitter excess (tachycardia, flushing, palpitations) only very rarely (< 5%),[49] when this occurs, the hemodynamic effects of such functional tumors can be dramatic.[51] Moreover, physical manipulation of nonfunctional tumors can occasionally result in the intravenous release of neurotransmitters and subsequent symptoms.[52]

As surgery is the most commonly employed treatment for these tumors, pre- and intraoperative anesthetic precautions for potential neurotransmitter release must be observed.[51] Such precautions include careful preoperative questioning regarding the intermittent occurrence of any symptoms referable to neurotransmitter release (tachycardia, palpitations, headache, flushing) and a detailed family history seeking to identify relatives with similar tumors or symptoms (see below). When potential symptoms of a functional tumor are suggested, preoperative screening should include the measurement of plasma and urinary levels of catecholamines as well as their metabolites (metanephrine, VMA).[51] The pre- and intraoperative use of α- and β-adrenergic blockade are important agents that can reduce the anesthetic risk associated with the treatment of these tumors.

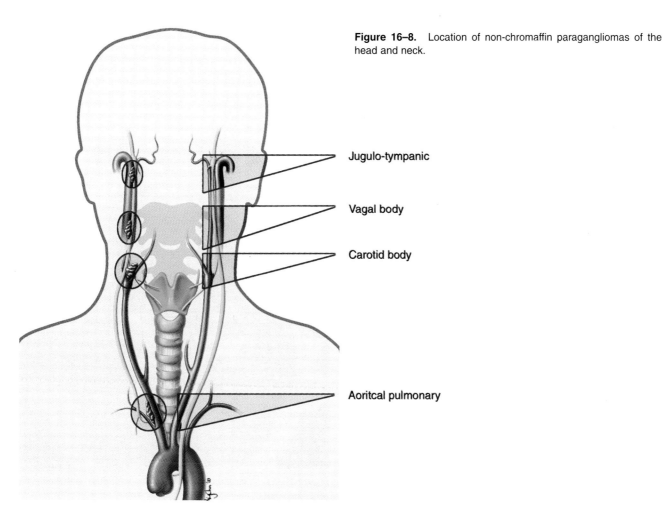

Figure 16–8. Location of non-chromaffin paragangliomas of the head and neck.

Jugulo-tympanic

Vagal body

Carotid body

Aoritcal pulmonary

An additional consideration in the treatment of patients with paragangliomas relates to the familial incidence of these tumors as well as the occurrence of multiple paragangliomas in the same patient. Although the vast majority of paragangliomas occur spontaneously, as many as 10 percent can occur as part of an autosomal dominantly-inherited condition with incomplete penetrance.[53] Recently, genetic linkage studies have suggested that the gene responsible for familial paragangliomas is located on the long arm of chromosome 11.[54,55] These familial paragangliomas, as compared to their sporadic counterparts, are more commonly bilateral, multicentric, and become clinically apparent at a younger age.[53,56,57]

Paragangliomas of the head and neck are commonly named according to the major neurovascular structures with which they are associated. Within the head and neck, three of the most common paragangliomas are the carotid body tumor, the glomus jugulare, and the glomus intravagale (Figure 16–8).

Carotid Body

Anatomy

The carotid body is a discrete paraganglion located in the adventitia of the posteromedial aspect of the carotid bifurcation.[58] It functions as a chemoreceptor, responding to changes in arterial oxygen, carbon diox-

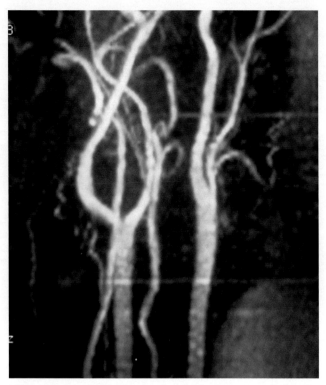

Figure 16–10. MRA showing carotid body tumor splaying the carotid arteries.

ide, and pH by regulating ventilation.[58,59] Individuals who live at high altitudes, chronically exposed to oxygen of a lower partial pressure than that at sea level,

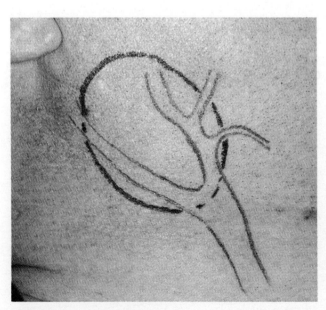

Figure 16–9. Carotid body tumor.

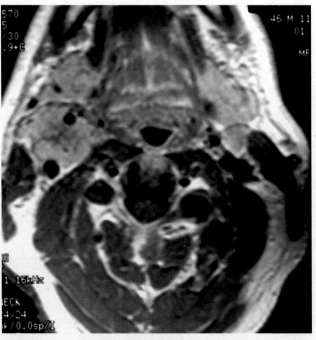

Figure 16–11. Carotid body MRI ("salt and pepper" enhancement with flow voids).

appear to have an increased risk of developing sporadic (non-familial) carotid body tumors.[59,60]

Diagnosis

A carotid body tumor most commonly presents as a painless neck mass with limited superior-inferior mobility, near the angle of the mandible, during the fifth decade of life (Figure 16–9).[58,59] Computed tomography (CT) and magnetic resonance imaging (MRI) characteristically reveal splaying of the internal and external carotid arteries (Figure 16–10). While intense contrast enhancement on CT is seen, a "salt and pepper" pattern on MRI may be appreciated secondary to the presence of flow voids within the tumor (Figure 16–11).[61,62] The pattern of displacement of the neurovascular structures in the vicinity of the mass, coupled with the clinical examination, usually is sufficient to confirm the diagnosis of a carotid body tumor.

Treatment

The treatment for carotid body tumors is surgical excision. The surgical approach to these tumors is via a horizontal neck incision at approximately the level of the carotid bifurcation. Meticulous hemostasis at all stages of the operative procedure, and the establishment of proximal and distal control of the carotid artery are mandatory, as is proficiency in vascular surgery (or assistance) if patch grafting or venous replacement become necessary. When preoperative evaluation suggests that carotid body tumor removal might require intraoperative interruption of carotid artery flow, balloon occlusion studies to assess the cerebral blood flow should be obtained.[63] Careful identification and preservation of the integrity of the marginal branch of the facial nerve and the lower cranial nerves is to be expected. Due to the location of the carotid body, a sub-adventitial plane of tumor dissection is required, a maneuver that does not appear to compromise the integrity of the artery.[64]

Surgical resection of these tumors with minimal morbidity should be the treatment goal. The structures most likely to be injured when resecting a carotid body tumor include the superior laryngeal nerve, vagus nerve, and the hypoglossal nerve.[58] In patients with bilateral carotid body tumors, surgical resection of the smaller tumor should be attempted first with a period of 3 to 6 months elapsing prior to resection of the contralateral tumor. Patients undergoing bilateral carotid body resection may demonstrate markedly labile postoperative blood pressure, a phenomenon thought to be due to the complete loss of carotid sinus function as a secondary consequence of the dissection and removal of the carotid body tumors.[58] However, this lability diminishes with time as alternative blood pressure regulatory mechanisms appear to compensate.

While meticulously-performed surgical resection is unquestionably the treatment of choice for carotid body tumors, the use of radiotherapy as primary treatment for these neoplasms (particularly extensive tumors whose excision might be associated with significant morbidity) has been reported.[65] The rationale for such treatment derives from the fact that although these tumors are minimally radiosensitive, radiotherapy likely produces fibrosis of the tumor's vasculature and therefore can arrest tumor growth.[65]

Glomus Jugulare

The jugulotympanic region is the site of origin for two types of paragangliomas. The glomus tympanicum arises from either a branch of the vagus nerve (posterior auricular branch of Arnold) or a branch of the glossopharyngeal nerve (tympanic branch of Jacobson), while the glomus jugulare arises from the jugular bulb itself. As the majority of jugulotympanic tumors are of jugular bulb origin, the discussion that follows will focus exclusively on these tumors.[19]

Anatomy

The glomus jugulare tumor is a slow-growing lesion that arises from the paraganglionic tissue of the jugular bulb at the skull base.[48] Anatomically, this area of the cranial base is in close proximity to the internal carotid artery, cranial nerves IX, X, XI, XII, and the internal auditory canal. As lesions of the skull base are exceedingly difficult to appreciate clinically, these tumors are often not identified until they begin to cause some degree of cranial nerve dysfunction from expansile growth.[64]

Diagnosis

The most common presenting symptoms of a glomus jugulare tumor include tinnitus, hearing loss, vocal cord paralysis, diminished gag reflex, and tongue deviation.[67] On physical examination, the presence of a vascular mass medial to an intact tympanic membrane (due to tumor erosion of the bony hypotympanum) can be seen.[66] Radiographically, these tumors are best diagnosed and subsequently assessed by a combination of CT and MRI with contrast enhancement.[68] While CT imaging can best demonstrate the details of bony erosion at the skull base as well as the proximity of the tumor to the structures of the temporal bone (Figure 6–12), MRI can delineate the relationship of the tumor mass to adjacent neurovascular structures.[68]

Treatment

The optimal treatment of a glomus jugulare tumor depends upon a combination of both patient and tumor factors. The morbidity that can often accompany the surgical resection of these tumors primarily relates to paresis or paralysis of the facial nerve as well as the lower cranial nerves.[67] While the treatment of a particular tumor in a specific patient needs to be individualized, there is general agreement that the optimal treatment of this benign, slow-growing tumor of the skull base in older patients is nonsurgical.[67,68] In younger patients, however, the issue of what is the optimal treatment is unresolved.

Radiotherapy for glomus jugulare tumors, as is the case with carotid body tumors, is believed to cause fibrosis of the tumor's vascular elements, leading to growth arrest.[65,69] In an extensive review of 24 major series of glomus jugulare tumors treated by either primary surgery or radiotherapy, both modalities yielded similar rates of post-treatment persistent and recurrent disease (8% and 7% respectively).[70] While there was extensive variability among the studies with respect to follow-up and treatment modality selection, the similar results suggest that the morbidity of a particular treatment may be the most important determinant for treatment selection.

The surgical approach to glomus jugulare tumors requires adequate access and visualization of both the tumor and the vital neurovascular structures of

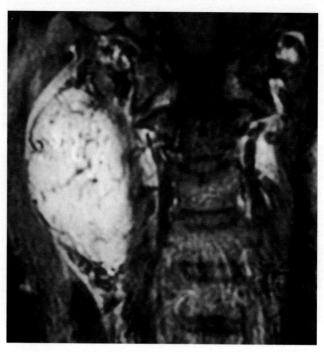

Figure 16–12. MRI showing Glomus jugulare at the base of the skull.

the cranial base. Based upon a careful review of preoperative imaging studies (CT, MRI, MRA), the likelihood of intraoperative interruption of carotid circulation needs to be assessed and, if deemed to be a significant risk, a preoperative balloon occlusion study should be obtained.

The most common approach for these tumors is some variation of the approach to the infratemporal fossa first described by Fisch.[71] In this approach, which includes exposure of the mastoid segment of the facial nerve and the upper lateral neck, the facial nerve is identified and then anteriorly translocated. While this approach permits safe access to both the internal carotid artery and the jugular bulb at the skull base, it can potentially result in paresis or paralysis of the facial mimetic musculature.[67,71]

The morbidity of surgical resection of glomus jugulare tumors, with paresis or paralysis of the lower cranial nerves (IX through XII), can be rehabilitated in order to improve postoperative function and quality of life. In particular, vocal cord paralysis that results from injury to the vagus nerve is frequently compensated for by the contralateral vocal cord over a period of months. However, in those cases where inadequate compensation is present with aspiration and/or incomplete adduction, the paralyzed vocal cord can be surgically medialized, restoring glottic closure.[72] Isolated paralysis of the spinal accessory nerve mandates the institution of an aggressive postoperative physical therapy regimen to minimize the development of significant shoulder pain and joint restriction.[73] While isolated paralysis of either the glossopharyngeal or hypoglossal nerves will not cause significant morbidity and may only require speech and swallowing therapy for rehabilitation, bilateral paralyses of these or the other nerves as well as combinations of nerve injuries (ie, simultaneous hypoglossal and vagus injuries) may cause significant problems with deglutition and/or respiration—necessitating tracheostomy, gastrostomy or both.

Glomus Intravagale

Anatomy

Glomera intravagale are tumors that arise from the paraganglionic tissue of the vagus nerve's perineurium.[48] These tumors usually present at approximately the level of the inferior vagal ganglion (nodosum) although tumors as far inferior as the carotid bifurcation and as far superior as the jugular foramen have been described.[48]

Diagnosis

Glomus intravagale frequently presents as a neck mass near the origin of the sternocleidomastoid muscle in association with paralysis of the ipsilateral vocal cord (Figure 16–13).[48,66] With progressive tumor growth, a Horner's syndrome frequently develops, as do multiple cranial neuropathies and pharyngeal pain secondary to irritation of the pharyngeal plexus.[66] Radiographic imaging demonstrates the presence of a mass in the posterior portion of the carotid sheath that displaces the carotid artery anteriorly (Figure 16–14). The differential diagnosis for a glomus intravagale includes neural tumors (neurofibromas and schwannomas) that arise from the lower cranial nerves or the cervical sympathetic chain. Unlike the other paragangliomas which manifest very low rates of malignant transformation and distant metastasis, glomus intravagale may

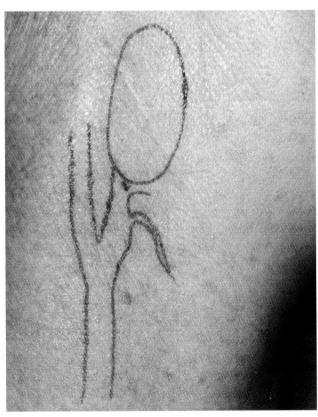

Figure 16–13. Glomus intravagale.

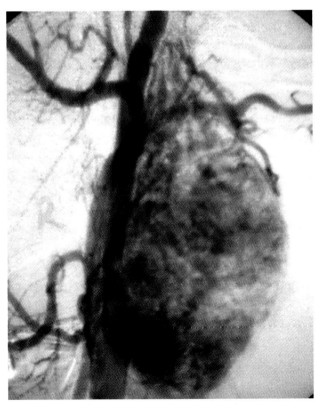

Figure 16–14. Glomus intravagale on angiogram, displacing carotid sheath structures.

metastasize in nearly 20 percent of cases with pulmonary metastases occurring most commonly.[66]

Treatment

The pretreatment considerations and surgical approaches for the treatment of glomus intravagale tumors mirror those mentioned previously for glomus jugulare. The major differences, however, are the fact that more than half of glomera intravagale present with nerve paralyses (compared to only about one-third of glomus jugulare), complete resection of a glomus intravagale necessitates sacrifice of the vagus nerve at or near the skull base. Glomus intravagale tumors do not manifest intracranial extension as commonly as jugulare tumors do.[66]

NEURAL TUMORS

Schwannoma

Anatomy

Schwannomas or neurilemmomas are solitary, predominantly benign, well-encapsulated tumors that arise from the Schwann cells of the peripheral nerve sheath.[74] While these tumors can arise from nerves throughout the body, as many as one-half occur within the head and neck,[75] and demonstrate a slight female predominance, presenting most commonly in the fourth and fifth decades.[19] Within the head and neck, schwannomas can arise from the eighth cranial nerve (acoustic neuroma), the vagus nerve, or the sympathetic chain, and less commonly from cranial nerves VII, IX, XI, XII, the cervical nerve roots, the brachial plexus, and the sinonasal tract (maxillary/ophthalmic branches of trigeminal nerve or autonomic ganglia)[19,74–80] As they grow, these tumors manifest a pushing pattern of expansion potentially permitting the separation and preservation of the integrity of the nerve from which they arise (Figure 16–15).[74,76] This review will focus on schwannomas that arise from neural structures in the neck. While a discussion of facial schwannomas and acoustic neuromas is beyond the scope of this review, the reader is referred to textbooks of otology and neurotology for a more comprehensive treatment of these tumors.

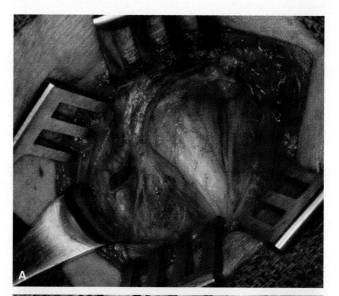
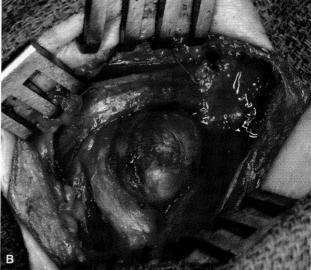
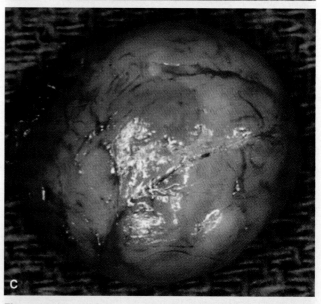

Figure 16–15. *A,* Schwannoma of the brachial plexus. *B,* Schwannoma attached to its nerve of origin. *C,* Surgical resection specimen.

Diagnosis

Clinically, schwannomas present as solitary, painless, lateral neck masses with evidence of either intact nerve function or only subtle dysfunction. For sinonasal schwannomas, endoscopic evidence of a polypoid mass with epistaxis and nasal obstruction may be present.[77–79] Radiographically, while no pathognomonic imaging features are apparent, a schwannoma will usually appear as a well-circumscribed, contrast-enhancing mass that is contiguous with an identifiable neural structure (particularly on MRI). The contrast enhancement on a CT scan is modest and not as intense as a paraganglioma, which is quite vascular. Additionally, a suggestion as to the nerve of origin may be offered by the pattern of displacement of contiguous structures that the schwannoma causes.

The diagnostic interpretation, by needle aspiration biopsy, of these benign spindle cell tumors can be difficult in the absence of tissue architecture and is frequently uninformative. Moreover, when this slow-growing mass has been present for a protracted period of time, cystic degeneration, hemorrhagic necrosis and calcification may be apparent in these so-called ancient schwannomas, further complicating cytologic diagnosis.[74] Histopathologically, schwannomas demonstrate two classic patterns of growth: the Antoni A pattern is composed of cells in a compact, orderly alignment, while the Antoni B pattern is much less cellular and has a myxoid type of appearance.[19,74] Additionally, schwannomas often demonstrate an orderly cellular alignment with nuclear palisading, referred to as Verocay bodies.[19]

Treatment

Schwannomas are most effectively treated by surgical excision; however, these benign tumors of minimal malignant potential grow in a manner that usually, but not always, permits separation and preservation of their nerve of origin. Therefore, considerations of surgical morbidity should be included when selecting a treatment modality.

Although clinical and radiographic information may suggest the diagnosis of a schwannoma, the precise nerve of origin may not be apparent until the tumor is surgically exposed. Consequently, the potential for postoperative nerve dysfunction resulting in vocal cord paralysis, Horner's syndrome, shoulder dysfunction, or other deficits must always be considered.[17]

Surgical exposure of the tumor and the presumed nerve of origin is usually obtained via a mid-neck horizontal incision with every attempt made to preserve the anatomic integrity of nerve branches that can be identified and separated from the tumor. The surgeon must be aware of the fact that, with some schwannomas that have attained a significant size, the chances

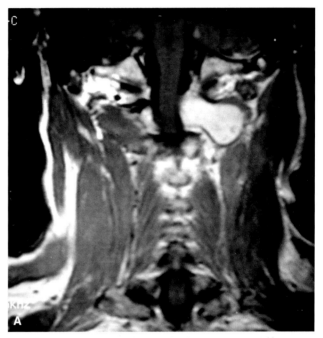

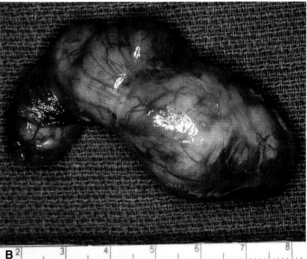

Figure 16–16. *A,* MRI showing a dumbbell neurofibroma of the neck. *B,* Surgical resection specimen of a dumbbell neurofibroma of the neck.

of compromise of adjacent neurovascular structures secondary to the surgical procedure (in addition to the nerve of origin) can add an additional element of potential morbidity to the operative procedure.

In the case of schwannomas arising from the cervical roots, a portion of the tumor may extend into the lateral neck while another component may pass within the intravertebral foramen. These tumors may thus adopt a dumbbell type configuration (Figure 16–16).[74] Such tumors may be optimally resected through neurosurgical/head and neck surgical collaboration. When a peripheral nerve sheath tumor is suspected of arising from any of the roots of the brachial plexus, the use of preoperative EMG for the assessment of subtle muscle dysfunction as well as the intraoperative use of nerve monitoring may be helpful.[80,81]

As previously noted, schwannomas are slow-growing tumors with approximate growth rates of 1 mm/year. Consequently, unless there is rapid recent growth suggestive of malignant transformation, careful clinical observation of a tumor whose surgical removal might result in significant morbidity has been advocated. Such a strategy of observation is most frequently advocated in the management of schwannomas in the elderly or patients who are poor surgical candidates. However, it must be recognized that the morbidity of surgical resection and the potential for incomplete tumor excision will likely increase with increased tumor size, therefore early intervention is preferable in most situations.

In addition to surgical excision and careful observation, there is a growing body of evidence (particularly with respect to schwannomas arising from the eighth cranial nerve), for the use of external beam radiotherapy (so-called stereotactic radiosurgery or the "gamma knife") for the treatment of schwannomas. Recently, the long-term results of the treatment of schwannomas of the eighth cranial nerve with radiosurgery have demonstrated excellent rates of tumor control with preservation of nerve function and minimal treatment-related morbidity (hearing loss).[82]

Malignant Schwannomas

While the majority of schwannomas are benign in their clinical behavior, approximately 5 percent of them manifest malignant clinical behavior with a

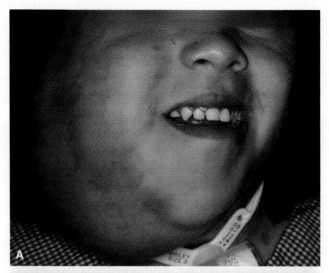

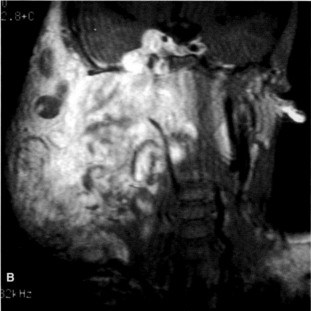

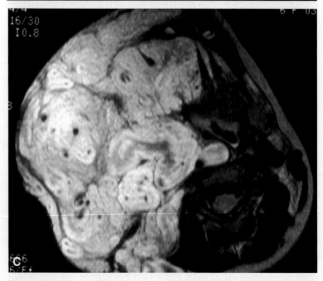

Figure 16–17.   *A,* Plexiform neurofibromat. *B* and *C,* MRI of plexiform neurofibromat.

small minority of these arising within the head and neck.[74,83] These malignant variants can demonstrate high mitotic activity, aggressive local infiltrative growth with a high recurrence rate, pulmonary metastases, and direct intracranial extension.[74,76,83,84] The prognosis of these tumors is quite poor (worse than at non-head and neck sites) and resembles that of many other head and neck soft tissue sarcomas.[84] An important consideration in the prognosis of these tumors is tumor size and whether complete tumor excision can be accomplished.[83,84] Accordingly, aggressive surgical resection is advocated for these lesions with radiotherapy and chemotherapy being of questionable benefit.[84]

Neurofibroma

Anatomy and Diagnosis

Neurofibromas are non-encapsulated, peripheral nerve sheath tumors that cause a fusiform dilatation of their nerve of origin.[19] While these tumors may occur as solitary, subcutaneous or submucosal masses, they more commonly present as multiple discrete tumor nodules or with extensive nerve sheath distortion (plexiform neurofibromatosis; Figure 16–17) in association with one of the two forms of neurofibromatosis (NF). Neurofibromatosis type 1 (NF-1), also known as von Recklinghausen's neurofibromatosis, is an autosomal dominantly-inherited disorder, occurring in 1 of 3,000 births, that is associated with the presence of multiple cutaneous, pigmented macules ("café au lait" spots; Figure 16–18) as well as skeletal, central nervous system and ocular lesions.[85–87] The neurofibromas that develop in patients with NF-1 are frequently multiple and can undergo malignant transformation in as many as 30 percent of cases.[74,85,86] Neurofibromas in NF-1 can also present as a so-called plexiform variant in which multiple, adjacent nerves are distorted by Schwann cell proliferation and the accumulation of a mucinous endoneurial matrix.[19,74,88] When this variant arises in the head and neck, its clinical behavior may be more aggressive.[89]

In neurofibromatosis type 2 (NF-2), the incidence of neurofibromas is much lower than in NF-1 and these tumors only rarely undergo malignant degeneration.[85] While NF-2 also demonstrates an autosomal dominant mode of transmission, it is seen in only 1 of 50,000 births with bilateral acoustic neuromas (schwannomas) and meningiomas being the most common associated tumors.[85]

In the absence of either the stigmata of neurofibromatosis or a suspicious family history, a solitary subcutaneous or submucosal mass cannot be diagnosed as a neurofibroma without a tissue biopsy. In its sporadic form, a neurofibroma frequently presents as a raised, nodular, subcutaneous mass arising from the end of a cutaneous nerve (Figure 16–19A). These neurofibromas are composed of a haphazard collection of spindle cells that microscopically resemble flags flapping in the wind.[76]

Treatment

Surgery is the only definitive treatment for neurofibromas that are not associated with neurofibromatosis. However, the fusiform growth pattern of these neoplasms invariably requires sacrifice of the nerve of origin if total tumor removal is to be achieved (Figure 16–19B and C). Consequently, although complete surgical excision is recommended, in certain circumstances, these benign neurofibromas may be clinically observed with surgical excision offered only in the case of rapid growth suspicious for

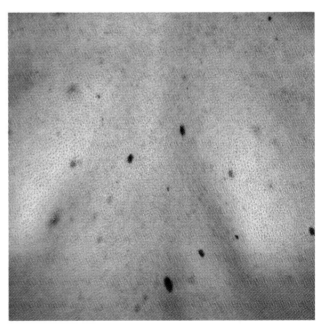

Figure 16–18. "Café au lait" lesions of neurofibromatosis.

malignancy and/or the development of significant functional or cosmetic sequelae.

In the case of multiple tumors that develop in patients with NF-1 or plexiform neurofibromas that can massively distort facial structures and/or compromise function, the risk of malignant transformation must be balanced against the morbidity of surgery and the recognition that NF-1 is a systemic disorder whose patients have a life-long propensity for tumor development.[88]

Esthesioneuroblastoma

Anatomy and Diagnosis

Esthesioneuroblastoma or olfactory neuroblastoma is a malignant tumor of the superior nasal vault that arises from the olfactory neuroepithelium and has a bimodal age distribution with peaks in the second and sixth decades.[90] These rare tumors can cause vague symptoms that include epistaxis, nasal obstruction, and headache, with expansile and invasive growth leading to malar swelling, dental pain, proptosis, diplopia and increased intracranial pressure.[19]

While these tumors exert the majority of their morbidity via direct extension and invasion into surrounding structures, they can metastasize to regional lymph nodes, the lungs or bone in as many as 10 to 20 percent of cases.[91,92] Endoscopically, a polypoid mass can often be observed in the superior nasal cavity (Figure 16–20) while radiographic imaging (CT/MRI) demonstrates a contrast-enhancing lesion that has both expansile and destructive growth patterns (Figure 16–21).[17,93] Esthesioneuroblastomas are composed of small, round cells and may need to be differentiated from melanoma, lymphoma, and sinonasal undifferentiated carcinoma (SNUC) on the basis of architecture (formation of neural rosettes) and immunohistochemical markers of neural differentiation (neuron-specific enolase; NSE).[19] Recently, esthesioneuroblastoma cells have been shown to have a characteristic chromosomal translocation as well as an extensive series of chromosomal gains and losses that may further permit their accurate identification.[94,95]

A clinical staging system for esthesioneuroblastoma was originally proposed by Kadish, with numerous modifications subsequently proposed.[96–98]

In the Kadish staging system, group A is composed of tumors confined to the nasal cavity, group B includes tumors that extend to the paranasal sinuses, and group C is composed of tumors that extend beyond the paranasal sinuses (into the orbit, intracranial, infratemporal fossa).[96]

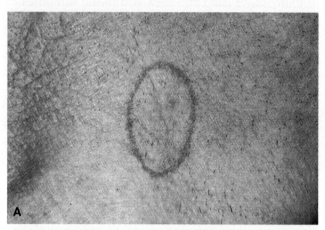

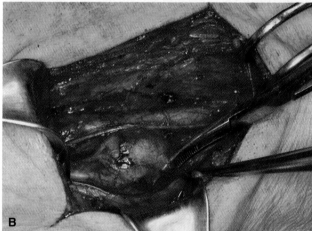

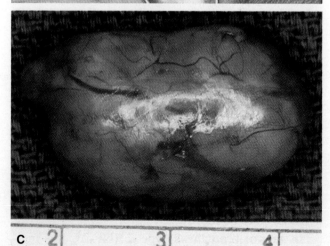

Figure 16–19. *A*, Neurofibroma. *B*, Neurofibroma causing fusiform dilatation of nerve. *C*, Neurofibroma surgical specimen.

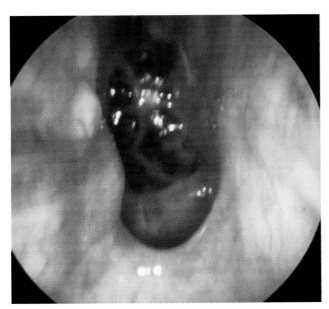

Figure 16–20. Esthesioneuroblastoma.

Treatment

Determining the optimal treatment for olfactory neuroblastoma is complicated somewhat by the variable clinical course that these tumors can adopt. Some demonstrate a very prolonged clinical course with relapses and recurrences over many years, while others grow in a much more aggressive pattern with rapid and massive local, regional, and distant disease recurrence.[92] In spite of this unpredictable clinical behavior, the treatment of choice for

esthesioneuroblastoma is surgical resection via an anterior craniofacial approach.[99,100] Such an approach can be expected to result in 10-year survival for approximately two-thirds of patients.[98,99]

Radiotherapy and chemotherapy, in a variety of combinations, have also been employed in the treatment of esthesioneuroblastoma.[101–104] While over one-half of these tumors demonstrate a brief objective clinical response to a number of single-agent chemotherapeutics, even tumors demonstrating intracranial extension are potential candidates for surgical resection with acceptable morbidity.[100,101] Therefore, chemotherapy for esthesioneuroblastoma should be considered only in those tumors that demonstrate distant metastasis or tumors that are deemed to be surgically unresectable due to major morbidity or inability to completely encompass them with clear margins.

The role for radiotherapy in the treatment of esthesioneuroblastoma is mainly in a postoperative setting where microscopic positive margins are present, or when a local recurrence arises whose resection would involve major surgical morbidity.[98] In these clinical situations, the recent introduction and future application of intensity-modulated radiotherapy (IMRT) may allow for the delivery of higher doses of radiation to the anterior cranial base while minimizing the dose received by surrounding structures.[105,106]

REFERENCES

1. Waner M, Suen JY, Dinehart S. Treatment of hemangiomas of the head and neck. Laryngoscope 1992;102:1123–32.
2. Batsakis JG, Rice DH. The pathology of head and neck tumors: vasoformative tumors, part 9A. Head Neck Surg 1981;3:231–9.
3. Stal S, Hamilton S, Spira M. Hemangiomas, lymphangiomas, and vascular malformations of the head and neck. Otolaryngol Clin North Am 1986;19(4):769–95.
4. Mulliken JB, Glowacki J. Hemangiomas and vascular malformations in infants and children: a classification based on endothelial characteristics. Plast Reconstr Surg 1982;69:412–22.
5. Batsakis JG. Vasoformative tumors. In: Batsakis JG, editor. Tumors of the head and neck: clinical and pathological considerations. 2nd ed. Baltimore (MD): Williams and Wilkins; 1979.
6. Myer CM. Congenital neck masses. In: Paparella MM, Shumrick DA, Gluckman JL, Meyerhoff WL, editors. Otolaryngology. 3rd ed. Philadelphia (PA): W.B. Saunders Co.; 1991.
7. Batsakis JG. Neoplasms of the larynx. In: Batsakis JG, editor. Tumors of the head and neck: clinical and pathologi-

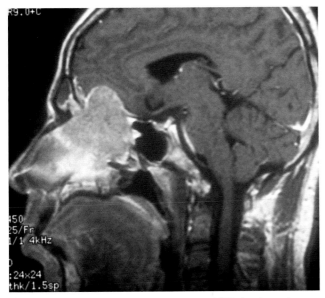

Figure 16–21. Esthesioneuroblastoma on MRI showing enhancement and bone destruction.

cal considerations. 2nd ed. Baltimore (MD): Williams and Wilkins; 1979.

8. Myer CM, Cotton RT. Congenital abnormalities of the larynx and trachea and management of congenital malformations. In: Paparella MM, Shumrick DA, Gluckman JL, Meyerhoff WL, editors. Otolaryngology. 3rd ed. Philadelphia (PA): W.B. Saunders Co.;1991.

9. Frieden IJ. Which hemangioms to treat and how? Arch Dermatol 1997;133(12):1593–5.

10. Hoeve LJ, Kuppers GL, Verwoerd CD. Management of infantile subglottic hemangioma: laser vaporization, submucous resection, intubation, or intralesional steroids? Int J Pediatr Otorhinol 1997;42(2):179–86.

11. Folkman J. Seminars in medicine of the Beth Israel Hospital, Boston: clinical applications of research on angiogenesis. N Engl J Med 1995;333:1757–63.

12. Greinwals JH Jr, Burke DK, Bonthius DJ, et al. An update on the treatment of hemangiomas in children with interferon α-2a. Arch Otolaryngol Head Neck Surg 1999;125(1):21–7.

13. Blei F, Isakoff M, Deb G. The response of parotid hemangiomas to the use of systemic interferon α-2a or corticosteroids. Arch Otolaryngol Head Neck Surg 1997;123(8):841–4.

14. Lieken S, Verbeken E, Vandeputte M, et al. A novel animal model for hemangiomas: inhibition of hemangioma development by the angiogenesis inhibitor TNP-470. Cancer Res 1999;59(10):2376–83.

15. Kennedy TL. Cystic hygroma-lymphangioma: a rare and still unclear entity. Laryngoscope 1989;99:1–10.

16. Ricciardelli EJ, Richardson MA. Cervicofacial cystic hygroma. Arch Otolaryngol Head Neck Surg 1991;117:546–53.

17. Calcaterra TC, Wang MB, Sercarz JA. Unusual tumors. In: Myers EN, Suen JY, editors. Cancer of the head and neck. 3rd ed. Philadelphia (PA): W.B. Saunders Co.; 1996.

18. Emory PJ, Bailey CM, Evans JM. Cystic hygroma of the head and neck: a review of 37 cases. J Laryngol Otol 1984;98:613–9.

19. Wenig BM, editor. Atlas of head and neck pathology. Philadelphia (PA): W.B. Saunders Co.; 1993.

20. DelGaudio JM, Garetz SL, Bradford CR, Stenson KM. Hemangiopericytoma of the oral cavity. Otolaryngol Head Neck Surg 1996:114:339–40.

21. Sabini P, Josephson GD, Yung RT, Dolitsky JN. Hemangiopericytoma presenting as a congenital midline nasal mass. Arch Otolarynol Head Neck Surg 1998;124(2):202–4.

22. Batsakis JG, Rice DH. The pathology of head and neck tumors: vasoformative tumors, part 9B. Head Neck Surg 1981;3:326–39.

23. Eichhorn JH, Dickersin GR, Bhan AK, Goodman ML. Sinonasal hemangiopericytoma: a reassessment with electron microscopy, immunohistochemistry, and long-term follow-up. Am J Surg Pathol 1990;14(9):856–66.

24. Robb PJ, Singh S, Hartley RB, Shaheen OH. Malignant hemangiopericytoma of the parapharyngeal space. Head Neck Surg 1987;9:179–83.

25. Carew JF, Kraus DH, Huvos AG. Hemangiopericytoma of the cheek. Pathologic quiz case 1. Arch Otolaryngol Head Neck Surg 1996;122(4):440–2.

26. Daniels RL, Haller JR, Harsberger HR. Hemangiopericytoma of the masticator space. Ann Otol Rhinol Laryngol 1996;105(2):162–5.

27. Tran LM, Mark R, Meier R, et al. Sarcomas of the head and neck: prognostic factors and treatment strategies. Cancer 1992;70:169–77.

28. Mira JG, Chu FCH, Fortner JG. The role of radiotherapy in the management of malignant hemangiopericytoma: report of eleven new cases and review of the literature. Cancer 1977;39:1254–60.

29. Cohen Y, Lichtig CH, Robinson E. Combination chemotherapy in the treatment of metastatic hemangiopericytoma. Oncology 1972;26:180–7.

30. Radkowski D, McGill T, Healy GB, et al. Angiofibroma: changes in staging and treatment. Arch Otolaryngol Head Neck Surg 1996;122:122–9.

31. Economou TS, Abemayor E, Ward PH. Juvenile nasopharyngeal angiofibroma: an update of the UCLA experience, 1960–1985. Laryngoscope 1988;98:170–5.

32. Chandler JR, Goulding R, Moskowitz L, Quencer RM. Nasopharyngeal angiofibromas: Staging and management. Ann Otol Rhinol Laryngol 1984;93:322–9.

33. Sessions RB, Bryan RN, Naclerio RM, Alford BR. Radiographic staging of juvenile nasopharyngeal angiofibroma. Head Neck Surg 1981;3:279–83.

34. Witt TR, Shah JP, Sternberg SS. Juvenile nasopharyngeal angiofibroma: a 30 year clinical review. Am J Surg 1983;146:521–5.

35. Spector JG. Management of juvenile angiofibromata. Laryngoscope 1988;98:1016–26.

36. Ungkanont K, Byers RM, Weber RS, et al. Juvenile nasopharyngeal angiofibroma: an update of therapeutic management. Head Neck 1996;18:60–6.

37. Deschler DG, Kaplan MJ, Boles R. Treatment of large juvenile nasopharyngeal angiofibroma. Otolaryngol Head Neck Surg 1992;106:278–84.

38. Li JR, Qian J, Shan XZ, Wang L. Evaluation of the effectiveness of preoperative embolization in surgery for nasopharyngeal angiofibroma. Eur Arch Otorhinolaryngol 1998;255(8):430–2.

39. Gates GA, Rice DH, Koopman CF, Schuller DE. Flutamide-induced regression of angiofibroma. Laryngoscope 1992;102(6):641–4.

40. Fagan JJ, Snyderman CH, Carrau RL, Janecka IP. Nasopharyngeal angiofibroma: selecting a surgical approach. Head Neck 1997;19:391–9.

41. Kamel RH. Transnasal endoscopic surgery in juvenile nasopharyngeal angiofibroma. J Laryngol Otol 1996;110(10):962–8.

42. Kasper ME, Parsons JT, Mancuso AA, et al. Radiation therapy for juvenile angiofibroma: evaluation by CT and MRI, analysis of tumor regression, and selection of patients. Int J Radiat Oncol Biol Phys 1993;25:689–94.

43. Cummings BJ, Blend R, Keane T, et al. Primary radiation therapy for juvenile nasopharyngeal angiofibroma. Laryngoscope 1984;94(12 Pt 1):1599–1605.

44. Herman P, Lot G, Chapot R, et al. Long-term follow-up of juvenile nasopharyngeal angiofibromas: analysis of recurrences. Laryngoscope 1999;109:140–7.

45. Makek MS, Andrews JC, Fisch U. Malignant transformation of a nasopharyngeal angiofibroma. Laryngoscope 1989;99:1088–92.

46. Patel SG, See ACH, Williamson PA, et al. Radiation induced

sarcoma of the head and neck. Head Neck 1999;21: 346–54.

47. Goepfert H, Cangir A, Lee YY. Chemotherapy for aggressive juvenile nasopharyngeal angiofibroma. Arch Otolaryngol Head Neck Surg 1985;111:285–9.

48. Batsakis JG. Paragangliomas of the head and neck. In: Batsakis JG, editor. Tumors of the head and neck: clinical and pathological considerations. 2nd ed. Baltimore (MD): Williams and Wilkins; 1979.

49. Ikejiri K, Muramori K, Takeo S, et al. Functional carotid body tumor: report of a case and a review of the literature. Surgery 1996;119(2):222–5.

50. Patel SR, Winchester DJ, Benjamin RS. A 15-year experience with chemotherapy of patients with paraganglioma. Cancer 1995;76(8):1476–80.

51. Jensen NF. Glomus tumors of the head and neck: anesthetic considerations. Anesth Analg 1994;78:112–9.

52. Jackson CG. Basic surgical principles of neurotologic skull base surgery. Laryngoscope 1993;103 Suppl 60:29–44.

53. Sobol SM, Daly JC. Familial multiple cervical paragangliomas: report of a kindred and review of the literature. Otolaryngol Head Neck Surg 1990;102:382–90.

54. Milunsky J, DeStefano AL, Huang XL, et al. Familial paragangliomas: linkage to chromosome 11q23 and clinical implications. Am J Med Genet 1997;72(1):66–70.

55. van Schothorst EM, Beckman M, Torremans P, et al. Paragangliomas of the head and neck region show complete loss of heterozygosity at 11q22-q23 in chief cells and the flow-sorted DNA aneuploid fraction. Hum Pathol 1998;29(10):1045–9.

56. Shedd DP, Arias JD, Glunk RP. Familial occurrence of carotid body tumors. Head Neck 1990;12:496–9.

57. Grufferman S, Gillman MW, Pasternak LR, et al. Familial carotid body tumor: case report and epidemiologic review. Cancer 1980;46:2116–22.

58. Netterville JL, Reilly KM, Robertson D, et al. Carotid body tumors: a review of 30 patients with 46 tumors. Laryngoscope 1995;105:115–25.

59. Mitchell RO, Richardson JD, Lambert GE. Characteristics, surgical management, and outcome in 17 carotid body tumors. Am Surg 1996;12:1034–7.

60. Rodriguez-Cuevas S, Lopez-Garza J, Labastida-Almendaro S. Carotid body tumors in inhabitants of altitudes higher than 2,000 meters above sea level. Head Neck 1998; 20:374–8.

61. Win T, Lewin JS. Imaging characteristics of carotid body tumors. Am J Otolaryngol 1995;16(5):325–8.

62. Stein AM, Lewin JS, Maniglia AJ. Value of magnetic resonance angiography in the evaluation of head and neck neoplasms. Otolaryngol Head Neck Surg 1996;114(1):125–30.

63. Anand VK, Alemar GO, Sanders TS. Management of the internal carotid artery during carotid body tumor surgery. Laryngoscope 1995;105:231–5.

64. Witterick IJ, Gullane PJ, Keller MA. Postoperative carotid body tumor evaluation: analysis using MR angiography. Laryngoscope 1995;105:764–7.

65. Guedea F, Mendenhall WM, Parsons JT, Million RR. Radiotherapy for chemodectoma of the carotid body and ganglion nodosum. Head Neck 1991;13:509–13.

66. Gulya AJ. The glomus tumor and its biology. Laryngoscope 1993;103 Suppl 60:7–15.

67. Green JD, Brackmann DE, Nguyen CD, et al. Surgical management of previously untreated glomus jugulare tumors. Laryngoscope 1994;104:917–21.

68. Jackson CG. Diagnosis for treatment planning and treatment options. Laryngoscope 1993;103 Suppl 60:17–22.

69. Cole JM, Beiler D. Long-term results of treatment for glomus jugulare and glomus vagale tumors with radiotherapy. Laryngoscope 1994;104:1461–5.

70. Carrasco V, Rosenman J. Radiation therapy of glomus jugulare tumors. Laryngoscope 1993;103 Suppl 60:23–7.

71. Fisch U. The infratemporal fossa approach for glomus tumors of the temporal bone. Ann Otol Rhinol Laryngol 1982;91:474–9.

72. Netterville JL, Civantos FJ. Rehabilitation of cranial nerve deficits after neurotologic skull base surgery. Laryngoscope 1993;103 Suppl 60:45–54.

73. Roberts WL. Rehabilitation of the head and neck cancer patient. In: McGarvey CL, editor. Physical therapy for the cancer patient. New York: Churchill Livingstone; 1990.

74. Batsakis JG. Tumors of the peripheral nervous system. In: Batsakis JG, editor. Tumors of the head and neck: clinical and pathological considerations. 2nd ed. Baltimore (MD): Williams and Wilkins; 1979.

75. Das Gupta TK, Brasfield RD, Strong EW, Hajdu SI. Benign solitary schwannomas (neurilemmomas). Cancer 1969; 24:355–66.

76. Bruner JM. Peripheral nerve sheath tumors of the head and neck. Semin Diagn Pathol 1987;4(2):136–49.

77. Hasegawa SL, Mentzel T, Fletcher CDM. Schwannomas of the sinonasal tract and nasopharynx. Mod Pathol 1997;10(8):777–84.

78. Donnelly MJ, Al-Sader MH, Blayney AW. View from beneath: pathology in focus. Benign nasal schwannoma. J Laryngol Otol 1992;106:1011–5.

79. Younis RT, Gross CW, Lazar RH. Schwannomas of the paranasal sinuses. Arch Otolaryngol Head Neck Surg 1991;117:677–80.

80. Lusk MD, Kline DG, Garcia CA. Tumors of the brachial plexus. Neurosurg 1987;21:439–53.

81. Kline DG, Hackett ER, Happel LH. Surgery for lesions of the brachial plexus. Arch Neurol 1986;43:170–81.

82. Kondziolka D, Lunsford LD, McLaughlin MR, Flickinger JC. Long-term outcomes after radiosurgery for acoustic neuromas. N Engl J Med 1998;339:1426–33.

83. Bailet JW, Abemayor E, Andrews JC, et al. Malignant nerve sheath tumors of the head and neck: a combined experience from two university hospitals. Laryngoscope 1991; 101:1044–9.

84. Ducatman BS, Scheithauer BW, Piepgras DG, et al. Malignant peripheral nerve sheath tumors. Cancer 1986;57: 2006–21.

85. Costantino PD, Friedman CD, Pelzer HJ. Neurofibromatosis type II of the head and neck. Arch Otolaryngol Head Neck Surg 1989;115:380–3.

86. White AK, Smith RJH, Bigler CR, et al. Head and neck manifestations of neurofibromatosis. Laryngoscope 1986;96: 732–6.

87. De Varebeke SJ, De Schepper A, Hauben E, et al. Subcutaneous diffuse neurofibroma of the neck: a case report. J Laryngol Otol 1996;110:182–4.

88. Krueger W, Weisberger E, Ballantyne AJ, Goepfert H. Plexiform neurofibroma of the head and neck. Am J Surg 1979;138:517–20.

89. Needle MN, Cnaan A, Dattilo J, et al. Prognostic factors in the surgical management of plexiform neurofibroma: The Children's Hospital of Philadelphia experience, 1974–1994. J Pediatr 1997;131:678–82.

90. Elkon D, Hightower SI, Lim ML, et al. Esthesioneuroblastoma. Cancer 1979;44:1087–94.

91. Levine PA, McLean WC, Cantrell RW. Esthesioneuroblastoma: The University of Virginia experience (1960–1985). Laryngoscope 1986;96:742–6.

92. Shah JP, Feghali J. Esthesioneuroblastoma. Am J Surg 1981; 142:456–8.

93. Schuster JJ, Phillips CD, Levine PA. MR of esthesioneuroblastoma (olfactory neuroblastoma) and appearance after craniofacial resection. AJNR Am J Neuroradiol 1994; 15(6):1169–77.

94. Whang-Peng J, Freter CE, Knutsen T, et al. Translocation t(11;22) in esthesioneuroblastoma. Cancer Genet Cytogenet 1987;29:153–7.

95. Szymas J, Wolf G, Kowalczyk D, et al. Olfactory neuroblastoma: detection of genomic imbalances by comparative genomic hybridization. Acta Neurochir 1997;139(9): 839–44.

96. Kadish S, Goodman M, Wang CC. Olfactory neuroblastoma: a clinical analysis of 17 cases. Cancer 1976;37:1571–6.

97. Biller HF, Lawson W, Sachdev VP, Som P. Esthesioneuroblastoma: surgical treatment without radiation. Laryngoscope 1990;100:1199–201.

98. Dulgerov P, Calcaterra T. Esthesioneuroblastoma: the UCLA experience (1970–1990). Laryngoscope 1992;102:843–9.

99. Shah JP, Kraus DH, Bilsky MH, et al. Craniofacial resection for malignant tumors involving the anterior skull base. Arch Otolaryngol Head Neck Surg 1997;123(12):1312–7.

100. Bilsky MH, Kraus DH, Strong EW, et al. Extended anterior craniofacial resection for intracranial extension of malignant tumors. Am J Surg 1997;174(5):565–68.

101. Wade PM, Smith RE, Johns ME. Response of esthesioneuroblastoma to chemotherapy. Cancer 1984;53:1036–41.

102. Levine PA, Debo RF, Meredith SD, et al. Craniofacial resection at the University of Virginia (1976–1992): survival analysis. Head Neck 1994;16:574–7.

103. Eden BV, Debo RF, Larner JM, et al. Esthesioneuroblastoma. Long-term outcome and patterns of failure—the University of Virginia experience. Cancer 1994; 73(10):2556–62.

104. McElroy EA Jr, Buckner JC, Lewis JE. Chemotherapy for advanced esthesioneuroblastoma: the Mayo Clinic experience. Neurosurgery 1998;42(5):1023–7.

105. Kuppersmith RB, Greco SC, Teh BS, et al. Intensity-modulated radiotherapy: first results with this new technology on neoplasms of the head and neck. ENT Ear Nose Throat J 1999;78(4):238–51.

106. Woo SY, Grant WH, Bellezza D, et al. A comparison of intensity modulated conformal therapy with a conventional external beam stereotactic radiosurgery system for the treatment of single and multiple intracranial lesions. Int J Radiat Oncol Biol Phys 1996;35(3):593–7.

17

Soft Tissue and Bone Tumors

SNEHAL G. PATEL, MD, FRCS

JATIN P. SHAH, MD, FACS

Soft-tissue sarcoma (STS) is the generic name used to describe a wide variety of tumors of mesenchymal origin that have widely diverse clinical characteristics and biologic behavior. Approximately 8,700 new cases are projected to occur in the United States in adults during 2001[1] with less than 10 percent of all sarcomas arising in the head and neck region.[2] Soft-tissue sarcomas of the head and neck (STSHN) are especially difficult to treat because aggressive treatment may cause unacceptable physiologic, functional and cosmetic sequelae. This inability to deliver aggressive treatment may in part explain why these tumors have historically been associated with poor outcome. Tumors of the craniofacial bones are even more rare. In addition to neoplasms of skeletal origin, the teeth-bearing bones of the head and neck are susceptible to odontogenic tumors. A detailed description of all these lesions is clearly beyond the scope of this book, and only some of the more common lesions and their management will be briefly discussed.

ANATOMY

Within the head and neck region, STS commonly involves the neck, the soft tissue of the upper aerodigestive tract, or one of the potential spaces such as the parapharyngeal space or infratemporal fossa. Bone tumors involve the mandible or maxilla more frequently than other extragnathic bones. The detailed anatomy of these structures has been described under the relevant sections in this book and the reader is referred to one of the several excellent anatomic texts for detailed features of individual bones. Instead, information that may be of practical importance in diagnosis and management is presented here.

As a generalization, the bones that constitute the floor of the middle and posterior cranial fossae ossify in cartilage while the bones above (cranial vault) and below (face) ossify in membrane. Some bones such as the occipital and temporal bones derive from both sources. Most of the separate bones of the skull and face are ossified by the time of birth but others do not do so until later, and this must be considered in treatment planning to minimize deformities associated with growth defects.

The bones of the facial skeleton transmit vital neurovascular structures that may be involved by tumor or its treatment. Involvement of nerves results in symptoms that may aid clinical diagnosis of tumors located in clinically inaccessible areas (Table 17–1).

Risk Factors and Etiology

Soft-tissue sarcoma of the head and neck (STSHN) is a disease most prevalent in adults and none of the risk factors commonly associated with squamous cell carcinoma are known to be involved in the pathogenesis of these tumors. Epidemiologic studies have identified genetically predisposed groups of individuals such as those suffering from neurofibromatosis who are at risk of malignant peripheral nerve sheath tumor (MPNT), people with the Li-Fraumeni syndrome and children with retinoblastoma who are at increased risk of rhabdomyosarcoma and osteosarcomas.[3] STSHN can also arise as a long-term complication of radiation therapy and can be a difficult problem to treat.[4] A viral etiology has been associated with Kaposi's sarcoma and chronic exposure to environmental carcinogens such as urethane and polycyclic hydrocarbons has been

Table 17–1. SYMPTOMS PRODUCED BY INVOLVEMENT OF THE NERVES TRANSMITTED BY THE CRANIAL BONES CAN BE A VALUABLE AID TO EARLY DIAGNOSIS

		Symptoms
Anterior cranial fossa		
Cribriform plate	Olfactory nerves/bulb	Altered sense of smell or anosmia
Middle cranial fossa		
Optic canal	Optic nerve	Visual field defects or blindness
Superior orbital fissure	III, IV, V1, VI nerves	Altered sensation over upper eyelid, forehead, conjunctiva, cornea, and nose; ptosis, external ocular muscle palsies and diplopia
Foramen rotundum	V2 (infraorbital nerve)	Altered sensation over midfacial skin, palate and upper teeth
Foramen ovale	V3 and inferior petrosal branch of IX	Altered sensation over external ear, skin of the temple, buccal and floor-of-mouth mucosa, and mandibular teeth
Posterior cranial fossa		
Hypoglossal canal	XII nerve	Paralysis of the tongue
Jugular foramen	IX, X and XI nerves	Vocal cord paralysis, difficulty swallowing and aspiration
Internal acoustic meatus	VII and VIII nerves	Facial paralysis, impaired hearing or deafness, tinnitus and vestibular symptoms

implicated in some STS. Trauma most often draws attention to an existing tumor, but there is no conclusive evidence to support the association of sarcomas to scar tissue. Risk factors for chondrosarcomas are thought to include the presence of pre-existing multiple chondromas or osteochondromas while predisposing factors for osteosarcoma include a history of retinoblastoma and genetic factors, Paget's disease of bone, fibrous dysplasia, and previous radiation therapy.

The Molecular Biology and Cytogenetics of Soft-Tissue Sarcoma

Research done in the past decade has significantly advanced our understanding of the molecular genetics of STS. As for most other cancers, alterations at the molecular level can result in either gain or loss of important gene function. The two main pathways are the p53 tumor suppressor pathway and the RB oncogene pathway, but new candidate genes are being constantly reported. Several cytogenetic and molecular abnormalities have been consistently reported in STS (Table 17–2). Many of these clonal aberrations are highly specific and have the potential to be used for differential diagnosis of tumors such as small round cell tumors (Ewing's sarcoma, alveolar rhabdomyosarcoma and desmoplastic round cell tumors) that are difficult to categorize on conventional histology and immunohistochemistry. In addition, some of these genetic abnormalities

may prove to be of prognostic importance, eg, alterations of the INK4A and INK4B genes have been significantly associated with a worse prognosis in adult STS5.[5] The routine clinical application of such techniques is likely to clear some of the existing controversies regarding the typing and grading of STS, and will also provide more reliable and objective indicators of prognosis in the future.

DIAGNOSIS

Clinical Features

STS have a biphasic age distribution: 80 to 90 percent affect adults while 10 to 20 percent are seen in the pediatric age group. The median age of presentation of STSHN at the Memorial Sloan-Kettering Cancer Center (MSKCC) was 49 years and there was a slight male preponderance.[6] Most patients present with a painless mass, but some tumors such as clear cell sarcoma, cutaneous leiomyosarcoma, and calcified synovial sarcoma can present as painful masses. Other symptoms depend upon the site of origin and local extent of the tumor, and can include visual disturbances, epistaxis, "chronic sinusitis," otalgia, etc. Tumors of the paranasal sinuses or base of the skull may present with no other symptoms except sensory or motor cranial nerve deficits (see Table 17–1). A detailed physical and head and neck examination is vital, and particular attention must be directed toward determining the relation of the mass to important structures in the vicinity. More often than not, the patient's symptoms and a thorough clinical exam are sufficient to form an impression of the extent of the lesion and to guide investigation. The investigative approach must rely on noninvasive methods to start with and a working stage of the lesion must be arrived at before an open biopsy is undertaken. This is important for two reasons: one, the process of staging may reveal findings that change the differential diagnosis and second, more crucially, tissue changes after open biopsy may hamper the ability of imaging studies to define the local extent of disease.

Radiologic Imaging

The imaging capabilities of computed tomography (CT) and magnetic resonance imaging (MRI) can yield vital three-dimensional information about the locoregional extent of the lesion and its relationship to important structures in the head and neck. Imaging can also improve diagnostic yield by allowing accurate placement of a percutaneous needle for biopsy of relatively inaccessible or large, necrotic lesions. Treatment planning is greatly facilitated by imaging if bony resection and reconstruction are anticipated. The risk of bleeding after needle biopsy of a highly vascular lesion can be minimized if the nature of the lesion is apparent on a contrast-enhanced CT or MRI. The individual advantages of CT and MRI can be used to complement each other in evaluation of tumors involving the complex anatomy of the head and neck region. However, the superior soft-tissue resolution of MRI and its multiplanar capabilities may provide additional information, especially in certain situations such as tumors involving the base of the skull.[7] Serial imaging using baseline scan(s) for comparison may be helpful in following patients who have had prior treatment, but differentiating posttreatment fibrosis from recurrent tumor has been found to be more reliable using the [18]FDG-PET scan.[8]

Plain radiography is of limited value in imaging tumors of the craniofacial skeleton which are best imaged using CT, MRI or both. The typical radiologic features of individual tumors are described later in this chapter. Other investigations such as bone scintigraphy are nonspecific and are generally not recommended. Undue reliance on any one radiologic or pathologic finding can lead to misinterpretation, and close interdisciplinary cooperation between the surgeon, the radiologist and the pathologist is crucial to accurate diagnosis and optimal treatment of these tumors.

Pathology

Noninvasive imaging can reliably diagnose some soft-tissue lesions such as lipomas, benign vascular tumors, and fibromatosis. For most other tumors, histologic examination of a biopsy specimen is currently the only reliable technique that can lead to a definitive diagnosis. Several techniques are in common use: fine-needle aspiration (FNA), core needle biopsy, incisional biopsy and excisional biopsy. FNA is the easiest to perform and can be safely undertaken at the first clinic visit of a patient presenting with an accessible mass that is clinically non-pulsatile. Although the tissue obtained is almost invariably inadequate for identification of tumor grade, its usefulness lies in its being able to identify other more common tumors like squamous cell carcinoma, thereby guiding further evaluation. Core needle biopsy, on the other hand, provides good tissue for diagnosis and grade can be determined in virtually all specimens.[9] Lesions of the paranasal sinuses and nasal cavity may be visualized using modern endoscopic techniques but obtaining a representative biopsy specimen from these tumors may be difficult.

Excisional biopsy of a suspected malignant mass should be avoided because foci of tumor have been

Table 17–2. SOME EXAMPLES OF TUMOR-SPECIFIC GENETIC ABNORMALITIES THAT HAVE BEEN IDENTIFIED IN SOFT TISSUE SARCOMA

Histologic Diagnosis	Genetic Abnormality	Gene Fusion Product
Synovial sarcoma	t(x;18) (p11;q11)	SYT-SSX
Ewing's sarcoma /	t(11,22) (q24;q12)	EWS-FL11
Primitive	t(21,22) (q12;q22)	EWS-ERG
neuroectodermal tumor	t(7,22) (p22;q12)	EWS-ETV1
Desmoplastic small	t(11,22) (q13;q12)	EWS-WT1
round cell tumor		
Liposarcoma	t(12,16) (q13;p11)	CHOP-TLS
Dermatofibrosarcoma	t(17,22) (q22;q13)	PDGFB-COL1A1
Myxoid chondrosarcoma	t(9,22) (q31;q12)	EWS-TEC
Alveolar	t(2,13) (q35-37;q14)	PAX3-FKHR
rhabdomyosarcoma	t(1,13) (p36;q14)	PAX7-FKHR

shown to persist in the patient after such a procedure.[10] Instead, an incisional biopsy allows for adequate sampling of viable tumor tissue under direct vision and ensures optimal hemostasis. The incision is planned directly over a point where the tumor feels closest to the skin and is oriented to allow its excision if a subsequent definitive procedure becomes necessary. Careful dissection should minimize opening up tissue planes and a sufficient wedge of viable, non-necrotic tissue must be sampled to be sent to the pathology laboratory in containers suitable for appropriate studies. If wound drainage is required after meticulous hemostasis, drains should exit either through or very close to the incision. Frozen-section analysis of the biopsy specimen can be used to confirm that diagnostic tissue has been sampled, but otherwise its role in establishing accurate histologic diagnosis is limited.

A positive smear from an FNA of osteogenic sarcoma and other bony sarcomas has been reported to be very reliable, but open biopsy is mandatory for negative or indeterminate smears.[11] The extraosseous soft-tissue component of a bony lesion may be adequately biopsied using a core biopsy needle such as the Jamshidi needle. Open biopsy of bone lesions is generally not recommended for craniofacial tumors as it contaminates tissue planes and may ultimately increase the extent of definitive resection.

Soft-Tissue Tumors

Histologic typing and grading of STS is often difficult and a considerable degree of inter-observer variability exists even among expert pathologists with a reported diagnostic discrepancy in as many as 25 to 40 percent of lesions.[12] The routine use of immunohistochemical stains has facilitated histologic classification, but these techniques are by no means definitive, and considerable experience is required in interpreting results. More objective methods such as cytogenetic, molecular and biochemical analysis may help resolve some of these diagnostic difficulties in the future.[13]

Mesenchymal tumors are a heterogeneous and biologically diverse group of tumors and some peculiar features in individual tumor types may require special consideration in treatment planning as described below.

Fibrosarcomas (FS) were the most common STS until better recognition of lesions such as malignant fibrous histiocytoma (MFH), and the fibromatoses resulted in reclassification of up to 50 percent of all cases.[14] Currently, FS constitute only 5 to 10 percent of all STS, and only 2 to 20 percent of all FS involve the head and neck.[15] They most frequently involve the face, neck, scalp, and paranasal sinuses and commonly affect adults, probably with no predilection for any particular gender. The tumor presents as a painless, slowly growing mass that on histologic examination shows spindle-shaped fibroblasts arranged in a "herringbone" pattern. The nuclei are generally uniform and if many large and bizarre giant cells are seen, the possibility of MFH must be considered. Histologic grading of FS has prognostic implications in adults, but not in children. Differential diagnosis of FS from tumors like MFH, synovial sarcoma, fibromatosis and malignant peripheral nerve sheath tumor may be difficult, especially when analyzing a limited biopsy specimen. Until the advent of immunocytochemistry and, more recently, molecular markers, accurate diagnosis would have been impossible. Two major series of head and neck FS in the 1960s and 1970s may have included patients with these diagnoses,[16,17] and their 5-year survival rates of 30 to 75 percent cannot be considered valid for comparison today. More recent reports indicate a 5-year survival rate of around 60 percent.[18] Fibrosarcomas of the jaws are extremely rare and may be either endosteal or periosteal. Endosteal or intramedullary lesions metastasize via the hematogenous route and consequently have a worse prognosis as compared to the periosteal lesion that generally invades along fascial planes to invade the bone from outside. These tumors are radioresistant and aggressive surgical excision is the treatment of choice.

Malignant fibrous histiocytoma (MFH) is the most common STS in adults, but only 1 to 3 percent of all MFH involve the head and neck.[19] Most patients are between 50 and 70 years of age and there is a slight male preponderance. The cell of origin is thought to be the fibroblast that differentiates into a variety of histologic patterns.[20] Distinguishing these tumors from other sarcomas such as liposarcoma and rhabdomyosarcoma can sometimes be difficult without ancillary methods such as immunohistochemistry, cytogenetics or molecular genetic analysis. Of the many histologic subtypes, the storiform-pleomorphic or myxoid variants are more common in the head and neck. About a third of cases involve the sinonasal tract, and up to 15 to 20 percent involve the larynx, craniofacial bones, neck, salivary glands and oral cavity each.[21] Adverse prognostic factors include advanced age, male gender, size greater than 6 cm and tumors arising from bone. The overall 5-year survival in MFH of the head and neck has been reported around 50 percent but the presence of distant metastases carries a dismal prognosis.[22] Although radiation and adriamycin-based chemotherapy have been used, wide surgical resection with adequate margins and neck dissection for palpable nodes is the treatment of choice.

Dermatofibrosarcoma protuberans, which constitute about 7 to 15 percent of STSHN are nodular cutaneous tumors with a high propensity for local recurrence after simple excision. The cell of origin and etiology of these tumors remain unknown. They usually present as an elevated, firm, solitary, slowly enlarging painless mass in the scalp or neck (Figure 17–1) of a 30- to 40-year-old man. The gross appearance of the tumor is deceptive because it appears well-encapsulated, but microscopic extensions may project up to 3 cm or more laterally, and invasion of the deep fascia is not uncommon. Histologically, the tumor is a low-grade sarcoma with sparse vasculature, moderate mitotic activity, little nuclear pleomorphism and rare necrosis. Adequate excision generally requires margins of about 2.5 to 3 cm from the edge of the tumor with the underlying deep fascia, as resections with margins less than 2 cm are highly prone to local failure.[23] Addition of postoperative radiation therapy may enhance local control in incompletely resected tumors or where adequate resection is impossible because of cosmetic or functional concerns. The outcome of adequately treated cases is excellent and an overall 5-year survival of 94 percent has been reported.[24]

Liposarcomas (LS) represent about 1 percent of STSHN and only about 80 cases have been reported in the literature. Most patients present in the seventh decade and males outnumber females 1.7 to 1. The neck is the single most common site but about 40 percent of tumors involve the larynx and/or pharynx.

Within the larynx the supraglottis is the most commonly affected site. Overall 5-year survival has been reported at 67 percent and prognosis is significantly related to the histologic grade of the tumor.[25] Liposarcomas of the larynx and scalp have a better prognosis as compared to those of the oral cavity.

Synovial sarcomas are believed to arise from undifferentiated or pluripotential mesenchymal cells[26] and fewer than 90 cases have been reported in the literature. The typical patient is a 20- to 30-year-old male who presents with a painless neck mass. The tumor may be located high in the superior aspect of the neck, in the prevertebral area, or in the retropharyngeal and parapharyngeal areas.[27] Compression of the upper aerodigestive tract or its nerves may cause hoarseness, dysphagia, or dyspnea. Histologic examination shows a fibroblastic spindle-cell stroma containing scattered pale epithelial-like cells arranged in glandular formations, nests, or cleft-like spaces. Microcalcification, seen in 30 to 60 percent of cases, is a favorable prognostic sign. Although up to 20 percent of these tumors spread to the nodes, routine elective neck dissection is not recommended in the absence of palpable nodes. Most synovial sarcomas of the extremities are relatively radioresistant, but postoperative radiation is advocated in tumors of the head and neck for improving local control rates. Five-year survival rates around 40 to 50 percent have been reported, the main cause of death being bloodborne metastases to the lungs.[28]

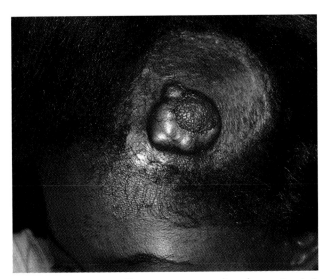

Figure 17–1. Dermatofibrosarcoma presenting as an elevated, firm, solitary, slowly enlarging mass most commonly on the scalp.

Angiosarcoma (AS) accounts for less than 0.1 percent of all head and neck malignancies, but approximately half of all AS occur in the head and neck region. Most patients are elderly white men who present with an ulcerating, nodular or diffuse dermal lesion of the scalp or face. The lesion looks like dermal ecchymosis or subcutaneous hematoma (Figure 17–2). Etiologic associations with prior irradiation, exposure to vinyl chloride and thorium, trauma and solar exposure have been reported. Unlike other sarcomas, grade is not a significant prognosticator, probably because the vast majority of AS are high-grade tumors. These tumors tend to spread laterally throughout the dermis, and their size is therefore a significant determinant of outcome.[29] About 10 to 15 percent of patients will develop neck node metastases, but elective treatment of the neck is not recommended. Postoperative radiation therapy may enhance local control and survival in patients with locally extensive disease and in those with adverse histology such as multicentricity, positive margins, or deep extension. Complete surgical excision is an important predictor of long-term survival, but these tumors are often relentless and despite aggressive management, only a third of the patients survive 5 years.[30] Experimental treatment modalities include anti-angiogenic therapy and intra-arterial chemotherapy using doxorubicin. In contrast to AS of the scalp, tumors arising in facial bones or other soft tissues are relatively less virulent, and a better outcome may be expected.

Neurogenous sarcomas or malignant schwannomas arise from the sheath of peripheral nerves and are now classified as malignant peripheral nerve sheath tumors (MPNST). Although benign neurogenous tumors commonly affect the region, only 6 to 16 percent of MPNST involve the head and neck.[31] They can present as a solitary mass or may arise as a result of malignant degeneration of a neurofibroma in 5 to 15 percent of patients. Malignant degeneration of an otherwise asymptomatic mass generally occurs in older patients and may be heralded by nerve dysfunction or pain. Previous irradiation has also been shown to predispose to MPNST with a mean postradiation latent period of 16.9 years.[32] In one report the majority of MPNST were reported to arise in the head[33] while another study reported a predilection for the neck.[34] Tumors of the major nerves present as a fusiform or nodular infiltration of the nerve that may involve the adjacent soft tissue, and imaging with gadolinium-enhanced MRI may demonstrate perineural extension of tumor. Lymph node metastases are rare but almost 50 percent of patients fail locally and pulmonary metastases are not uncommon.[33] Prognosis in patients with solitary neurogenous sarcoma is better (50 to 75%, 5-year survival) than that for malignant degeneration in individuals with neurofibromatosis (30%, 5-year survival).[35] Other adverse prognostic factors include size larger than 5 cm, radiation-induced tumors, and glandular or rhabdomyomatous differentiation. Complete surgical resection with negative margins is not always possible and postoperative radiation therapy should be used to improve local control.

Rhabdomyosarcoma (RMS) is a malignant tumor of striated muscle origin that is overwhelmingly seen in the pediatric population in whom it is the most common STS. The most common sites affected are the orbit, paranasal sinuses, nasal cavity and nasopharynx, and the middle ear.[36] The neck is rarely involved. Rhabdomyosarcoma have traditionally been classified into embryonal, alveolar and pleomorphic types. The first 2 variants are common in pediatric patients while the pleomorphic variant is more common in adults though rarely seen in the head and

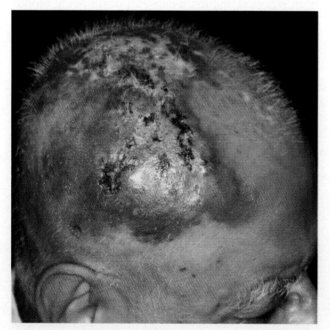

Figure 17–2. Angiosarcoma of the scalp seen as a diffuse, ecchymotic lesion with superficial ulceration.

neck.[37] Early metastases, both regional as well as systemic, are common and pretreatment evaluation must include imaging using CT or MR. Staging is different from other STSHN because it is done after biopsy and often after definitive surgery. The Intergroup Rhabdomyosarcoma Group system classifies patients into 4 groups based on the extent of their disease, the resection status, and metastatic status at onset.[38] Overall, patients with orbital tumors have a better prognosis while those arising in parameningeal sites including the nasopharynx and paranasal sinuses do not fare as well due to their propensity to invade the central nervous system.[39] Primary surgical resection is used either for small lesions in accessible locations or to reduce tumor bulk. There is no role for mutilating radical surgery as chemotherapy and radiation result in excellent control of disease with better function and cosmesis. Children treated with nonsurgical modalities need to be followed closely because of the risk of long-term complications.[40] Five-year survival rates reported from the Intergroup Rhabdomyosarcoma Study range from 81 to 93 percent for Group I patients to 20 percent for Group IV with an overall survival of 55 percent.[41]

Bone Tumors

Bone tumors are generally classified according to the matrix that their constituent cells produce: eg, tumors that produce a cartilaginous matrix are classified as chondrosarcomas, those that produce osteoid are classified as osteosarcomas and others that lack a distinct matrix may be classified as fibrosarcomas. Chondrosarcomas and osteosarcomas are by far the most common sarcomas involving the facial skeleton, but other rarer types such as Ewing's sarcoma and peripheral primitive neuroectodermal tumor (pPNET), malignant fibrous histiocytoma (MFH), vasoformative tumors such as angiosarcoma, and chordoma are also found.

Chondrosarcomas (CS) are a heterogeneous group of malignant tumors of cartilaginous origin. At the Memorial Sloan-Kettering Cancer Center (MSKCC), only 28 (5%) of 557 chondrosarcomas involved the head and neck.[42] Young males in the third or fourth decades of life are more commonly affected and the maxilla, cervical vertebrae and mandible are the most frequently involved sites (Figure 17–3). Most patients present with a painless swelling but there may be other site-specific symptoms. The pathologic spectrum ranges from a well-differentiated benign-looking cartilaginous tumor to a high-grade aggressive malignancy. Except for CS of the larynx that are known to be well-differentiated, slow-growing, localized tumors, the anatomic site of origin does not impact on the outcome. Surgical excision with histologically clear margins is the most effective treatment, and adjuvant radiotherapy may be added as indicated.

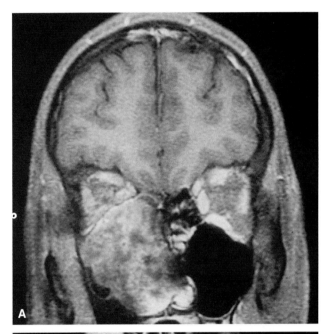
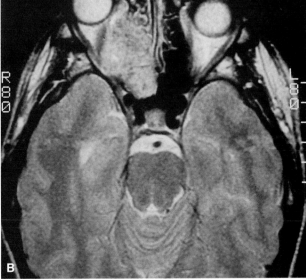

Figure 17–3. *A*, Coronal MRI appearance of a large chondrosarcoma of the right maxilla. *B*, Axial section demonstrating tumor invasion into the orbit.

Aggressive treatment of local failures is warranted because the median interval between recurrence and death is 2 years. The reported survival rates range from 44 to 81 percent. Distant metastases occur infrequently and the most common cause of death is local recurrence that invades the base of the skull.

Osteosarcoma (OS) is a tumor composed of malignant spindle-shaped or round cells that produce osteoid or primitive bone and they are generally classified according to the pattern of proliferation of their malignant cells (Table 17–3). Approximately 7 percent of 1,095 patients treated for OS at MSKCC between 1921 and 1979 had tumors involving the craniofacial bones.[43] Osteosarcomas of the jaws arise in older patients and tend to metastasize later in their natural course compared to OS of the long bones. The mandible (49%) is more frequently affected than the maxilla (37%), while other extragnathic bones are less commonly involved (14%).[44] Within the head and neck, the histologic distribution varies according to the site of the tumor.[47] Most OS of the head and neck are high-grade tumors but some lesions such as periosteal and juxtacortical OS may be of low grade. Local pain is a common symptom that leads to the patient seeking dental treatment, and a jaw lesion may be discovered subsequent to dental extraction. Radiologically (Figure 17–4), most OS tend to be osteolytic except those of the mandible where about 50 percent are osteoblastic.[45] Computed tomography, which is the imaging modality in routine use, reliably demonstrates calcification and cortical involvement, but MRI is more effective in detecting intramedullary and extraosseous soft-tissue extension. Unlike extremity

Table 17–3. THE CLASSIFICATION OF OSTEOSARCOMAS
Conventional osteosarcomas
Osteoblastic
Chondroblastic
Fibroblastic
Epithelioid
Giant cell
Small cell osteosarcoma
Telangiectatic osteosarcoma
Parosteal osteosarcoma
Periosteal osteosarcoma
Juxtacortical osteosarcoma
High grade
Low grade
Secondary osteosarcoma
Radiation-induced
Paget's sarcoma

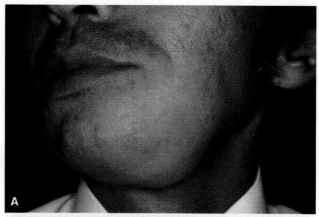
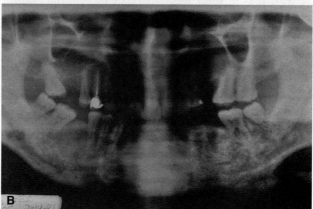
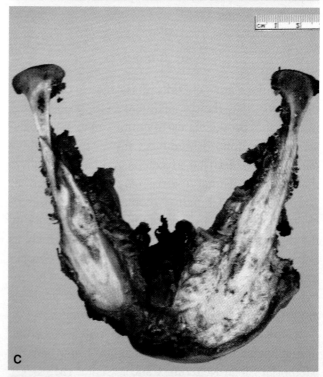

Figure 17–4. *A*, Clinical appearance of a patient presenting with an osteosarcoma of the left mandible. *B*, Panorex clearly demonstrating that the lesion was considerably more extensive than appreciated clinically. *C*, Complete surgical excision necessitated a total mandibulectomy and cut section of the specimen validated the radiologic findings.

OS, there is currently no data from randomized controlled trials on the role of chemotherapy in treatment of OS of the head and neck, but 2 meta-analyses based on nonrandomized published data have reported conflicting conclusions.[43,46] Adequate surgical resection remains the mainstay of treatment and adjuvant chemotherapy and/or radiation may be considered in appropriate situations. Osteosarcoma of the extragnathic craniofacial bones[47] and those arising in the background of Paget's disease[48] are generally associated with a poorer outcome. Although the overall 5-year survival of patients with head and neck OS was only 37 percent in a meta-analysis of 173 patients,[43] smaller individual series have reported better survival of up to 59 percent at 10 years.[49,50] Recurrences are usually local, but distant metastases, most commonly pulmonary, have been reported in 30 to 50 percent of patients.[51]

Ewing's sarcoma/peripheral primitive neuroectodermal tumor are now thought to represent a spectrum of tumors arising from the primitive neuroectoderm and characterized not only by certain common ultrastructural findings but also by a specific genetic translocation t(11;22) (q24; q11.2–12).[52] Immumohistochemical and cytogenetic studies are useful in distinguishing these tumors from other "small, blue, round cell tumors." Ewing's sarcoma of the jaw more commonly involves the mandible and most often presents with pain and swelling. It tends to affect individuals in their teens and seems to have no predilection for either sex. Imaging shows an osteolytic lesion but the classic "onion peel" appearance due to periosteal reaction is rarely seen. Ewing's sarcoma is considered a systemic disease even if only a single lesion is demonstrable, and treatment consists of multimodality treatment including chemotherapy, surgery and radiation. This approach has improved the 5-year survival of patients from around 15 percent to 74 percent.[53]

Odontogenic cysts (Table 17–4) ***and tumors*** (Table 17–5) arise from the teeth-producing tissue or its remnants and comprise a wide spectrum of lesions (see Chapter 2). Both ectodermal and mesenchymal odontogenic tissues can undergo neoplastic change giving rise to a myriad of lesions. The diverse clinical behavior of these tumors can generally be predicted by their histologic appearance. Therefore, adequate biopsy must be undertaken and the precise

Table 17–4. THE MSKCC STAGING SYSTEM FOR SOFT TISSUE SARCOMAS		
Factors	Favorable	Unfavorable
Size	< 5 cm	> 5 cm
Depth	Superficial	Deep
Grade	Low grade	High grade
	Good differentiation	Poor differentiation
	Hypocellularity	Hypercellularity
	Dense stroma	Minimal stroma
	Hypovascular	Hypervascular
	Minimal necrosis	Significant necrosis
	< 5 mitoses / 10 high-power fields	> 5 mitoses / 10 high-power fields
Stage Grouping		
Stage 0	3 favorable signs	
Stage I	2 favorable signs	
Stage II	1 unfavorable sign	
Stage III	1 favorable, 2 unfavorable signs	
Stage IV	3 unfavorable signs Distant metastasis	

Data from Hajdu S, et al. The role of the pathologist in the management of soft tissue sarcomas. World J Surg 1988;12:326–31.

histologic diagnosis of the lesion must be used to guide treatment. Tumors at the benign end of the spectrum such as ameloblastic fibromas, ameloblastic fibro-odontomas and cementoblastomas may be treated by enucleation with or without curettage. More aggressive lesions such as ameloblastoma, calcifying epithelial odontogenic tumor and ameloblastic odontoma require wider margins of excision while malignant tumors may require adjuvant treatment in addition to radical surgery.

Ameloblastomas are among the most common odontogenic tumors and are thought to arise from either the remnants of the dental lamina, the enamel organ or basal cells of the surface epithelium. They can also originate in the epithelium of odontogenic cysts such as dentigerous cysts. The mean age at diagnosis is about 38 years and there seems to be no predilection for either sex.[54] The mandible is more commonly affected than the maxilla, and most tumors

Table 17–5. ODONTOGENIC CYSTS OF THE JAWS
Periapical or radicular cyst
Residual cyst
Lateral periodontal cyst
Glandular odontogenic cyst
Dentigerous cyst
Odontogenic keratocyst
Calcifying odontogenic cyst

arise in a posterior location. Early lesions remain asymptomatic and may be incidentally picked up on dental radiographs as a radiolucency without any calcified components. However, most patients present with a slow-growing, painless swelling that may be associated with loose teeth, malocclusion, or ill-fitting dentures. Radiologically, the lesion may be either unilocular or multilocular (Figure 17–5). Conventional ameloblastomas have a tendency to infiltrate the bony trabeculae so that enucleation or curettage is associated with high failure rates.[55] Radical surgical resection is associated with a recurrence rate of only 4.5 percent while enucleation and curettage fails in as many as 59 percent and radiotherapy in 42 percent of cases.[56] Malignant odontogenic tumors are rare and may arise in one of three settings: (1) conventional ameloblastoma without cytologic features of malignancy that is designated *malignant ameloblastoma* because of histologically documented distant metastasis of well-differentiated ameloblastoma, (2) malig-

nant transformation of ameloblastoma with features of poorly differentiated carcinoma, *ameloblastic carcinoma,* and (3) *primary intra-alveolar carcinoma* that is thought to develop from residual odontogenic epithelium within the jaws so that it exhibits features of squamous cell carcinoma without any continuity with the surface epithelium. Malignant ameloblastomas almost always involve the mandible and have been reported to metastasize to lungs (75%) and lymph nodes (15%) with a median post-treatment disease-free interval of 9 years.[57] Ameloblastic carcinoma signifies the presence of poorly-differentiated elements within a primary well-differentiated ameloblastoma and/or its metastases. Most tumors involve the mandible and metastasize to the lungs, lymph nodes, liver or bones, and most patients with dedifferentiated tumors succumb to their disease within 2 years of detection of metastases.[58]

Primary intraosseous carcinoma is an aggressive disease that is best treated like squamous carcinoma of the oral cavity that has invaded bone. Surgical resection of malignant odontogenic tumors may need to be combined with radiation therapy for locoregional control and chemotherapy with or without radiation therapy may be necessary for management of distant metastases.

Metastatic tumors are usually diagnosed in patients between 50 and 70 years of age. The most common site of the primary in women is the breast followed by the adrenal, colon, female genital tract and thyroid. In men, the most common primary site is the lung followed by prostate, kidney, bone and adrenal gland. The mandible is the most commonly involved bone and about a third of patients present with an oral lesion as the first sign of their malignancy.[59]

Staging

Three staging systems have been in common use for adult STS: the American Joint Committee for Cancer/ International Union Against Cancer (AJCC/UICC) system, the Memorial Sloan-Kettering Cancer Center (MSKCC) system and the Enneking system. All 3 systems agree in general on the two most important prognostic variables: histologic grade and presence of metastatic disease. They disagree however, on the exact weight of importance that should be

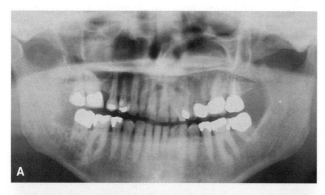

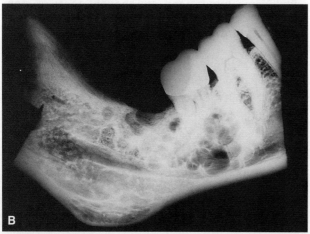

Figure 17–5. *A,* Panorex of the mandible showing a loculate lesion of the posterior aspect of the body of the right hemimandible. *B,* The extent of involvement of the bony trabeculae is clearly evident on this radiograph of the segmental mandibulectomy specimen.

given to size, site and anatomic extent. The AJCC/UICC staging system applies to all STS except Kaposi's sarcoma, dermatofibrosarcoma and desmoid type of fibrosarcoma grade 1.

Staging of STSHN using these systems is difficult, but the MSKCC system (Table 17–6) is more practical and easier to adapt in staging STSHN. It divides tumors into 2 categories—favorable and unfavorable. Grades include low and high, and the grouping into 5 stages depends upon the number of unfavorable factors.

TREATMENT GOALS AND TREATMENT ALTERNATIVES

The management of mesenchymal tumors of the head and neck in adults is primarily surgical, and adjuvant radiation therapy is used as indicated. Although chemotherapy has been effective for childhood STSHN such as rhabdomyosarcoma, its usefulness in the treatment of tumors in adults remains unproven.

FACTORS AFFECTING CHOICE OF TREATMENT

Tumor Factors

Complete surgical resection with an adequate margin of normal tissue forms the mainstay of treatment of mesenchymal head and neck tumors. The tight anatomic confines within the head and neck region dictate the extent of surgical excision and the same definitions of so-called adequate margins obviously cannot be held as relevant in head and neck tumors as for other locations. Adequate surgical excision of these tumors most often depends on the ability of the surgeon to do so without causing unacceptable cosmetic and/or functional disability. Many series have shown the increased propensity of high-grade lesions to recur locally, and such tumors should be resected more aggressively if possible. If the anatomic setting makes it impossible to achieve tumor-free margins, the patient must be offered postoperative radiation therapy. Locally advanced tumors that infiltrate vital structures such as the carotid artery in the neck, optic nerve at the orbital apex, or cranial nerves at the skull base may be treated with neoadjuvant chemotherapy with or without radiation therapy prior to excision.

Host Factors

Radiation and chemotherapy have the potential to adversely affect growing bones, causing craniofacial growth deformities when used in the treatment of tumors in children. The majority of adult tumors are treated surgically, but patients with significant comorbidity may undergo nonsurgical treatment. For instance, surgical resection of tumors that involves sacrifice of multiple cranial nerves at the skull base may be functionally intolerable in a patient with significant co-morbidity.

Physician Factors

Tumors in some locations such as the skull base require special technical skills and close interdisciplinary cooperation, eg, for craniofacial resection. Neurogenous tumors that extend via a dumbbell

---

Table 17–6. THE WHO HISTOLOGIC CLASSIFICATION OF ODONTOGENIC TUMORS

Benign
A. Odontogenic epithelium without odontogenic ectomesenchyme.
    Ameloblastoma
    Squamous odontogenic tumor
    Calcifying epithelial odontogenic tumor (Pindborg tumor)
    Clear cell odontogenic tumor
B. Odontogenic epithelium with odontogenic ectomesenchyme, with or without dental hard-tissue formation
    Ameloblastic fibroma
    Ameloblastic fibrodentinoma (dentinoma) and ameloblastic fibro-odontoma
    Odontoameloblastoma
    Adenomatoid odontogenic tumor
    Calcifying odontogenic cyst
    Complex odontoma
    Compound odontoma
C. Odontogenic ectomesenchyme with or without included odontogenic epithelium
    Odontogenic fibroma
    Odontogenic myxoma
    Benign cementoblastoma

Malignant
A. Odontogenic carcinomas
    Malignant ameloblastoma
    Primary intraosseous carcinoma
    Malignant variants of other odontogenic tumors
    Malignant changes in odontogenic cysts
B. Odontogenic sarcomas
    Ameloblastic fibrosarcoma
    Ameloblastic fibrodentinosarcoma and ameloblastic fibro-odontosarcoma
    Odontogenic carcinosarcoma

WHO = World Health Organization. Data from Kramer IRH, et al. Histological typing of odontogenic tumors. 2nd ed. New York: Springer-Verlag; 1992.

configuration into the spinal canal may be excised in cooperation with a spinal surgeon.[60] Optimal results following resection require the services of an expert reconstructive plastic surgeon, and rehabilitation may involve multidisciplinary input from other experts such as the maxillofacial prosthodontist, speech and swallowing therapist, and nutritionist.

SURGICAL TREATMENT

Surgical access and the extent of resection depend upon the location of the tumor, and a few examples will be used to illustrate the general principles of surgical treatment (Figures 17–6 to 17–9).

Histologic types associated with a higher than usual risk of lymphatic metastasis include embryonal rhabdomyosarcoma, epithelioid sarcoma, clear cell sarcoma, synovial cell sarcoma and vascular sarcoma. However, in view of the overall low risk of lymph node metastasis, neck dissection is indicated only in the presence of palpable nodes, or if the neck needs to be entered for resection of the primary lesion.

A particularly difficult problem is the patient referred with no gross clinical findings after unplanned excision of a mass that turned out to be a sarcoma on histopathologic examination. A recent study reported a 59 percent incidence of microscopic residual disease in 95 STSs that were re-excised following inadequate surgery elsewhere; 4 out of 5 head and neck tumors in this report had residual disease.[61] Re-resection followed by postoperative radiotherapy is generally indicated in such a situation, but for some tumors of the head and neck where one does not expect to gain extra margins, the dilemma is whether to subject the patient to the morbidity of another operation. The decision for reoperation, as opposed to radiotherapy alone, will in most instances be guided by the treating surgeon's impression of the adequacy of the original operation, appropriate radiologic eval-

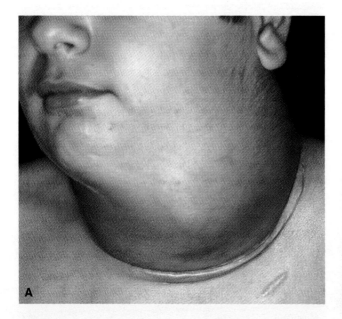

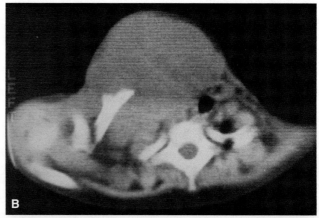

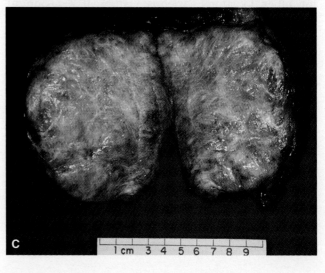

Figure 17–6. *A*, A 12-year-old boy presented with a large, firm, diffuse swelling of the left neck which had been diagnosed as a desmoid tumor on previous biopsy. *B*, CT scan of the neck showed an avascular, homogeneous mass pushing the viscera of the central compartment over to the opposite side and obliterating the internal jugular vein. *C*, The patient underwent exploration and excision of the mass that was found to have invaded the left internal jugular vein, vagus and hypoglossal nerves. These structures had to be sacrificed but the mass could be dissected off the common carotid artery and the brachial plexus, leaving gross residual disease for which afterloading brachytherapy catheters were placed. The tumor was fleshy and relatively avascular on cut section and histopathologic examination confirmed the diagnosis of a fibrosarcoma.

uation, the anatomic site of the lesion, the histologic grade, its predicted radiosensitivity, and its proximity to neurovascular structures. In the final analysis, the risks of recurrence and/or morbidity have to be weighed against the benefits of excision on an individual basis.

NONSURGICAL TREATMENT

Radiation Therapy

Radiation therapy alone is rarely successful in achieving local control of STSHN. Some authors have advocated a preference for preoperative radiation for extremity STS citing lower dose and smaller tumor volumes with results equivalent to postoperative radiation as reasons.[62] The problem with using this approach in the head and neck is the proximity of many of these lesions to bone

and/or major neural structures and the very real concern of wound complications following radical radiation therapy.

In contrast, the beneficial role of adjuvant postoperative radiotherapy (PORT) in improving local control after surgery has been demonstrated in a number of retrospective studies of STSHN. At the University of California, Los Angeles, local control after surgery (52%) improved to 90 percent with the addition of postoperative radiation. As would be expected, the impact of PORT was even greater in patients with positive surgical margins: 75 percent local control versus only 26 percent if no additional treatment was given.[63] Almost all major retrospective series have reported equivalent survival rates for surgery alone and surgery with PORT: the addition of radiation therapy to surgery improves local control in the selected group of poor prognosis patients who are offered PORT because of adverse features

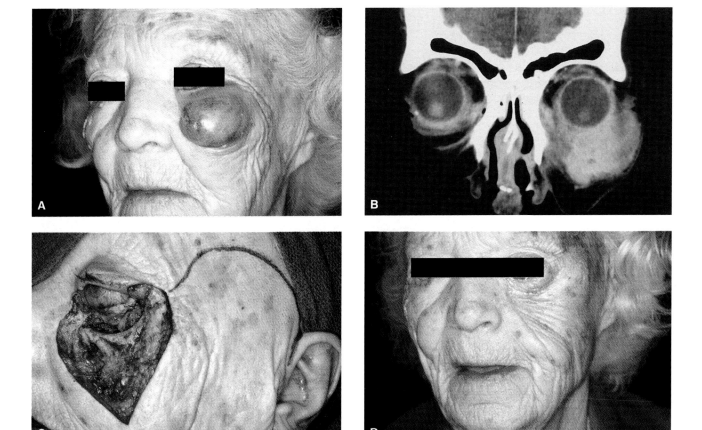

Figure 17–7. *A,* An 86-year-old woman presented with a malignant fibrous histiocytoma of the left infraorbital region that had recurred following previous excision. *B,* CT scan was suspicious of intraorbital extension. *C,* The lesion and the lower eyelid were excised down to the infraorbital rim which was grossly uninvolved, and the wedge-shaped soft-tissue defect was reconstructed using a Mustarde type advancement flap. *D,* Six months following surgery the patient maintained good function of the left eye with an acceptable cosmetic result.

of their tumors.

A prospective randomized trial from the MSKCC has shown the benefit of adding brachytherapy to surgery for high-grade lesions of the extremity and superficial trunk.[64] This may be a useful approach in selected patients with STSHN who have minimal postoperative residual disease in areas such as the skull base. Good results have been reported for neutron therapy in the treatment of gross residual disease after resection of extremity STS.[65] The major disadvantages of fast neutrons are the increased risk of complications and the technical inability to shape and control the beam, which limits their safe use in critical areas of the head and

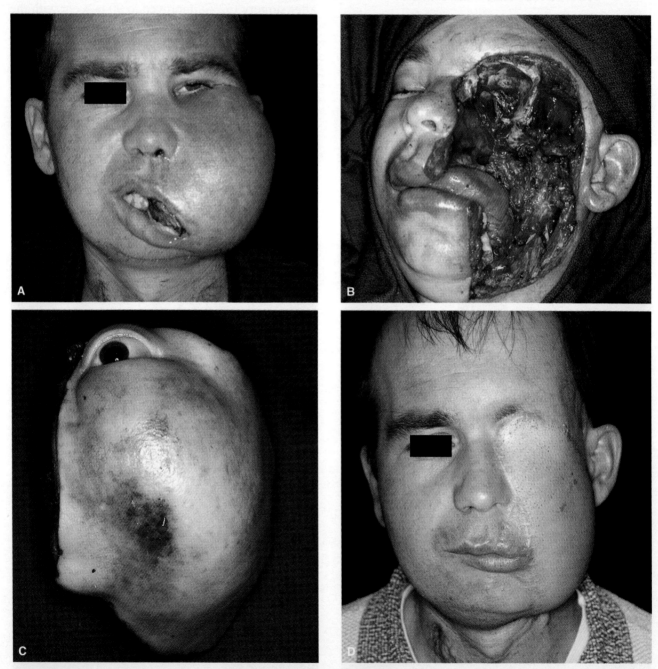

Figure 17–8.   *A,* The clinical appearance of a 30-year-old man presenting with an extensive osteosarcoma of the left maxilla that had not responded to chemotherapy and radiation. *B,* The patient underwent radical surgical excision of the tumor including orbital exenteration, total maxillectomy and hemimandibulectomy. *C,* The specimen included the tumor with the contents of the left orbit and the maxilla and left hemimandible. *D,* The extensive surgical defect was reconstructed with microvascular tissue transfer using the rectus abdominis muscle with its overlying subcutaneous tissue and skin.

neck. In contrast, techniques such as intensity modulated beam radiotherapy (IMRT) can deliver very precisely controlled dosages of photons to the tumor or its bed while minimizing radiation to vital structures such as the optic chiasm.[66] Improved local control using adjuvant radiation therapy has, however, not translated into better survival as patients succumb to distant metastases. This fact underscores the need to develop more effective systemic treatment.

Chemotherapy

The results of adjuvant chemotherapy in the treatment of STSHN have, on the whole, been disappointing. Doxorubicin and ifosfamide, which are the two most active agents, have reported response rates of only about 25 percent, and most of these responses are short-lived.[67] A meta-analysis of 1,568 patients of extremity STS from 14 trials using doxorubicin-based adjuvant chemotherapy in localized resectable STS of adults reported a 6 percent absolute benefit in

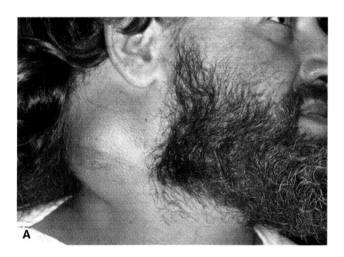

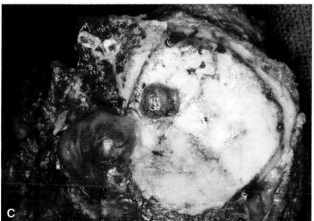

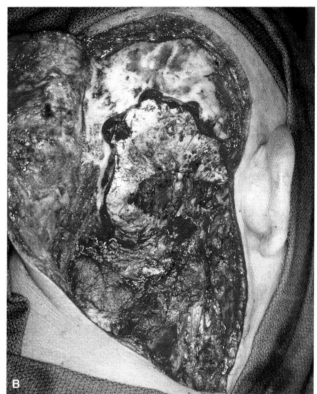

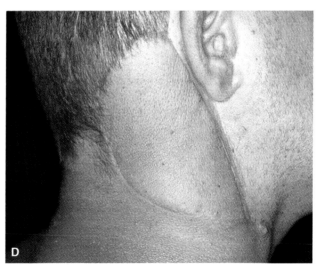

Figure 17–9. *A*, A 34-year-old man presented with a tumor of the right upper neck that had increased in size progressively over the preceding months. Clinical and radiologic examination was consistent with fixation of the mass to the adjacent mastoid process and occipital bone. Biopsy of the mass had been reported to show a spindle-cell lesion. *B*, The patient underwent wide excision of the tumor with a posterolateral neck dissection.*C*, At operation, the tumor was grossly adherent to the adjacent occipital bone so that its outer table had to be resected to secure tumor-free deep margins of excision. Histopathologic examination of the specimen revealed low-grade myxoid fibrosarcoma. *D*, The surgical defect was reconstructed using a pedicled trapezius flap with an acceptable cosmetic result.

local control and only 4 percent in terms of overall survival from adjuvant chemotherapy.[68] Chemotherapy may have a role in the management of distant metastases, but the relative inefficacy of currently used drugs is highlighted by the observation that as many as 30 to 40 percent of patients with extremity sarcomas who are controlled locally using multimodality treatment will develop distant metastases despite preoperative chemotherapy.[69]

The T-12 chemotherapy protocol for pediatric extremity osteosarcoma (OS) at the MSKCC consists of preoperative high-dose methotrexate and adriamycin to select patients who would benefit from postoperative adjuvant chemotherapy based on the histologic response to neoadjuvant treatment. The potential advantages of such therapy include reduction in tumor size and vascularity, increasing tumor-free surgical margins, elimination of micrometastases, and providing prognostic information. Unfortunately, OSs of the craniofacial skeleton in adults have not shown the same response and the use of chemotherapy in these tumors must be considered experimental.

Newer approaches such as high-dose chemotherapy with GM-CSF support, liposome-encapsulated anthracycline therapy and differentiation therapy for liposarcoma are being evaluated. There are about 32 ongoing clinical trials at this time on STS[70] and although only a few of these involve head and neck sarcomas specifically, information from some of the trials may prove useful in the management of STSHN.

SEQUELAE, COMPLICATIONS AND THEIR MANAGEMENT

Excision of STS of the neck has the potential for spinal accessory nerve damage and shoulder dysfunction in addition to other cranial nerve dysfunction. As for radical neck dissection, disability may be decreased by postoperative rehabilitation. Other cranial nerve disabilities such as dysphonia and aspiration, facial paralysis and tongue paralysis more commonly complicate resection of tumors high in the neck or at the skull base. The presence of multiple cranial nerve dysfunction can be debilitating and if such a situation is anticipated, alternative nonsurgical treatment may be considered for patients with poor performance status. Apart from speech and swallowing therapy,

rehabilitation of patients with chronic aspiration may necessitate surgical procedures such as vocal cord medialization, laryngoplasty, tracheostomy, feeding gastrostomy and occasionally even laryngectomy. Treatment for tumors involving the orbit or its surroundings has the potential for impairment of vision either due to direct involvement of the globe or due to dysfunction of the optic nerve and nerves to the extraocular muscles. Radiation therapy fields must be planned very carefully to avoid exposure of the optic nerve or chiasm, and complications can be minimized by using accurate delivery techniques such as IMRT. Facial nerve paralysis can result in exposure keratitis which may be avoided by anticipating the need for gold weight implants or tarsorrhaphy. Radiation therapy, especially in young individuals, can cause craniofacial growth defects, cataracts, hearing loss, hypopituitarism, and can also induce subsequent malignant tumors. Long-term multidisciplinary follow-up of these individuals is important for appropriate management of such side effects.

Rehabilitation and Quality of Life

In spite of improved reconstructive techniques, the cosmetic and functional rehabilitation of most major postsurgical facial deformities is far from optimal. It is easy to underestimate the value of a skillfully fabricated facial prosthesis in this era of sophisticated free microvascular transfer, however the services of an expert maxillofacial prosthetist can be invaluable. The psychologic, physical and social impact of major cosmetic disfigurement and functional disability, especially in young individuals, can be devastating and the treatment team must be able to provide comprehensive support to these patients. Advances in speech and swallowing therapy, physical therapy and nursing have been vital in improving outcome after major head and neck surgery and it is crucial for the treating surgeon to involve these experts in the management of the patient as early as possible—preferably before the resection.

Outcomes and Results of Treatment

Overall 5-year survival rates in STSHN range from 32 to 87 percent, local control rates from 52 to 90 percent, and disease-free survival from 27 to 66 percent (Table 17–7). Analysis of some major series in the literature for the impact of various prognostic factors (Table 17–8) is remarkable for a lack of consistency which is most likely due to the fact that all except two of these studies have analyzed patients accumulated over a long period of time. Apart from advances in diagnosis, management policies have evolved and surgical technique has greatly improved over the years, making the inferences from such series suspect. In an effort to overcome these deficiencies, a Head and Neck Sarcoma Registry was established by the Society of Head and Neck Surgeons in 1986 with the purpose of classifying these lesions and correlating results with other series. Retrospective data was collected from protocols that were mailed out to active members, and the results of analysis of the initial 214 patients treated from 1982 to 1990 were reported in early 1992.[71] The majority of patients (84%) underwent wide local resection of their tumors. Seventeen percent of these patients had microscopically positive margins of resection and most were treated with adjuvant radiation with or without chemotherapy. The overall median survival was 127 months and the estimated 5-year overall survival was 70 percent. The median disease-free survival was 75 months with a 57 percent 5-year disease-free survival. The T stage was reported to have no significant impact on survival, but the histology of the tumor did have a significant prognostic impact (Figure 17–10). Patients with dermatofibrosarcoma protuberans and chondrosarcoma had an excellent survival rate—approaching 100 percent, patients with malignant fibrous histiocytoma and fibrosarcoma had intermediate survival (60 to 70%) while those with osteosarcoma, angiosarcoma and rhabdomyosarcoma had poor survival (< 45%). There was insufficient information on grade of the tumor to analyze it for prognosis. Multivariate analysis of the data showed only two significant independent predictors: pediatric age group and clear margins of surgical resection.

Tumors of the head have been reported to have a better prognosis as compared to those of the neck,[72] but this is not a universal observation,[14,73] and indeed the reverse has also been reported.[74] Some of this confusion may be explained by the relative number of tumors such as angiosarcoma included in each series. Other factors such as local extension to neurovascular structures, bone[2] or skin have been reported to impact significantly on local control, distant metastases and survival.[75]

Univariate analysis of prognostic factors in 60 patients recently treated at the MSKCC revealed that patients with high-grade sarcomas or positive surgical margins are at greatest risk for local recurrence, but only margin status was significant in predicting local control based on a Cox proportional hazards model.[6] The size of the tumor, its histologic type or previous treatment did not appear to affect local recurrence or survival. Invasion of bone was an adverse prognostic sign on univariate analysis in a previous study from our institution[2] (Table 17–9). Based on these findings, patients with low-grade STSHN and no other adverse features can be treated with wide local excision alone. Adjuvant radiation therapy is indicated in all patients with high-grade

Table 17–7. SURVIVAL RATES OF PATIENTS WITH STSHN REPORTED IN RECENT LITERATURE

Author	Year	No. of Patients*	Overall 5-Year Survival (%)	5-Year Disease-free Survival (%)
Farr[81]	1981	285 (119)	32	–
Litttman et al[82]	1983	32 (9)	75	–
Wharam et al[83]	1984	72 (27)		78
Weber et al[14]	1986	188 (155)	29	27 (Median follow-up 29 months)
Greager et al[74]	1985	53 (46)	–	54
Figueiredo et al[84]	1988	94 (79)	39	–
Freedman et al[85]	1989	352 (216)	67	–
Farhood et al[2]	1990	176 (134)	55	–
Tran et al[63]	1992	164 (121)	66.5	45
Eeles et al[72]	1993	103	50	47
Le Vay et al[75]	1994	52 (49)	63	49
Kowalski and San[73]	1994	128 (90)	47.8	34.8
Kraus et al[6]	1994	60	71	60

* Numbers in ( ) indicate no. of patients in each study if diagnoses of embryonal rhabdomyosarcoma, osteosarcoma and chondrosarcoma were excluded.

Table 17–8. SUMMARY OF PROGNOSTIC FACTORS FROM LITERATURE ON STSHN

Authors	Length of Study (yrs)	No. of Patients	Local Recurrence			Survival		
			Grade	Margin	Size	Grade	Margin	Size
Greager et al, 1985[74]	15	53	x	x	x	+	x	+
Weber et al, 1986[14]	23	188	x	x	x	+	+	+
Freedman et al, 1989[85]	21	254 adult	x	x	x	x	x	x
Farhood et al, 1990[2]	26	176	x	x	x	+	+	+
Tran et al, 1992[63]	34	164	+	+	+	+	+	+
Eeles et al, 1993[72]	45	103	–	(+)	–	–	(+)	–
Kowalski and San, 1994[73]	33	128	x	–	–	x	–	–
Kraus et al, 1994[6]	8	60	+	+	–	+	+	–
Le Vay et al, 1994[75]	9	70	–	+	–	–	–	–

x = not reported; + = statistically significant prognostic factor; – = no prognostic impact; (+) = positive prognostic factor, statistically not significant.

tumors and in patients with low-grade tumors with positive surgical margins.

About 10 to 12 percent of patients with STSHN will develop distant metastases.[2] Of patients with distant metastases, 75 percent have pulmonary metastases while the rest involve the lymph nodes, bone, other soft tissue and the liver. Pulmonary metastases occur early with high-grade STS, but unfortunately even low-grade tumors can metasta-

size. The presence of nodal disease also increases the risk of distant metastasis. Treatment options for pulmonary metastases include surgical resection with or without multi-agent chemotherapy. Patients with pulmonary metastases from head and neck cancers can be successfully resected if locoregional control of their disease has been obtained.[76] Whether the metastases are surgically resected generally depends upon the status of the primary tumor,

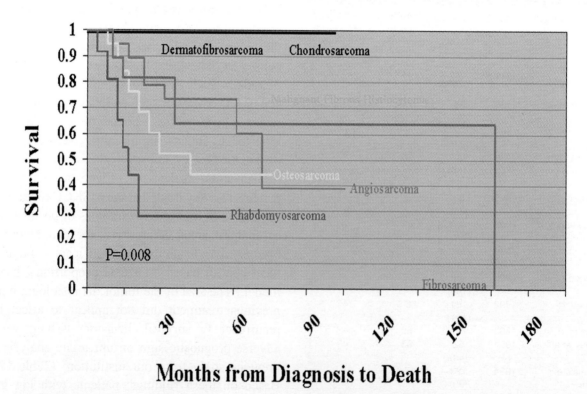

Figure 17–10. The overall survival has been correlated to histologic type: patients with dermatofibrosarcoma protuberans and chondrosarcoma have the best overall prognosis, those with malignant fibrous histiocytoma and fibrosarcoma fall in the intermediate range, and those with osteosarcoma, angiosarcoma and rhabdomyosarcoma have the worst outcome. Adapted from Wanebo et al. Head and neck sarcoma: report of the Head and Neck Sarcoma Registry. Head Neck 1992;14:1–7.

absence of other metastases, general medical condition, and resectability of the lesions. Complete resection, long disease-free interval before metastasis, absence of preceding local recurrence, and age less than 50 years have been identified as independent factors predictive of a favorable outcome.[77] In the largest single institution experience reported from the MSKCC, median survival after complete resection (19 months) was significantly better than incomplete resection (10 months) and no operation (8 months).[78] As discussed earlier, osteosarcoma of the head and neck metastasize to the lungs later in their natural course as compared to osteosarcoma of the extremities, but as many as 30 to 50 percent patients ultimately develop pulmonary metastases.

SUMMARY

Soft tissue and bone sarcomas comprise a group of tumors with varying morphology and clinical behavior. The histologic classification of these tumors has been in a state of flux, and as the molecular and genetic events leading to their development become clearer, a better understanding may be expected. The management of these tumors is essentially surgical with postoperative radiation therapy as indicated. Surgical excision poses a challenge to the head and neck surgeon because of the limited anatomic margins available without causing unacceptable cosmetic and functional morbidity. A rational treatment plan can be formulated based on our knowledge of prognostic factors, and although current local control rates are reasonable, improvements in outcome will have to await the development of more effective systemic therapy.

REFERENCES

1. Greenlee RT, Hill-Harman MB, Murray T, Thun M. Cancer Statistics, 2001. CA Cancer J Clin 2001;51:15–36.
2. Farhood A, Hajdu S, Shiu M, Strong E. Soft tissue sarcomas of the head and neck in adults. Am J Surg 1990;160:365–9.
3. Zahm S, Fraumeni J Jr. The epidemiology of soft tissue sarcoma. Semin Oncol 1997;24:504–14.
4. Patel SG, See ACH, Williamson PA, et al. Radiation induced sarcoma of the head and neck. Head Neck 1999;21:346–54.
5. Orlow I, Drobnjak M, Zhang Z, et al. Alterations of INK4A and INK4B genes in adult soft tissue sarcomas: effect on survival. J Natl Cancer Inst 1999;91:73–9.
6. Kraus D, Dubner S, Harrison L, et al. Prognostic factors for recurrence and survival in head and neck soft tissue sarcomas. Cancer 1994;74:697–702.
7. Kraus D, Lanzieri C, Wanamaker J, et al. Complementary use of computed tomography and magnetic resonance imaging in assessing skull base lesions. Laryngoscope 1992;102:623–9.
8. McGuirt WF, Greven K, Williams D III, et al. PET scanning in head and neck oncology: a review. Head Neck 1998;20:208–15.
9. Heslin M, Lewis J, Woodruff J, Brennan M. Core needle biopsy for diagnosis of extremity soft tissue sarcoma. Ann Surg Oncol 1997;4:425–31.
10. Giuliano A, Eilber F. The rationale for planned reoperation after unplanned total excision of soft tissue sarcomas. J Clin Oncol 1985;3:1344–8.
11. Hajdu SI. Aspiration biopsy of primary malignant bone tumors. Front Radiat Ther Oncol 1975;10:73–81.
12. Coindre JM, Trojani M, Contesso G, et al. Reproducibility of a histolopathologic grading system for adult soft-tissue sarcoma. Cancer 1986;58:306–9.
13. Graadt van Roggen JF, Bovee JVMG, Morreau J, Hogendoorn PCW. Diagnostic and prognostic implications of the unfolding molecular biology of bone and soft tissue tumours. J Clin Pathol 1999;52:481–9.
14. Weber R, Benjamin R, Peters L, et al. Soft tissue sarcomas of the head and neck in adolescents and adults. Am J Surg 1986;152:386–92.
15. Scott SM, Reiman HM, Pritchard DJ, Ilstrup DM. Soft tissue fibrosarcoma: a clinicopathologic study of 132 cases. Cancer 1989;64:925–31.
16. Conley J, Stout AP, Healey WV. Clinicopathologic analysis of eighty-four patients with an original diagnosis of fibrosarcoma of the head and neck. Am J Surg 1967;114:564–9.

Table 17–9. ANALYSIS OF PROGNOSTIC FACTORS IN TWO SERIES OF STSHN AT MEMORIAL HOSPITAL

		5-year Survival and p Value	
		1990[2] (Univariate Analysis)	1994[6] (Multivariate Analysis)
No. of patients		176	60
Size	< 5cm	65%	
	> 5cm	38% p < 0.0001	Not significant
Margins	–ve	85%	Significant
	+ve	28% p < 0.0001	p = 0.01
Grade	Low	90%	Significant
	High	32% p < 0.0001	p = 0.03
Bone	Invaded	18%	–
	Free	75% p < 0.0001	
Recurrence	–	67%	–
	+	45% p < 0.0001	
Metastasis	–	78%	–
	+	28% p < 0.0001	
Histologic type			Not significant
Previous treatment			Not significant

17. Swain RE, Sessions DG, Ogura JH. Fibrosarcoma of the head and neck: a clinical analysis of forty cases. Ann Otol 1974;83:439–44.

18. Mark RJ, Sercarz JA, Tran L, et al. Fibrosarcoma of the head and neck. Arch Otolaryngol Head Neck Surg 1991;117:396–401.

19. Weiss SW, Enzinger FM. Malignant fibrous histiocytoma: an analysis of 200 cases. Cancer 1978;41:2250–66.

20. Wood GS, Bekstead JH, Turner RR, et al. Malignant fibrous histiocytoma tumor cells resemble fibroblasts. Am J Surg Pathol 1986;10:323–5.

21. Barnes L, Kanbour A. Malignant fibrous histiocytomas of the head and neck. A report of 12 cases. Arch Otolaryngol Head Neck Surg 1988;114:1149–56.

22. Blitzer A, Lawson W, Biller H. Malignant fibrous histiocytoma of the head and neck. Laryngoscope 1977;87:1479–99.

23. Gayner SM, Lewis JE, McCaffrey TV. Effect of resection margins on dermatofibrosarcoma protuberans of the head and neck. Arch Otolaryngol Head Neck Surg 1997;123:430–3.

24. Mark RJ, Bailet JW, Tran LM, et al. Dermatofibrosarcoma protuberans of the head and neck. A report of 16 cases. Arch Otolaryngol Head Neck Surg 1993;119:891–6.

25. Golledge J, Fisher C, Rhys Evans PH. Head and neck liposarcoma. Cancer 1995;76:1051–8.

26. Batsakis J. Tumors of the head and neck: clinical and pathological considerations. Baltimore (MD): Williams & Wilkins; 1979. p. 357.

27. Roth J, Enzinger F, Tannenbaum M. Synovial sarcoma of the neck: a follow-up study of 24 cases. Cancer 1975;35:1243–53.

28. Bukachevsky RP, Pincus RL, Shechtman FG, et al. Synovial sarcoma of the head and neck. Head Neck 1992;14:44–8.

29. Aust MR, Olsen KD, Lewis JE, et al. Angiosarcomas of the head and neck: clinical and pathologic characteristics. Ann Otol Rhinol Laryngol 1997;106:943–51.

30. Lydiatt WM, Shaha AR, Shah JP. Angiosarcoma of the head and neck. Am J Surg 1994;168:451–4.

31. Toriumi D, Atiyah R, Murad T, et al. Extracranial neurogenic tumors of the head and neck. Otolaryngol Clin N Am 1986;19:609–17.

32. Ducatman BS, Scheithauer BW. Post-irradiation neurofibrosarcoma. Cancer 1983;51:1028–33.

33. Conley J, Janecka IP. Neurilemomma of the head and neck. Trans Am Acad Ophthalmol Otol 1975;80:459–64.

34. Das Gupta T, Brasfield R. Solitary malignant schwannoma. Ann Surg 1970;171:419–28.

35. Ghosh BC, Ghosh L, Huvos AG, Fortner JG. Malignant schwannoma: a clinicopathologic study. Cancer 1973;31:184–90.

36. McGill T. Rhabdomyosarcoma of the head and neck: an update. Otolaryngol Clin North Am 1989;22:631–6.

37. Feldman B. Rhabdomyosarcoma of the head and neck. Laryngoscope 1982;92:424.

38. Maurer HM, Beltangady M, Gehan EA, et al. The Intergroup Rhabdomyosarcoma Study: a preliminary report. Cancer 1977;40:2015–26.

39. Tefft M, Fernandez C, Donaldson M, et al. Incidence of meningeal involvement by rhabdomyosarcoma of the head and neck in children: a report of the Intergroup Rhabdomyosarcoma Study (IRS). Cancer 1978;42:253–8.

40. Fromm M, Littman P, Raney RB, et al. Late effects after treatment of twenty children with soft tissue sarcomas of the head and neck. Experience at a single institution with a review of the literature. Cancer 1986;57:2070–6.

41. Maurer HM, Beltangady M, Gehan EA, et al. The Intergroup Rhabdomyosarcoma Study: I. A final report. Cancer 1988;61:209–20.

42. Ruark D, Schlehaider U, Shah J. Chondrosarcomas of the head and neck. World J Surg 1992;16:1010–6.

43. Huvos AG. Osteogenic sarcoma of the craniofacial bones. In: Huvos AG, editor. Bone tumors: diagnosis, treatment, and prognosis. 2nd edition. Philadelphia (PA): W.B. Saunders Company; 1991. p. 179–200.

44. Kassir RR, Rassekh CH, Kinsella JB, et al. Osteosarcoma of the head and neck: meta-analysis of non-randomized studies. Laryngoscope 1997;107:56–61.

45. Lee YY, Van Tassel P, Nauert C, Raymond AK, Edeiken J. Craniofacial osteosarcomas: plain film, CT and MR findings in 46 cases. Am J Roentgenol 1988;150:1397–402.

46. Smeele LE, Kostense PJ, van der Waal I, Snow GB. Effect of chemotherapy on survival of craniofacial osteosarcoma: a systematic review of 210 patients. J Clin Oncol 1997;15:363–7.

47. Nora FE, Unni KK, Pritchard DJ, Dahlin DC. Osteosarcoma of extragnathic craniofacial bones. Mayo Clin Proc 1983;58:268–72.

48. Huvos AG, Sundaresan N, Bretsky SS, et al. Osteogenic sarcoma of the skull. Cancer 1985;56:1214–21.

49. Van Es RJ, Keus RB, van der Waal I, et al. Osteosarcoma of the jaw bones. Long-term follow up of 48 cases. Int J Oral Maxillofac Surg 1997;26:191–7.

50. Ha PK, Eisele DW, Frassica FJ, et al. Osteosarcoma of the head and neck: a review of the Johns Hopkins experience. Laryngoscope 1999;109:964–9.

51. Caron AS, Hajdu SI, Strong EW. Osteogenic sarcoma of the facial and cranial bones. Am J Surg 1971;122:719–25.

52. Batsakis JG, Mackay B, El-Naggar AK. Ewing's sarcoma and peripheral primitive neuroectodermal tumor: an interim report. Ann Otol Rhinol Laryngol 1996;105:838–43.

53. Wood RE, Nortje CJ, Hesseling P, et al. Ewing's tumor of the jaw. Oral Surg Oral Med Oral Pathol 1990;69:120–7.

54. Small IA, Waldron CA. Ameloblastomas of the jaws. Oral Surg 1955;8:281.

55. Sehdev MK, Huvos AG, Strong EW, et al. Proceedings: ameloblastoma of maxilla and mandible. Cancer 1974;33:324–33.

56. Becker R, Pertl A. Zur Therapie des Ameloblastoms. Deutsch Zahn-Mund Kieferheilkd Zentralbl Gesamte 1967;49:423–36.

57. Laughlin EH. Metastasizing ameloblastoma. Cancer 1989;64:776–80.

58. Slootweg PJ, Muller H. Malignant ameloblastoma or ameloblastic carcinoma. Oral Surg 1984;57:168–76.

59. Hirshberg A, Leibovich P, Buchner A. Metastatic tumors to the jawbones: analysis of 390 cases. J Oral Pathol Med 1994;23:337–41.

60. Patel SG, Sarkar S, Mehta AR. Dumbbell tumors of the neck: the posterior operative approach. J Surg Oncol 1995;59:209–10.

61. Goodlad J, Fletcher C, Smith M. Surgical resection of primary soft-tissue sarcoma. Incidence of residual tumour in 95 patients needing re-excision after local resection. J Bone Joint Surg Br 1996;78:658–61.

62. Suit H, Mankin H, Wood W, Proppe K. Preoperative, intraoperative, and postoperative radiation in the treatment of primary soft tissue sarcoma. Cancer 1985;55:2659–67.

63. Tran L, Mark R, Meier R, et al. Sarcomas of the head and neck: prognostic factors and treatment strategies. Cancer 1992;70:169–77.

64. Harrison L, Franzese F, Gaynor J, Brennan M. Long-term results of a prospective randomized trial of adjuvant brachytherapy in the management of completely resected soft tissue sarcomas of the extremity and superficial trunk. Int J Radiat Oncol Biol Phys 1993;214:328–38.

65. Stannard C, Vernimmen F, Jones D, et al. The neutron therapy clinical programme at the National Accelerator Centre (NAC). Bull Cancer Radiother 1996;83 Suppl:87–92.

66. Kuppersmith RB, Greco SC, Teh BS, et al. Intensity-modulated radiotherapy: first results with this new technology on neoplasms of the head and neck. Ear Nose Throat J 1999;78:238–46.

67. Edmonson J. Chemotherapeutic approaches to soft tissue sarcomas. Semin Surg Oncol 1994;10:357–63.

68. Sarcoma Meta-analysis Collaboration. Adjuvant chemotherapy for localised resectable soft-tissue sarcoma of adults: meta-analysis of individual data. Lancet 1997;350:1647–54.

69. Engel C, Eilber F, Rosen G, et al. Preoperative chemotherapy for soft tissue sarcomas of the extremities: the experience at the University of California, Los Angeles. In: P. H. Verwiej J, Suit HD, editors. Multidisciplinary treatment of soft tissue sarcomas, Boston (MA): Kluwer Academic; 1993. p.135–141.

70. PDQ Clinical Trials Database. htttp://cancernet.nci.nih.gov/cgi-bin/cancerform.

71. Wanebo H, Koness R, MacFarlane J, et al. Head and neck sarcoma: report of the Head and Neck Sarcoma Registry. Head Neck 1992;14:1–7.

72. Eeles R, Fisher C, A'Hern R, et al. Head and neck sarcomas: prognostic factors and implications for treatment. Br J Cancer 1993;68:201–7.

73. Kowalski L, San C. Prognostic factors in head and neck soft tissue sarcomas: analysis of 128 cases. J Surg Oncol 1994;56:83–8.

74. Greager J, Minu K, Briele H, et al. Soft tissue sarcomas of the adult head and neck. Cancer 1985;56:820–4.

75. Le Vay J, O'Sullivan B, Catton C, et al. An assessment of prognostic factors in soft-tissue sarcoma of the head and neck. Arch Otolaryngol Head Neck Surg 1994;120:981–6.

76. Liu D, Labow DM, Dang N, et al. Pulmonary metastasectomy for head and neck cancers. Ann Surg Oncol 1999;6:572–8.

77. Billingsley K, Lewis J, Leung D, et al. Multifactorial analysis of the survival of patients with distant metastasis arising from primary extremity sarcoma. Cancer 1999;85:389–95.

78. Gadd M, Casper E, Woodruff J, et al. Development and treatment of pulmonary metastases in adult patients with extremity soft tissue sarcoma. Ann Surg 1993;218:705–12.

79. Hajdu S, Shiu MH, Brennan MF. The role of the pathologist in the management of soft tissue sarcomas. World J Surg 1988;12:326–31.

80. Kramer IRH, Pindborg JJ, Shear M. Histological typing of odontogenic tumors. 2nd ed. New York: Springer-Verlag; 1992.

81. Farr H. Soft part sarcomas of the head and neck. Semin Oncol 1981;8:185–9.

82. Littman P, Raney B, Zimmerman R, et al. Soft-tissue sarcomas of the head and neck in children. Int J Radiat Oncol Biol Phys 1983;9:1367–71.

83. Wharam M Jr, Foulkes M, Lawrence W Jr, et al. Soft tissue sarcomas of the head and neck in childhood: non-orbital and nonparameningeal sites. Cancer 1984;53:1016–9.

84. Figueiredo M, Marques L, Campos-Filho N. Soft-tissue sarcomas of the head and neck in adults and children: experience at a single institution with a review of the literature. Int J Cancer 1988;41:192–200.

85. Freedman A, Reiman H, Woods J. Soft-tissue sarcomas of the head and neck. Am J Surg 1989;158:367–72.

18

General Principles of Reconstructive Surgery for Head and Neck Cancer

JOSEPH J. DISA, MD
ERIC SANTAMARIA, MD
PETER G. CORDEIRO, MD, FACS

Current treatment of head and neck cancer follows a multidisciplinary approach. The principle of this combined approach is to provide the patient with the optimal cancer treatment for the stage of disease, and to maximize the quality of life for the patient, with preservation or restoration of form and function. Reconstructive surgical procedures developed over the past several decades have substantially contributed to attain these objectives. Currently, reconstructive surgery is considered an integral part of the multidisciplinary treatment of patients with cancer of the head and neck.

Excision of head and neck tumors may result in exposure of vital structures such as the brain, eye, aerodigestive tract or major neurovascular structures. If inadequately reconstructed, such defects may result in significant complications and/or impairment in the performance of routine daily functions, such as speech and swallowing. In addition, esthetic disfigurement may be very significant to the patient's self-image and social adaptability. Adequate reconstruction after tumor excision is therefore the first step to rehabilitating the head and neck cancer patient—aiming to preserve and restore preoperative activity and quality of life.

Reconstructive Principles

Ideally, reconstruction of a surgical defect should be performed immediately—at the time of tumor resection. Immediate reconstruction prevents retraction and fibrosis of the defect, allows administration of adjuvant therapy, minimizes the number of surgical procedures and favors psychologic rehabilitation. Some authors, claiming easier identification of tumor recurrence, have advocated delayed reconstruction, which might otherwise be difficult to monitor if the cancer defect is covered with a flap. With development of better diagnostic techniques (ie, computed tomographic scanning, magnetic resonance imaging and positron emission tomography), delayed reconstruction to detect tumor recurrence earlier is no longer valid.[1] Likewise, it is not acceptable to favor delayed reconstruction, arguing better appreciation of the oncologic defect by the patient.

The basic tenets of reconstructive surgery include restoration of form and function while minimizing donor site deformity. Whenever possible, this should be accomplished with similar tissue rather than allografts or synthetic materials.[2] An additional principle in head and neck reconstruction is to respect facial esthetic units or subunits by placing scars following a crease or transition skin in the face[3,4] (Figure 18–1). Although sacrificing adjacent normal tissue occasionally is necessary, final results are more esthetic when adhering to this basic principle.

Surgical options for head and neck reconstruction have been described schematically as a ladder: starting from direct closure and skin grafting and moving forward to local flaps, regional cutaneous and myocutaneous pedicled flaps, and finally to the wide variety of microvascular free flaps (Figure 18–2). Historically, it

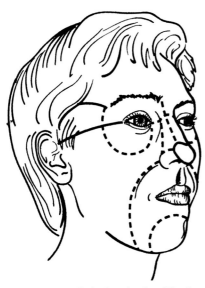
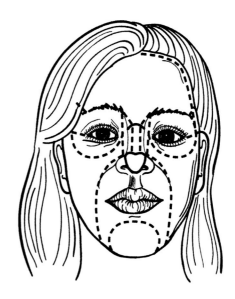

Figure 18–1. Esthetic subunits of the face.

has been recommended to start from the simplest method and if required, or the first option fails, to move over to the next step on the reconstructive ladder.[2,5] The current approach, however, is to select the reconstructive option which best provides the patient with the ideal reconstruction, thus maximizing functional and esthetic results primarily. For example, a young, healthy patient with a mandibular defect is best reconstructed using an osteocutaneous free flap at the time of tumor resection, instead of using a reconstruction plate covered with a pedicled myocutaneous flap (Figure 18–3). One-stage microvascular reconstruction of the mandible allows the surgeon to replace bone and soft tissue primarily with like tissue. Osseointegrated dental implants can be inserted on a secondary basis to optimize oro-facial rehabilitation. Alternatively, a local or regional flap is generally preferred over a free flap when there is no significant functional or esthetic advantage of the latter.[2] In general, regional flaps and free flaps are equally reliable as experienced surgeons accomplish free tissue transfer with success rates higher than 95 percent.[6] However, regional flaps often demand less technical expertise and operating time.

In selecting the best option for reconstruction of head and neck defects, these basic principles should always be followed for a successful outcome. In addition, other issues such as age, functional status, concomitant medical conditions and extent of disease must be taken into account.[7]

RECONSTRUCTIVE OPTIONS

Primary Closure

Many defects that result from excision of small skin cancers may be closed primarily with excellent esthetic results. The skin in the face and neck is very elastic and its laxity allows extensive undermining and direct closure, particularly in elderly patients. In order to minimize the visible scar, the excision should be designed to fall within the relaxed skin tension lines (Figure 18–4). Whenever possible, primary closure should be used for repair of defects of the eyelids and lips. Up to one-third of the eyelid and lip can be resected in a V fashion, with primary closure.[5]

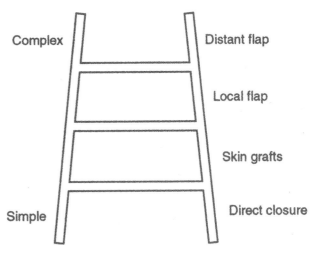

Figure 18–2. The reconstructive ladder.

Straight-line repair perpendicular to the lid or lip margin will result in the best esthetic and functional result (Figure 18–5). These critical areas are difficult to reconstruct using distant tissue that is different both structurally and functionally. When the defect becomes larger, adjacent or distant tissue should be used to restore form and function.[2]

Skin Grafts

Skin grafts may be either split-thickness (ie, including the epidermis and only a portion of the dermis) or full-thickness (including the entire dermis and epi-

dermis). Skin grafts lack their own blood supply and therefore can only be used for resurfacing well-vascularized soft tissues, periosteum and perichondrium. Exposed bone and cartilage will not allow skin grafts to take. Heavily irradiated, unstable or contaminated tissues are also less likely to permit skin graft adhesion, and must therefore be covered with well-vascularized tissues or débrided sufficiently to allow granulation tissue formation before skin grafting.

Split-thickness grafts are used to resurface large defects and may be meshed to further increase the surface area they can cover. They contract more, are less durable once healed, become more prominent and

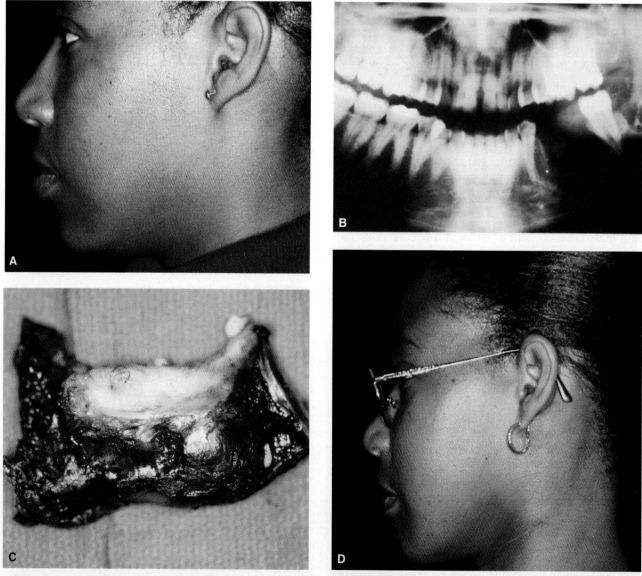

Figure 18–3. *A,* Preoperative view of patient with ameloblastoma of lateral mandible. *B,* Panorex showing lucency in lateral mandible. *C,* Surgical specimen—lateral mandible. *D,* Postoperative appearance after free fibula mandible reconstruction. Note natural appearance of jaw line.

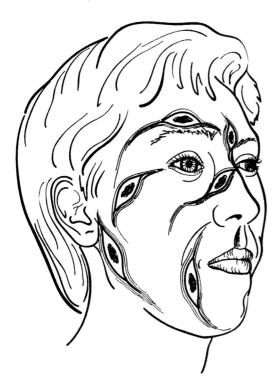

Figure 18–4. Elliptical incision planned in the relaxed skin tension lines will minimize visible scars.

recover less sensation than full-thickness skin grafts. Split-thickness skin grafts provide simple and reliable coverage for cutaneous defects of the head and neck, but because of color and contour mismatch they are generally considered inferior to full-thickness grafts and soft-tissue flaps. Split-thickness skin grafts are a useful option to provide temporary coverage of facial or scalp defects, which are later replaced with tissue expansion or a cutaneous flap (Figure 18–6).

Full-thickness skin grafts are suitable only for small defects because their donor sites must be closed primarily. Color match and texture of full-thickness skin grafts is better, particularly in the Caucasian patient.[8] Within the head and neck, they are a good choice for resurfacing eyelids and small nasal skin defects (Figure 18–7). Usual donor sites for full-thickness skin grafts are the forehead, preauricular, postauricular, contralateral eyelid and supraclavicular regions.

Skin grafts have also been used to resurface intraoral defects confined to the floor of the mouth, lateral aspect of the tongue, retromolar trigone or cheek mucosa.[9] Due to unpredictable scarring and contraction of skin grafts used intraorally, it is imperative that such defects be limited to achieve the best results.

FLAPS

A flap is a full-thickness segment of tissue that has its own blood supply. Depending upon the type of tissue or tissues, these flaps can be cutaneous, fasciocutaneous, muscle, musculocutaneous, osseous or osteocutaneous. According to their location (donor site), flaps are classified as local, regional or distant. The method of mobilization of the tissue defines it as a rotation, transposition, advancement or free (tissue transplantation) flap. Finally, flaps have been described by the blood supply they receive: random (based on local subdermal blood supply), axial (containing a discrete vascular pedicle), or free (containing a discrete vascular pedicle which is detached and transplanted to new recipient vessels). A combination of these terms is used to describe the type of flap that is used for reconstruction. For example, a forehead flap used for nasal reconstruction is a local cutaneous flap with an axial blood supply that is rotated based on the supratrochlear vessels. A pectoralis major flap is a regional myocutaneous pedicled flap that may be either rotated or advanced to reconstruct a head and neck defect. A fibula flap used for mandible reconstruction may be either an osseous or osteocutaneous free flap.

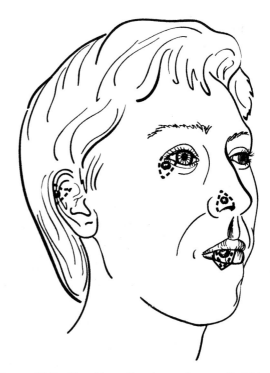

Figure 18–5. V-excision with primary closure will yield optimum results when planned perpendicular to the margin of the ear, eyelid, lip, and nasal ala.

Local Flaps

Local flaps consist of tissue that is mostly detached from surrounding tissue but retains enough connec-tion to preserve an adequate blood supply to the entire flap. These are mostly cutaneous flaps that are used very often for reconstruction of small- to mod-erate-sized cutaneous defects of the head and neck.[10] Local flaps may be transposed, rotated or advanced, and the donor site closed primarily. Examples of local flaps frequently used for reconstruction of facial defects include the Limberg or rhomboid (transposition), V-Y (advancement) and Imre (rota-tion) flap (Figure 18–8). Rearrangement of existing tissue in one area (ie, Z-plasty) is another technique frequently used to change the orientation of a scar or lengthen a scar contracture (Figure 18–9).

Moderate-sized composite defects requiring spe-cialized tissues, such as those of the eyelids or lips, can often be reconstructed using switch flaps from their opposite, intact counterparts.[11,12] The borrowed tissue is mobilized and left attached to the defect for 3 weeks. At this time collateral neovascularization to

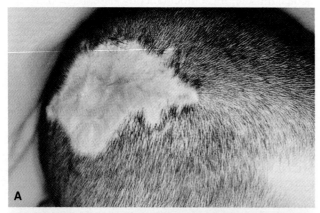
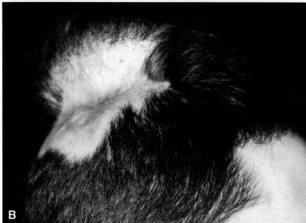
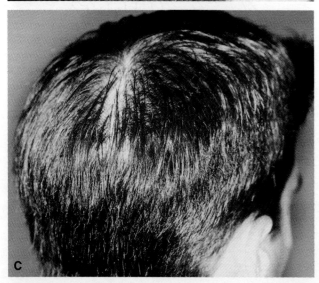

Figure 18–6. *A*, A patient with dermatofibrosarcoma of the scalp was reconstructed with pericranial flap and split-thickness skin graft which have healed well. *B*, Tissue expander in place and scalp fully expanded. *C*, Appearance after excision of skin graft, removal of tis-sue expander and advancement of expanded scalp.

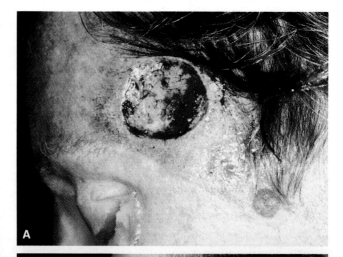
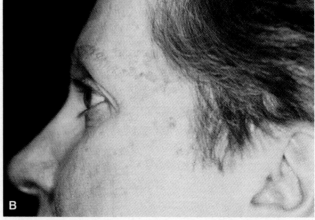

Figure 18–7. *A*, Defect in temporal region. *B*, Late follow-up after repair with full-thickness skin graft. Note reasonable color match.

the flap is developed at the recipient site, the original vascular pedicle is divided and both defects closed primarily (Figure 18–10).

Random Flaps

A random flap is a cutaneous flap (ie, skin and subcutaneous tissue) that receives its blood supply through the subdermal capillary plexus rather than from named vessels. Random flaps for head and neck reconstruction are transposition, rotation or advancement flaps that are used mostly to resurface superficial defects after excision of skin cancers. Due to the nonspecific blood supply, these flaps tend to have a marginal viability at the distal tip; thus its length-to-width ratio limits the size of a random flap. According to experimental studies, this ratio should be no larger than 3 to 1 so that the entire flap can survive.[13] Occasionally, the flap vascularity may be augmented using a so-called delay procedure, which consists of partially raising the skin flap and suturing it back to its vascular bed for 2 to 3 weeks.[14,15] Although the mechanism of the delay phenomenon is not completely understood, it is felt that partially elevating the flap results in a degree of local ischemia which in turn augments the remaining blood supply to the tissue. In general, delaying a flap allows for the successful transfer of a larger flap with an increased length-to-width ratio. Expanding adjacent tissue to obtain larger skin flaps with the same color and texture as the recipient site functions also as a gradual delay phenomenon. Tissue expansion has been extremely useful for head and neck reconstruction achieved in a delayed fashion[16] (see Figure 18–2).

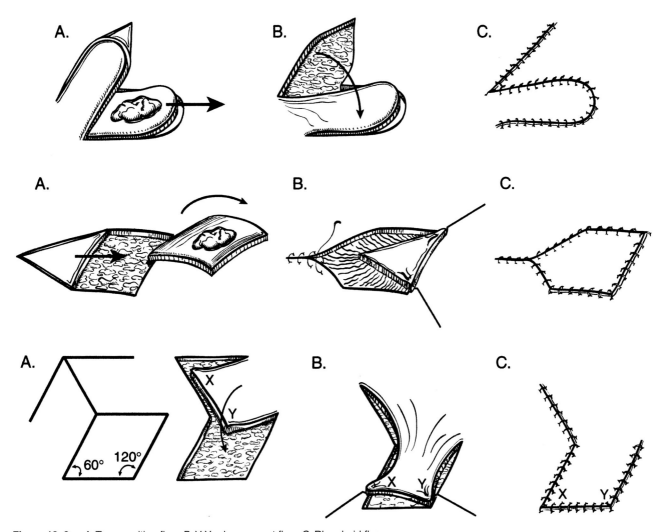

Figure 18–8. *A*, Transposition flap. *B*, V-Y advancement flap. *C*, Rhomboid flap.

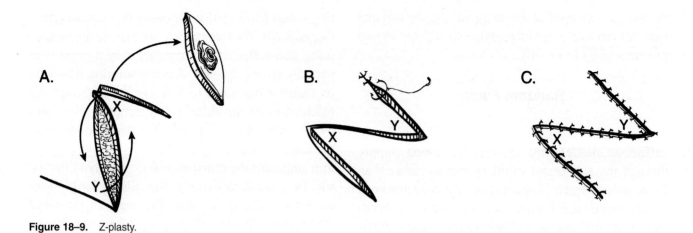

Figure 18–9.   Z-plasty.

Axial Flaps

Axial flaps are skin and subcutaneous tissue segments designed to parallel the major axis of a named vessel. If required, an axial flap may be designed such that all tissue may be raised, except at the connection with the vascular pedicle. This allows further mobilization of the cutaneous segment, as opposed to a random flap that has a more significant soft-tissue attachment to the donor site. Due to an identifiable blood supply,

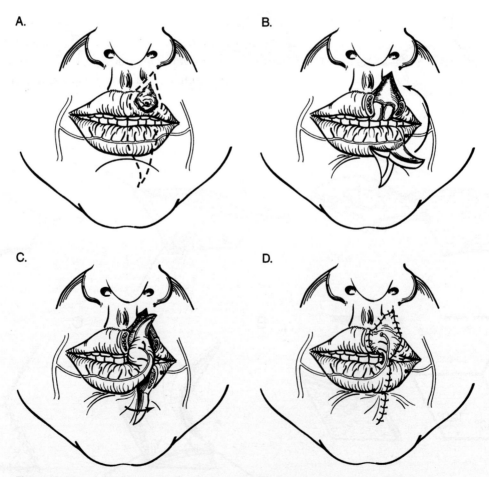

Figure 18–10.   *A,* Design of excision of lip lesion and lip switch flap for repair. *B, C,* Flap elevated and transposed into defect. *D,* Flap inset into upper lip. Pedicle is left attached for 10 to 21 days.

length-to-width ratio of axial flaps is not a concern and survival is increased when compared to random flaps.

Axial flaps most frequently used for head and neck reconstruction are based on the supratrochlear vessels (median or paramedian forehead flap) and the labial marginal artery and vein (nasolabial flap). Following are examples of axial flaps used in head and neck reconstruction.

Scalp and Frontal Flaps

Nearly the entire scalp and forehead may be divided and raised into different hair-bearing, cutaneous or composite flaps. These flaps are based on the superficial temporal vessels, the supratrochlear vessels and/or the occipital vessels.

Hair-bearing flaps are used for reconstruction of moderate-sized defects in the frontal or occipital region. The Orticochea triple scalp flap consists of two flaps based on the superficial temporal vessels on each side and a larger third flap based on both occipital arteries.[17] The flaps are elevated in the loose areolar tissue plane between the pericranium and the galea aponeurotica. Many parallel incisions are made in the aponeurosis of the flaps to increase mobilization. The flaps are then advanced and sutured to each other over the defect (Figure 18–11).

Flaps based on the parietal branch of the superficial temporal artery include only hair-bearing skin (the temporoparietooccipital flap). This flap may be used for reconstruction of the anterior hairline, eyebrow, and mustache. Flaps based on the frontal branch of the superficial temporal artery may include hair-bearing skin and the forehead (scalping flap), or the entire forehead unit (frontal flap). If based on both superficial temporal arteries, a visor flap may be raised. Scalping and frontal flaps have been used for reconstruction of the nose, midface and the intraoral lining (Figure 18–12). An important disadvantage of the scalping of frontal flap is that the donor site has to be skin grafted.[18]

Paramedian Forehead Flap

This axial flap is commonly used for external coverage in nasal reconstruction. It is based on the supratrochlear artery and vein, running on the undersurface of the flap.[19] The flap is designed using a precise template of the missing nasal subunits and is placed on the contralateral forehead. Usually the distal third of the flap is elevated subcutaneously; the middle third includes part of the frontalis muscle, and from 1 cm above the supraorbital rim, flap elevation is in the subperiosteal plane. The flap is rotated 180 degrees and remains attached to the

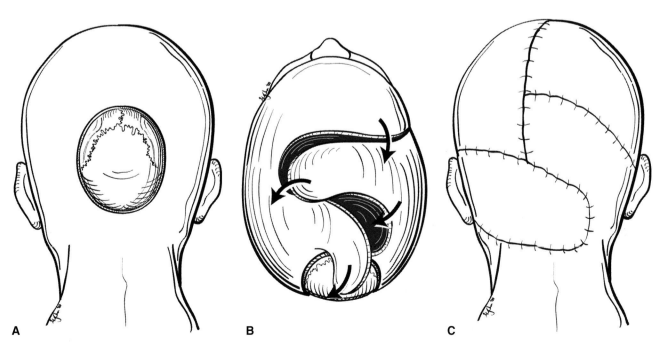

A   **B**   **C**

Figure 18–11. Reconstruction of scalp defect using the orticochea 4-flap technique.

pedicle for 3 to 6 weeks, to allow development of collateral circulation, before division of the feeding vessels (Figure 18–13). The forehead donor defect is generally closed primarily. When the donor site cannot be completely closed, healing by secondary intention of the remaining defect produces good esthetic results (Figure 18–14).

Nasolabial Flaps

The skin parallel to the nasolabial fold can be raised as an axial cutaneous flap. Depending upon flap design (either superiorly- or inferiorly-based), the

blood supply is provided by branches of the facial, infraorbital and angular vessels. Superiorly-based nasolabial flaps are more useful for reconstruction of small-sized nasal defects, due to easier transposition. The inferiorly-based pedicle flap is often advanced in a V-Y fashion for cheek or upper lip defects (Figure 18–15).[20] Nasolabial flaps are usually elevated in a superficial subcutaneous plane that excludes the main vascular pedicle. The donor site is usually closed primarily, with the scar concealed within the skin fold. Sometimes a secondary revision may be needed. Bilateral nasolabial flaps, based on the facial artery and vein, have been used to resurface floor of mouth and intraoral defects.[21,22]

Deltopectoral Flap

The deltopectoral flap was the workhorse for intraoral, cheek and neck reconstruction in the 1960s and 1970s.[23–25] The flap is based on the first, second, and third perforators of the internal mammary artery and associated venae comitantes. The base of the flap is located at 2 cm from the sternal edge, where the perforators pierce. Cranial incision follows the infraclavicular line and the caudal incision parallels the cranial incision. The flap extends to the shoulder or even the upper arm. However, depending upon the

A.
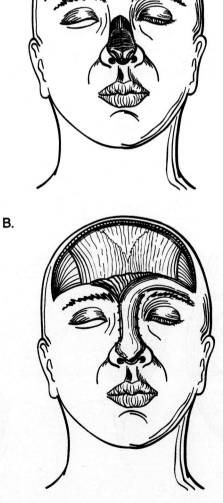
B.

Figure 18–12.   Nasal reconstruction with the Converse scalping flap.

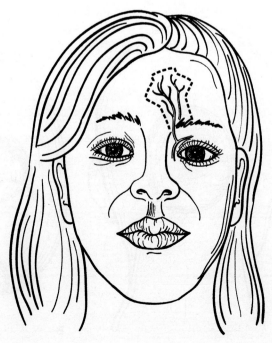

Figure 18–13.   Design of the paramedian forehead flap.

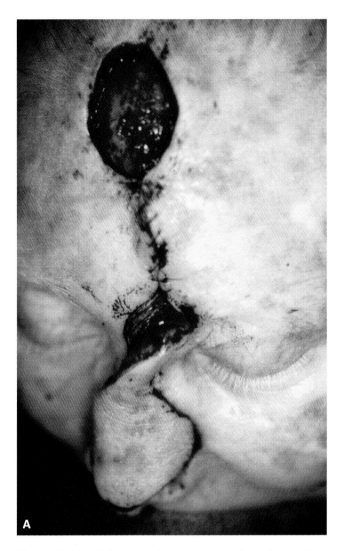

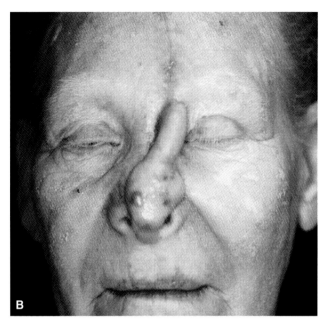

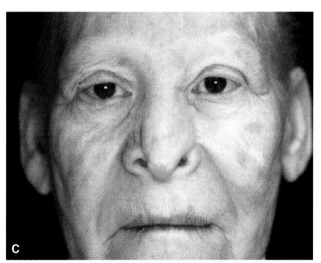

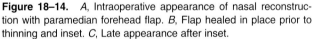

Figure 18–14. *A*, Intraoperative appearance of nasal reconstruction with paramedian forehead flap. *B*, Flap healed in place prior to thinning and inset. *C*, Late appearance after inset.

size of the flap needed, one or more delays may be required prior to transfer.[24] The deltopectoral flap has been used to resurface defects of the neck, face, and oral cavity (Figure 18–16). The donor site must be skin grafted, resulting in a significant disfigurement.

MUSCLE AND MUSCULOCUTANEOUS FLAPS

The development of muscle and musculocutaneous flaps resulted from an understanding of the blood supply to muscles and their overlying skin segments.[26,27] This development in reconstructive surgery has significantly maximized flap survival and allowed reconstruc-

tion of larger head and neck defects that could not be covered with local flaps alone.[28] A complete muscle or a muscle segment may be rotated or transposed into a defect, based on its own inherent blood supply. The muscle surface may be either skin grafted or an overlying skin paddle may be included with the muscle as a myocutaneous unit. The cutaneous territory of the flap is perfused by a system of perforating vessels from the main vascular pedicle that runs through the muscle component. Myocutaneous flaps revolutionized head and neck reconstruction in the 1970s. The pectoralis major myocutaneous flap rapidly became the workhorse for reconstruction of intraoral and cheek defects and for covering synthetic materials used for mandible

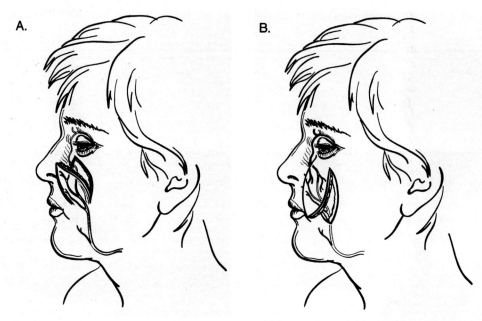

Figure 18–15. Inferiorly- and superiorly-based nasolabial flaps.

reconstruction.[29,30] Other myocutaneous pedicled flaps used less often for reconstruction of posterior or lateral defects in the head and neck region include the temporalis muscle, latissimus dorsi, trapezius, sternocleidomastoid and platysma muscles.[28,31–34] Although regional muscle and myocutaneous flaps are useful options for head and neck reconstruction, they often cannot reach the defect due to a limited arc of rotation (imposed by the vascular pedicle), and may result in incomplete survival of the skin island. In addition, donor sites are very noticeable, particularly when skin grafting of the defect is required.

Temporalis Muscle Flap

The temporalis muscle originates from the temporal fossa and inserts into the coronoid process of the mandible. It is surrounded by the galea and frontalis fascia and incorporates the underlying pericranium.[31] If required, the outer table of the parietal bone may be incorporated together with the muscle. Its blood supply is provided by the deep temporal vessels. These vessels run deep to the pterygoid muscles and penetrate the undersurface of the temporalis muscle near the insertion. Elevation of the temporalis muscle flap

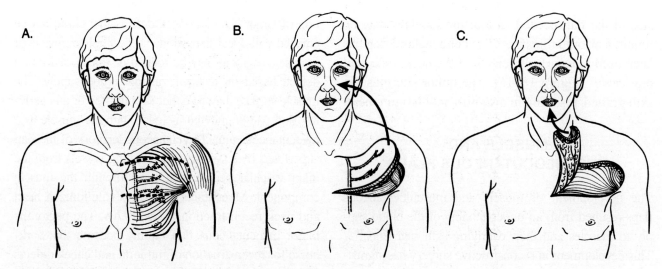

Figure 18–16. Design and arc of rotation of the standard deltopectoral flap.

is simple; however, the temporal branch of the facial nerve is at risk for injury during flap harvest. Functional loss from use of this flap is minimal and the donor site can be closed primarily. The main drawback with this flap is the donor site contour deformity.[35]

The temporalis muscle flap may be transferred as a turnover flap using the coronoid process as rotation pivot. To maximize flap excursion, the central portion of the zygomatic arch should be temporarily removed and fixed back after elevating the muscle.[36] Its main utility is to cover cheek, palatal and pharyngeal defects.[36–38] It is a good option for obliteration of the orbit through the lateral orbital wall, and it is useful to cover exposed dura or cranial bone (Figure 18–17).

Pectoralis Major Flap

The pectoralis major (PM) myocutaneous flap is the most frequently used pedicled flap for head and neck reconstruction.[29,39–41] The PM muscle originates from the clavicle, the first five ribs, the xiphoid, and from the upper abdominal muscles. It inserts on the humerus. Its blood supply is provided by branches of the thoracoacromial trunk, which pierces the clavipectoral fascia medial to the tendon of the pectoralis minor muscle. Multiple perforators run through the muscle in the subcutaneous fat, supplying the overlying skin with direct cutaneous vessels. The skin paddle can be located anywhere over the muscle pedicle. However, the design used most often is a vertical paddle up to 8 x 17 cm raised over the sternal origin of the muscle, which provides thin skin and allows primary closure of the donor defect. The skin island may extend into the inframammary fold and multiple skin paddles can be carried on the same muscle pedicle.[42]

The PM flap has been used to resurface cervical, facial, intraoral and pharyngeal defects (Figure 18–18).[39–44] Although it can reach as far as the orbit, the most distal part of the flap may be compromised due to limited arc of rotation. In addition, it is often too bulky for intraoral reconstruction where thin, pliable tissue is needed to replace intraoral lining. The donor site may be closed primarily; however, a very noticeable scar and nipple-areola distortion is often observed. Large or multiple skin islands may result in the need for donor site skin grafting.

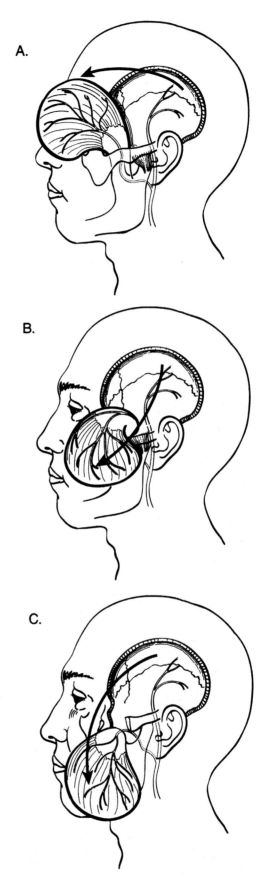

Figure 18–17. Arc of rotation of the temporalis muscle flap.

Latissimus Dorsi Flap

The latissimus dorsi (LD) muscle originates from the six caudal thoracic spines and fascia, the lumbar spines and fascia, and the posterior iliac crest. It inserts into the humerus. Its blood supply is from the thoracodorsal artery, accompanied by the thoracodorsal vein and nerve. The neurovascular pedicle enters the undersurface of the muscle 6 to 11.5 cm distal to the origin of the subscapular artery and 1.0 to 4.0 cm medial to the anterior border of the muscle. The thoracodorsal artery divides into a medial and lateral branch. The medial branch parallels the upper border and the lateral runs 2.5 cm from the lateral edge of the LD. Secondary smaller branches come from the dorsal branch of the ninth, tenth, and eleventh intercostal arteries and the four lumbar arteries. The overlying skin is supplied in the upper portion by large myocutaneous perforators and in the middle by smaller perforators and by lateral dorsal branches of the intercostal and lumbar vessels entering 8 cm from the midline. One or more skin islands with different orientation may be outlined over the muscle (Figure 18–19). A maximum size of 12 x 35 cm allows direct closure. For head and neck reconstruction, it is advisable to design the skin island distally over the lateral border of the muscle in order to reach the defect.[45] The flap is transferred to the head and neck through a tunnel either subcutaneously or beneath the pectoralis muscle.[46–48] As a pedicled flap it is a useful option for neck and cheek defects that do not extend beyond the buccomandibular subunit (Figure 18–20). The donor site is usually closed primarily. The main shortcoming of the LD flap is that simultaneous resection/reconstruction of the head and neck region is not feasible, due to the need for patient repositioning in order to harvest the flap and close the donor site. Due to a limited arc of rotation,

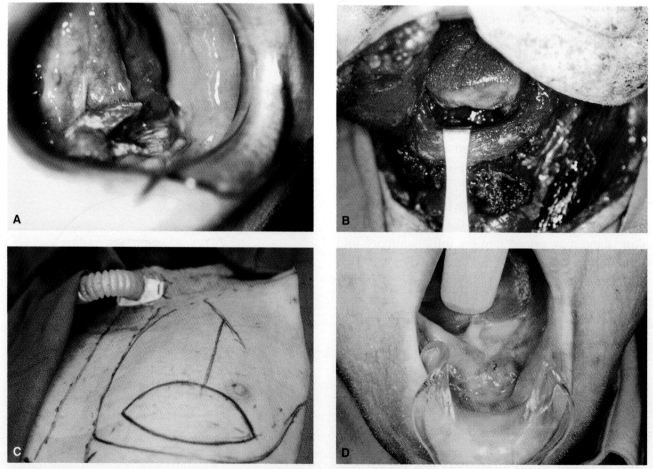

Figure 18–18. *A,* Squamous cell carcinoma of anterior floor of mouth. *B,* Intraoperative appearance after tumor resection, marginal mandibulectomy and neck dissection. *C,* Design of pectoralis major flap. *D,* Late appearance of flap healed in anterior floor of mouth.

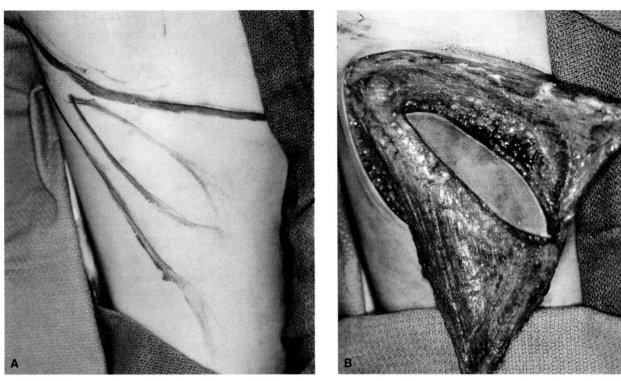

Figure 18–19. *A*, Design of latissimus dorsi flap with skin island. *B*, Flap elevated with skin island.

this flap is often transferred as free tissue. Its large diameter vessels (2.0 to 3.0 mm) and length (8.0 to 12.0 cm) allow the performance of anastomoses with neck vessels safely (see below). It is not as bulky as the rectus abdominis myocutaneous flap and therefore can be folded more easily.

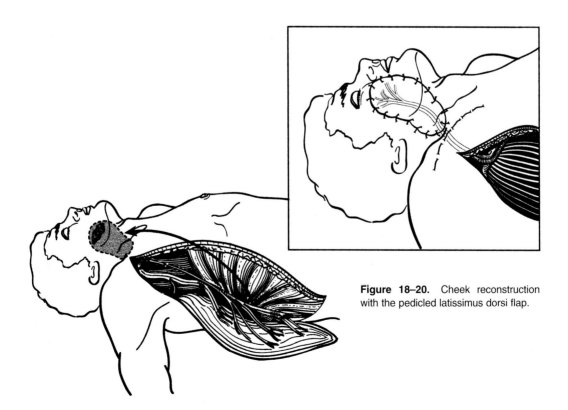

Figure 18–20. Cheek reconstruction with the pedicled latissimus dorsi flap.

Trapezius Flap

The trapezius muscle originates from the occipital bone and the lateral processes of the seventh cervical and all thoracic vertebrae. It inserts into the scapular spine, acromion, and lateral third of the clavicle. The trapezius myocutaneous flap may be transferred as a horizontal, lateral or vertical flap.

The horizontal myocutaneous trapezius flap (7 × 30 cm) receives its blood supply from a branch of the occipital artery in the uppermost part, and by a direct cutaneous descending branch, lying on the semispinalis between the sternocleidomastoideus and the trapezius.[49] This flap has a large arc of rotation and has been used for reconstruction of the floor of mouth, cheek, temporal fossa and occiput (Figure 18–21).[49–51] Closure of the donor site requires a skin graft. The lateral trapezius flap is based on the transverse cervical artery, arising from the subclavian artery. The skin island is centered over the acromioclavicular joint, and the muscle may carry the scapular spine. This flap has been used for reconstruction of floor of mouth, midfacial and mandibular defects with poor results.[50]

The vertical trapezius flap has a wider range of transfer in the head and neck area than other flaps (see Figure 18–21). Its blood supply comes from the dorsal scapular artery, originating from the descending branch of the transverse cervical artery, near the cranial border of the scapula or emerging directly from the subclavian artery. It descends vertically midway between the vertebral column and the medial border of the scapula, where the skin island of the flap usually is centered. Its caudal end may extend beyond the muscle and has a random blood supply. The skin island may be as large as 9 x 20 cm. The donor site may be closed primarily if it is less than 9.0 cm wide; however donor site healing in this area is frequently associated with seroma formation and a very noticeable scar. This flap has been used for reconstruction of defects centered around the orbit and upward to the skull, across the midline, or for intracranial reconstruction. Although color match and texture of the trapezius flap is good for use in the neck, it is not ideal when used for the face. Similar to the latissimus dorsi flap, intraoperative repositioning of the patient is usually required. Additionally, this flap is not an option in the setting of an ipsilateral

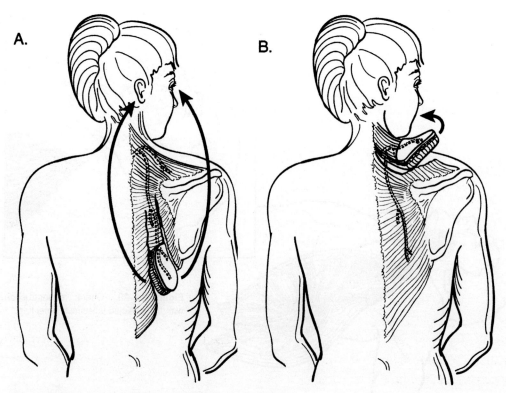

Figure 18–21.   Arc of rotation of the trapezius muscle flap.

radical neck dissection, due to sacrifice of the transverse cervical vessels.

FASCIOCUTANEOUS FLAPS

Fasciocutaneous flaps were described after recognition of certain patterns of cutaneous blood supply. The blood supply of the deep fascia appears to consist of both a deep and a superficial fascial plexus.[52] These fascial vessels connect both: to perforating vessels from the underlying muscles, and to the subcutaneous tissue vessels above them. In some areas, fascia supplies overlying subcutaneous tissue and skin in a more direct fashion. Direct branches from major vessels course through intermuscular septa to reach the deep fascia. These septocutaneous perforators supply the overlying skin and subcutaneous tissue. At least three types of fasciocutaneous flaps exist according to their blood supply configuration.[53] Type A flaps are those fed by multiple small, longitudinal vessels that course with the deep fascia. This type of flap must be raised with a base of a certain width to ensure its vascular supply and therefore cannot be raised as an island. The majority of type A fasciocutaneous flaps have been described on the lower leg. Type B flaps are those fed by a single major vessel within the fascia (scapular or lateral arm flap). Type C flaps are those supplied by multiple perforating segments from a major vessel that courses through intermuscular septa (eg, radial forearm flap) (Figure 18–22). Both type B and C flaps can be raised as island flaps or can be transferred as free tissue. All fasciocutaneous flaps described for head and neck reconstruction can only be transferred as free flaps.

FREE FLAPS

Perhaps the most significant contribution to the management of head and neck cancer patients in the past 3 decades is the development of microsurgical free tissue transfer.[54,55] Different specialized tissues receiving blood supply from specific vessels are totally detached from the donor site and the artery and vein are reconnected at the recipient site by performing vascular anastomoses with the aid of magnification systems. Success rates using microvascular reconstruction techniques have been reported to

be ≥ 95 percent in most major medical centers.[6,56,57] Although many free flaps have been described for head and neck reconstruction, a review of 716 free flaps performed in our institution revealed that only four free flaps are required for reconstructing 95 percent of head and neck defects in the oncologic patient.[6] These include radial forearm flap, rectus abdominis, fibula and jejunum. Some of the other free flaps occasionally used for head and neck

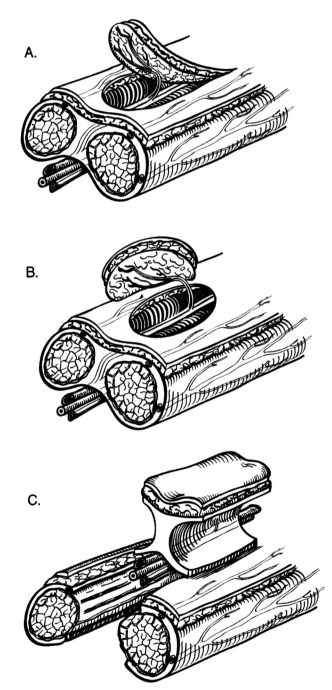

Figure 18–22. Types A,B,C fasciocutaneous flaps.

reconstruction are the scapula, latissimus dorsi, lateral arm, iliac crest and anterolateral thigh flaps. The versatility of some of these free flaps is reflected in their ability to include different tissues from the same donor site based on one single pedicle, and therefore to harvest composite tissue which can then be used for reconstruction of complex defects, as described below.

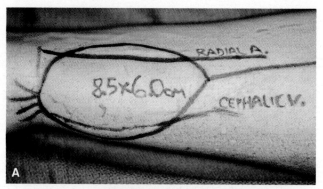

Cutaneous and Fasciocutaneous Free Flaps

Radial Forearm Free Flap

The forearm free flap is a fasciocutaneous free flap, based on the radial artery and cephalic vein or venae comitantes. It consists of thin, pliable skin with minimal soft tissue and a very long pedicle with a large diameter. In addition, a sensory nerve over the anterior forearm skin (lateral antebrachial cutaneous nerve) can be included within the flap, to provide sensory recovery at the recipient site. These characteristics have made it a very useful flap for intraoral, pharyngeal and cutaneous facial defects (Figure 18–23).[58–62] Two or more skin islands can be designed with the flap. The folded flap is used for reconstruction of full-thickness defects in the cheek, with one skin island for inner lining and the other for external coverage (Figure 18–24).[63]

The radial forearm free flap can be designed to include tendons, muscle, or a vascularized segment of bone up to 12 cm in length, based on the same vascular pedicle. As a tendocutaneous unit, the radial forearm free flap has been used for reconstruction of total lower lip and cheek defects (Figure 18–25). The radial forearm osteocutaneous free flap has been very useful for reconstruction of maxillary and mandibular defects (Figure 18–26).[64,65]

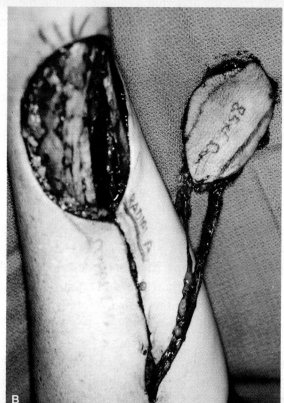

Lateral Arm

The lateral arm flap is a useful free flap for head and neck reconstruction due to the following advantages: there is no need to sacrifice an artery that may be essential to the vascularity of the distal upper extremity (as compared to the radial forearm free flap), and in many patients it is possible to close the donor defect primarily.[66–68]

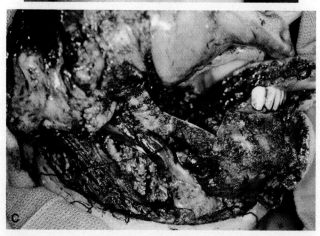

Figure 18–23. *A,* Design of radial forearm free flap. *B,* Flap elevated on radial artery pedicle. *C,* Defect after composite resection of lateral floor of mouth and marginal mandibulectomy which is suitable for reconstruction using this flap.

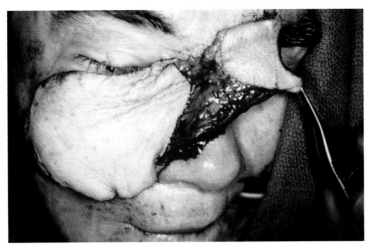

Figure 18–24. Radial forearm free flap with two skin islands used for external skin and intranasal reconstruction.

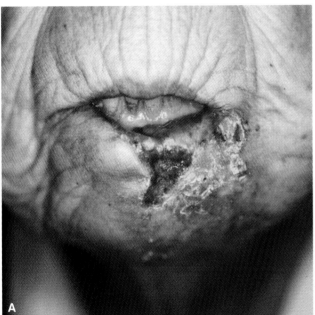

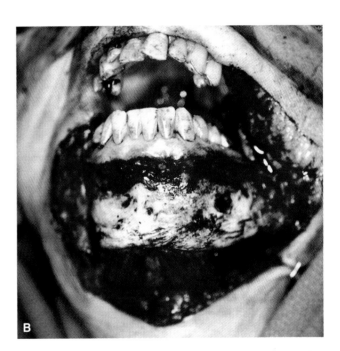

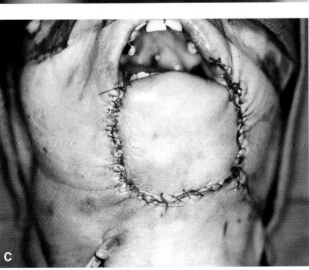

Figure 18–25. *A,* Squamous cell carcinoma of lower lip. *B,* Defect of surgical resection of tumor. *C,* Lower lip reconstruction with radial forearm free flap folded over palmaris longus tendon sling.

The lateral arm free flap may be transferred either as a fascial or fasciocutaneous flap based on the posterior radial collateral artery, a terminal branch of the profunda brachii artery. The vascular pedicle runs parallel to the lateral intermuscular septum and anastomoses with the recurrent interosseous artery distally. The maximum dimensions of the cutaneous paddle are 18 × 11 cm; however, in most cases the width of the flap is limited to 6 to 8 cm, in order to allow primary closure of the posterior aspect of the arm (Figure 18–27). The skin paddle is moderately pliable and the recovery of sensation is made possible by anastomosing the posterior cutaneous nerve of the arm to a recipient nerve in the head and neck. This sensate lateral arm flap has been used for restoration of the oral cavity and for partial glossectomy defects.[60,68] In addition, the lateral arm flap is used to resurface facial defects and less often for through and through cheek defects.[67]

Muscle and Musculocutaneous Free Flaps

Rectus Abdominis

Various designs of musculocutaneous flaps may be transferred as free flaps based on the rectus abdominis muscle, supplied by the deep inferior epigastric artery and vein and the periumbilical perforators[69] (Figure 18–28). The rectus abdominis muscle is flat and thin, with a large skin island over the muscle that may be oriented in a vertical transverse or oblique fashion. In addition, one or more cutaneous paddles may be used to cover multiple surfaces of complex multidimensional defects in the head and neck.[70] In obese patients, however, the flap may be too bulky and therefore it is preferable to transfer the muscle alone, covered with a split-thickness skin graft.

The deep inferior epigastric artery and vein are vessels with a large caliber (2 to 3 mm) and length (8 to 10 cm). If required, the length of the vascular pedicle may be extended to up to 18 cm by dissecting the lateral branch of these vessels within the muscle.[71]

Another advantage of the rectus abdominis flap for head and neck reconstruction is the possibility of harvesting the flap at the same time the ablative procedure is being performed, without needing to change the position of the patient.

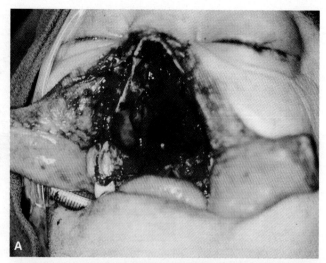

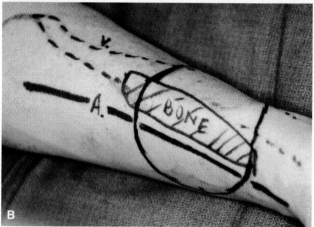

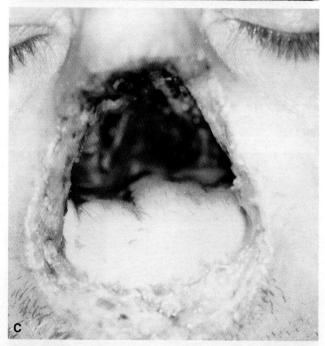

Figure 18–26.   *A,* Defect after total rhinectomy and anterior maxillectomy. *B,* Design of osseocutaneous radial forearm flap. *C,* Flap inset so that osseous component bridges maxillectomy defect; two skin islands are used to resurface floor of nasal cavity and roof of mouth.

A.   B.

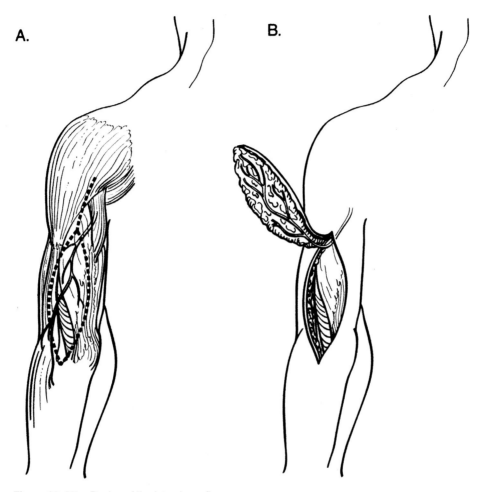

Figure 18–27. Design of the lateral arm flap.

The rectus abdominis free flap is without question the first choice for defects that require a large amount of skin coverage and soft tissue. Such requirements are usually observed after wide excision of scalp or skull base tumors,[71,72] total maxillectomy and midfacial defects,[38] orbitomaxillectomy, and composite resections of mandible and soft tissue[73,74] (Figure 18–29).

Latissimus Dorsi

The latissimus dorsi may be used as a free muscle or musculocutaneous flap for head and neck reconstruction. Anatomic details of the latissimus dorsi muscle were described in the pedicle flap section. In this section, it is important to emphasize that the vascular anatomy of this flap is extremely consistent and reliable for performing microvascular anastomoses with neck vessels or the superficial temporal artery and vein. The latissimus dorsi is a broad and flat muscle that is very useful to reconstruct extensive scalp defects, especially following resection of large tumors or débridement of calvaria for osteoradionecrosis[75,76] (Figure 18–30). The muscle is covered with a split-thickness skin graft, and once it atrophies a very stable wound is achieved. As a musculocutaneous flap the latissimus dorsi free flap is used for reconstruction of extensive orbitomaxillary or skull base defects that require minor soft-tissue fill and a cutaneous surface.[77] For more complex defects of the midface that require two epithelial surfaces, the latissimus dorsi may be harvested with two skin paddles; the intervening bridge of skin is de-epithelized and the muscle folded to repair the inner mucosal lining and the overlying skin.[78]

One of the few shortcomings of the latissimus dorsi free flap for head and neck reconstruction is the impossibility of harvesting the flap at the same time the ablative procedure is taking place. Unfortunately, the

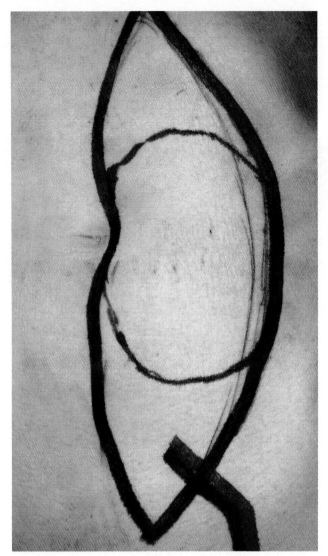

Figure 18–28.   Design of vertical rectus abdominis free flap.

fibula osseocutaneous free flap has been described for reconstruction of maxillary defects alone or in combination with mandible defects.[81]

Approximately 22 to 25 cm of bone can be harvested from the fibula. This thick cortical long bone receives its endosteal and periosteal blood supply from the peroneal artery and veins which run along

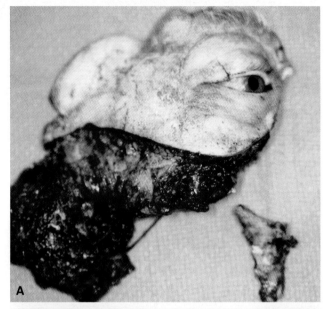

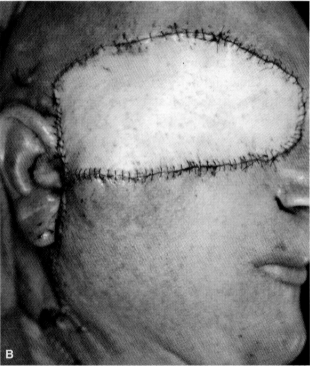

Figure 18–29.   *A,* Surgical specimen after anterior skull base resection with orbital exenteration. *B,* Reconstruction with vertical rectus abdominis myocutaneous free flap.

patient needs to be repositioned several times during surgery, thus significantly increasing the surgical time.

Osseous and Osseocutaneous Free Flaps

Fibula

The fibula can be transferred as a free osseous or free osseocutaneous flap. Since introduced first for mandible reconstruction in 1989, the fibula free flap has been applied for reconstruction of challenging defects in the head and neck.[79] However, the primary application of the fibular donor site is in the reconstruction of segmental defects of the mandible, as described elsewhere in this text.[80] In addition, the

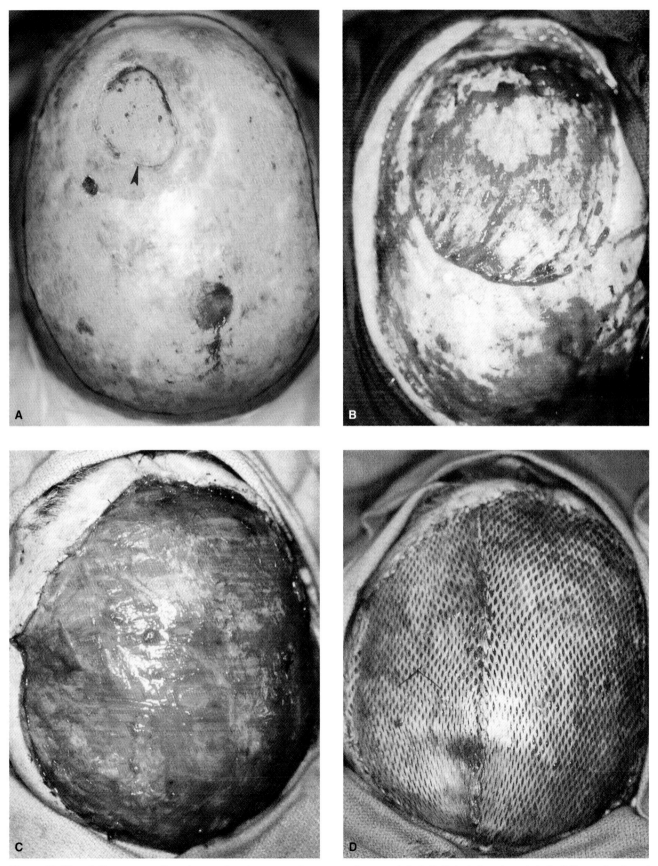

Figure 18–30. *A*, Squamous cell carcinoma of scalp—arrow shows area of exposed skull. *B*, Defect of scalp and skull. *C*, Reconstruction of scalp with latissimus dorsi free flap. *D*, Split-thickness skin graft over flap.

the entire length of the fibula.[82] The excellent periosteal circulation permits multiple osteotomies with reliable perfusion on each bony segment; thus allowing shaping and remodeling of the bone to duplicate the inferior border of the mandible. The skin over the lateral aspect of the calf is supplied by either septocutaneous or musculocutaneous perforators arising from the peroneal artery and vein[83] (Figure 18–31). In spite of the skin island of the fibula free flap being considered initially unreliable in 10 percent of cases due to unpredictable vascular supply,[79] it is now acknowledged that identification and inclusion of one single septocutaneous perforator can adequately perfuse a skin island as large as 10 × 22 cm.[82] This skin island may be used to reconstruct oromandibular defects that include the external skin, inner lining or both[82–84] (Figure 18–32). The flexor hallucis longus muscle may be transferred with the bone as well to provide some soft-tissue fill for the submental region.

Additional advantages of the fibula for reconstruction of the mandible include the ability to dissect the flap with the patient supine (allowing a two-team approach), and adequate bone stock for incorporating osseointegrated dental implants.[85] Donor site morbidity is usually minimal. The leg defect may be closed primarily when a narrow skin island (less than 4 cm in width) is included with the flap; otherwise a skin graft

is necessary to close the donor site. Some patients may experience transitory stiffness in the ankle joint, however, no physical limitations are usually observed.[80]

Scapula

Studies of the vascular anatomy of the subscapular system have dramatically expanded the versatility of this donor site and its range of applications to the head and neck. Large separated skin islands, muscle or musculocutaneous units and bone may be transferred based on one single pedicle, providing the most freedom for reconstruction of any composite defect (Figure 18–33).

The length of bone that can be harvested from the lateral border of the scapula ranges from 10 to 14 cm, depending on the sex of the patient.[86] The thickness of this bone, however, is not enough to place osseointegrated dental implants and therefore it is selected only for reconstruction of mandibular defects that involve the ascending ramus and require moderate to large amounts of soft-tissue fill and skin replacement over the cheek (see related chapter). As an osseocutaneous composite flap the scapular flap also has been used to reconstruct maxillectomy and midfacial defects.[86–88] The floor of the orbit or palate is reconstructed with the bony segment and one or two skin islands are used for inner lining and/or skin

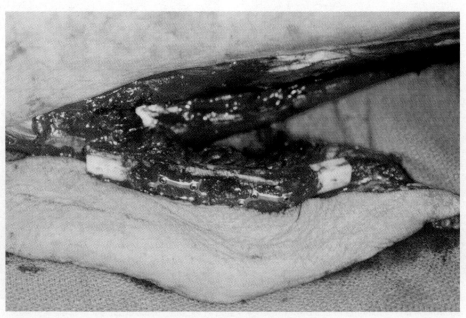

Figure 18–31. In situ appearance of fibula free flap with skin island.

coverage. Potential pitfalls with the scapular flap for reconstruction of such defects include: difficulty placing the different tissue components, a short pedicle that cannot reach the neck vessels and therefore vein grafts are required, and the need to reposition the patient during surgery.

Visceral Free Flaps

Jejunum

Transfer of jejunal free graft was the first microsurgical flap reported in the literature.[89] Currently the jejunal free graft is used as a mucosal tube or mucosal patch (depending on the configuration of the defect) for reconstruction of the hypopharynx or cervical esophagus.[90] The jejunal free flap has proved

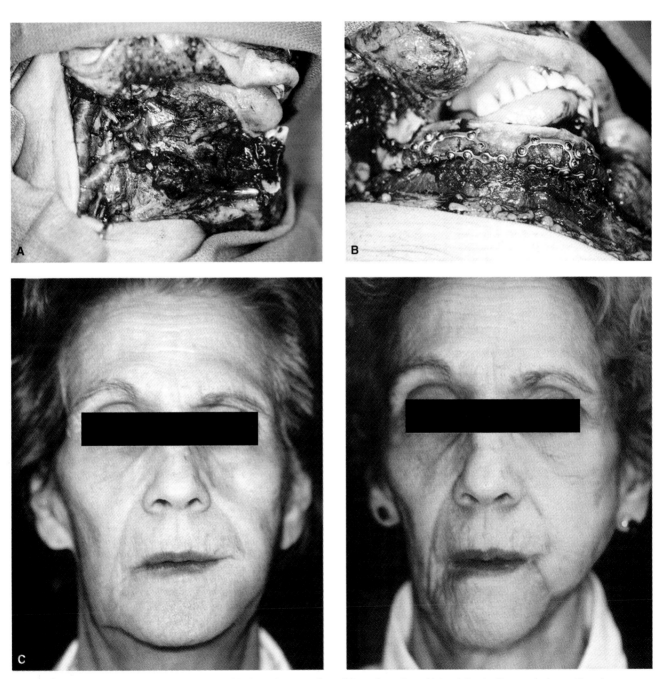

Figure 18–32. *A*, Defect of anterolateral mandible, lateral tongue, lateral floor of mouth and lateral cheek after surgical resection of squamous cell carcinoma. *B*, Mandible reconstruction with fibula osseocutaneous free flap prior to inset of skin island. *C*, Preoperative appearance. *D*, Postoperative appearance after reconstruction and external beam radiation therapy.

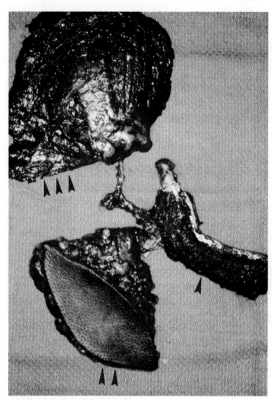

Figure 18–33. Composite scapula flap demonstrating osseous component (single arrow), cutaneous component (double arrow), latissimus muscle component (triple arrow) all based upon single vascular pedicle.

to be superior to pedicled visceral flaps such as stomach or colon that are transferred to reconstruct the cervical esophagus. Advantages of microsurgical transplantation of a jejunal segment, over the gastric pull-up procedure to reconstruct defects of the upper aerodigestive tract, include no limitations on reaching the neck and a predictable blood supply. In addition, there is no need for extensive abdominal and thoracic dissections, which are often fraught with complications. Finally, postoperative adjuvant radiotherapy can be administered without significant risk of complication.[91]

The caliber of the jejunum lumen matches the esophagus in most individuals. However, for reconstruction of pharyngoesophageal defects the pharynx opening may be considerably larger. For such defects, the cephalad portion of the free jejunum can be opened along its antimesenteric border to increase the caliber.[90]

The small intestine segment to be transferred is usually 40 cm distal to the ligament of Treitz. The isolated portion of bowel is supplied by a single vas-

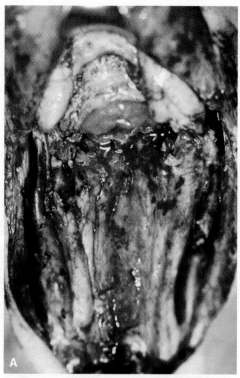

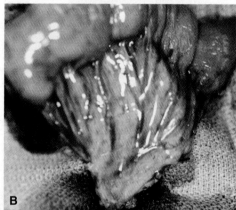

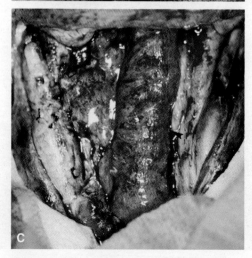

Figure 18–34. *A,* Defect after total laryngopharyngectomy. *B,* Jejunal free flap. *C,* Pharynx reconstruction with jejunal free flap.

cular arcade arising from large nutrient vessels coming from the superior mesenteric artery and vein (Figure 18–34). Due to limited tolerance of the jejunum to ischemia, it is advisable to prepare the recipient vessels before dividing the vascular pedicle and to complete the vascular anastomoses in less than 120 minutes.

Postoperative monitoring of the blood supply to the jejunal segment buried under the neck flaps is facilitated by exteriorizing a small segment of jejunum that remains attached to the large segment of bowel except through its vascular connections to the main vascular pedicle. The exteriorized jejunum is divided under local anesthesia 5 to 7 days after surgery. A barium swallow is usually performed between day 7 and 12 postoperatively, to assess permeability of the jejuno-esophageal anastomoses. Recently, the utility of this routine study has been questioned in our institution and is not considered 100 percent accurate.[92]

Complications at the donor site have been reported to occur in approximately 5.8 percent of patients.[93] These include bowel obstruction, abdominal wound dehiscence, gastrointestinal hemorrhage, G-tube leakage and prolonged ileus.

REFERENCES

1. Kroll SS, Marchi M. Immediate reconstruction. Current status in cancer management. Tex Med 1991;87:67.
2. Hidalgo DA, Disa JJ. Plastic surgical reconstruction. In: Scientific American Inc. 1998;X,1–18.
3. Gonzalez-Ulloa M. Restoration of the face covering by means of selected skin in regional aesthetic units. Br J Plast Surg 1956;9:212.
4. Burget GC, Menick FJ. The subunit principle in nasal reconstruction. Plast Reconstr Surg 1985;76:239.
5. Place MJ, Herber SC, Hardsty RA. Grabb and Smith plastic surgery. Basic techniques and principles in plastic surgery. 5th ed. Philadelphia (PA): Lippincott-Raven; 1997. p. 2, 13.
6. Hidalgo DA, Disa JD, Cordeiro PG, et al. A review of 716 consecutive free flaps for oncologic surgical defects: refinements in donor-site selection and technique. Plast Reconstr Surg 1998;102:722.
7. Singh B, Cordeiro PG, Santamaria E, et al. Factors associated with complications in microvascular reconstruction of head and neck defects. Plast Reconstr Surg 1999;103:403.
8. Edgerton MT, Hansen FC. Matching facial color with split thickness skin grafts from adjacent areas. Plast Reconstr Surg 1960;25:455.
9. Schramm VL, Myers EN. Skin grafts in oral cavity reconstruction. Arch Otolaryngol 1980;106:528.
10. Jackson IT. General principles. In: Local flaps in head and reconstruction. St. Louis (MO): C.V. Mosby Co.; 1989. p. 1–34.
11. McGregor I. Eyelid reconstruction following subtotal resection of upper or lower lid. Br J Plast Surg 1973;26:346.
12. Burget GC, Menick FJ. Aesthetic restoration of one-half of the upper lip. Plast Reconstr Surg 1986;78:583.
13. Milton SH. Pedicled skin-flaps: the fallacy of the length: width ratio. Br J Surg 1970;57:502.
14. Callegari PR, Taylor GI, Caddy CM, et al. An anatomical review of the delay phenomenon: 1 Experimental studies. Plast Reconstr Surg 1992;89:397.
15. Taylor GI, Corlett RJ, Caddy CM, et al. An anatomical review of the delay phenomenon: II. Clinical applications. Plast Reconstr Surg 1992;89:408.
16. Argenta LC, Watanabe MJ, Grabb WC. The use of tissue expansion in head and neck reconstruction. Ann Plast Surg 1983;11:31.
17. Orticochea M. New three-flap scalp reconstruction technique. Br J Plast Surg 1971;24:184.
18. Lewis MB, Rememsnyder JP. Forehead flap for reconstruction after ablative surgery for oral and oropharyngeal malignancy. Plast Reconstr Surg 1978;62:59.
19. McCarthy JG. The median forehead flap revisited: the blood supply. Plast Reconstr Surg 1985;76:866.
20. Cameron RR, Lathan WD, Dowling JA. Reconstructions of the nose and upper lip with nasolabial flaps. Plast Reconstr Surg 1973;52:145.
21. Cohen IK, Theogaraj SD. Nasolabial flap reconstruction of the floor of the mouth after extirpation or oral cancer. Am J Surg 1975;130:479.
22. Elliot RA Jr. Use of nasolabial skin flap to cover intraoral defects. Plast Reconstr Surg 1976;58:201.
23. McGregor IA, Jackson IT. The extended role of the deltopectoral flap. Br J Plast Surg 1970;23:173.
24. Bakamjian VY, Long M, Rigg B. Experience with the medially based deltopectoral flap in reconstructive surgery of the head and neck. Br J Plast Surg 1971;24:174.
25. Daniel RK, Cunningham DM, Taylor GI. The deltopectoral flap: an anatomical and hemodynamic approach. Plast Reconstr Surg 1975;55:275.
26. Mathes SJ, Nahai F. Classification of the vascular anatomy of muscles: experimental and clinical correlation. Plast Reconstr Surg 1981;67:177.
27. McCraw JB, Vazcones LO. Musculocutaneous flaps: principles. Clin Plast Surg 1980;7:9.
28. Ariyan S, Cuono CB. Myocutaneous flaps for head and neck reconstruction. Head Neck Surg 1980;2:321.
29. Ariyan S. The pectoralis major myocutaneous flap. A versatile flap for reconstruction in the head and neck. Plast Reconstr Surg 1979;63:73.
30. Cordeiro PG, Hidalgo DA. Soft tissue coverage of mandibular reconstruction plates. Head Neck Surg 1994;2:112.
31. McGregor IA. Temporal flap in intraoral cancer: its use in repairing the post-excisional defect. Br J Plast Surg 1963;16:318.
32. Futrell JW, et al. Platysma myocutaneous flap for intraoral reconstruction. Am J Surg 1978;136:504.
33. McCraw JB, Magee WP, Kawaic H. Uses of the trapezius and sternomastoid myocutaneous flaps in head and neck reconstruction. Plast Reconstr Surg 1979;63:49.

34. Coleman JJ III, Nahai F, Mathes SJ. Platysma musculocutaneous flap: Clinical and anatomic consideration in head and neck reconstruction. Am J Surg 1982;144:477.

35. Cordeiro PG, Wolfe SA. The temporalis muscle flap revisited on its centennial: advantages, newer used and disadvantages. Plast Reconstr Surg 1996;98:980.

36. Koranda FC, McMahon MF. The temporalis muscle flap for intraoral reconstruction: technical modifications. Otolaryngol Head Neck Surg 1988;98:315.

37. Bradley P, Brockbank J. The temporalis muscle flap in oral reconstruction. J Maxillofac Surg 1981;9:139.

38. Cordeiro PG, Santamaria E, Krause DH, et al. Reconstruction of total maxillectomy defects with preservation of the orbital contents. Plast Reconstr Surg 1998;102:1874.

39. Magee WP Jr, et al. Pectoralis "paddle" myocutaneous flaps. The workhorse of head and neck reconstruction. Am J Surg 1980;140:507.

40. Baek S-M-, Lawson W, Biller HF. An analysis of 133 pectoralis major myocutaneous flaps. Plast Reconstr Surg 1982;69:460.

41. Kroll SS, et al. Analysis of complications in 168 pectoralis major myocutaneous flaps used for head and neck reconstruction. Ann Plast Surg 1990;25:93.

42. Palmer JH, Batchelor AG. The functional pectoralis major musculocutaneous island flap in head and neck reconstruction. Plast Reconstr Surg 1990;85:363.

43. Shah JP, Haribhakti V, Loree TR, et al. Complications of the pectoralis major myocutaneous flap in head and neck reconstruction. Am J Surg 1990;160:352.

44. Fabian R. Pectoralis major myocutaneous flap reconstruction of the laryngopharynx and cervical esophagus. Laryngoscope 1988;98:1227.

45. Quillen CG. Latissimus dorsi myocutaneous island flaps in head and neck reconstruction. Plast Reconstr Surg 1979;63:664.

46. Barton FE Jr, Spicer TE, Byrd HS. Head and neck reconstruction with the latissimus dorsi myocutaneous flap: Anatomic observations and report of 60 cases. Plast Reconstr Surg 1983;71:199.

47. Sabatier RE, Bakamjian VY. Transaxillary latissimus dorsi flap reconstruction in head and neck cancer. Limitations and refinements in 56 cases. Am J Surg 1985;150:427.

48. Davis JP, et al. The latissimus dorsi flap in head and neck reconstructive surgery: a review of 121 procedures. Clin Otolaryngol 1992;17:487.

49. Urken ML, et al. The lower trapezius island musculocutaneous flap revisited. Report of 45 cases and a unifying concept of the vascular supply. Arch Otolaryngol Head Neck Surg 1991;117:502.

50. Nicher LS, et al. The trapezius musculocutaneous flap in head and neck reconstruction. Potential pitfalls. Head Neck Surg 1984;7:129.

51. Demergasso F, Piazza MV. Trapezius myocutaneous flap in reconstructive surgery for head and neck cancer: An original technique. Am J Surg 1979;138:533.

52. Taylor GI, Palmer JH. The vascular territories (angiosomes) of the body: Experimental study and clinical applications. Br J Plast Surg 1987;40:113.

53. Lamberty B, Cormack G. The arterial anatomy of skin flaps. 2nd ed. New York: Churchill Livingstone; 1993. p.

54. Conley J. Use of composite flaps containing bone for major repairs in the head and neck. Plast Reconstr Surg 1972; 49:522.

55. Shestak KC, Myers EN, Ramasastry SS, et al. Vascularized free-tissue transfer in head and neck surgery. Am J Otolaryngol 1993;14(3):148.

56. Cordeiro PG, Santamaria E. Experience with the continuous microvascular anastomosis in 200 consecutive flaps for head and neck reconstruction. Transactions from the Annual Meeting: The Society of Head and Neck Surgeons. April 1997.Cancun, Mexico. p.55–6.

57. Schusterman MA, Miller MJ, Reece GP, et al. A single center's experience with 308 free flaps for repair of head and neck cancer defects. Plast Reconstr Surg 1994;93:472.

58. Boyd B, Mulholland S, Gullane P, et al. Reinnervated lateral antebrachial cutaneous neurosome flaps in oral reconstruction: are we making sense? Plast Reconstr Surg 1994;93:1350.

59. Santamaria E, Wei FC, Chen I-H. Sensation recovery on innervated radial forearm flap for hemiglossectomy reconstruction by using different recipient nerves. Plast Reconstr Surg 1999;103:450.

60. Cordeiro PG, Schwartz M, Neves RI, et al. Recipient site sensation in free tissue reconstruction of the oral cavity. Ann Plast Surg 1997;39:461.

61. Urken ML, Weinberg H, Vickery C, Biller HF. The neurofasciocutaneous radial forearm flap in head and neck reconstruction: a preliminary report. Laryngoscope 1990;100: 161.

62. Soutar DS, McGregor IA. The radial forearm flap in intraoral reconstruction: The experience of 60 consecutive cases. Plast Reconstr Surg 1986;78:1.

63. Freedman AM, Hidalgo DA. Full-thickness cheek and lip reconstruction with the radial forearm free flap. Ann Plast Surg 1990;25:287.

64. Soutar DS, Widdowson WP. Immediate reconstruction of the mandible using a vascularized segment of radius. Head Neck 1996;8:232.

65. Zenn MR, Hidalgo DA, Cordeiro PG, et al. Current role of the radial forearm free flap in mandibular reconstruction. Plast Reconstr Surg 1997;99:102.

66. Katsaros J, Schustermann M, Beppu M, et al. The lateral upper arm flap: anatomy and clinical applications. Ann Plast Surg 1984;12:489.

67. Sullivan MJ, Carroll WR, Kurloff DB. Lateral arm free flap in head and neck reconstruction. Arch Otolaryngol Head Neck Surg 1992;118:1095.

68. Matloub H, et al. Lateral arm free flap in oral cavity reconstruction: a functional evaluation. Head Neck 1989;11: 205.

69. Taylor GI, Corlett RJ, Boyd JB.The versatile deep inferior epigastric (inferior rectus abdominis) flap. Br J Plast Surg 1984;37:330.

70. Kroll SS, et al. Comparison of the rectus abdominis free flap with the pectoralis major myocutaneous flap for reconstructions in the head and neck. Am J Surg 1992;164:615.

71. Cordeiro PG, Santamaria E. The extended pedicle rectus abdominis free flap for head and neck reconstruction. Ann Plast Surg 1997;39:53.

72. Jones N, Sekhar L, Schramm V. Free rectus abdominis mus-

cle flap reconstruction of the middle and posterior cranial fossa. Plast Reconstr Surg 1986;78:471.

73. Disa JJ, Cordeiro PG. Efficacy of the rectus abdominis free flap in reconstruction of composite resections of the mandible. Proceedings from the 1999 Annual Meeting of the American Society of Reconstructive Microsurgery p.88.

74. Cordeiro PG, Santamaria E. Primary reconstruction of complex midfacial defects with combined lip-switch procedures and free flaps. Plast Reconstr Surg 1999;103:1850.

75. Earley MJ, Green M, Milling M. A critical appraisal of the use of free flaps in primary reconstruction of combined scalp and calvarial cancer defects. Br J Plast Surg 1990; 43:283.

76. Pennington D, Stern H, Lee K. Free flap reconstruction of large defects of the scalp and calvarium. Plast Reconstr Surg 1989;83:655.

77. Baker S. Closure of large orbital maxillary defects with free latissimus dorsi myocutaneous flaps. Head Neck 1984; 6:828.

78. Stueber K, Saloman M, Spence T. The combined use of the latissimus dorsi musculocutaneous free flap and split-rib grafts for cranial vault reconstruction. Ann Plast Surg 1985;15:155.

79. Hidalgo DA. Fibular flap: a new method of mandibular reconstruction. Plast Reconstr Surg 1989;84:71.

80. Cordeiro PG, Disa JJ, Hidalgo DA, et al. Reconstruction of the mandible with osseous free flaps: A ten year experience with 150 consecutive patients. Plast Reconstr Surg 1999;104:1314.

81. Sadove R, Powell L. Simultaneous maxillary and mandibular reconstruction with one free osteocutaneous flap. Plast Reconstr Surg 1993;92:141.

82. Cordeiro PG, Hidalgo DA. Conceptual considerations in mandibular reconstruction. Clin Plast Surg 1995;22:61.

83. Hidalgo DA. Aesthetic improvements in free-flap mandible reconstruction. Plast Reconstr Surg 1991;88:574–85.

84. Wei FC, Seah CS, Tsai YC, et al. Fibula osteoseptocutaneous flap for reconstruction of composite mandibular defects. Plast Reconstr Surg 1994;93:294.

85. Frodel JL, Funk GF, Capper DT, et al. Osseointegrated implants: a comparative study of bone thickness in four vascularized bone flaps. Plast Reconstr Surg 1993;92: 449.

86. Swartz WM, et al. The osteocutaneous scapular flap for mandibular and maxillary reconstruction. Plast Reconstr Surg 1986;77:530.

87. Granick MS, Ramasastry SS, Newton ED, et al. Reconstruction of complex maxillectomy defects with the scapular free flap. Head Neck Surg 1990;12:377.

88. Thoma A, et al. The free medial scapular osteofasciocutaneous flap for head and neck reconstruction. Br J Plast Surg 1991;44:477.

89. Seidenberg B, et al. Immediate reconstruction of the cervical oesophagus by revascularized isolated jejunal segment. Ann Surg 1959;149:162.

90. Theile DR, Robinson DW, Theile DE, et al. Free jejunal interposition reconstruction after pharyngolaryngectomy: 201 consecutive cases. Head Neck 1995;17:83.

91. Schusterman MA, Shestak K, de Vries E, et al. Reconstruction of the cervical esophagus: free jejunal transfer versus gastric pull-up. Plast Reconstr Surg 1990; 85:16.

92. Cordeiro PG, Shah K, Santamaria E, et al. Barium swallows after free jejunal transfer: Should they be performed routinely? Plast Reconstr Surg 1999;103:1167.

93. Coleman JJ III, et al. Jejunal free autograft: analysis of complications and their resolution. Plast Reconstr Surg 1989;84:589.

19

Mandible Reconstruction

PETER G. CORDEIRO, MD, FACS
ERIC SANTAMARIA, MD
JOSEPH J. DISA, MD

Mandible reconstruction remains one of the most challenging problems faced by the reconstructive plastic surgeon. Major advances in reconstruction of the jaw were derived from extensive clinical experiences centered around 2 historical events: (1) treating traumatic injuries to the face during World Wars I and II, and (2) increased experience with surgical treatment of tumors involving the mandible. In addition, development of better bony fixation techniques and prosthetic rehabilitation encouraged reconstructive surgeons to look into newer methods of mandible reconstruction.

Techniques to reconstruct the mandible were initially developed around the turn of the twentieth century, using nonvascularized autologous bone grafts. Donor sites included iliac crest, rib, and tibia. During World War I, external fixation and secondary delayed mandible reconstruction was described.[1] During the Second World War, both internal wiring to stabilize bone grafts and antibiotics further contributed to our ability to reconstruct mandibles.[2] The iliac crest gained increasing popularity as an elective donor site.[3] Nonvascularized bone grafts became the preferred method for mandible reconstruction until the mid-1960s. As surgeons became trained in radical surgery for oncologic problems, mandibular defects increased in extent, and with postoperative radiation therapy a significant challenge to reconstruction was now encountered.[4] Various authors reported increasing failures after immediate reconstruction in patients with defects due to malignant disease.[4,5]

The major problems with nonvascularized bone grafts were inadequate soft-tissue cover and poor tolerance to infection, especially when grafts were used to reconstruct defects after cancer surgery via an intraoral approach.[6] Bone graft resorption after irradiation was another lesson learned from this reconstructive period, and surgeons began to advocate the use of a prosthetic mandible instead of primary bone grafting.[7]

A variety of reconstructive efforts using mandibular autografts proved to be unsuccessful. Alloplastic implants were therefore introduced to reduce problems with antigenic response and donor sites. These materials included stainless steel, titanium, and chrome-cobalt steel. The use of nonvascularized bone grafts and a supporting tray for mandible reconstruction was introduced in the 1960s.[8] The rationale was to provide better fixation while tissue ingrowth and neovascularization were taking place. Because cancellous bone chips could develop more rapid vascular ingrowth, a combination of these autografts with the alloplastic material were used. Trays made of different metals (titanium, Vitalium, tantalum) or Dacron, Silastic and Teflon were tried, and although good restoration of mandibular continuity and cosmetic results were reported, long-term results were poor.[8–10] Failure rate was higher after immediate reconstruction for malignant disease, due to wound contamination from saliva and from hardware exposure.

Further development of rigid fixation methods helped to improve mandibular reconstruction in the early 1980s. Metal reconstruction plates, titanium plates with or without a nonvascularized bone graft were used, with unsatisfactory functional results—an overall failure rate as high as 30 percent and a complication rate of 45 percent.[11,12]

Myocutaneous flaps for reconstruction of head and neck defects were introduced at the end of the 1970s. Some of these flaps included an underlying bony segment based on periosteal blood supply from the muscle. Pectoralis major flap with ribs, sternocleidomastoid with clavicle, trapezius with scapula, and temporalis muscle with parietal bone were used with marginal success. Bone resorption was reduced with introduction of osteomyocutaneous flaps; however, flap failure, functional and cosmetic results and prosthetic rehabilitation were still far from optimal.[12]

The use of vascularized bone grafts for mandible reconstruction was first reported in the late 1970s.[13] The iliac crest became widely used and a variety of other flaps including the groin flap with iliac crest, the dorsalis pedis flap with the second metatarsal bone and scapula were also described.[14–16] Although functional and cosmetic results were acceptable, success rates using microvascular reconstruction were comparable to those reported with the use of pedicled myocutaneous flaps. Further developments including the radial forearm and fibula osteocutaneous flaps increased the microsurgeon's armamentarium for mandible reconstruction. As microvascular techniques and success rates have improved, these flaps have become the techniques of choice for mandibular reconstruction with success rates over 95 percent and outstanding function and esthetic outcomes.[19]

INDICATIONS FOR MANDIBULAR RECONSTRUCTION

The mandible is essential to maintain adequate mastication, deglutition and speech. A mandibular defect, particularly if it involves the lower border of the mandible, will result in a significant deformity. Functional deficits after mandibulectomy depend upon the extent and location of the resection. Patients with lateral segmental defects are less likely to develop functional deficits if dental alignment can be maintained. Anterior mandibular defects must be reconstructed because these patients have very severe functional problems and can become oral cripples. Thus, most mandibular defects should be reconstructed if technically possible. It is only the very poor medical risk patient or the patient with advanced disease who is not likely to survive for more than a couple of months should they be denied a mandible reconstruction. Even if the patient's survival period is low (6 months to 1 year), we feel that the quality of life gained from mandible reconstruction is worth the additional time of surgery. The hospitalization time and the cost of care for these patients can be dramatically reduced by reconstructing the mandible.

Timing of Reconstruction

In the past, most mandibular reconstructions were delayed because of the inability to transfer tissue immediately. A rationalization for this approach included the idea that sufficient time should be allowed to get through the period for highest risk of local recurrence. This is now considered purely an excuse for inadequate reconstructive techniques. The idea that one should wait to see if the cancer recurs prior to performing the reconstruction is also invalid since contemporary techniques of accurate radiologic assessment and frozen-section controls at the time of surgery ensure adequate resection. These methods, coupled with adjuvant radiotherapy, have reduced the risk of local recurrence to an irreducible minimum.

It is essential to reconstruct the segmental mandibular defect immediately because if the resected ends of the mandible are allowed to scar and fibrose, one can never restore the native mandible to its proper position. Postoperative radiation therapy compounds the problem with contracture, and creates a functional trismus that can never be corrected. The refinement of microsurgical techniques has allowed the reconstructive surgeon to immediately and reliably transfer well-vascularized bone and soft tissue in a single operation. Immediate replacement of the tissue that is lost contributes significantly to primary wound healing. This decreases hospital stay and also helps the patient's psychological status by restoring their sense of well-being and body image. The ability to initiate radiotherapy/chemotherapy early after surgery is a further benefit of primary reconstruction. Thus immediate reconstruction generally provides the optimal esthetic and functional result and is indicated for most patients.

Objectives of Reconstruction

With any type of reconstruction it is important to restore both function and form. The mandible is the principal component of the infrastructure of the lower face and has several important functions. It supports the tongue and structures of the floor of the mouth which are essential for mastication, speech and swallowing. Restoring the continuity of the mandibular arch therefore is critical for preservation of oral function. In addition, the mandible maintains the vertical height, transverse width and projection of the lower face. Any deviation from the normal contour of the lower border of the mandible will result in a very significant deformity. Restoration of form is a crucial objective of mandible reconstruction, since it maintains the patient's ability to interact with other members of society. The esthetic and functional objectives of reconstruction are best achieved by addressing the bone, soft-tissue and skin requirements of the defect.

Bony Reconstruction

Restoration of the continuity of bone after segmental resection of the mandible is essential to maximize both esthetic and functional outcomes. The location of the defect has varying impact on form and function. Bony reconstruction of the anterior defect prevents the so-called Andy Gump deformity (and the development of an oral cripple) by supporting the structures of the floor of the mouth. Reconstruction of lateral bony defects is not critical with regard to function but is very important in order to minimize deformity. Patients with lateral segment resections can develop deviation of the mandible which can subsequently lead to functional malocclusion, difficulty using dentures, and an inability to masticate.

Soft Tissue Reconstruction

Many patients that undergo mandible resection for cancer have significant soft-tissue involvement of the floor of mouth and the tongue by tumor. Resection of the intraoral mucosal lining can lead to scarring and immobility of the remaining portion of tongue, which can create significant functional problems. Recreation of an adequate buccal sulcus will allow use of dentures postoperatively, and will maintain space for placement of osseointegrated implants. Loss of soft tissue in the submental region and the cheek can also lead to a significant cosmetic deformity. Thus, replacement of soft tissue and intraoral mucosa is often as important as reconstruction of the bony defect.

Skin replacement

Segmental mandibular resections that include external skin create the most extensive defects because these are usually cancers that involve bone and skin as well as intraoral lining. These patients have major functional and esthetic deformities. In general, it is essential to replace both external skin as well as intraoral lining. Reconstruction of such a defect in one operation with a single free-tissue transfer can be highly challenging, because of the composite tissue requirements.

Preoperative Evaluation

Most mandibular resections with immediate reconstruction are formidable procedures. All patients should be carefully evaluated preoperatively in order to maximize both esthetic and functional results. Many patients with head and neck cancers are elderly with multiple co-morbid conditions.[20] These patients should undergo full medical evaluations by pulmonary and cardiology services, if at all indicated.

With any reconstruction it is important to establish the extent of the defect preoperatively. Although panorex, CT scan or MRI will often help to evaluate the size of tumor and involvement of bone, the best predictor of the margins of resection is the oncologic surgeon.[21] It is essential to have a good working relationship with the head and neck surgeon in order to establish the quantity of bone, mucosa, and soft tissue and external skin that will be resected. Each defect has different requirements and the type of flap selected usually will be dictated by the extent of resection. In some circumstances, patient-specific factors may dictate the type of reconstruction. Thus the presence of donor vessels for a free flap that will require anastomoses to the contralateral neck may dictate the choice of flap. Similarly, previous radiation, neck dissection, as well as donor site availability are very important factors that need to be assessed. In some patients, for example, a fibula flap may not be an option because of peripheral vascular disease. A patient who is massively obese or extremely thin may similarly provide inappropriate amounts of a certain type of tissue necessary for the desired reconstruction.

We usually obtain a 1:1 CT scan of the mandible in order to identify the angles of the osteotomies made in the reconstructed mandible. This allows simultaneous shaping of the mandible at the donor site, prior to transfer to the neck, which minimizes ischemia time.[22] A lateral cephalogram will provide the template for the angle of osteotomy at the angle of the mandible. We only rarely obtain an angiogram of the donor leg to evaluate whether a fibula can be used. Clinical evaluation of the patient will dictate whether an angiogram of the leg is needed.[23] We have not found angiograms of the neck vessels to be useful, since arterial blood supply is almost never a problem. A branch of the external carotid artery system is almost always accessible, in addition to the transverse cervical vessels. Angiograms do not provide a good evaluation of the venous structures in the neck. If the internal and external jugular veins are known to be obliterated, it is safer to use the vessels in the opposite neck. Patients are evaluated by the dental service preoperatively in order to determine the status of dentition, any need for extractions, and to establish the status of preoperative occlusion, as well as to discuss options for future dental restoration with the patient. Nursing staff should counsel the patient and family in order that they have a good understanding about their perioperative course, and to psychologically prepare them for this very extensive procedure.

Intraoperative Considerations

There are multiple issues that should be addressed intraoperatively, in order to improve the success of the operation and to maximize functional and esthetic results. Since these are very extensive procedures, great care is taken with regard to positioning of the patient under anesthesia. All pressure points are protected with silicon gel pads, in order to prevent pressure sores and neuropraxia. To reduce surgical time, we try to initiate the reconstructive procedure simultaneously with ablative procedure.

The concept of a two-team approach to head and neck reconstruction is now well accepted. The flap dissection is started as soon as the bone, skin, and muscle requirements are established. In most cases a small excess of tissue is taken with the flap to meet with contingencies in order to eliminate the possibility of having inadequate tissue for reconstruction.

Minimizing flap ischemia is crucial to success of the operation. We will usually shape the mandible and make osteotomies at the donor site using templates. Vessel dissection is also performed at the donor site, in order to minimize ischemia time. Prior to disconnecting the flap, we make sure that the recipient vessels in the neck are completely dissected and of adequate length. This minimizes the use of vein grafts, which can increase thrombosis rates. All patients with intact dentition are placed into intermaxillary fixation in order to achieve perfect postoperative alignment of the upper and lower jaws prior to insetting the reconstructed mandible. We use only rigid fixation of the reconstructed mandible with miniplates in order to prevent postoperative deviation and malocclusion. Watertight closure of the intraoral skin island is essential in order to avoid plate exposure and potential plate infection. While multiple free flaps can be used to provide bone reconstruction as well as intraoral lining, such procedures add significantly to the length of the operation, as well as the likelihood of developing complications. This can almost always be avoided by careful prediction of the surgical defect, appropriate donor site selection and flap design.

RECONSTRUCTIVE OPTIONS

Although a variety of surgical techniques have been described for mandible reconstruction, the techniques that are commonly used include: (1) nonvascularized bone grafts, (2) reconstruction plates with and without soft-tissue pedicled flaps, and (3) vascularized osteocutaneous flaps.

Nonvascularized Bone Grafts

Nonvascularized bone grafts have been used for many years to reconstruct partial mandibular defects from small segmental resections. However, in reported large series, success rates have ranged from

17 to 22 percent.[5,24] Nonvascularized bone grafts therefore should be used only for very small, partial or segmental mandibular defects. Benign tumors of dental origin are often simply cureted leaving a large dead space and only a thin shell of cortex. Nonvascularized bone grafts (usually in the form of cancellous bone chips) will often aid to increase the rapidity of bone healing and decrease chances of fracture. Similarly, short mandibular defects (< 5.0 cm) which are not likely to require radiation, can be reconstructed adequately with block cortical nonvascularized bone grafts. It is essential in all these cases that there be no mucosal or soft-tissue deficit. Nonvascularized bone grafts should never be used when the patient has had or is to undergo radiation therapy. Nonvascularized bone grafts have a high success rate only when placed through an external approach, and in nonirradiated tissues. Most studies have demonstrated that the adjuvant radiation will decrease success rates and greatly increase complication rates and bony resorption.

Reconstruction Plates

Alloplastic materials were introduced to prevent collapse of remaining mandibular segments and to provide soft-tissue support. A variety of materials have been used including medical polymers, ceramics and metals. The ideal material should be inert, easy to bend and contour, reliable, and strong enough to withstand the forces of mastication. Most centers currently use either stainless steel or titanium reconstruction plates. Titanium plates are more expensive than stainless steel, but bending and contouring is easier. The THORP reconstruction plate system uses a perforated hollow titanium screw that allows bone ingrowth and osseointegration which, in theory, increases the stability of the bone-screw interface.[25]

There are several large series describing the use of reconstruction plates for mandible reconstruction after tumor resection.[11,26] The success of these plates is variable and depends on the amount of bone resected and the location of the defect. These plates are successful only if they are used for reconstruction of short lateral segmental defects. Plate extrusion rates increase greatly when soft-tissue/mucosa is resected or if the plate is placed in the anterior position. Mandibular reconstruction plates are indicated only for reconstruction of short lateral segments, in patients who have no mucosal or soft-tissue resection, and who are not likely to undergo radiation. Success rates with osteocutaneous flaps are so much higher that mandibular reconstruction plates should be used only in patients with a very poor prognosis or those who are unable to tolerate a longer, more complicated, microvascular procedure.

Mandibular Reconstruction Plates plus Soft-tissue Flaps

Many authors have combined the use of reconstruction plates with soft-tissue flaps. The pedicled myocutaneous pectoralis major flap has been combined with reconstruction plates with variable success rates.[26,27] Recently, soft-tissue free flaps have been used in combination with reconstruction plates with higher success rates.[27] When used in the anterior position however, these plates are more likely to fracture and extrude. As microvascular techniques have improved, the combination of a metal plate with a soft-tissue free flap saves only a small amount of time as compared with an osteocutaneous flap. Given the high reliability of osteocutaneous flaps, a few additional hours of surgery is a small price to pay for the significant advantages gained by this technique. Thus a mandibular reconstruction plate in combination with a soft-tissue free flap is indicated only for a patient with inadequate osteocutaneous flap donor sites, or one in whom the soft-tissue defect is so massive (ie, large intraoral as well as external skin requirement) that 2 free flaps are necessary (radial forearm plus rectus abdominis) and therefore less indicated.

Vascularized Osteocutaneous Flaps

The development of microsurgery and further refinement of techniques in mandible reconstruction have revolutionized our ability to reconstruct the defect from a resected mandible. Since we can transfer large quantities of highly vascularized bone, soft tissue and skin with a single flap, almost any defect of the mandible can be reconstructed with one operation. Although vascularized tissue transfers are highly complex and time-consuming, their advantages far outweigh their disadvantages. Immediate reconstruction with one operation is clearly the major advantage of free flaps. Vascularized bone will heal within a period of 2 to 3 months, even with preoperative or postoperative radiation. The high bone union rates (> 98%) using this technique have made it the reconstructive option of choice.[28] The ability to transfer healthy muscle, soft tissue, and large quantities of skin with the bone segment further supports the indications for its use. Well-vascularized bone serves as an excellent bed for placement of osteointegrated implants, which maximizes both functional and esthetic results. Thus a vast majority of patients with segmental mandibular defects will benefit from the use of a vascularized bone flap.

Choice of Osteocutaneous Free Flap

The 4 osteocutaneous flaps most commonly used are the (1) radial forearm, (2) iliac crest, (3) scapula and

(4) fibula (Figure 19–1). Each flap has its distinct advantages and disadvantages.[28] Table 19–1 evaluates each flap with regard to ease of dissection, length of pedicle, amount of available bone, soft tissue and skin, potential for osseointegrated implants, as well as donor site morbidity. The choice of flap is dependent on a combination of these different factors but is most commonly dictated by the amount of bone and skin that is required to reconstruct a given defect.[19] Other parameters such as donor site availability, patient choice, ease of dissection, and the patient's overall medical condition may, in a rare case, override the tissue requirements.

Radial Forearm Osteocutaneous Flap

The radial forearm osteocutaneous flap is based on the radial artery, its venae comitantes, and the cephalic vein. This flap has the best available donor site vessels, with excellent length as well as diameter.

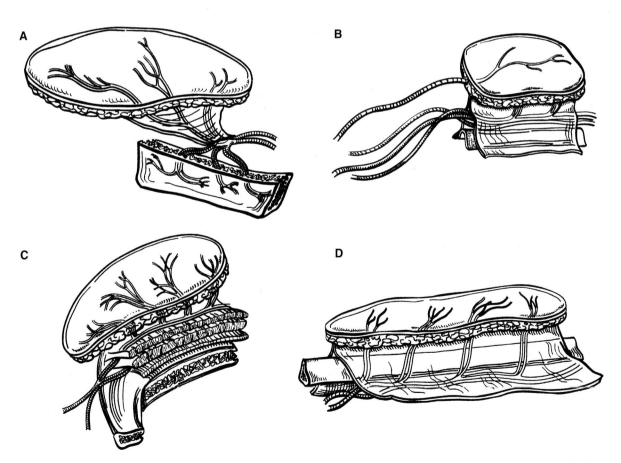

Figure 19–1. Osteocutaneous donor sites for mandible reconstruction drawn to the same scale: *A*, scapula, *B*, radius, *C*, ilium, *D*, fibula. Note the differences in tissue characteristics, with regard to quantity and configuration of the available bone and soft tissue, as well as type of blood supply and the vascular pedicle.

Table 19–1. COMPARISON OF OSTEOCUTANEOUS FREE FLAP DONOR SITES

	Tissue Characteristics			Donor Site Characteristics		
	Bone	Skin	Vessels	Two-teamable	Donor Site Morbidity	Osseointegration
Radial forearm flap	+	+++	+++	++	++	–
Iliac crest	+++	+	+	++	+++	+++
Scapula	++	++	++	–	+	+
Fibula	+++	++	++	+++	–	+++

Flap characteristics are rated excellent (+++) to poor (+) and negative (–).

It also provides a skin island which is highly reliable, well-vascularized, and that is thin and pliable. It is thus perfectly suited for repair of mucosal lining of intraoral defects.[29] One can usually harvest up to 8 to 10 cm of unicortical bone that is thin and cannot be reliably osteotomized. It also provides only minimal soft-tissue bulk, although a segment of the brachioradialis muscle can be harvested to yield a small amount of extra bulk. The major disadvantages of this flap are inadequate bone, and a significantly high morbidity of the donor site if the radius fractures. We have resorted to bone grafting the donor site primarily in order to increase the amount of bone that can be harvested. The radial forearm osteocutaneous flap is best suited to reconstruct defects that require a large amount of intraoral skin and small amounts of bone in a lateral location (Figure 19–2). This area usually does not require osseointegration.

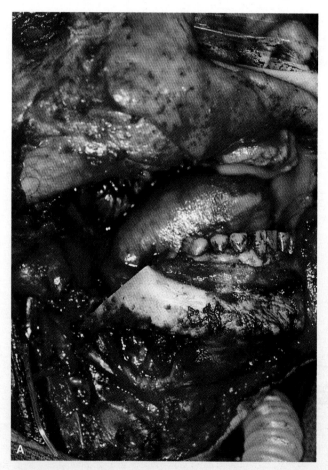
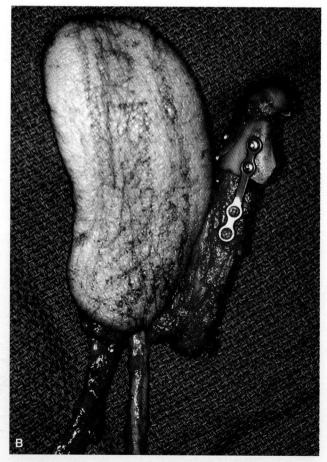

Figure 19–2. *A,* A 62-year-old man with an intraoral carcinoma involving the ascending ramus of the mandible, who underwent segmental mandibulectomy with large mucosal resection. *B,* Radial forearm osteocutaneous flap with the patient's condyle autotransplanted and rigidly fixed to the flap. Note large, thin, pliable skin island and long vascular pedicle in this flap.

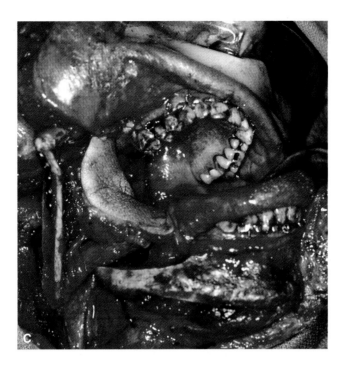

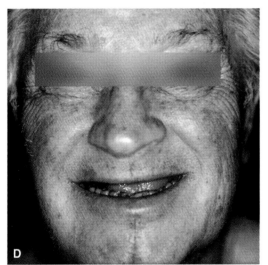

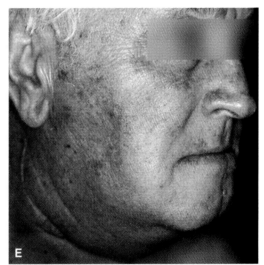

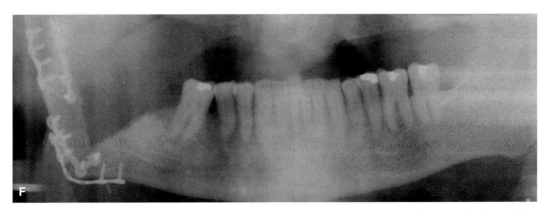

Figure 19–2. *C,* Flap inset. The skin island has been used to resurface the retromolar trigone and palate, and the radius fixed to the remaining mandible. *D,* and *E,* Postoperative photos 4 months after surgery showing good lower face contour and esthetic result. *F,* Panoramic roentgenograph showing adequate bony healing and symmetry, when compared with the contralateral side.

Thus patients with large intraoral tumors involving the lateral pharyngeal wall, tonsillar pillar, soft palate or retromolar trigone who require resection of the ascending ramus of the mandible should have reconstruction with the forearm flap.[19,29] We do not advocate its use for the anterior arch or even a mid-body lateral segment defect of the mandible.

Iliac Crest

The iliac crest was the workhorse for reconstruction of the mandible in the 1980s. As use of the fibula has become more common, there is only a very rare indication for harvesting the iliac crest. The blood supply for this flap is based on the deep circumflex iliac artery and vein. The iliac crest was initially selected for use because of its similarity in shape to the hemimandible.[30] The vessels tend to be short and often of small diameter. A large quantity of thick bicortical bone can be harvested with this flap. Iliac bone is very well suited to osseointegration; however, the principal disadvantage of this flap is that the bone lacks segmental perforators, and osteotomies can devascularize distal segments. Thus highly accurate shaping of the reconstructed mandible is not possible.

The functional and esthetic deformities of the donor site are also a disadvantage. Many patients complain of numbness of the anterior hip region as well as the bulging due to hernia of the internal oblique muscle. Although a version of this flap has been described using the inner cortex,[31] this variation provides inadequate bone with regard to osseointegration, and remains limited with regard to shaping and osteotomies. The skin island of the iliac crest is unreliable and often provides too much bulk for either intraoral or external skin defects. Thus the iliac crest is indicated only in the rare case where fibula or scapula is unavailable[19] (Figure 19–3).

Fibula Flap

The fibula has become the flap of choice for reconstruction of most segmental mandibular defects (Figure 19–4). The flap is based on the peroneal artery and vein. It is usually harvested with the flexor hallucis longus muscle, which provides good soft-tissue bulk. The skin island can be designed to include a majority of the lateral leg and can be positioned either intraorally or externally. In the rare case it can be de-epithelized and used both intraorally and externally. The vessel quality is usually good, with regard to both length and diameter. This flap can provide up to 27 cm of bone. Because it receives both a segmental and intraosseous blood supply, multiple osteotomies can be made without devascularizing the bone.[18,22,32] Since this long bicortical bone provides excellent quality bone for osseointegration, it can be used for both lateral segment and anterior arch reconstruction.[19] Its position in the leg allows for very easy simultaneous dissection at the time of resection. It also allows for shaping of the bone at the leg prior to insetting at the mandible. The main disadvantage of the fibula is the "unreliability" of the skin island. Although up to 10 percent of patients in cadaver studies have shown lack of perfusion to this area based on the peroneal vessels, our experience has been significantly better. With increasing experience, survival of the skin island can be maximized.[33,34] The superior soft-tissue, bone and skin characteristics of the fibula make this donor site the most versatile choice for reconstructing an anatomically accurate mandible defect (see Figure 19–4). In our experience, it has been employed in over 90 percent of mandible reconstructions.[19] We advocate its use for short and long, lateral and anterior segment reconstructions as well as reconstruction of the hemimandible—thus minimizing ischemia time. Donor site morbidity is minimal if at least 7 to 8 cm of bone at the ankle and 3 to 4 cm of bone at the knee are preserved. These patients return to full ambulation in 2 months.

Scapula Flap

This flap is based on the circumflex scapular artery and vein. The vessels are usually of adequate length and diameter. It provides up to 14 cm of bone of poor quality. Although it can accept osseointegrated implants, it is not as good as the fibula or iliac crest for this indication. The scapular flap provides a large amount of very well vascularized skin island, with moderate soft-tissue bulk.[16] The bone and skin segments originate from different vessels relative to the pedicle and can therefore be oriented in different three-dimensional positions. Although donor site

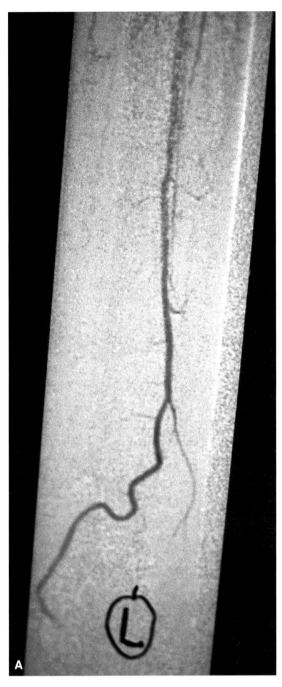

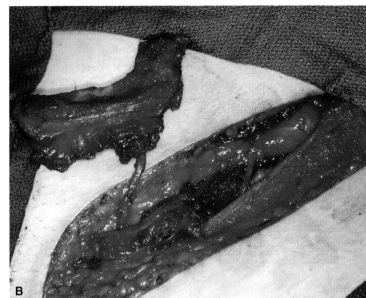

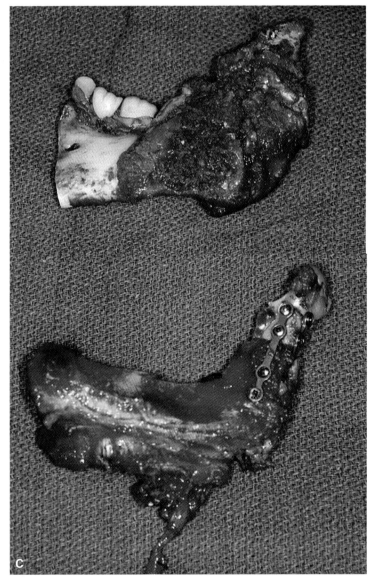

Figure 19–3. *A,* A 46-year-old woman with an osteosarcoma of the mandible who underwent left hemimandibulectomy. Preoperative arteriogram of the leg revealed the presence of a single artery (peroneus magnus malformation), which precluded use of the fibula. The iliac crest was therefore selected for immediate reconstruction of the mandible. *B,* Iliac crest osseous flap in situ. *C,* Left hemimandibulectomy specimen alongside the reconstructed mandible. The condyle has been mounted on the iliac crest. Note the similarities between the shapes of the iliac crest and the hemimandible, without any osteotomy.

morbidity is usually minimal, patients with radical neck dissections are more likely to develop a stiff shoulder. The bone cannot be osteotomized safely without devascularizing the distal segment. A major drawback of this flap is the fact that harvest of the flap cannot be performed simultaneously with the ablative procedure. We therefore avoid this flap for reconstruction of most defects in the head and neck. The scapula provides large quantities of soft tissue and skin with marginal quality bone; consequently,

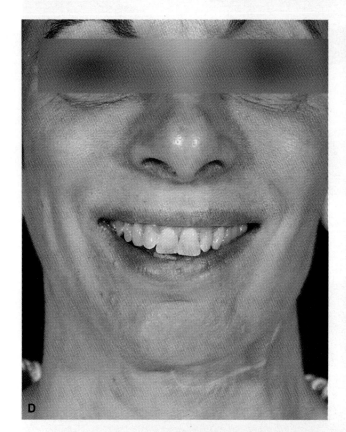

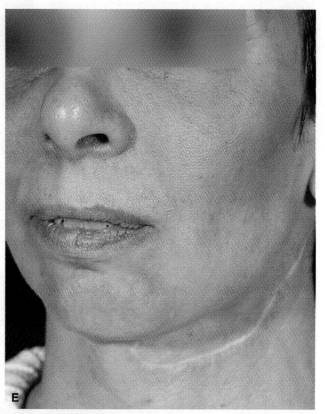

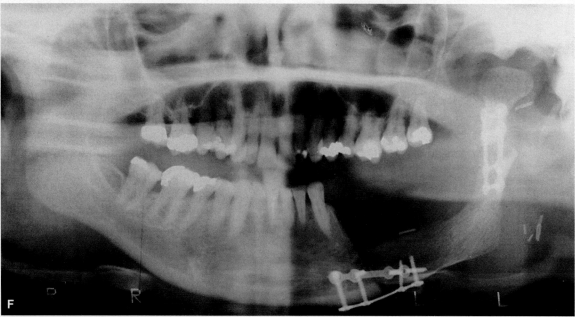

Figure 19–3.   *D* and *E,* Postoperative photos 10 months after surgery showing an excellent result. *F,* Panoramic roentgenograph showing adequate contour and height of the reconstructed mandible.

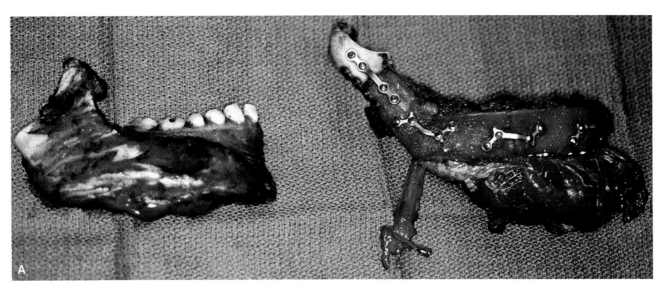

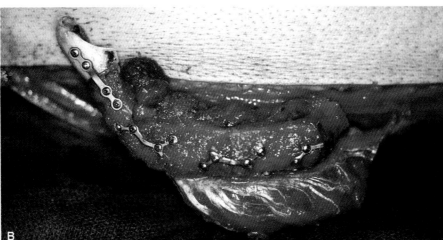

Figure 19–4. *A,* Right hemimandibulectomy specimen alongside the reconstructed mandible. *B,* Shaping of the fibula and condyle fixation was performed at the leg donor site, in order to minimize ischemia time. *C,* The reconstructed mandible rigidly fixed in situ with titanium miniplates and screws.

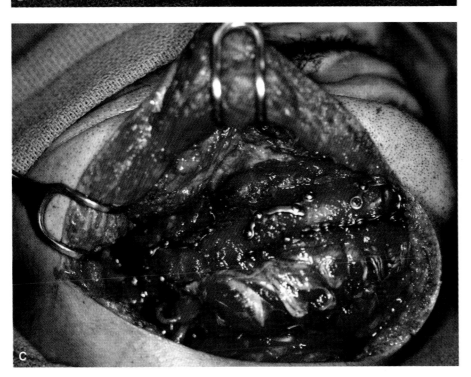

it is indicated only for those defects which require a short segment of bone with no osteotomies and large external and soft-tissue defects.[19] We have found this to be useful for defects involving the ascending ramus of the mandible in combination with large external soft tissue and skin resections of the posterior cheek (Figure 19–5). Thus recurrent parotid malignancies that require resection of cheek skin and ascending ramus are best suited to the qualities of this flap.

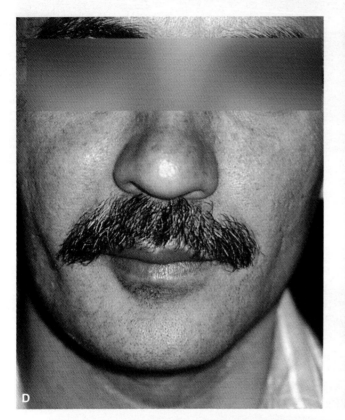

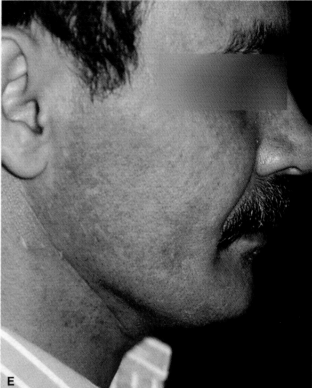

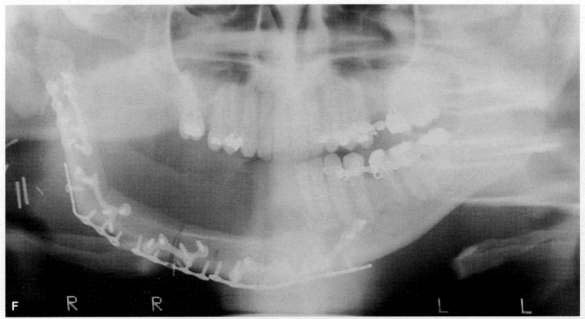

Figure 19–4. *D* and *E* A typical early postoperative result showing an excellent result. *F*, Panoramic roentgenograph showing osteotomies and rigid fixation of the reconstructed mandible to native mandible with titanium miniplates.

Condylar Reconstruction

The condyle is sometimes resected in combination with the ramus and angle of the mandible for tumors which originate in the lateral pharynx, external skin, or parotid gland. In cases where the condyle is not involved with tumor it is preferable to transplant the proximal 2.0 to 2.5 cm of condyle back onto the reconstructed mandible using titanium plates and screws.[35] An intraoperative frozen section of the

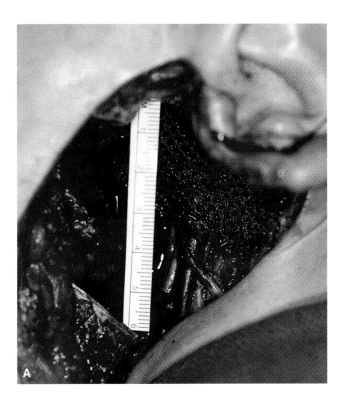

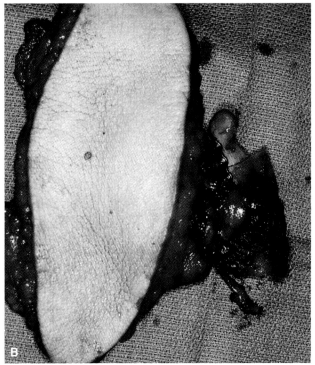

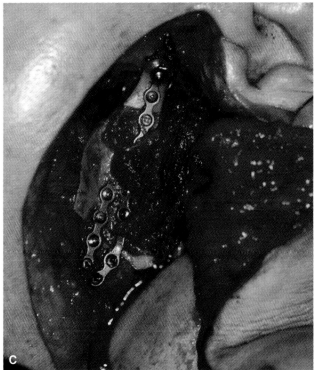

Figure 19–5. *A,* A 49-year-old woman with a recurrent parotid tumor after receiving radiation therapy. She underwent resection of the cheek skin, parotid gland, facial nerve, masticatory muscles and the ascending ramus of the mandible. *B,* The defect was reconstructed using an osteocutaneous scapular free flap. Note that this flap provides an extensive amount of skin and subcutaneous tissue, in conjunction with the lateral border of the scapula, which is used for reconstruction of the ascending ramus of the mandible. C, Inset of the vascularized bone graft with the condyle mounted and rigidly fixed to the native mandible.

marrow from the condylar margin of resected mandible is obtained to avoid the possibility of transferring tumor back into the patient (Figures 19–2B, 19–3C, 19–4B and 19–5C). Autotransplantation usually is the most effective method of condylar reconstruction and reliably produces the best functional results with minimal complications. If it is necessary to resect more than 1 to 2 cm above the

angle of the mandible, then it is easier to disarticulate the condyle with the specimen and to transplant it back onto the reconstructed mandible. Exposure of this area of the mandible and condyle risks injury to the facial nerve and makes application of plates and screws practically impossible. Condylar disarticulation and reimplantation provides the simplest and safest solution.

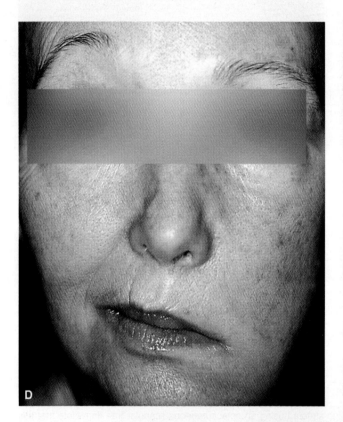

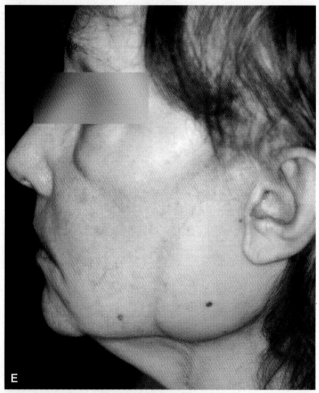

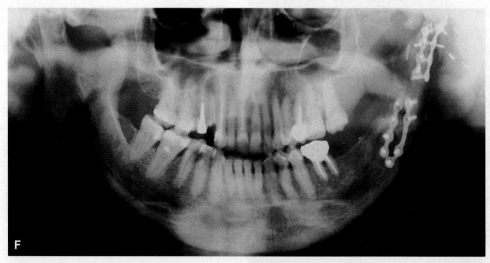

Figure 19–5. *D* and *E,* Postoperative result at 2 years. Although an excellent mandibular contour is observed, the esthetic result was considered fair, due to facial palsy and poor external skin color match. *F,* Panoramic roentgenograph showing adequate position of the bone graft.

When condyle transplantation is oncologically unsafe, the proximal end of the reconstructed mandible can be shaped and rounded to mimic a condyle (with fascia used as a spacer), or a 1 cm gap can simply be left in the temporomandibular joint. The potential for ankylosis or some dislocation of the jaw to the side of the defect is higher with this type of reconstruction, but most patients function remarkably well with only one intact temporomandibular joint. This is essentially the equivalent of a condylar resection for a shattered condyle after trauma. Although prosthetic condylar implants have been used, potential extrusion or erosion of these implants into the temporal fossa is a serious complication that should be avoided if at all possible. Thus we do not advocate the use of these prostheses.

Dental Rehabilitation and Osseointegration

Mandible reconstruction has been refined to the point that esthetic and functional results approach normal. Preoperative occlusion is usually restored and most patients will have normal jaw opening. The lateral and anterior vestibules can be reconstructed effectively with skin and soft tissue. For many patients, a simple dental prosthesis can be used in areas that are not involved with mastication. Thus, posterior and lateral defects can be adequately rehabilitated with a prosthesis that is attached to the remaining dentition. This provides an esthetic rather than functional benefit, since the patient will usually chew with their intact dentition and not with the denture. In patients who require replacement of anterior teeth or who are edentulous preoperatively, a denture will not restore normal function. In these cases, osseointegrated implants will provide the best functional and esthetic results.

Free tissue transfers provide well vascularized bone that will easily tolerate the stresses of mastication. The fibula or iliac crest will provide enough bone stock for osseointegration.[36] Osseointegrated implants were initially developed for the edentulous patient, and these techniques have been successfully applied to the reconstructed mandible. Success rates in these cases are over 95 percent and most patients with osseointegrated implants will be restored to normal function. Implants are usually placed on a delayed basis. This allows the osteotomies to heal. After plates and screws are removed, implants can then be placed in the optimal position (Figure 19–6). Although immediate placement of osseointegrated implants has been advocated by some authors,[37] this approach can compromise bone viability, extends an already lengthy procedure and will often result in implant positioning that is not biomechanically ideal.

To date, osseointegration in irradiated bone remains largely antecdotal and we therefore generally do not recommend use of implants in these scenarios.[38] We would recommend placement of implants in irradiated reconstructed mandible only after treatment with hyperbaric oxygen. Thus osseointegration is best indicated in the anterior segment reconstructions, non-radiation-treated patients and those with inadequate dentition for attachment of a prosthesis.

The Algorithm For Reconstruction of Mandibular Defects

Our experience clearly indicates that osseous free flaps have a very high success rate and should be used for most primary mandible reconstructions. The functional and esthetic outcomes are good-to-excellent for the majority of patients. The algorithm for flap selection is driven principally by the extent and site of bone and skin/soft tissue loss. (Figure 19–7). The fibula donor site should be the first choice for a vast majority of patients, particularly those with large bony defects requiring anterior reconstruction and multiple osteotomies. The radius is sometimes a better alternative for the rare patient that requires a large quantity of thin pliable skin for intraoral lining and/or who has a small lateral bony defect (though donor site morbidity is high). Patients with extensive skin and soft-tissue defects with minimal bone defects that do not require osteotomy tend to be the best candidates for the scapula flap. The ileum is recommended only when no other options are available. Osseointegration is recommended in cases where bone is not irradiated and particularly for patients with anterior defects.

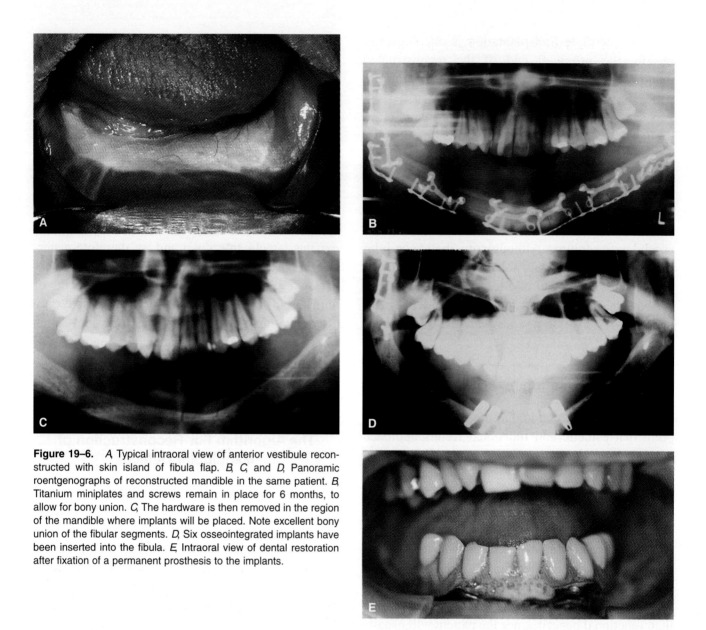

Figure 19–6. *A,* Typical intraoral view of anterior vestibule reconstructed with skin island of fibula flap. *B, C,* and *D,* Panoramic roentgenographs of reconstructed mandible in the same patient. *B,* Titanium miniplates and screws remain in place for 6 months, to allow for bony union. *C,* The hardware is then removed in the region of the mandible where implants will be placed. Note excellent bony union of the fibular segments. *D,* Six osseointegrated implants have been inserted into the fibula. *E,* Intraoral view of dental restoration after fixation of a permanent prosthesis to the implants.

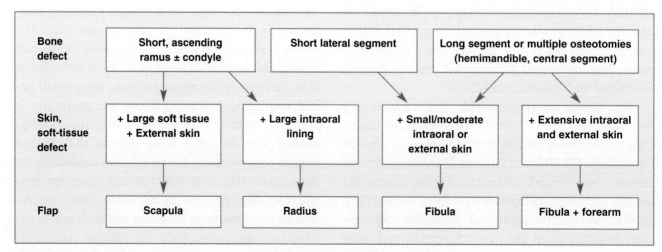

Figure 19–7. Algorithm for reconstruction of mandibular defects using osteocutaneous free flaps.

REFERENCES

1. Ivy R, Epes BM. Bone grafting for defects of the mandible. Mil Surg 1927;60: 286–300.

2. Blocker TC, Stout RA. Mandibular reconstruction, World War II. Plast Reconstr Surg 1949;4:153.

3. Millard RD, Deane M, Garst WP. Bending an iliac bone graft for anterior mandibular arch repair. Plast Reconstr Surg 1976;48:600–1.

4. Philips C. Primary and secondary reconstruction of the mandible after ablative surgery. Am J Surg 1967;114:601–4.

5. Kudo K, Fujikoka Y. Review of bone grafting for reconstruction of discontinuity defects of the mandible. J Oral Surg 1978;36:791–3.

6. Obwegeser HL. Simultaneous resection and reconstruction of parts of the mandible via the intraoral route in patients with and without gross infections. Oral Surg Oral Med Oral Pathol 1966;21:693–704.

7. Lawson W, Loscalzo L, Baek S, et al. Experience with immediate and delayed mandibular reconstruction. Laryngoscope 1981;92:5.

8. Bown JB, Fryer MP, Kollias P, et al. Silicon and Teflon prostheses, including full jaw substitution: laboratory and clinical studies of Etheron. Ann Surg 1963;157:932–43.

9. Leake DL, Rapport M. Mandibular reconstruction bone induction in an alloplastic tray. Surgery 1972;72:332–6.

10. Terz JJ, Bear E, Brown P, et al. An evaluation of the wire mesh prosthesis in primary reconstruction of the mandible. Am J Surg 1978;135:825–7.

11. Chow J, Hill J. Primary mandibular reconstruction using the A-O reconstruction plate. Laryngoscope 1986;96:768–73.

12. Snyder C. Mandibulofacial restoration with live osteocutaneous flaps. Plast Reconstr Surg 1983;64:14–9.

13. Ostrup LT, Fredrickson JM. Reconstruction of mandibular defects after radiation using a free living bone graft transferred by microvascular anastomosis. Plast Reconstr Surg 1975;55:563–72.

14. Franklin JD, Shack BR, Stone J, et al. Single-stage reconstruction of mandible and soft tissue defects using a free osteocutaneous groin flap. Am J Surg 1980;140:492–8.

15. MacLeod AM, Robinson DW. Reconstruction of defects involving the mandible and floor of mouth by free osteocutaneous flaps derived from the foot. Br J Plast Surg 1982;35:239–46.

16. Schwartz WM, Banis JC, Newton EO, et al. The osteocutaneous scapular flap for mandibular and maxillary reconstruction. Plast Reconstr Surg 1986;77:530.

17. Soutar DS, Widdowson WP. Immediate reconstruction of the mandible using a vascularized segment of radius. Head Neck Surg 1986;8:232–46.

18. Hidalgo DA. Fibular flap: a new method of mandibular reconstruction. Plast Reconstr surg 1989;84:71–77.

19. Cordeiro PG, Disa JJ, Hidalgo DA, et al. Reconstruction of the mandible with osseous free flaps: a ten year experience with 150 consecutive patients. Plast Reconstr Surg 1999;104:1314.

20. Singh B, Cordeiro PG, Santamaria E, et al. Factors associated with complications in microvascular reconstruction of head and neck defects. Plast Reconstr Surg 1999;103:403.

21. Shaha AR. Preoperative evaluation of the mandible in patients with carcinoma of the floor of mouth. Head Neck 1991;13:398–402.

22. Hidalgo DA. Aesthetic improvements in free-flap mandible reconstruction. Plast Reconstr Surg 1991;88:574–85.

23. Disa JJ, Cordeiro PG. The current role of preoperative arteriography in fibula free flaps. Plast Reconstr Surg 1998; 102:1083–8.

24. Tiwari RM, van der Waal I, Snow GB. Reconstruction of the mandible with conventional bone grafts: an evaluation. J Laryngol Otol 1994;108:969–72.

25. Vuillemin T, Raveh J, Sutter F. Mandibular reconstruction with the titanium hollow screw reconstruction plate (THORP) system: evaluation of 62 cases. Plast Reconstr Surg 1998;82:804.

26. Schusterman MA, Reece KP, Kroll SS, et al. Use of the A-O plate for mandibular reconstruction in cancer patients. Plast Reconstr Surg 1991;88:588–93.

27. Cordeiro PG, Hidalgo DA. Soft tissue coverage of mandibular reconstruction plates. Head Neck 1994;16:112–5.

28. Cordeiro PG, Hidalgo DA. Conceptual considerations in mandibular reconstruction. Clin Plast Surg 1995;22:61.

29. Zenn MR, Hidalgo DA, Cordeiro PG, et al. Current role of the radial forearm free flap in mandibular reconstruction. Plast Reconstr Surg 1997;99:102.

30. Taylor GI. Reconstruction of the mandible with free composite iliac bone grafts. Ann Plast Surg 1982;9:362.

31. Shenaq SM, Klebuc MJ. The iliac crest microsurgical free flap in mandibular reconstruction. Clin Plast Surg 1994; 21:37.

32. Hidalgo DA, Rekow A. Review of 60 consecutive fibula free flap mandible reconstructions. Plast Reconstr Surg 1995;96:585.

33. Wei FC, Seah CS, Tsai YC, et al. Fibula osteoseptocutaneous flap for reconstruction of composite mandibular defects. Plast Reconstr Surg 1994;93:294.

34. Schusterman MA, Reece GP, Miller MJ, et al. The osteocutaneous free fibula flap: Is the skin paddle reliable? Plast Reconstr Surg 1992;90:787.

35. Hidalgo DA. Condyle transplantation in free flap mandible reconstruction. Plast Reconstr Surg 1994;93:770.

36. Frodel JL Jr, Funk GF, Capper DT, et al. Osseointegrated implants: a comparative study of bone thickness in four vascularized bone flaps. Plast Reconstr Surg 1993;92: 449.

37. Zlotolow IM, Huryn JM, Piro JD, et al. Osseointegrated implants and functional prosthetic rehabilitation in microvascular fibula free flap reconstructed mandibles. Am J Surg 1992;165:677.

38. Chang Y-M, Santamaria E, Wei F-C, et al. Primary insertion of osseointegrated dental implants into fibula osteoseptocutaneous free flap for mandible reconstruction. Plast Reconstr Surg 1998;102:680.

20

Dental Oncology and Maxillofacial Prosthetics

IAN M. ZLOTOLOW, DMD

GENERAL CONSIDERATIONS

Treatment of head and neck cancers has oral sequelae and treatment-related toxicities requiring intervention by dentists. Dental team intervention should begin prior to radiation therapy, surgical resection, and/or chemotherapy. For optimal post-treatment oral functional outcomes, regardless of cancer therapies, a comprehensive dental assessment is paramount.[1] The multidisciplinary team should encompass trained dentists with interests and training in comprehensive oral/dental care of the patient. A comprehensive dental team includes the maxillofacial prosthodontist, oral and maxillofacial surgeon and dental oncologist, all of whom can contribute to quality of life issues such as restoring oral defects and facial deformities, eliminating or decreasing the intensity of dental disease and/or complications of cancer treatment.

Oral sequelae of treatment can vary from patient to patient even with the same modality of treatment and stage of disease. Generally, surgical resections can, but may not always, compromise oral function. Many, if not most of these resections, (eg, soft palate, hard palate, mandible, tongue, floor of mouth, or a combination of these) can be restored adequately by means of intervention with maxillofacial prostheses[2] alone or combined with surgical reconstruction.

Complications related to radiation therapy for head and neck cancers can vary with a range of sequelae including caries, mucositis, trismus, xerostomia, fungal infections and, rarely, osteoradionecrosis, all of which can be minimized, and many of which can be prevented with pretreatment intervention.[3]

A comprehensive oral/dental evaluation should include clinical and radiographic surveys to identify potential sources of dental infection and elimination of ongoing dental caries, symptomatic periapical lesions, calculus and plaque, and clinical and symptomatic periodontal disease. Dental screening at least 2 weeks before commencement of radiation therapy and/or chemotherapy is recommended. This period generally allows for appropriate healing of extraction sites (10 to 14 days), recovery of soft-tissue manipulations and restoration of key teeth, all of which are elements critical in maintaining an overall mucosal integrity during and after treatment. The initial dental evaluation should include a thorough prophylaxis, scaling and root planing, unless there is a visible or palpable tumor at the site of anticipated dental manipulation. The dentist should establish pretreatment baseline data against which subsequent examinations and treatments can be compared. During the initial appointment, the patient's dentition should be checked for carious lesions and defective restorations which are sources of potential irritation to the oral mucosa and should be replaced. In addition, the periodontium and the vitality of the pulp must be evaluated. Periodontal status is a major consideration with pocket-depth measurements and assessment of furcation and mobility included as a pretreatment routine. Eliminating symptomatic periodontal disease including plaque, gingival hemorrhage or dental pocket probing are very helpful in describing the treatment plans regarding dental intervention such as pre-radiation extractions.

To eliminate extractions, the patient must possess motivation to maintain dentition properly and to comply completely with prescribed oral hygiene and preventive measures. Principal maintenance of teeth (if possible), prevention of extractions after radiation therapy and prevention of mucosal or gingival ulcerations are the dentist's primary goals.

Discussion with the referring head and neck surgeon, radiation oncologist or medical oncologist is paramount in decision making. The subsequent rendered dental treatment should correlate with the overall prognosis of the patient. Each TMN classification, anatomic subset and cancer treatment modality has a unique effect on both the short (acute) and long-term (chronic) oral sequelae. The patient's dental awareness and previous dental compliancy is as much a major factor as tumor prognosis for subsequent dental treatment.[4] Patient and family education, counseling and motivation are essential for successful dental preventive strategies.

RADIATION THERAPY

Radiation therapy delivered for tumors of the oral cavity, oropharynx, nasopharynx, paranasal sinuses, base of skull, to salivary gland tumors, or to the neck for unknown primaries will have a sequelae to the oral cavity. On the other hand, radiation therapy for tumors of the thyroid, larynx and hypopharynx lead to minimal or possibly no direct effect on the teeth, periodontium, or mucous membranes of the oral cavity. However, if levels I and II of the neck are included in the radiation portal, the posterior body of the mandible, submandibular glands and mandibular canal are exposed to radiation and thus have a potential clinical significance and oral sequelae. Such exposure can lead to mucositis, xerostomia, radiation caries, advancement of pre-existing periodontal disease, temporary loss of taste, trismus from fibrosis of muscles of the temporomandibular joint and possibly, but not usually, osteoradionecrosis. Acute incidents of focal infection, such as periodontal or periapical infection, may necessitate an adjustment or an interruption of the radiation therapy schedule.

Most preventive procedures described in the literature are based on clinical experience and observation and are empirically prescribed, resulting in diverse treatment policies and preventive approaches in daily dental practices. Usually each institution has its own protocol and treatment guidelines, which are considered extremely precise.

Screening patients at least 2 weeks before radiation therapy allows adequate time for fabrication of radiation-protective mouthguards for those patients who have extensive metal fillings (gold, gold-based, or amalgam) which the direct beam of radiation will pass through. Such mouthguards potentially decrease scatter radiation to adjacent non-keratinizing mucous membranes. In addition, a minimum of 2 weeks usually allows wound healing from possible dental extractions, periodontal surgery and/or restorations, and root canal therapy for symptomatic teeth (Figure 20–1).

A lack of patient motivation should lead to a decision to extract those questionable teeth before radiation therapy. Radiation exposure, type, field, and dosage also are parts of the decision formula regarding extraction of teeth. Usually not all of the mandibular teeth are included in the radiation portal. For example, teeth and anterior mandible between the mental foramen in radiation for base of tongue tumors receive less than 3,000 cGy, (absorbed bone dosage), and are thus at a very low risk for osteoradionecrosis. On the other hand, posterior mandibular teeth receive a much higher dose of radiation.

Extraction of teeth is usually indicated in the following circumstances: (1) Advanced carious lesions with questionable pulp status or pulpal involvement that are non-restorable; (2) advanced or symptomatic periodontal disease, especially with advanced bone loss, mobility, and/or root furcation involve-

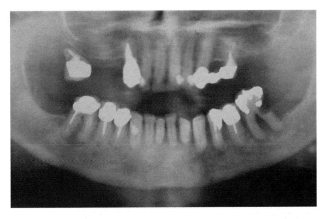

Figure 20–1. Panorex demonstrates non-salvageable posterior left molars and advanced periodontal disease requiring pre-radiation extraction.

ment; (3) residual root tips not fully covered by alveolar bone or showing radiolucency; and (4) symptomatic impacted or incompletely erupted teeth that are not covered fully by the alveolar bone. Deeply impacted teeth usually are left without risk of later problems. Alveolectomy and primary soft-tissue wound closure are suggested to eliminate sharp ridges and bony spicules that could project to the overlying soft tissues[5] (Figure 20–2). This issue is particularly important for later prosthetic considerations, especially in the beam portals involving the mandible because negligible bone remodeling can be expected after bone absorption dosages that are greater than 6,500 cGy.

Asymptomatic nonvital teeth located in the portal fields without periapical radiolucencies can be treated endodontically.[6] In restorable mandibular molars that are not periodontally involved, endodontics with retrograde fillings are preferred over extractions. Teeth which are important for retentive abutments for maxillofacial prostheses (obturators), but with small, moderate periapical granulomas or radiolucencies without periodontal involvement can be treated with apicoectomy.

Patient Education, Home-Care Instructions, Fluoride Application

Oral hygiene procedures including scaling, polishing, sub-gingival root planing and curettage should be performed and home-care instructions and fluoride prescriptions given between the initial screening appointment and commencement of external beam radiation therapy (EBRT).[7] In addition, overhanging and faulty restorations should be removed and replaced appropriately. Ill-fitting partial and/or complete dentures should be corrected during this period. Temporary soft liners should be removed and changed (relined) to a permanent acrylic resin (less porous material) to decrease the risk to surrounding soft tissues by a potential nidus for chronic candidiasis.

Patients are instructed about effective daily plaque removal and are instructed to use soft toothbrushes and high-potency fluoride applications. Instructions are given to floss daily and brush the teeth at least 3 to 4 times daily. A neutral 1 percent sodium fluoride gel, either as a 5,000 ppm brush-on with a toothbrush or self-applied every night for 5 minutes in a mouthguard carrier, or a 5,000 ppm fluoride mouth rinse used routinely is prescribed. Usually, acidulated gels are not prescribed because they might lead to significant decalcification without sufficient remineralization potential in the presence of xerostomia. Sodium fluoride preparations are preferred to stannous fluoride because the latter has unpleasant side effects such as a bad taste, sensitivity of teeth and gingiva, and the staining of arrested lesions. Daily compliance in the use of high-potency fluoride for the rest of the patient's life is more important than the type of fluoride or the modality of fluoride application.[8]

Many recent studies of long-term survivors report lack of compliance with a fluoride regimen (Figure 20–3). It has been reported that 75 to 95 percent of patients who receive head and neck radiation probably use a standard dentifrice as their only means of oral hygiene. Trays have been reported as being inconvenient, time consuming, and cumbersome.

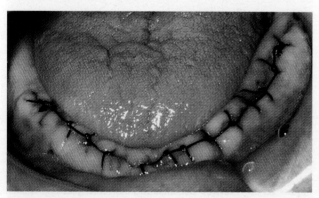

Figure 20–2. Full mouth extractions post-radiation therapy with alveolectomy and primary closure.

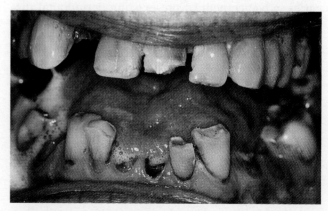

Figure 20–3. Advanced caries. Lack of fluoride compliancy.

They are particularly not used during acute episodes of mucositis. It is difficult to persuade patients who are sore and depressed to continue complicated prophylactic dental care.[9,10] In addition, patients who have undergone surgical resections 4 to 6 weeks before radiation therapy, find fluoride application via mouthguard carriers difficult, if not impossible, during the immediate postoperative period.

Patients should be monitored weekly during their radiation therapy for compliance with fluoride application and oral hygiene. Monitoring should continue on a monthly basis for the first 6 months post-treatment. The frequency of these visits is necessary because of the quick-acting nature of radiation caries, and the sequence establishes a pattern for continuity of care, possibly reducing the frequency and severity of oral complications from cancer therapy.

Several long-term oral complications can result from head and neck radiation therapy. Many of these adversely affect the patient's quality of life, of which xerostomia is probably the most prevalent and disabling major sequela of the irradiated oral cavity.[11] Radiotherapy causes loss of parenchyma and atrophy of glandular elements with development of fibrosis, and lack of saliva production. Severity depends on total radiation dosage, source and fractionation as well as location of tumor, portion of exposed salivary glands. Concurrent chemotherapy further aggravates the situation. Xerostomia affects speech, oral comfort, eating, fit of prostheses, and increases the risk of caries which can ultimately lead to osteoradionecrosis. Some recent clinical investigations concerning xerostomia have not correlated actual caries development via measuring decayed, missing, or filled (DMF) rates of tooth surfaces.[12] Many potentially carious bacterial measurements are increased (*Streptococcus* mutant and *Lactobacillus* sp.) but can be transient. Salivary dysfunction might not affect caries development in the fluoride-compliant patient particularly if three-dimensional conformal radiation or electron beam radiation is used, minimizing the radiation dosage to contralateral salivary glands. Xerostomia is best relieved by frequent use of water. Pilocarpine as a sialagogue has been reported to provide subjective relief in some patients, however, its efficacy is unpredictable.

Treatment-related sequelae of head and neck irradiation also include soft-tissue fibrosis and oblit-erative endarteritis. These changes become more pronounced over time and may include trismus and non- or slow-healing mucosal ulcerations. The muscles of mastication located within the field of radiation can lose their elasticity over time and become fibrotic with clinical symptoms (trismus). During the post-radiation period, exercising with trismus appliances (eg, tongue depressors taped together or an acrylic resin cork screw) 10 to 15 times a day for 10 minutes can decrease or even prevent the severity of this sequela.

Osteoradionecrosis (ORN) is a relatively uncommon clinical condition. However, its risk increases if the radiation dosage is greater than 6,500 cGy to any portion of the mandible[13] (Figure 20–4). The maxilla is rarely affected due to its inherent rich blood supply. Radiotherapy causes endothelial damage to blood vessels within the mandible, causing fibrosis and ischemia, increasing the risk of necrosis of hypovascular or avascular bone when exposed to the insult of bacterial infection. It can be devastating and may even develop many years after completion of radiation therapy. As many as 30 percent of cases of ORN are reported to be of a spontaneous origin. However, most reports in the literature focus on caries and extraction sites as precipitating factors. Acute and chronic periodontal disease and mandibulotomy sites can also be a focus of origin for ORN. Traditional and conservative treatment of ORN consists of antibiotics (when symptoms are present), surgical débridement and curettage; all of which can be effective in early disease. In advanced and extensive ORN, the use of hyperbaric oxygen (HBO) as an adjunct to aggressive surgical approach, to boost

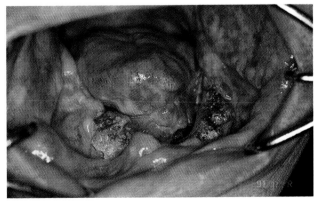

Figure 20–4. Osteoradionecrosis of mandible.

tissue oxygenation and promote angiogenesis in damaged irradiated bone is advocated. However, controversy exists in the literature regarding use of HBO, and conservative surgery versus resection and reconstruction of the mandible.[14,15] No controlled, prospective clinical trials have assessed the efficacy of HBO, and all reports attesting to its effectiveness are anecdotal. Further well-designed studies are needed to verify the positive clinical outcomes claimed by Marx in 1983 and 1985. Individual cases of osteoradionecrosis usually are complicated by so many etiologic and treatment-related variables that separating the efficacy of hyperbaric oxygen alone becomes difficult. Routine advocacy of HBO should not be a standard of care until it undergoes unbiased investigations, the methodology and results of which must survive vigorous scientific analysis and scrutiny.[16] Decisions to use HBO should be made on a case by case basis. It must, however, be emphasized that necrotic bone with a sequestrum will not heal with HBO. Angiogenesis stimulated by HBO is most beneficial in soft-tissue necrosis and in ischemic but viable bone at risk of necrosis.

Radiation therapy protective devices, or shields, can be fabricated and used to optimize delivery of radiation while reducing morbidity. Lead-lined mouthguards can prevent scatter radiation (radiation reflecting off gold and amalgam tooth restorations) to the tongue, cheek, and floor of mouth regions (Figure 20–5).

CHEMOTHERAPY

Most patients receiving chemotherapy for head and neck cancer have previously undergone radiation therapy or receive concomitant radiation therapy. Chemotherapy-related toxicities can exhibit several different clinical presentations including mucous membrane inflammation and ulceration, oral candidiasis, and/or viral or bacterial oral infections (Figure 20–6). When or if ulcerations occur, dental intervention can be instituted to reduce the debilitating symptoms associated with mucous membrane lesions such as secondary systemic bacterial or fungal infections (septicemia and fungemia). Chemotherapy-induced toxicities are reflected in the mouth by changes in color, contour, character, and continuity of the

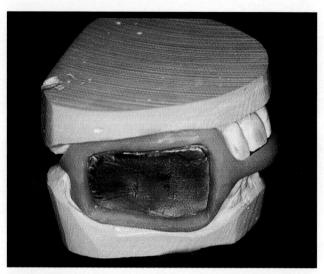

Figure 20–5. Lead-lined shield to protect scatter radiation to tongue and hard palate.

mucosa. These oral complications from chemotherapy (usually a stomatitis) can vary in pattern, direction, intensity, and progression.[18] Oral complications and manifestations from chemotherapy are well documented and more common for hematologic diseases (leukemia, lymphoma), but have not frequently been reported for head and neck cancers.

Lockhart and Clark examined 82 patients receiving chemotherapy with stage III or IV head and neck disease to determine the incidence and severity of oral sequelae.[19] Taste alteration (37%), mucositis (30%), ulceration (22%), xerostomia, weight loss, dysphagia, hemorrhage and infection were encountered. However, these reported sequelae could have originated with previous radiation therapy.

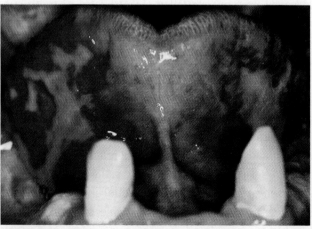

Figure 20–6. Grade IV mucositis from concomitant radiation and chemotherapy.

Some of the agents used most commonly for head and neck tumors (eg, methotrexate, bleomycin, cisplatin, and 5-fluorouracil) are considered stomato-toxic when used alone, and in combination they likely can result in dose-limiting stomatitis. Lockhart and Clark's study suggested no significant increase in incidence or severity of complications with each successive cycle of chemotherapy. The number of patients for whom second and third cycle data were available was too small for statistical assessment. Nearly one-third of the chemotherapy cycles resulted in at least mild mucositis and ulceration or in problems with nutrition.

In general, current regimens of chemotherapy for head and neck cancer result in less frequent and less severe oral complications than seen in hematologic disease. In the future, intensification of chemotherapy to obtain increased response rates could result in more frequent and severe mucositis as a sequela. This outcome has been especially true when patients received concomitant radiation therapy and chemotherapy or when radiation therapy follows chemotherapy within a short time period.

All patients receiving head and neck chemotherapy are advised to visit a dentist at least 10 days before commencement of chemotherapy. The hematologic status should be reviewed with the oncologist in regard to platelets, neutrophils, total white blood cell count, partial thromboplastin time, and prothrombin time. Home-care hygiene initiatives and caries control are also commenced. Third-molar pathology is evaluated and addressed appropriately. All potential oral sources of bacteremia, including advanced or acute periodontal disease, should be eliminated. If symptomatic teeth with periapical lesions are present, pulpotomies or extractions should be considered.[20]

Stage III or IV head and neck patients might not desire or require the so-called ideal dental treatment due to guarded or poor tumor prognosis. Asymptomatic but periodontally involved teeth might be salvaged with alternate dental treatment plans. Retaining asymptomatic anterior teeth (maxillary and mandibular) could be considered even in the presence of periodontal disease, caries, or periapical pathology. Considerations for this patient population could be maintenance of mandibular cuspids and first bicus-

pids for abutment retention of a mandibular anterior stay-plate prosthesis instead of full-mouth extractions. Control of carious teeth with an intermediate restorative material instead of more definitive restorations (crowns, fixed bridges, onlays) might suffice until all chemotherapy cycles are completed.

During chemotherapy for head and neck cancer, the dental team should emphasize oral hygiene with frequent saline and baking soda oral rinses and toothbrushing. Unlike chemotherapy for hematologic diseases, bleeding usually does not occur from brushing the gingival surfaces with a soft toothbrush.

Many medical decisions about the type and timing of cancer therapy are based on the dental-oral findings and recommendations are made at the time of referral or at periodic oral examinations.

HEAD AND NECK SURGICAL RESECTIONS REQUIRING MAXILLOFACIAL PROSTHETICS

Head and neck patients requiring surgical resections often require maxillofacial prosthetic rehabilitation, an integral component of head and neck cancer care. Restoration of speech, swallowing, control of saliva, mastication, and restoration of facial deficits are goals of maxillofacial prosthetic rehabilitation. Consultation between surgeon and maxillofacial prosthodontist during treatment planning can eliminate many unwanted sequelae. In many instances, proper surgical planning, and precise surgical technique or additional surgery can improve the existing anatomic structures that would make the maxillofacial prosthesis more successful.[21] This process could include creating lingual, buccal, and labial sulci (vestibuloplasty) to free a tongue, or osseointegrated implants in a microvascular free flap that restore the mandibular continuity to increase masticatory function.

Maxillary Defects and Obturators

Tumors that require maxillary resection will create defects of the maxilla, palate, or adjacent soft tissue. They can range from small perforations of the hard or soft palate to extensive resections (eg, the maxilla, the soft palate, and such adjacent structures as the orbit and cheek). Defects of these regions can lead to a variety of sequelae. Hypernasality renders speech unintelligible. Mastication can be difficult, particularly for the edentulous patient, because dental structures and dental-bearing tissue surfaces are lost. Swallowing can be awkward because food and liquids sometimes are forced out the nasal cavity; the nasal mucous membranes become desiccated by abnormal exposure; controlling nasal and sinus secretions that collect in the defect area may be difficult; and facial disfigurement can result from lack of midface bony support or resection of a branch of the facial nerve.

Rehabilitation after resection of the hard and soft palate is usually best accomplished prosthodontically.[21] Traditionally, a temporary or immediate surgical obturator is placed at the time of surgery. The purpose of a maxillary obturator prosthesis is to restore the physical separation between the oral and nasal cavities, thereby restoring speech and swallowing to normal function and providing support for the lip and cheek.[22] During the healing period, an interim obturator prosthesis is adjusted periodically, with temporary soft denture liners to compensate for the tissue changes secondary to organization and contracture of the wound. When the defect has healed and is dimensionally stable (usually 3 to 4 months after surgery), a definitive obturator prosthesis is constructed. If, however, the patient receives radiation therapy postoperatively, this healing period can last approximately 6 months.

Fabricating a functional obturator follows use of conventional principles of removable prosthetics: retention, stability and support. The remaining teeth, therefore, are valuable for optimal functional rehabilitation. The head and neck surgeon can improve the prosthetic prognosis by considering the following principles or modifications at the time of ablative surgery:[23]

1. A split-thickness skin graft should be used to line the cheek surface of the defect. This skin graft provides a keratinized surface to support the prosthesis and forms a scar contracture at the junction of the skin graft and buccal cheek mucosa, forming an undercut with which the lateral wall of the obturator can engage for increasing stability and support.

2. The surgeon should save a portion of the medial palatal mucosa, if possible, to cover the medial cut margin of the palatal bone. If this palatal margin of the defect is covered with keratinized mucosa, the prosthesis may engage this surface more completely, thus decreasing potential ulcerations at the margins from a fulcrum effect due to compression of tissue during mastication.

3. Attempts should be made to save as much of the maxilla as possible for support of the obturator. Retaining the premaxilla segment is particularly advantageous. If the patient is dentulous in the anterior region, esthetics can be enhanced also with appropriate clasping using cuspids and bicuspids instead of incisors.

4. The transalveolar bone resection should be made as far as is feasible from the tooth adjacent to the proposed defect. This requires extracting the distal tooth and making the transalveolar resection at the center of the previously extracted tooth socket. This approach allows more supporting bone against the abutment tooth, thus potentially making this tooth less susceptible to destructive periodontal forces of clasp retention.

5. If the soft palate does not retain the ability to bring about palatopharyngeal closure, it should be resected. If a posterior, nonfunctioning band of soft palate remains after surgery, it often prevents proper placement of the pharyngeal bulb portion of the obturator into the nasopharynx, thus limiting the bulb's effectiveness of eliminating hypernasality.

6. In edentulous patients, the placement of osseointegrated implants into appropriate maxillary-mandibular bone sites should be considered. These implants can be used later to aid in retention of a future obturator prosthesis.

Immediate Surgical Obturator Prosthesis

The immediate coverage of a palatal defect with a surgical obturator will simplify the patient's postoperative course (Figure 20–7). The surgical obturator provides a support on which the surgical packing can be placed, minimizes contamination of the wound in the immediate postoperative period, and enables the patient to speak and swallow immediately after surgery. Use of the surgical obturator can eliminate the need for nasogastric tube feeding in most situations. The surgical obturator prosthesis is worn for approximately 7 to 10 days. Prosthesis design is determined by the surgical boundaries of

resection, which can be marked by the operating surgeon preoperatively on a dental cast model. The surgical obturator, fabricated in autopolymerizing methyl methacrylate resin, is sterilized and ligated interdentally to remaining teeth using 24-gauge stainless steel pre-stretched wires. If the patient is edentulous, the prosthesis is ligated through the alveolar ridge and palatal shelf on the non-resected side in addition to other available structures (zygomatic arch, anterior nasal spine, etc.).[22]

Interim Obturator Prosthesis

An interim obturator prosthesis replaces the surgical obturator in 7 to 10 days postoperatively. The interim prosthesis, in addition to 18-gauge wrought-wire claspings to engage abutment teeth, can have denture teeth and a flange for lip and cheek support.[24] Its purpose is to facilitate mastication and anterior cosmesis, to restore normal contour of the palate, cheeks, and lips, to prevent food and liquids from escaping through the defect out the nasal cavity, and to provide normal non-nasal speech. A previously worn, removable partial denture or maxillary complete denture can be modified appropriately and used during this interim period as an interim obturator. Speech and swallowing usually are restored during this time, which is important for improving psychologic well-being. A soft lining material usually is appropriate for forming the obturator of the defect and might require four to five trial impressions before success. The obturator portion is hollowed to reduce its weight, thereby providing better retention. As the healing progresses, the obturator is relined periodically—usually every other week for the first 6 to 8 weeks after surgery.

Definitive Obturator Prosthesis

The definitive obturator prosthesis, usually fabricated 4 to 6 months after all cancer therapy is completed, should extend maximally along the lateral wall of the defect.[25] The higher the lateral extension of the bulb, the greater is the increase in lateral stability of the prosthesis.[26] When the definitive obturator prosthesis is completed, speech and swallowing are restored to normal limits (Figures 20–8 and 20–9). The patient is

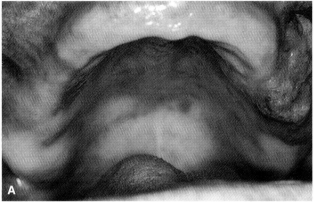
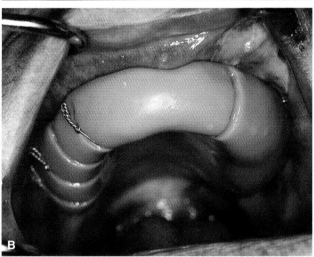
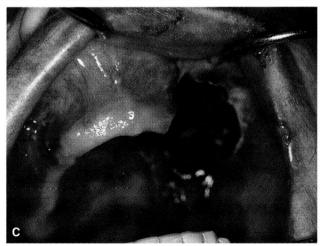

Figure 20–7. *A,* Preoperative squamous cell carcinoma—posterior alveolar ridge. *B,* Surgical obturator ligated to non-resected alveolus and palate with 24-gauge stainless steel wires. *C,* Immediate postoperative partial maxillectomy defect.

recalled periodically for adjustments and examination for recurrent disease by the multidisciplinary surgical team. Home-care instructions and cleaning (irrigation) of the defect area are essential.

Soft-Palate Speech Bulb Prostheses

Defects of the soft palate usually require maxillofacial prosthetic intervention. Palatopharyngeal closure normally occurs when the soft palate elevates and contracts the lateral and posterior pharyngeal walls of the nasopharynx.[27] When a portion of soft

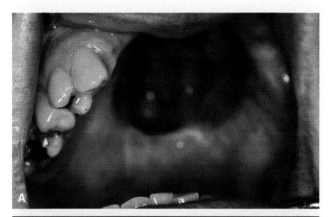

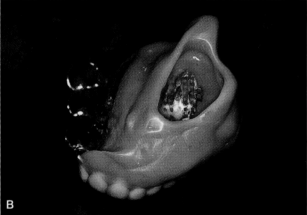

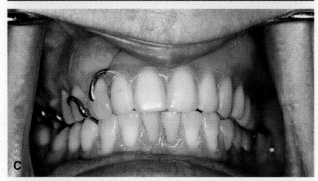

Figure 20–8. *A*, Six months post-maxillectomy. *B*, Definitive obturator. *C*, Definitive obturator in occlusion.

palate is excised or when the soft palate is perforated, scarred, or neurologically impaired, complete palatopharyngeal closure cannot occur. Speech becomes hypernasal, and normal swallowing is compromised. With a pharyngeal speech bulb obturator, the patient may be able to reestablish palatopharyngeal closure. The speech bulb obturator must not interfere with breathing, impinge on soft tissue during postural movements, or interfere with the tongue during swallowing and speech. During the breathing and production of nasal sounds, the space around the speech bulb reflects a potential for muscular contraction. During the production of speech sounds, the sphincter muscular network moves into contact with the stationary acrylic resin speech bulb portion, establishing palatopharyngeal closure. A correctly constructed and positioned speech bulb can provide non-hypernasal and intelligible speech and functional swallowing for patients with acquired soft-palate defects.[28]

Optimally restoring the acquired soft-palate defect is probably one of the most difficult intraoral challenges for a maxillofacial prosthodontist. One must consider approaches for restoration of a soft-palate resection in conjunction with newer surgical interventions for head and neck cancer. Many tumors can originate from the retromolar trigone, oropharynx, base of the tongue, posterior buccal mucosa, palatal minor salivary glands, extension of paranasal sinus tumors posteriorly, and not the soft palate alone. Many resections of the soft palate include a segmental mandibulectomy, a base-of-tongue resection, or a partial glossectomy, pharyngectomy, cheek mucosa resection, palatectomy and maxillectomy (partial, subtotal, or total).[29]

Similar to the interim hard palate obturator prosthesis, an interim soft palate speech bulb obturator uses acrylic resin and 18-gauge wrought-wire clasps (when appropriate) for retention. If a musculocutaneous flap is used for reconstruction of the lateral border of the soft palate, only minimum contact of the speech bulb should be attained against the flap. Many of these flaps and grafts provide bulk and do not provide physiologic movement in any direction. If a defect is present posterior to this flap, a properly placed speech bulb component into the nasopharynx can extend laterally and come in close approximation with the torus tubarius, thus improving speech intelligibility while not interfering with breathing. Impressions of the soft-palate defect usually take place approximately 10 days after surgery. An extended dental tray with dental compound and wax can be safely used at this time with an irreversible hydrocolloid impression material.

Reconstruction with regional or free flaps in this region will necessitate a variety of speech bulb shapes, each individually formed for functional results (Figure 20–10). Difficulty in obtaining speech phonemes is not necessarily related to the size of the speech bulb but rather to the location of the defect and reconstruction.

For this patient population, separating or differentiating resonance, articulation, hypernasality, and hyponasality is sometimes difficult. Factors affecting speech and swallowing will vary, including location of the defect, surgical flap reconstruction, compromised or nonfunctional adjacent anatomic structures and assessment at different postoperative time intervals.

During the postoperative period, if the soft palate resection includes a neck dissection, gastric pull-up procedure or reconstructed flap to the residual base of the tongue or pharynx, edema of the tongue will ensue, thus adjacent buccal spaces can be compromised. During this period the patient can experience

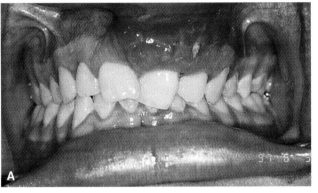
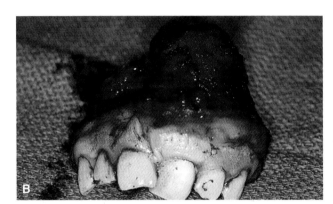
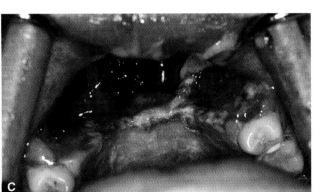
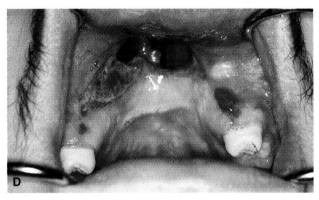
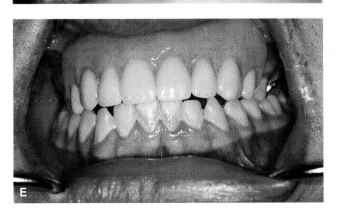

Figure 20–9. *A,* Osteogenic sarcoma-maxillary anterior gingiva. *B,* Surgical specimen. *C,* Anterior defect at surgery (anterior maxillary resection). *D,* Anterior defect 2 months post surgery. *E,* Definitive obturator in occlusion—4 months after surgery.

difficulty in obtaining maximum physiologic movement to complete the velopharyngeal complex.

In summary, rehabilitation of the soft-palate resection can have a variety of subjective successes. Modified barium swallow, cinefluoroscopy and nasal endoscopic studies can be used to show abnormal muscular movements in a wide range of functional activities.[30] Defining objective measurements (length, width and height) for proper speech bulb prosthesis placement is difficult. Reduction and

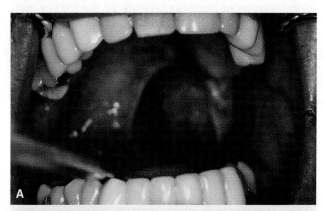

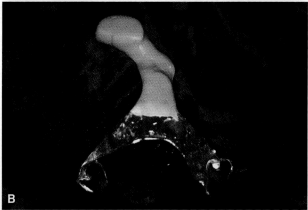

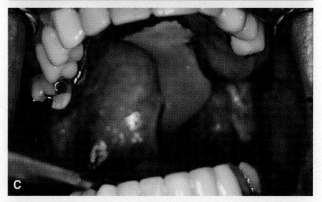

Figure 20–10. *A,* Soft-palate defect with microvascular radial free-flap reconstruction of the lateral pharyngeal wall. *B,* Speech bulb extension on denture base extended into the nasopharynx. *C,* Speech bulb prosthesis in place.

elimination of hypernasality does not necessarily correlate with elimination of leakage of liquids or foods through the nasal cavity. Head position and tongue maneuvering can contribute to the effectiveness of the speech bulb. Variation in the healing of the surgical margins is the rule rather than the exception. A lateral cephalometric radiograph can demonstrate the appropriate extension of the speech bulb in the nasopharynx and its position with the anterior tubercle of the atlas.

Rehabilitation of the soft palate is an ongoing treatment consideration. Other factors will contribute to improvement of speech and swallowing over time; hence, multiple prosthetic modifications and continued evaluation are necessary to achieve long-term functional success. Objective measurement of speech is difficult for the patient who has palatal insufficiency after soft-palate resection in addition to resection of adjacent hard and soft oral and oropharyngeal tissues. Nasality thus remains a perceptual phenomenon, the definition of which is elusive. Thus, each patient must be analyzed on an individual basis via means of voice interpretation and reading ability. The speech bulb prosthesis is effective in rehabilitating soft-palate defects and should be considered and discussed with the patient prior to resection.

Palatal Augmentation Prostheses

Patients who have undergone glossectomies with or without microvascular free-flap (radial forearm) reconstruction can improve consonant speech phonemes [k,g] and swallowing ability with the aid of a palatal augmentation (tongue) removable prosthesis (Figure 20–11). This can be considered when the remnant dorsum of the tongue (or reconstructed tongue with a flap) cannot make contact with the junction of the hard and soft palate. For optimal results, the patients will benefit with additional speech and swallowing therapy from a speech pathologist after being fitted with the palatal augmentation prosthesis.[31] The success of a palatal augmentation prosthesis usually depends on the location and function of the residual tongue, degree of other resected adjacent entities (eg, mandible, floor of mouth, soft palate and especially base of tongue), along with the degree of the patient's motivation and family support.[32]

Mandibular Defects

Malignant tumors associated with the lower gum, floor of mouth and adjacent structures also represent a difficult challenge for the prosthodontist with regard to rehabilitation after treatment. The disabilities resulting from such resections would include impaired speech articulation, difficulty in swallowing, deviation of the mandible during functional movements, and poor control of salivary secretions.[33] Cosmetic disfigurement also can be present. These patients present a far more difficult rehabilitation problem than do patients with maxillary sur-

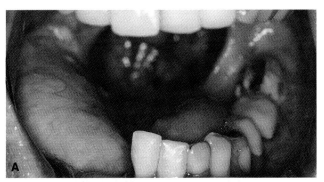

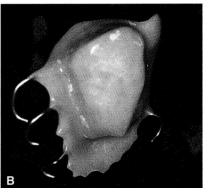

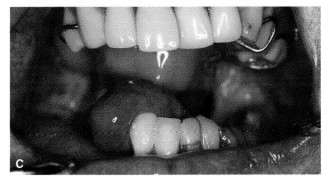

Figure 20–11. *A,* Subtotal glossectomy—microvascular radial free flap reconstruction. *B,* Palatal augmentation prosthesis. *C,* Palatal augmentation prosthesis allowing contact of residual tongue against junction of hard and soft palate for swallowing and [k,g] phoneme improvement.

gical defects, particularly if a significant portion of the tongue is also resected.

Recently, advances in the reconstruction of such defects by means of microvascular free flaps have allowed the maxillofacial prosthodontist to rehabilitate these patients more effectively. With proper multidisciplinary pretreatment planning and postoperative treatment, osseointegrated implants can be strategically placed in patients with reconstructed mandibles to restore occlusal and masticatory functions.[34–40]

For the mandibular resection patient, most emphasis previously has been placed on the amount of mandible resected and the number of teeth remaining in the non-resected portion of the mandible. Equally important are the quantity and position of adjacent structures lost, including tongue, floor of mouth, and the buccal and lingual vestibules. The degree to which mastication is affected depends somewhat on the amount of mandible removed, but equally significant is the status of the tongue in function.[41] The tongue must be able to place the food bolus on the occlusal surface of the teeth for mastication to take place. The tongue—which, in many instances has limited mobility and strength—is also required to balance the position of these removable prostheses.

Following segmental mandibulectomy an unrestored mandible becomes retruded and deviates toward the surgical site.[42] When the mandible opens and closes, previous vertical movements are replaced by an oblique or diagonal motion controlled by the unilateral temporomandibular joint apparatus. Loss of one temporomandibular joint leads to less precise movements of the mandible. Loss of muscles of mastication in the resected side also forces the mandible to rotate upward upon closure if the coronoid process is present owing to the pull of the temporalis musculature. The severity and permanence of this mandibular deviation are unpredictable. Loss of the adjacent soft tissue and primary closure of the defect without flap reconstruction contribute to severe functional disability.

Closure of composite resections with soft-tissue flaps or grafts is desirable. Musculocutaneous flap closure can decrease the deviation of the mandible, making mandibular guide therapy more effective.

Traditionally, if mandibular continuity is not restored surgically, mandibular guide appliances, hemidentures, or palatal ramps on maxillary prostheses are used to decrease mandibular functional disabilities. Sometimes these prosthetic appliances are cumbersome and do not provide a presurgical degree of functional mastication.

If mandibular continuity is not restored, a number of methods can reduce the degree of mandibular deviation. These methods include intermaxillary fixation (IMF) at the time of surgery, mandibular guide-bar restorations, and palatal-based guidance restorations. If IMF is not employed, the patient should be placed into an exercise program as early as possible after surgery. On maximum opening, the mandible is displaced by hand as forcefully as possible toward the non-resected side. These movements tend to lessen scar contracture, reduce trismus and improve maxillomandibular relationships. Exercises should be carefully demonstrated to the patient and notes made periodically to record the degree of progress (via Boley gauge). The earlier the mandibular guidance is initiated, the more successful is the result.

If the patient is dentulous in the non-resected maxillary and mandibular quadrants, a cast mandibular resection prosthesis is appropriate. This prosthesis consists of a removable partial denture framework with a metal flange extending 7 to 10 mm laterally and superiorly on the buccal aspects of the maxillary bicuspids and molars on the unresected side. The non-resected quadrants of the maxilla and mandible must be periodontally stable and caries-free and should have enough bony support to absorb diagonal forces. The guide flanges engage the maxillary buccal bicuspid and molar surfaces during initial mandibular opening and closure, thereby directing the mandible to an appropriate intercuspal position. In the postoperative setting, mandibular guidance appliances are usually delayed until healing is complete (2 to 3 months).

Because many patients receive radiation therapy after mandibular resections, the oral mucosa is usually atrophic and fragile, predisposing it to soft-tissue irritation. Chronic alcohol abuse and poor nutrition may further compromise oral mucous membranes. The diminished output and thick mucinous nature of saliva after radiation can impair retention and may be inadequate to lubricate the denture-mucosal interface. Deviation of the mandible can create abnormal maxillo-mandibular relationships that may prevent ideal placement of the denture teeth and flanges over their supporting structures.[44] In the resected mandible patient, most consequential is the impairment of the motor and sensory control of tongue, lip, and cheek, limiting the ability of the patient to control dentures during function. The integrated neuromuscular balance between tongue, lips, and cheeks contributes to limited success of edentulous resection appliances. Microvascular free-flap mandibular reconstruction via a fibula has a success rate of 95 percent.[43] By use of free-flap mandibular reconstruction followed by osseointegrated implants on selected patients, occlusal function can be restored.

Thus, as one readily can appreciate, osseointegrated implant-supportive resection appliances can overcome many of the aforementioned difficulties, particularly those associated with compromised retention, stability, or support. Osseoimplants in the resected reconstructed irradiated mandible in selected patients, both with and without hyperbaric oxygen, have proven to be successful[45] (Figure 20–12; see also Figures 19–6, D and E).

Osseointegrated implants are strategically placed in the fibula approximately 1 year after completion of all cancer therapy (Stage I). Using placement and surgical techniques described by Branemark and colleagues, 4 to 6 months for osseointegration is suggested prior to abutment placement (Stage II).

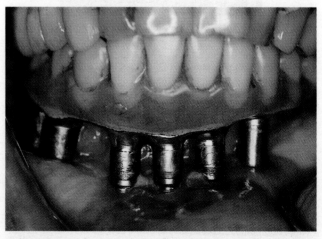

Figure 20–12.   Osseointegrated fixed implants prosthesis in fibula free-flap mandibular reconstruction (6 years after surgery).

Bicortical integration is required, utilizing at least 10 mm implants into the fibula. A variety of occlusal schemes can be utilized with attention focused on providing maximum tongue movement for efficiency of mastication.

Facial Defects

Restoration of the facial defect is a difficult challenge for both the surgeon and the maxillofacial prosthodontist. It is not uncommon for an advanced head and neck cancer to require a rhinectomy, orbital exenteration, loss of an ear or cheek, or a midface resection (nose, lip, palate). Both surgical reconstruction and prosthetic restoration have distinct limitations. The surgeon is limited by the availability of tissue and by damage to the local tissue bed. The maxillofacial prosthodontist is limited by the materials available for facial restoration, the mobile tissue beds, difficulty in retaining large prostheses, and the patient's willingness to accept the result.[46] Whatever the mode of rehabilitation, the patient should be fully informed about advantages and disadvantages of the expected quality of the final result. In patients with extensive facial tumors requiring resection, the method of facial restoration should be considered before surgery. The patient should be involved in this discussion and participate in the decision-making process (Figures 20–13 and 20–14).

The choice between surgical reconstruction and prosthetic restoration of large facial defects is difficult and complex and depends on the size and etiology of the defect and on the patient's desires. Surgical reconstruction of small facial defects is possible in most cases—and preferable. Many patients prefer masking a defect with their own tissue rather than with a prosthesis. It is difficult (if not impossible) for the surgeon to fabricate a facial part that is as successful in appearance as a well-made prosthesis. However, not everyone will accept an artificial part, and many would rather have a permanent, though perhaps less esthetic, nose or ear.

The application of osseointegrated implants in facial deformities has, in part, changed patient perceptions about facial prostheses because of improved retention.[47,48] Even when surgical reconstruction is deemed possible, significant delay (up to a year) in reconstruction may be necessary to ensure control of the tumor. The challenge of the maxillofacial prosthodontist is to fabricate a cosmetically pleasing restoration. Successful use of the restoration may depend on the patient's psychologic acceptance of it.

At present, materials used for facial prostheses exhibit excellent and acceptable properties. How-

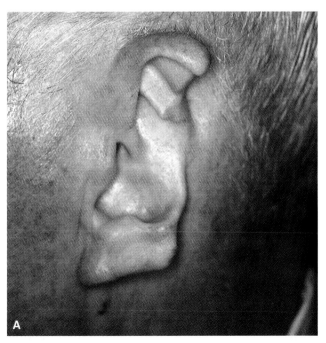 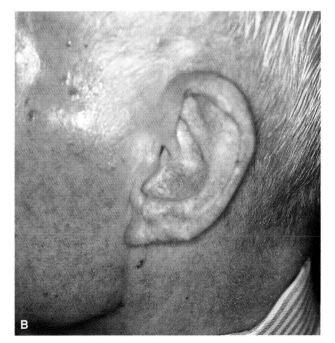

Figure 20–13. *A,* Partial ear resection post-basal cell carcinoma. *B,* Silicone auricular prosthesis.

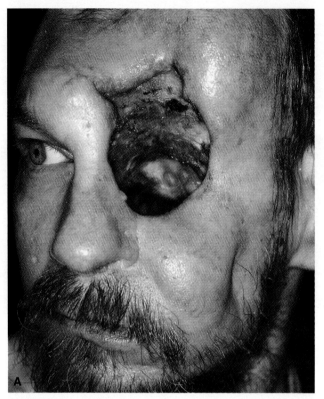 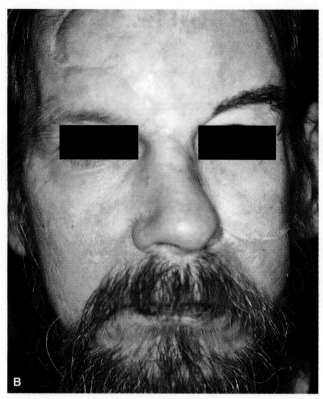

Figure 20–14.   *A,* Orbital exenteration and cranial resection for squamous cell carcinoma ethmoid sinus. *B,* Orbital-cranial silicone prosthesis.

ever, all materials possess some undesirable characteristics. Most materials are constructed from silicone elastomers, of which MDX 4-4210 (Dow Corning, Kalamazoo, MI) has been shown to be the material most clinically accepted for the past 25 years and has achieved acceptance worldwide.[49–51]

Preoperatively, a presurgical moulage is helpful, especially if a total rhinectomy or ear resection is anticipated. Impressions of the defect usually are obtained with elastic impression materials, taking care not to displace the tissues being recorded. The contours of the replaced anatomy are sculpted in wax, both on the cast and on the patient. Surface characteristics, appropriately contoured, and coloration and margin placement are equally important factors to be considered for a successful, acceptable facial prosthesis. Extrinsic coloring of the prosthesis varies with the type of base materials used.

Midfacial (Combined Oral and Facial) Defects

Large combination defects of the oral cavity and the external face create a challenge for the patient and the maxillofacial prosthodontist. Many of these patients previously have had numerous minor surgical removals and have had these tumors over a long period of time. In addition, when the integrity of the oral cavity has been compromised, food and air escape during swallowing, speech often is unintelligible, and saliva control is difficult[52] (Figures 20–15 and 20–16).

Many facial defects currently are reconstructed with a combination of microvascular free flaps, tissue expanders, and the use of a maxillofacial prosthesis. The microvascular surgeon can incorporate techniques that create concavities that allow a facial prosthesis to maintain as much normal anatomy as possible in replacing the lost orbital contents, nasal structures, or auricular components (Figure 20–17).

Percutaneous osseointegrated implants placed in the superior or lateral orbital rim, inferior base of nasal bones and temporal bone are acceptable treatment modalities.[53,54] Even in irradiated tissue beds, properly placed osseoimplants have been shown to be successful in many studies with 5-year follow-up.[55] Consideration of tumor prognosis is an important factor in this patient population for selection of osseointegrated implant placement.

In the absence of osseointegrated implants, conventional retention of facial prostheses usually relies on skin adhesives. They are placed daily on the inner surface of the prosthesis and on the skin margins. Currently, silicone materials usually last up to 2 years if maintained properly, and if the skin margins are cleansed daily.

Patients requiring facial prostheses are recalled by the maxillofacial prosthodontist approximately every 6 months. Additional tinting can be applied, and hygiene instructions are reinforced at this time.

A duplicate prosthesis is usually fabricated with the same mold so that, if deterioration or color wear occurs, the second prosthesis can be tinted easily for patient satisfaction.

Quality of life issues can be addressed adequately with well-informed patients and their families during and after fabrication of facial prostheses. A comfortable, well-fitting and esthetic facial prosthesis will help restore a patient's self-image and allow them to return to society without loss of dignity.[56,57]

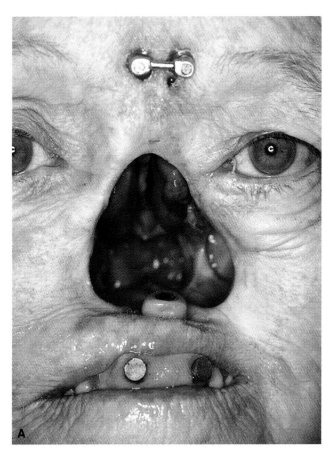
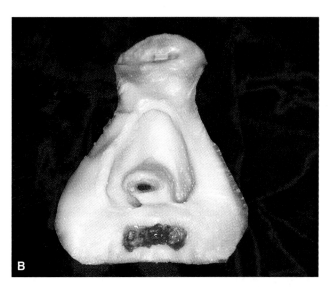
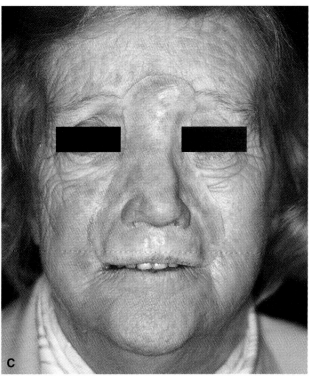

Figure 20–15. *A,* Total rhinectomy and anterior maxillectomy with obturator with magnet retention and cranial osseoimplant Hader Bar. *B,* Midfacial appliance with magnets and connecting clip bar attachments. *C,* Midfacial appliance in place.

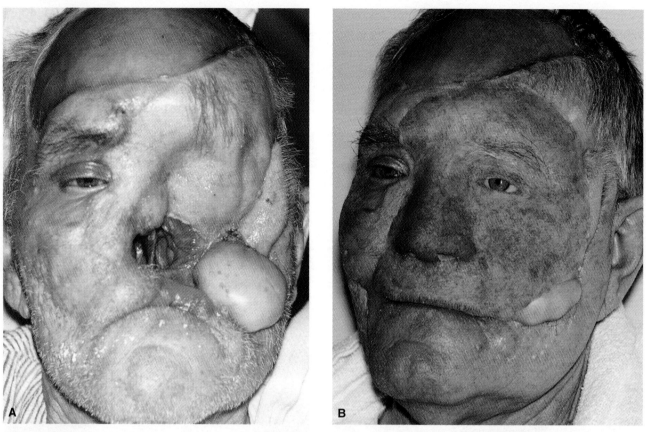

Figure 20–16.   *A,* Combined forehead and myomusculocutaneous flap reconstruction for a large resection of basosquamous cell carcinoma of the face. *B,* Silicone combined orbital-nasal cheek facial appliance.

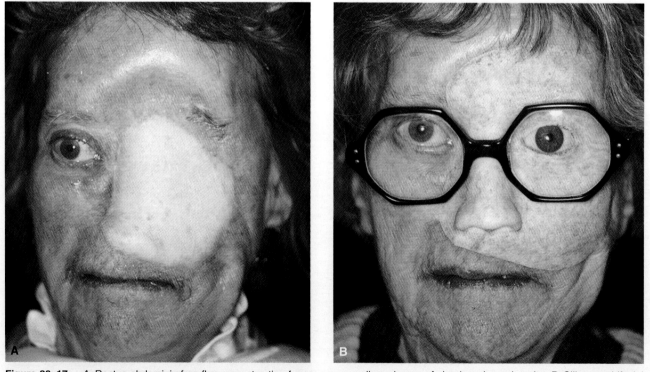

Figure 20–17.   *A,* Rectus abdominis free flap reconstruction for squamous cell carcinoma of cheek and nasal cavity. *B,* Silicone midfacial prosthesis post-microvascular reconstruction.

CONCLUSION

Availability, accessibility and visibility of the members of the dental team and their integral relationship with head and neck surgeons, radiation oncologists and medical oncologists are the keys to preventing and limiting oral complications and sequelae from cancer therapies for head and neck tumors. Preventive dentistry becomes medically necessary and dental intervention, regardless of modality of cancer treatment and required dental modality (eg, maxillofacial prosthetics, oral surgery, endodontics, periodontal therapy, restorative dentistry and oral medicine), is an integral component of multidisciplinary control, treatment, and rehabilitation of the head and neck cancer patient.

An ongoing dialogue between physicians (oncologists), dentists and patients is essential for improving quality of life. Minimizing oral sequelae complications of head and neck cancer treatment is a reality.

REFERENCES

1. USDHHS. Consensus Statement: Oral complications of cancer therapies. NIH Consensus Development Conference—Proceedings; [Monograph] 1990; Washington (DC): NIH Publication No. 89–3081, 1990;9:4–15.
2. Beumer J, Curtis T, Marunick M, editors. Maxillofacial rehabilitation—prosthetic and surgical considerations. St. Louis (MO): Ishiyaku Euro America; 1996. p. 225–33.
3. Beumer J, Curtis T, Nishimura R. Radiation therapy of head and neck tumors. In: Beumer J, Curtis T, Marunick M, editors. Maxillofacial rehabilitation—prosthodontic and surgical considerations. St. Louis (MO): Ishiyaku Euro America; 1996. p. 43–112.
4. Beumer J, Brady F. Dental management of the irradiated patient. Intl J Oral Surg 1978;7:208.
5. Dreizen S, Brown LR, Daly TE, et al. Prevention of xerostomia-related dental caries in irradiated cancer patients. J Dent Res 1977;56:99–104.
6. Seto BG, Beumer J, Kagawa T, et al. Analysis of endodontic therapy in patients irradiated for head and neck cancer. Oral Surg Oral Med Oral Pathol 1985;60:540–5.
7. Toth BB, Martin JW, Fleming TJ. Oral and dental care associated with cancer therapy. Cancer Bull 1991;43:397–402.
8. Zlotolow IM. Clinical manifestations of head and neck irradiation: compendium of continuing education dentistry—Special Issue 1997;18(2):51–6.
9. Billings RJ, Meyerowitz C, Featherstone JDB, et al. Retention of topical fluoride in the mouths of xerostomia subjects. Caries Res 1988;33:306–10.
10. Lockhart PB. Oral complications of radiation therapy. In: Peterson DE, Elias EG, Sonis ST, editors. Head and neck management of the cancer patient. Boston (MA): Martinus Nijhoff; 1986. p. 429–49.
11. Markitziu A, Zaficopolous G, Tsalikis L, Cohen L. Gingival health and salivary function in head and neck-irradiated patients. Oral Surg Oral Med Oral Pathol 1992;73:427–33.
12. Keene HJ. Cariogenic microflora in patients with Hodgkin's disease before and after mantle field radiotherapy. Oral Surg Oral Med Oral Pathol 1994;78:5.
13. Beumer J, Harrison R, Sanders B, Kurrasch M. Postradiation dental extractions: a review of the literature and a report of 72 episodes. Head Neck Surg 1983;6:581–6.
14. Marx RE. A new concept in the treatment of osteoradionecrosis. J Oral Maxillofac Surg 1983;41:351–7.
15. Shaha A, Cordeiro P, Hidalgo D, et al. Resection and immediate microvascular reconstruction in the management of osteoradionecrosis of the mandible. Head Neck Surg 1997;19(5):406–11.
16. Schwartz HC. Treatment of osteoradionecrosis with measures other than hyperbaric oxygen. Proceedings of First International Congress on Maxillofacial Prosthetics; April 1994. New York: Memorial Sloan-Kettering Cancer Center; 1995.LOC 95–78016.
17. Gulbransen HJ. Radiation stents and splints. Proceedings of First International Congress on Maxillofacial Prosthetics; April 1994. New York: Memorial Sloan-Kettering Cancer Center; 1995. LOC 95–78016.
18. Sonis ST. Oral complications of cancer therapy. DeVita VT, Hellman S, Rosenberg SA, editors. Cancer: principles and practice of oncology. 4th ed. Philadelphia (PA): JB Lippincott; 1993. p. 2385–94.
19. Lockhart P, Clark J. Oral complications following neoadjuvant chemotherapy in patients with head and neck cancer. Oral Development Conference—Proceedings; [Monograph] 1990; Bethesda (MD): NIH Publication No. 89–3081, 1999;9:99–101.
20. Zlotolow I. [review]; Toth BB, et al. Minimizing oral complications of cancer treatment. Oncology 1995;9:858–64.
21. Curtis T. Restoration of acquired hard palate defects. In: Beumer J, Curtis T, Marunick M, editors. Maxillofacial rehabilitation—prosthodontic and surgical considerations. St. Louis (MO): Ishiyaku Euro America; 1996.
22. Huryn JM, Piro JD. The maxillary immediate surgical obturator prosthesis. J Prosthet Dent 1989;61:343–7.
23. Beumer J, Zlotolow I, Sharma A. Rehabilitation. In: Silvermans, Ed. Oral cancer. 4th Ed. Toronto: American Cancer Society; 1996.
24. Martin JW, Lemon JC. Prosthetic rehabilitation in head and neck surgery. In: Bailey BJ, editor. Otolaryngology. Philadelphia (PA): JB Lippincott; 1993. p. 1431–40.
25. Desjardin RP. Obturator prosthesis design for acquired maxillary defects. J Prosthet Dent 1978;39:424.
26. Brown KE. Peripheral considerations in improving obturator retention. J Prosthet Dent 1968;20:176.
27. Kantner CE, West R. Phonetics. New York: Harper and Brothers; 1941
28. Aram A, Subtelny JD. Velopharyngeal function and cleft palate prosthesis. J Prosthet Dent 1959;9:149.
29. Zlotolow IM, Huryn JM. Restorations of the acquired soft palate deformity with surgical resection and reconstruction. In: Proceedings of First International Congress on Maxillofacial Prosthetics; April 1994. New York: Memorial Sloan-Kettering Cancer Center; 1995. LOC 95–78016.

30. Logeman JA. Swallowing physiology and pathophysiology. Otolaryngol Clin N Am 1988;84:71–9.

31. Robbins KT, Bowman JB, Jacob RF. Postglossectomy deglutitory and articulating rehabilitation with palatal augmentation prostheses. Arch Otolaryngol Head Neck Surg 1987;113:1214–8.

32. Cantor R, Curtis TA, Shipp L, et al. Defects. J Prosthet Dent 1969;22:253.

33. Curtis TA, Cantor R. The forgotten patient in maxillofacial prosthetics. J Prosthet Dent 1974;31:662.

34. Hidalgo DA. Fibula free flap: a new method of mandible reconstruction. Plast Reconstruct Surg 1989;84:71–9.

35. Zlotolow IM, Huryn JM, Piro JD, et al. Osseointegrated implants and functional prosthetic rehabilitation in microvascular fibula free flap reconstructed mandibles. Am J Surg 1992;164:677.

36. Cordeiro PG. General principles of reconstructive surgery for head and neck cancer. In: Harrison LB, Sessions RB, Hong WK, editors. Head and neck cancer, a multidisciplinary approach. Philadelphia (PA): Lippincott-Raven; 1999. p. 197–216.

37. Keller EE, Tolman DE, Zuck SL, Eckert SE. Mandibular endosseous implants and autogenous bone grafting in irradiated tissue: a 10-year retrospective study. Int J Oral Maxillofac Implants 1997;12:800–13.

38. Ganstrom G, Tjellstram A, Branemark PI. Bone-enhanced reconstruction of the irradiated head and neck cancer patient. Otolaryngol Head Neck Surg 1993;108:334–43.

39. Keller EE. Mandibular discontinuity reconstruction surgical implant placement in free bone grafts. Proceedings of First International Congress on Maxillofacial Prosthetics; April 1994. New York: Memorial Sloan-Kettering Cancer Center; 1995. LOC 95–78016.

40. Roumanas ED, Markowitz B, Lorant J, et al. Reconstruction of mandible defects: Conventional prosthodontics vs. use of implants. Proceedings of First International Congress on Maxillofacial Prosthetics; April 1994. New York: Memorial Sloan-Kettering Cancer Center; 1995. LOC 95–78016. p. 81–6.

41. Marunick M, Mathes B, Klein B. Masticatory function in hemimandibulectomy patients. J Oral Rehabil 1992;19:289–95.

42. Beumer J, Marunick M, Curtis T, Roumanas E. Acquired defects of the mandible. In: Beumer J, Curtis T, Marunick M, editors. Maxillofacial rehabilitation—prosthodontic and surgical considerations. St. Louis (MO): Ishiyaku Euro America; 1996. p. 113–224.

43. Hidalgo D. Fibula free flap mandibular reconstruction. Clin Plast Surg 1994;21:25.

44. Curtis T, Taylor R, Rositano J. Physical problems in obtaining records of the maxillofacial patient. J Prosthet Dent 1975;34:539.

45. Keller EE. Placement of dental implants in the irradiated mandible. A protocol without adjunctive hyperbaric oxygen. J Oral Maxillofac Surg 1997;55:972–80.

46. Beumer J, Ma T, Marunick M, et al. Restoration of facial defects. In: Beumer J, Curtis T, Marunick M, editors. Maxillofacial rehabilitation—prosthodontic and surgical considerations. St. Louis (MO): Ishiyaku Euro America; 1996. p. 377–454.

47. Nishimura R, Roumas E. Implant-retained facial prostheses: rhinectomy defects. Proceedings of First International Congress of Maxillofacial Prosthetics; April 1994. New York: Memorial Sloan-Kettering Cancer Center; 1995. LOC 95–78016. p. 120–5.

48. Parel S, Tjellstrom A. The United States and Swedish experience with osseointegration and facial prostheses. Int J Oral Maxillofac Implants 1991;6:75–9.

49. Moore DJ, Glaser ZR, Togacco NJ, Linebaugh MD. Evaluation of polymeric materials for maxillofacial prosthetics. J Prosthet Dent 1977;38:319–26.

50. Andres CJ, Haug SP, Munoz CA, Bernal G. Effects of environmental factors on maxillofacial elastomers. Part 2, Survey of currently used elastomers. J Prosthet Dent 1992;68;519–22.

51. Polyzois GL, Oilo G, Dahl JE. Tensile bond strength of maxillofacial adhesives. J Prosthet Dent 1993;69(4):374–7.

52. Marunick M, Harrison R, Beumer J. Prosthetic rehabilitation of mid-facial defects. J Prosthet Dent 1985;54:533.

53. Henry P. Mid-facial defects. Proceedings of First International Congress of Maxillofacial Prosthetics; April 1994. New York: Memorial Sloan-Kettering Cancer Center; 1995.LOC 95–78016, p. 132–6.

54. Beumer J, Calcaterra T. Prosthetic restoration of large midfacial defects. Laryngoscope 1976;86:280.

55. Jacobson M, Tjellstrom A, Fine L, Andersson H. A retrospective study of osseointegrated skin penetrating titanium fixtures used to retain facial prostheses. Int J Oral Maxillofac Implants 1992;7:523.

56. Shafritz L. Face valve. Los Angeles (CA): Linda Shafritz; 1994.

57. Zlotolow IM. Dental oncology and maxillofacial prosthetics. In: Harrison LB, Sessions RB, Hong WK, editors. Head and neck cancer, a multidisciplinary approach. Philadelphia (PA): Lippincott-Raven; p. 151–68.

21

Head and Neck Radiation Oncology

LANCEFORD M. CHONG, MD

THE BASIC SCIENCES OF RADIATION ONCOLOGY—RADIATION PHYSICS

Definition of Radiation

Radiation is energy which is emitted from atoms and is transmitted through space.[1] It is the capture of this energy emanating from physical reactions occurring at an atomic level and its application to cellular material which results in biologic change that forms the scientific basis of the specialty of radiation oncology. There is a broad spectrum of radiation types, however the particular one of clinical interest is known as ionizing radiation. This is defined as radiation of sufficient energy that when applied to an atom is capable of dislodging an orbiting electron that can subsequently cause a biologic effect when it interacts with cellular components such as H_2O or DNA.

Types of Therapeutic Radiation

There are two main categories of ionizing radiation and each contains several subtypes of clinical importance: (1) electromagnetic radiation (photons): x-rays, gamma rays, and (2) particulate radiation: electrons, neutrons, protons.

The electromagnetic radiation subtypes do not differ in any physical characteristic or in their biologic action. The only distinction is in how they are each produced. X-rays are created by linear accelerators and involve an electrical input that causes a filament to become heated and which serves as a source of electrons. These electrons are then accelerated and are administered to a patient as particulate radiation or are directed to strike a tungsten target which results in the production of x-rays. Gamma rays are produced by materials such as cobalt 60 that are undergoing radioactive decay, resulting in the emission of gamma ray photons. Photons interact with atoms through three processes that depend on the energy of the incident photon and on the characteristics of the absorbing material: (1) photoelectric effect, (2) Compton effect, and (3) pair production.

Photons used in radiation oncology have a wide range of energies. The choice of which energy or teletherapy unit to employ will depend on the clinical characteristics of a particular case, including the depth of penetration required. Superficial and orthovoltage x-rays are not very penetrating and can be selected for more superficial lesions. Supervoltage gamma rays and megavoltage x-rays are extremely penetrating and are used for deep-seated tumors (Table 21–1).

Particulate radiation all cause ionization and each subtype has its own mechanism of absorption. In clinical head and neck radiation oncology, electrons are the most important type while neutrons and protons have limited roles.

Electrons used in clinical practice range from 6 MeV to 20 MeV electrons and are produced in linear accelerators. The determination of the desired depth of penetration will dictate the selection of the

Table 21–1. RADIATION ONCOLOGY TREATMENT UNITS

Photon Energy	Teletherapy Unit
40 to 100 kV	Superficial
250 kV	Orthovoltage
1.25 MV	Supervoltage (cobalt 60)
4 to 25 MV	Megavoltage (linear accelerator)

appropriate electron energy. Electrons deposit their energy relatively superficially as opposed to supervoltage gamma rays and megavoltage x-rays which are deeply penetrating. Electrons have a fixed depth of penetration which is estimated in centimeters by the electron energy divided by one half. Another important clinical estimate is the depth in centimeters where 80 percent of the maximum dose is deposited, and this is approximately one-third of the electron energy. Electrons are particularly useful in head and neck radiation oncology for skin cancers and regions over the spinal cord.

Neutrons are located in the nucleus of atoms, carry no charge, and are highly penetrating in tissue. These particles are produced by cyclotrons and can have a maximum energy of 50 MeV. They have no dose distribution advantages over photons. However, neutrons have a higher relative biologic effectiveness ranging from 3.0 to 3.3 compared to an equivalent dose fraction of cobalt gamma rays. These neutrons are more efficacious in producing biologic effects per unit dose than photons. While this may be helpful in treating malignant cells, one must be quite vigilant with respect to this increased biologic response of neutrons on normal tissues as this can potentially result in major complications. Neutrons are indicated in the treatment of unresectable primary and recurrent salivary gland tumors because of their superior local control rates compared to that of photons.

Protons are also found in the atomic nucleus but carry a positive charge. They are produced by cyclotrons for therapeutic usage. These particles have a characteristic dose distribution known as the Bragg peak that confers a major treatment planning advantage through significant control of the depth of penetration. Their use is indicated in the treatment of chordomas and chondrosarcomas in the base of the skull. Protons and photons have roughly equivalent relative biologic effectiveness.

MOLECULAR AND CELLULAR RADIATION BIOLOGY

Mechanisms of Radiation Cellular Kill

The most significant radiation-induced damage that results in the death of the cell occurs in the DNA molecule. X-rays or gamma rays interact with the orbiting electrons of an atom, causing their excitation and ejection as fast electrons. These in turn will react with water molecules with the formation of highly reactive free radicals, which in turn cause DNA damage known as an indirect action. Alternatively, the fast electrons can directly damage DNA and this is known as a direct action. Many of the DNA damages can be repaired, however certain lesions are not rectified and this results in the cell undergoing perhaps one or two subsequent cellular divisions before entering a stage where it cannot undergo further mitosis and thus cannot reproduce, a condition defined as cell death.

Another notable radiation effect that can result in cell death involves changes occurring in the cellular membrane in particular and perhaps also with the nuclear DNA, which ultimately results in programmed cell death known as apoptosis.[2]

Irradiated cells that cannot undergo mitosis are dead and either undergo cellular lysis or enter a postmitotic state by forming giant cells which are not capable of tumor regeneration.

Cell Survival Curve

Exponential Cell Survival

The relationship between the dose of radiation administered and the percentage of surviving cells is characteristic for a given radiation quality (low linear energy transfer versus high linear energy transfer), dose size, environmental conditions (oxygenated versus hypoxic) and cell line. Cell survival is exponential and is expressed graphically in the cell survival curve (Figure 21–1) which plots the logarithm of cell survival along one axis versus radiation dose on the other axis. The resultant shape of the curve will vary in the width of the initial shoulder and in the slope of the subsequent curve depending on the characteristics noted above. The cell survival after a conventional fraction dose of 200 cGy can vary from 20 to 80 percent depending on the histology, and this finding may explain some of the differences in radiosensitivity between the various types of tumors.

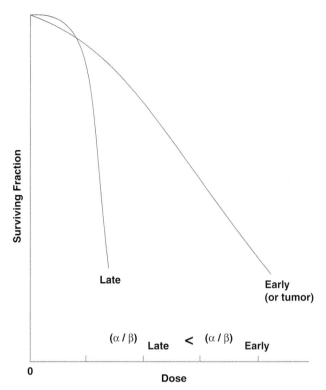

Figure 21–1. Cell survival curves contrasting the differences between early versus late responding tissues.

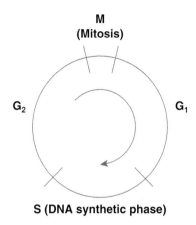

Figure 21–2. Cell cycle showing the mitotic stages for actively growing cells. M is mitosis, G1 and G2 are gaps (periods of inactivity), S is DNA synthesis.

Relationship of Cell Cycle and Ionizing Radiation

The cell cycle (Figure 21–2) has four phases that are distinctly sequenced and describe the life cycle of cells: (1) **Synthesis (S)**: DNA synthesis, (2) **Gap (G2)**: a period of apparent cellular inactivity, (3) **Mitosis (M)**: cellular division into two daughter cells, (4) **Gap (G1)**: a period of apparent cellular inactivity. Cells vary in their sensitivity to ionizing radiation and this is dependent on their position within the cell cycle at the time of the exposure to the radiation (Figure 21–3). The most sensitive phases are G2 and M. The medium sensitivity phases include G1 and early S. The least sensitive phase is late S (Table 21–2).

In a given volume of tissue, its cells are asynchronously distributed within the various phases of the cell cycle. Each cell will progress through the cycle at its own individual rate. When exposed to ionizing radiation, the surviving cells will undergo partial synchronization. This occurs as a consequence of G2 arrest which delays cells in a more radiosensitive phase. Also, other surviving cells may progress into the next phase which may be more radiosensitive.

Oxygen Effect

The ability of ionizing radiation to cause biologic change is very much dependent on the amount of oxygen present in the tissue environment. Oxygen is the most potent radiosensitizer known at this time. Cells in a 100 percent oxygen environment are 3 times more radiosensitive than cells in complete anoxia. It is the oxygen that reacts with the DNA damage and prevents its repair which ultimately leads to cellular death.

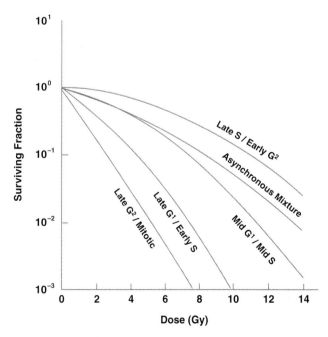

Figure 21–3. Cell survival curves for differing mitotic stages showing the variation of radiosensitivity.

Table 21–2. CELL CYCLE VARIATION OF RADIOSENSITIVITY	
Radiosensitivity	Cell Cycle Phase
Most	G2, M
Intermediate	G1, early S
Least	Late S

The Radiobiologic Basis of Fractionation

Improving the Therapeutic Ratio

The use of multiple fractions over many weeks of radiation therapy is based on the principle of improving the therapeutic ratio between normal tissues and tumors (Table 21–3). The goal is to maximize the cell death of tumors and to minimize unacceptable damage to normal cells. The radiobiologic mechanisms involved with causing cell death are similar for both normal and malignant cells. It is the differential ability of ionizing radiation to sterilize tumor while avoiding excessive normal tissue damage that forms the basis of clinical radiation oncology. This is accomplished through the use of multiple fractions and is explained by the four radiobiologic processes: (1) repair, 2) re-oxygenation, (3) redistribution, and (4) repopulation.

Repair

Both normal and malignant cells suffer radiation-induced DNA damage of three types: lethal, potentially lethal, sublethal. Each category of damage has its own distinctive potential for repair. Although many of the DNA modifications can undergo repair, certain defects cannot be rectified and ultimately result in cell death. Repair may occur to a greater degree in slowly dividing normal tissue compared to tumors and this may contribute to a beneficial therapeutic ratio. Repair is depressed in selected tumors such as lymphomas and may be incomplete in previously irradiated tissues leaving them to possess a reduced tolerance to subsequent radiation treatments.

Re-oxygenation

Bulky tumors may have centers that are relatively hypoxic due to their location > 150 micrometers away from a blood vessel—the maximum diffusing distance of oxygen from a capillary.[3] Tumor cells

Table 21–3. COMPARATIVE FRACTIONATION SCHEDULE				
SCHEME	Dose/Fraction	No. of FX/Day	Total Dosage	Treatment Duration
Conventional Fractionation	180 – 200 cGy	1	6,500–7,000 cGy	6½ – 7½ weeks
Hyperfractionation				
University of Florida[9]	120 cGy	2	7,440–8,160 cGy	6–7 weeks
Accelerated Fractionation				
C.C. Wang[35]				
SHART = Split Hyperfractionated Accelerated Radiotherapy	160 cGy	2	6,400–6,720 cGy	6 weeks
MSKCC M.D. Anderson[3,109] Accelerated Fractionation with Concomitant Boost	180 cGy	1 (first 4 weeks)	7,000 cGy	6 weeks
	180 cGy (am tx) 150 – 160 cGy (pm boost)	2 (last 2 weeks)		
Hybrids				
Mt. Vernon Hospital (England)[110–112] CHART = Continuous Hyperfractionated Accelerated Radiotherapy	140 – 150 cGy	3	5,400 cGy	12 days
HARDE = Hyperfractionated Accelerated Radiotherapy with Dose Escalation[113]	120 cGy wk 1–2	2	7,600 cGy	5 weeks
	140 cGy wk 3–4	2		
	160 cGy wk 5	2		
	200 cGy wk 2–5 (Saturdays)	1		

FX = fraction.

located in this region would be more resistant to radiation due to the low oxygen tension. As fractionated radiation therapy is administered to the tumor, the better oxygenated malignant cells located at the outer regions of the mass are preferentially killed. Progressively, this process will result in tumor mass shrinkage and bring the previously hypoxic central cells closer to the blood vessels and thus allow their oxygenation, development of increased radiosensitivity and increased potential for their cell kill. This re-oxygenation of certain tumor areas can occur during treatment and may take between a few hours or up to a few days to occur.[4]

Tumor re-oxygenation can also occur through fluctuation of blood flow in tumor capillaries. Also, radiation damaged cells have a reduced oxygen utilization. Re-oxygenation is more extensive after large radiation doses (> 200 to 300 cGy).

Repopulation

In both tumors and normal tissues, there exist clonogens that can proliferate during a course of fractionated radiation therapy. As cell death occurs over the ensuing weeks of radiation therapy, an accelerated rate of cellular proliferation may occur which is called repopulation.

For tumors, this results in an increase in the number of malignant cells despite ongoing radiation therapy and thus reduces the net effect of treatment and ultimately will contribute to local treatment failure.[5]

For acutely-responding normal tissues, this phenomenon of repopulation during treatment is efficacious in the process of healing acute radiation reactions. However, late-responding normal tissues do not produce an early proliferative response to treatment due to their minimal cellular reproduction.

Redistribution

Many cell lines show a large variation of up to a factor of 3 in the radiosensitivity differential of the various phases of the cell cycle. When a tissue is irradiated, a certain percentage of the cells are killed and these are generally located in the more radiosensitive phases such as G2 and M. The surviving cells may go into a mitotic delay such as in G2 arrest, or may progress into the next phase of the cell cycle which may be more radiosensitive. The net effect is that there will be an increase in the percentage of cells in the more radiosensitive phase as part of this partial synchronization response.

CLINICAL PRACTICE OF HEAD AND NECK RADIATION ONCOLOGY

Multimodality Therapeutic Approach

Specialty Team Coordination

The practice of head and neck oncology requires a comprehensive multidisciplinary team of specialists dedicated to the treatment of these diseases. This will include the surgical specialists (head and neck surgeons, plastic and reconstructive surgeons, dentists and oral surgeons, neurosurgeons), radiation oncologists, medical oncologists, pathologists, radiologists, nutritionists, oncology nurses, psychologists and social workers. It is imperative that there is excellent communication and close interaction among the various specialties starting early on in the evaluation and care of the patient.

Radiation Oncology Consultation

The radiation oncologist will obtain a thorough history and perform a comprehensive physical examination that will include a detailed head and neck evaluation. This will involve a careful inspection and palpation of the patient's oral cavity, oropharynx, nasopharynx, larynx and neck. Indirect laryngoscopy and fiberoptic nasopharyngolaryngoscopy will be performed. In selected cases, it may be quite helpful to examine the patient under anesthesia with the surgeon. The primary lesion and palpable lymph nodes should be carefully described with respect to their specific anatomic location, diameter and depth, bulkiness, mobility and topography. A diagram of the primary tumor and lymphadenopathy lesion should be placed in the chart. Pertinent radiographs such as CT and MRI scans of the head and neck will be evaluated. After communication with the other physicians participating in this patient's care, a therapeutic plan is jointly developed and a schedule coordinated.

Clinical Preparation for Radiation Therapy

Patients who will undergo radiation therapy for head and neck cancer require a comprehensive pretreatment evaluation. For those who are scheduled to receive cisplatin chemotherapy, audiology testing, EKG and a 12-hour creatinine clearance evaluation is obtained in addition to our baseline blood studies that include a complete blood count, chemistry panel and thyroid function tests (including TSH). Patients undergoing treatment with a curative intent will require that their hematocrit be ≥ 30 percent. Significant anemia has been suggested to adversely affect the efficacy of radiation therapy in head and neck cancers.[6,7]

Patients in whom the radiation treatment volume will include the major salivary glands, mandible or teeth and gingiva are scheduled for consultation with the dental service. The radiation oncologist and dentist will discuss the proposed treatment portals, therapeutic plan and status of the oral cavity. Any teeth that are not felt to be salvageable are extracted. Customized mouth guards are designed in patients with significant tooth fillings to decrease the effect of their interaction with in order radiation which could cause focal sites of adjacent mucositis. A program in fluoride prophylaxis is prescribed for the patient. Routine periodic follow-up dental appointments are scheduled during and after completion of radiation therapy.

In selected patients where high doses of radiation therapy will include a portion of the orbits, consideration of a baseline ophthalmologic evaluation may be indicated. This can be important in patients being treated for nasopharyngeal carcinoma and malignancies of the nasal cavity and paranasal sinuses.

The nutritional status of the patient will require close attention. Any significant problems such as weight loss, dysphagia, odynophagia, and major trismus must be aggressively addressed. Special dietary supplements and perhaps placement of a percutaneous endoscopic gastrostomy tube may be required.

Patients who are still abusing alcohol will require specialized care. Those smoking cigarettes should be started on a smoking cessation program. Not only are these risk factors for head and neck cancer but their continued use during radiation therapy can exacerbate acute side effects.

Therapeutic Indications

Primary Therapy Decision Making

The decision as to whether a patient should undergo surgery, radiation therapy, or combined chemotherapy and radiation therapy with a curative intent as the primary treatment for their head and neck cancer will depend on the analysis of several clinical factors:

Patient status. Evaluation of the age, debility, pulmonary status, medical co-morbidities, psychological status, motivation, capability of self-care, family support, and rehabilitation potential is essential.

Primary Tumor Characteristics. Factors such as the anatomic site, tumor volume, topography (exophytic versus infiltrative), tumor extent (eg, bone involvement), and histopathology help determine which therapeutic modality may be best suited for that case.

Presence of Field Cancerization. For patients who present with widespread leukoplakia and/or carcinoma in situ, surgery is preferred for operable early local invasive lesions, with radiation therapy reserved for perhaps an anticipated more advanced future lesion. Such patients are usually plagued with multiple relentless regional recurrences of cancer, and the initial use of radiation therapy for a clearly operable early lesion may prevent its application at a later time when it may be efficacious for a more extensive lesion that may not be so amenable to surgery.

Anticipated Functional Sequelae of Treatment. While locoregional control is the most important consideration of therapy, this must be balanced with any functional compromise that may result from treatment such as dysphagia, aspiration, or loss of the ability to speak or swallow.

Post-therapy Cosmesis. With the latest techniques in plastic and reconstructive surgery as well as the artistic capabilities of maxilloprosthodontists, this factor becomes one of only relative importance but still merits critical analysis.

Prior Therapy. Previous high-dose radiotherapy to the region of concern may prevent the use of subsequent radiation therapy. There are highly selected patients who may be candidates for re-irradiation if surgery cannot be performed.

Single Modality Approach. For early stage primary head and neck tumors where both surgery or radiation therapy can be administered with equally good locoregional control and cosmetic and functional outcomes, it is our practice at Memorial Sloan-Kettering Cancer Center to select only one treatment that will address both the primary lesion and neck together.

Preoperative Radiation Therapy

Indications

A major indication for preoperative radiation therapy is to improve the operability of a primary lesion or a fixed lymph node. A corollary indication is the initial use of a so-called test dose of radiation in a patient in whom full course radiation therapy is being seriously considered yet in whom there is concern with the tumor characteristics suggesting a less than optimal response.

Strong[8] reported on one of the first randomized trials in head and neck cancer which evaluated patients with clinically positive neck nodes who were randomly assigned to either receive preoperative radiation (2,000 cGy) and then a radical neck dissection or a neck dissection alone. In patients in whom the pathologic neck specimen revealed one nodal level of involvement, the incidence of neck relapse was 28 percent with preoperative radiation compared to 37 percent with just neck dissection. When multiple nodal levels were involved, the incidence of neck relapse was 37 percent with preoperative radiation and 71 percent for those treated with a neck dissection alone. This study thus showed that preoperative radiation was beneficial in reducing the incidence of neck recurrence after a neck dissection in patients presenting with clinically positive neck nodes.

Benefits/Drawbacks

The benefits of preoperative radiation therapy include: (1) the allowance of time for patients to undergo vigorous supportive therapy (eg, nutritional, pulmonary, cardiac) to optimize their condition in preparation for subsequent surgery, (2) prevention of marginal recurrences, (3) prevention of wound implantation of tumor cells at surgery, and (4) control of subclinical disease at the primary site and in the lymph nodes.

Radiobiologically, the tumor cells are in their maximal state of oxygenation in a preoperative setting and this may confer a therapeutic advantage, as the malignant cells would be more radio-responsive. Postoperatively, with scarring and a disruption of the normal vasculature, any remaining malignant cells in the surgical bed may be in a suboptimal environment with respect to their oxygenation and thus may not respond as well to radiation.

Drawbacks to preoperative therapy include: delay of surgery by perhaps to $2^1/_2$ to 3 months; the radiation dosage may adversely impact on subsequent postoperative healing; radiation dose limitations.

Preoperative Dosage

Typically, preoperative radiation therapy is given at 180 to 200 cGy per fraction, one fraction per day 5 days per week, to a total dosage of 5,000 to 6,000 cGy. After completion of treatment, there is a 4 to 6 week break prior to surgery to allow for patient recovery, a decrease in the acute inflammatory reactions from radiation therapy, and to allow for a maximum clinical shrinkage of the tumor.

In cases where preoperative radiation is given as a "test dose," the tumor is treated to a dosage of around 5,000 cGy at a conventional fraction size of 180 to 200 cGy. At this point, the patient is reevaluated by both the radiation oncologist and the surgeon. If a reasonable amount of shrinkage has occurred, the patient will then be continued on radiation to completion using a curative dosage. For those patients whose tumors have had a poor clinical response to radiation, surgery is performed after a 4-week break. It should be noted that the initial extent of the tumor must be included within the resection volume, as viable malignant cells may still be present in the grossly normal-appearing tissues beside the residual tumor.

Postoperative Radiation Therapy

Indications

Postoperative radiation therapy is indicated when the estimated risk of locoregional recurrence of disease is > 20 percent.[9] Improvement in local control with postoperative radiation therapy for selected head and neck cancer cases is a clinical observation that has been confirmed in many retrospective reviews. A Memorial Sloan-Kettering Cancer Center study showed that postoperative radiation therapy for head and neck cancer in patients with nodal metastases at multiple levels decreased recurrences from 71 percent (surgery alone) down to 13 percent (surgery and postoperative radiation therapy).[10] However, it should be noted that there are no randomized studies available. Despite this fact, the place for postoperative radiation therapy is clinically well established and accepted.

Specific clinical indications for postoperative radiation therapy of the primary tumor bed include the following: (1) advanced T3 or T4 lesions, (2) positive or close margins of resection, (3) perineural/vascular invasion, (4) high-grade histology, and (5) concern of the surgeon with respect to the adequacy of the procedure, irrespective of the status of the surgical margins on final pathology review.

Surgical margins can be considered at high risk for recurrence with the presence of the following features: (1) invasive carcinoma, (2) carcinoma in situ, (3) margin < 5 millimeters,[11] (4) surgical margins initially positive but ultimately rendered negative with further resection,[12] and (5) tumor borders that are infiltrating rather than "pushing."[13] It is important to emphasize that even with a negative margin status noted on the pathology report, there is a potential for recurrence of up to 30 percent.[11]

The result of the previously cited study by Strong[8] on preoperative radiation provided the basis for the Radiation Therapy Oncology Group Trial 73-03[14] which evaluated preoperative versus postoperative radiation therapy for advanced squamous cell carcinoma of the head and neck. The overall locoregional control was significantly improved in all subsites with postoperative radiation (65% vs. 48%; p = .04). There also was a trend toward improved survival with postoperative radiation as well. The complication rates were similar between both approaches.

Benefits/Drawbacks

The benefits of postoperative radiation therapy include: (1) no delay in surgery, (2) no radiation dose limitations, (3) no influence on the extent of initial surgery, (4) no effect on wound healing, (5) allows for a full surgical and histopathologic evaluation of the extent of the tumor and lymph nodes, and (6) sterilization of residual microscopic disease which can result in improved local control.

A possible drawback to this approach would be the potential for delay in initiation of radiation therapy due to wound complications from surgery. Scarring and vascular modifications from surgery may decrease tissue oxygenation and thus adversely affect radiation tumor cell kill.

Indications for Postoperative Radiation Therapy for Cervical Node Metastasis

The indications for postoperative radiation therapy for cervical nodal metastasis include: (1) extracapsular extension, (2) lymph node size > 3 cm (N2a N3), (3) multiple ipsilateral lymph node involvement (N2b), (4) bilateral or contrlateral lymph node metastasis (N2c), (5) massive nodel metastases > 6 cm (N3), (6) surgical procedure (eg, excisional or incisional biopsy) prior to definitive surgery, and (7) perineural/vascular invasion.

The most important predictor of neck relapse is extracapsular extension, particularly with macroscopic disease.[15] Of note is the related finding that a desmoplastic lymph node growth pattern has been significantly correlated with extracapsular extension.[16]

If only one cervical lymph node is found to contain metastatic disease and it is ≤ 3 cm (N1) and without extracapsular extension, the overall risk for neck recurrence is approximately 10 percent (range of 5 to 15%). Therefore, uncomplicated N1 disease does not require postoperative neck radiation.[17]

The use of postoperative radiation therapy after radical neck dissection results in the following control rates:[18,19] (1) N1: 83 to 91 percent, (2) N2: 64 to 82 percent, (3) N3: 61 to 66 percent.

At Memorial Sloan-Kettering Cancer Center, comprehensive postoperative irradiation of the neck nodes would always include the cervical and supraclavicular nodes. Inclusion of the retropharyngeal nodes is important for these primary sites: (1) nasopharynx, (2) soft palate, (3) tonsils, (4) base of tongue, (5) posterior pharyngeal wall, (6) pyiform sinus, (7) thyroid.

Time Interval from Surgery to Radiation Therapy

The significance of the time interval from surgery to the commencement of radiation therapy for head and neck cancers has been evaluated by Vikram who initially found that a delay of 7 weeks or more was associated with an increased locoregional failure rate and decreased survival.[20] This was subsequently evaluated by Schiff and colleagues, who noted that in head and neck cancer patients who had a delay of 6 weeks or more from surgery to radiation therapy and subsequently developed a locoregional recurrence, 73 percent had received a suboptimal radiation dose of less than 5,600 cGy.[21] Of those patients who received doses of ≥ 6,000 cGy and who also had a greater than 6-week delay before initiation of treatment, only 12 percent experienced locoregional failure, which was similar to patients who started radiation therapy within the first 6 weeks after surgery. Further investigation by Vikram and colleagues revealed that the recurrence rate at the primary site was not influenced by the time interval between surgery and radiation therapy. However, a strong temporal correlation was found between delay in starting postoperative radiation therapy and subsequent failure in the cervical lymph nodes. However, the majority of these patients only received 5,000 cGy. Those that did start treatment within 6 weeks of surgery and still only received 5,000 cGy to the neck achieved a very high level of control.[10,22]

Our policy at Memorial Sloan-Kettering Cancer Center is to start postoperative radiation therapy within 6 weeks after surgery using adequate doses.

Postoperative Radiation Dosage

All patients undergoing postoperative radiation therapy for the high-risk indications noted previously for the primary tumor site and/or the neck lesion receive conventional fractionation of 180 to 200 cGy per fraction, one fraction per day, 5 days per week to a total dosage of 6,000 to 6,300 cGy to the high-risk areas, and 5,000 to 5,400 cGy for elective nodal irradiation. This is based on published data from a randomized prospective trial by Peters and colleagues from M.D. Anderson Cancer Center in 1993.[23]

Prevention of Tracheostomy Stomal Recurrence

Local recurrence in the tracheostomy stoma is a very ominous development whose overall incidence is 5 percent;[24] however, this risk increases in the subgroup with massive disease in the larynx or hypopharynx, particularly with subglottic extension and para-tracheal nodal metastasis. These patients may present with stridor and require an emergency tracheotomy. Such recurrences in the stoma may be the result of inferior submucosal extension or lymphatic spread including involvement of the para-tracheal lymph nodes.

Therefore, in these high risk patients, we recommend that the tracheostomy stoma undergo a local electron boost with a 0.5 cm bolus delivering 1,000 cGy in 5 fractions to the 90 percent isodose line, after the initial irradiation with photons to the low neck region including the para-tracheal and superior mediastinal nodes to 4,500 to 5,000 cGy. Also, treatment of the para-tracheal and superior mediastinal nodes is necessary.

THE ROLE OF RADIATION THERAPY ALONE FOR HEAD AND NECK TUMOR BY SITE

Lip

Surgery or radiation therapy can be considered for primary treatment of T1 to T2 lip cancers based on the specific anatomic location and size of the lesion. Local control rates with either modality range between 80 to 90 percent.[25]

Surgery can be used for T1 to T2 lesions that are small in size and located away from the commissure in which a V-shaped incision is employed. However, one must make sure that there will be no resultant major cosmetic deformity or functional debility. In such instances, radiation therapy should be considered.

Advanced T3 to T4 lesions with mandibular involvement and/or significant loss of soft tissue should be treated with radical resection and reconstruction. If there is bone involvement, radiation would not be successful in eradicating the tumor. Also, if there was massive soft tissue disease, major surgical reconstruction would be necessary after radical high-dose radiation therapy, but this would carry a significant risk of wound healing problems—thus the primary use of radiation is not recommended. Local control rates with radiation therapy in advanced lesions run between 40 to 60 percent.[29] Consideration of concurrent cisplatin chemotherapy with radiation for these advanced lesions would be discussed.

Radiation therapy is indicated for: commissure involvement, patients who refuse surgery, and superficial lip cancers involving less than one-third of the entire lip. Small lesions may involve the use of a temporary interstitial implant alone (Figures 21–4A, B and C). Larger lesions may require external beam radiation therapy with an interstitial boost. Local control rates are high at 80 to 90 percent.[25]

The risk for regional lymph node metastasis is small. For the upper lip, the lymphatic network is more extensive than the lower lip and so there is a 20 percent incidence of nodal metastasis. The lower lip carries a less than 10 percent risk for nodal metastasis. Elective nodal treatment is therefore not indicated. Clinically involved nodes, however, are treated in the usual fashion.

Oral Cavity

General Therapeutic Principles

For early T1 and T2 lesions, radiation therapy and surgery are equally effective in achieving local control. Superficial lesions that are ≤ 2 cm (T1) and are away from the bone can be considered for treatment with an interstitial implant alone. Lesions > 2 cm and ≤ 4 cm (T2) and without clinical lymphadenopathy may be treated with external radiation therapy (5,000 cGy) which would include the adjacent regional lymph nodes (submental, submandibular and jugulodigastric) and a temporary interstitiary implant (2,000 to 2,500 cGy).

For moderately advanced T2 to T3 lesions, full course external beam radiation therapy is used. However, for lesions in the floor of mouth and oral tongue, extension of disease deep into the musculature and into adjacent mandibular bone would best be treated with surgery and postoperative radiation therapy. A major concern in the primary use of radi-

ation therapy for T1 and T2 oral cancer regions is the potential for complications including soft tissue and bone necrosis as well as acute and long-term side effects such as mucositis and xerostomia. These concerns must be considered for early stage lesions

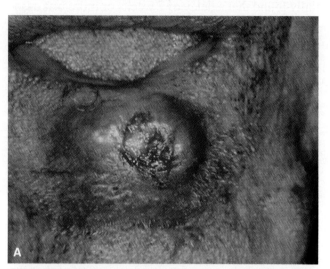

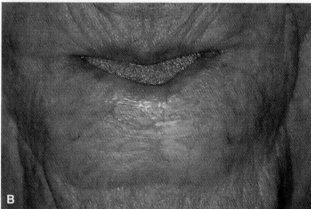

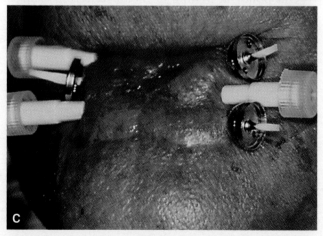

Figure 21–4.   A patient with T2N0 squamous cell carcinoma of the lower lip prior to (A) and several months after (B) brachytherapy. He was treated with a temporary afterloaded interstitial implant technique (C).

when evaluating a patient for treatment using primary surgery or radiation therapy. At Memorial Sloan-Kettering Cancer Center, we generally would favor proceeding with surgery for T1 and T2 lesions of the oral cavity where no significant functional sequelae would result. These lesions would be technically quite accessible surgically and this modality would carry a low complication rate.

While lymph node metastasis in head and neck cancer generally occur in an orderly predictable manner by spreading consecutively from level to level, oral cavity lesions can occasionally skip the first echelon of lymph nodes down to level III or IV with an overall incidence of around 5 percent.[27] Byers and colleagues[28] found that 15 percent of patients with primary oral tongue cancer exhibited skip metastases down to level IV. This should be kept in mind when one is considering a patient with oral cavity cancer for possible regional nodal irradiation.

Floor of Mouth

T1 and T2 lesions can be treated with surgery or radiation therapy. If there are clinically positive nodes, surgical resection of the primary lesion and a neck dissection is performed. Postoperative external beam radiation therapy may be indicated for close or positive margins in the primary site and/or nodal disease. If radiation is to be given, both the floor of mouth and nodes are treated within 6 weeks after surgery to a dosage of 6,300 cGy to the primary site and high-risk node levels as well as 5,000 to 5,400 cGy for elective nodal irradiation. Even with a clinically negative neck, primary surgery is favored, as one can often avoid acute and late side effects from radiation if no high-risk factors are found on the pathology evaluation.

If an early lesion extends to the ventral aspect of the oral tongue, radiation therapy may be preferred in that it can avoid any functional morbidity that may result from a surgical resection involving this area of the oral tongue.

Radiation therapy commonly would involve external beam radiation therapy and brachytherapy or brachytherapy alone. If the lesion is quite close to or actually involves the mucosa overlying the mandible, brachytherapy should be avoided as its use can be associated with an increased risk of osteoradionecrosis. For very small and superficial T1 lesions, a temporary interstitial implant alone (6,000 to 6,500 cGy) could be administered. For larger T1 and T2 lesions, we would use external beam radiation therapy (4,500 cGy) with a temporary interstitial implant boost to the tumor (2,500 cGy). The local control results of radiation therapy have been reported at 94 percent for T1 and 74 percent for T2 disease.[29]

T3 and T4 lesions are usually approached with surgery and postoperative radiation therapy in a similar manner as described above. Selected cases that are not amenable to surgery would be considered for investigational cisplatin chemotherapy concurrent with accelerated fractionation radiation therapy with a delayed concomitant boost. We do feel that results are better with surgery for these advanced lesions.

Oral Tongue

T1 and T2 local control rates are comparable between surgery and radiation therapy. For T1 lesions, there is a local control rate of 76 percent with surgery compared to 79 percent with radiation; for T2 lesions, the rate is 76 percent with surgery and 72 percent with radiation.[30] Surgery would generally be chosen as this approach is shorter, would obviate the acute and late side effects of radiation, and has a lower complication rate. Primary radiation therapy would include external beam irradiation of the oral tongue and regional nodes to a dosage of 4,000 cGy with a subsequent brachytherapy boost of 3,000 cGy. 5,000 to 5,400 cGy is administered for elective nodal irradiation.

Advanced T3 and T4 lesions are generally approached with surgery and postoperative radiation therapy within 6 weeks of the procedure. The tumor bed and high-risk nodal levels are treated to a dosage of 6,300 cGy with conventional fractionation while 5,000 to 5,400 cGy is administered for elective nodal irradiation. If the patient refuses surgery, is medically inoperable or would have prohibitive morbidity from the surgical procedure, we would treat the patient with combined cisplatin chemotherapy and concurrent radiation therapy using accelerated fractionation with a delayed concomitant boost under an investigational protocol.

Pharynx

Nasopharynx

Nasopharyngeal carcinoma is primarily a squamous carcinoma or a variant such as lymphoepithelioma. Lesions most commonly arise in the fossa of Rosenmüller. There is a 75 to 90 percent incident of lymph node metastasis that usually occurs in the upper level V and upper level II regions as well as the retropharyngeal nodes. They are frequently bulky and are bilateral in 30 to 50 percent of cases.

Because of the anatomic location of the nasopharynx, surgery is not used except to obtain a biopsy. Radiation therapy is the primary treatment modality for this very radiosensitive tumor.

For early disease—stage I/T1N0M0[3]—radiation therapy alone is administered as the primary treatment of choice. At Memorial Sloan-Kettering Cancer Center, we would use CT simulation techniques and intensity modulated radiation therapy treatment planning. This allows for a better homogenous dose distribution to the primary tumor and involved lymph nodes while reducing the dose to important adjacent structures.[31,31a] Accelerated fractionation with a delayed concomitant boost to a dosage of 7,000 cGy to the primary tumor and lymphadenopathy is administered; 5,000 to 5,400 cGy is administered for elective nodal irradiation. Local control rates based on conventional fractionation are high at 70 to 90 percent for T1 primary lesions[32–34] and regional nodal control is > 90 percent for N0 to N1 nodes.[32–35]

Advanced disease, stages II through IV[3], are treated with cisplatin chemotherapy concurrent with radiation therapy, based on the data from the randomized Intergroup Study 0099[36] published in 1998. This study revealed a significant improvement in 3-year progression-free survival with the chemotherapy-radiation therapy arm at 69 percent versus 24 percent with radiation therapy alone. The chemotherapy-radiation therapy arm had a 78 percent 3-year overall survival versus 47 percent with radiation therapy alone.

At Memorial Sloan-Kettering Cancer Center, stage II through IV disease is treated with cisplatin chemotherapy on days 1 and 22, concurrent with radiation therapy using accelerated fractionation with a delayed concomitant boost to a dosage of 7,000 cGy to the primary lesion and lymphadenopathy using intensity modulated radiation therapy treatment planning.[36a] 5,000 to 5,400 cGy is administered for elective nodal irradiation.

As opposed to other head and neck sites with lymphadenopathy, even large lymph nodes can usually be controlled with radiation therapy alone. Occasionally, a patient may require a post-radiation therapy neck dissection 2 to 3 months later for persistent adenopathy. Relapse in the neck without recurrence at the primary site is rare. Despite very good primary and nodal control rates with radiation therapy, the presence of extensive disease in the neck increases the risk for regional failure, metastatic disease and decreased survival. It has been reported that there is a distinct variation in the 5-year survival rates based on nodal stage: N0 to N1 60 to 75 percent, N2 to N3 40 to 50 percent.[33,37] Bilateral nodal metastases carry no major prognostic implications.

Oropharynx

Soft Palate

T1N0 or T2N0 lesions can be treated with either radiation therapy or surgery with equivalent excellent local control rates of 80 to 90 percent.[38,39] Primary radiation therapy involving external beam radiation and brachytherapy, brachytherapy alone in selected cases, or full course external beam radiation is favored in that it provides superior functional results. However, some would argue in favor of surgery in that these patients have a potential for field cancerization within condemned mucosa and thus a 30 percent risk for subsequent development of another cancer. Therefore, if the early soft palate lesion is treated surgically, radiation therapy would be saved for a more advanced lesion that may subsequently develop.

The necessity of a brachytherapy implant has not been absolutely proven. However, it can decrease the radiation dosage to adjacent structures including the parotid gland. Careful patient selection and physician expertise with the brachytherapy technique is mandatory. When external beam radiation is also used, a dosage of 4,500 to 5,000 cGy is administered in addition to the 2,000 to 3,500 brachytherapy boost.

For patients with early disease in whom full course external beam radiation is given, we would deliver the following doses: T1: 6,600 cGy; and T2: 6,800 to 7,000 cGy.

Advanced T3 to T4 lesions are treated with surgery and postoperative radiation therapy to doses of at least 6,300 cGy depending on the surgical findings, completeness of resection and pathology evaluation. The results with radiation therapy alone are poor with local control rates of 30 to 50 percent.[40] Unresectable patients would be considered for our investigational protocols including cisplatin concurrent with accelerated fractionation radiotherapy with a delayed concomitant boost to 7,000 cGy.

The overall risk for lymph node metastasis is high at 45 percent (10 to 30% for T1 to T2 and 60 to 70% for T3 to T4 disease). Both the clinically positive nodes and negative neck must be addressed in the usual fashion. Midline lesions can result in bilateral nodal metastasis.

Tonsillar Region

The most common locations for a primary tumor of the oropharynx are the anterior tonsillar pillar and the tonsillar fossa. Tumors of the tonsillar fossa present with more advanced stages than do tumors of the tonsillar pillars or soft palate. Tonsillar fossa lesions have a slightly lower recurrence rate than those arising from the anterior tonsillar pillar areas when comparing T1 to T2 lesions.

T1, T2 and selected exophytic T3 lesions can be treated very effectively with radiation therapy or surgery. Radiation is the preferred modality as the control rates are excellent and the functional results are better. Pre-radiation tonsillectomy is not indicated. The overall risk for lymph node metastasis is high (60 to 75% for tonsillar fossa; 45% for tonsillar pillar) and they must be addressed in the usual fashion. Contralateral lymph node metastasis in general is low (11% for tonsillar fossa; 5% for tonsillar pillar).

External beam radiation doses for early disease include the following: (1) T1: 6,600 cGy (180 cGy/Fx), (2) small T2: 6,800 to 7,000 cGy (180 cGy/Fx) and (3) large T2/selected exophytic T3: accelerated fractionation with a delayed concomitant boost to 7,000 cGy (primary tumor and involved nodes). Concurrent cisplatin chemotherapy for stage III an IV disease would be used.

Radiation therapy for well-lateralized T1 to T2, N0 to N1 primary tonsillar lesions without involvement of the base of tongue uses an ipsilateral treatment plan with a wedged pair directed to the involved tonsillar region with margin (2 cm) as well as anterior-posterior/posterior-anterior opposed portals to the ipsilateral cervical-supraclavicular nodes. Care is taken to avoid irradiating the contralateral parotid gland, in order to decrease the degree of xerostomia.

If the tonsillar mass extends medially to involve the soft palate and approaches the uvula or extends inferiorly to infiltrate the base of tongue, the gross tumor volume and margins will increase and bilateral right/left opposed portals must be used. This will provide good dosimetric coverage of the primary tumor with adequate margin. If the patient has N2a or higher stage nodal disease, they are at an increased risk for bilateral cervical lymph node metastasis and thus both sides of the neck must be irradiated. Consideration of a brachytherapy boost with involvement of the base of tongue may improve local control rates.[41]

Clinically involved lymph nodes > 2 cm will usually undergo post-radiation therapy neck dissection approximately 6 weeks after treatment. N1 nodes ≤ 2 cm can be boosted to 7,000 cGy with a high control rate using radiation therapy alone. If there is no palpable or radiographic evidence of residual adenopathy 6 weeks after irradiation, these patients may be followed rather than undergo a neck dissection.

T1 to T2 local control rates from radiation therapy alone are excellent. Remmler and colleagues[42] reported local control rates of 100 percent for T1 and 89 percent for T2 lesions.

Surgery for T1 and T2 lesions require an en bloc resection of the tonsillar mass with margin. Access is gained through a trans-oral or mandibulotomy approach depending on the size and anatomic extent of the tumor. A therapeutic neck dissection for clinically positive nodes or a staging dissection for a negative neck is performed as well. Local control rates of 80 to 90 percent have been reported and are comparable to similar stage lesions treated with radiation therapy alone.[42] Postoperative radiation therapy within 6 weeks of surgery may be indicated, depending on the primary margin status and nodal metastasis. Conventional fractionation at 180 cGy per fraction to a total dosage of 6,300 cGy for high-risk primary site and nodal levels are given in addition to 5, 000 to 5,400 cGy for elective nodal irradiation.

T3 and T4 lesions are poorly controlled with radiation therapy or surgery alone. A combined modality approach with radical surgery and postoperative radiation therapy is usually employed. The radiation therapy is administered within 6 weeks of surgery with conventional fractionation to total dosage of 6,300 cGy to high-risk primary and nodal regions with 5,000 to 5,400 cGy to administer for elective nodal irradiation.

However, our current preference would be to approach such advanced disease with cisplatin chemotherapy on days 1 and 22 concurrent with radiation therapy using accelerated fractionation with a delayed commitant boost to the primary site and lymphadenopathy to a dosage of 7,000 cGy; 5,000 to 5,400 cGy is administered for elective nodal irradiation. Current data suggests improved locoregional control and survival rates with chemoradiation (Figures 21–5A–C).

Base of Tongue

T1 and T2 lesions can be successfully treated by either surgery or radiation therapy. Both modalities have equivalent local control and survival rates. Local control rates of 80 to 90 percent for radiation[43] and 75 to 85 percent for surgery[44,45] have been reported. The therapeutic decision will need to be based on the morbidity of one treatment compared to the other. The majority of patients are usually treated with radiation therapy, as it provides a better functional outcome and quality of life with equivalent control rates. Surgery would be indicated for patients with endophytic, locally advanced lesions which may be difficult to control with radiation alone. In such cases, postoperative radiation therapy may be necessary. Such radiation would commence within 6 weeks following surgery using conventional fractionation delivering 6,300 cGy to the high-risk primary site and nodal levels, with 5,000 to 5,400 cGy administered for elective nodal irradiation.

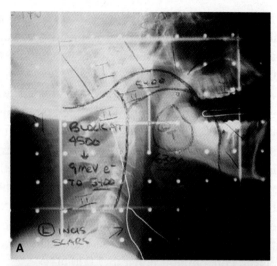

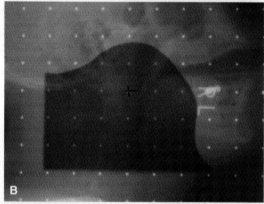

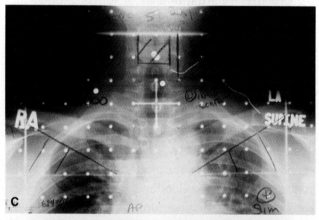

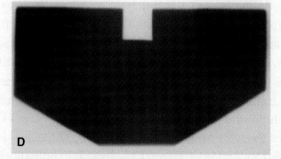

Figure 21–5.   Simulation (*A, C*) and corresponding port films (*B, D*) for a patient with a T3N2b squamous cell carcinoma of the tonsillar region.

At Memorial Sloan-Kettering Cancer Center, patients with T1 and T2 lesions would be considered for treatment with radiotherapy conventional fractionation with the primary lesion taken to 5,400 cGy, the involved neck nodes to 6,000 cGy and elective nodal irradiation to 5,000 to 5,400cGy (Figures 21–6A and B). Following a 3-week break, the patient would undergo a neck dissection for clinically positive nodes and an elective tracheotomy, as well as an iridium 192 temporary interstitiary implant to the base of the tongue delivering 2,400 to 3,000 cGy. Local control rates have been reported at up to 100 percent for the T1 and T2 lesions treated with this approach.[46–48] Also, such early T stage patients would be considered for full course accelerated fractionation external beam radiation with a delayed concomitant boost alone or with concurrent cisplatin chemotherapy with patients who have cervical adenopathy where neck dissection would generally follow.

Selected exophytic early T3 lesions may still be approachable with full course radiation therapy as described above. Local control rates of 80 percent have been obtained with this approach.[46–49]

Advanced T3 and T4 lesions often would require surgery with a partial or total glossectomy, possibly a total laryngectomy and neck dissection to be followed with postoperative radiation therapy. The results with surgery alone for these advanced lesions has been reported at a 27 percent 2-year local control and a 20 percent overall survival.[50] Radiation therapy alone has been reported to have a 50 percent local control rate. Combining surgery with postoperative radiation therapy has a local control rate of 75 to 90 percent.[45] In such cases, it is currently reasonable to consider a larynx preservation approach, with chemo-radiation

At Memorial Sloan-Kettering Cancer Center, very advanced or unresectable lesions are preferentially treated on our research protocol with cisplatin chemotherapy on days 1 and 22 concurrent with radiation therapy using accelerated fractionation with a delayed concomitant boost to a dosage of 7,000 cGy to the primary lesion and lymphadenopathy; 5,000 to 5,400 cGy is administered for elective nodal irradiation (Figures 21–7A and B). Patients with an initially positive neck would undergo a neck dissection approximately 6 weeks after treatment.

Hypopharynx

Pyriform Sinus

The pyriform sinus is the most common site of squamous cell carcinoma in the hypopharynx. The incidence of palpable lymph node metastasis is high at 75 percent. Upward of 10 to 14 percent of such patients will have bilateral or contralateral nodal disease.

Early stage disease, T1 and early T2 lesions with exophytic low bulk lesions, can be effectively treated with primary radiation therapy or surgery.

T1 lesions can be treated with radiation administered with conventional fractionation at 180 cGy to a dosage of 7,000 cGy. Likewise, larger volume T1 and selected T2 lesions can be treated with accelerated fractionation with a delayed concomitant boost to a dosage of 7,000 cGy to the primary lesion and lymphadenopathy. A larynx compensator is used to improve the dose homogeneity to that region. Comprehensive nodal irradiation is necessary in view of the high incidence of lymph node metastasis. 5,000 to 5,400 cGy is administered for elective nodal irradiation; 6,000 cGy is administered for clinically palpable lymphadenopathy, with subsequent neck dissection planned approximately 6 weeks after treatment. Such patients with advanced disease by virtue of the adenopathy would also be administered cisplatin chemotherapy concurrently. Mendenhall and colleagues[51,52] report local control rates of 88 percent for T1 and 80 percent for T2 lesions treated with radiation therapy alone. However, it should be noted that some feel that only exophytic, small lesions of the membranous portion of the pyriform sinus can be reliably treated with radiation and this should be considered in the therapeutic decision. Surgical salvage of radiation failure may be possible, however it may be associated with an increased complication rate.

Conservation surgery for T1 and T2 lesions can be considered as well and is associated with local control rates of 96 percent.[53] Various surgical procedures have been used based on the location and size of the lesion and include supracricoid hemilaryngopharyngectomy and a partial laryngopharyngectomy. Postoperative radiation therapy may be indicated particularly for large T2 lesions and with nodal metastasis.

Advanced disease, stage T3 and T4, can be treated with a larynx preservation approach using chemotherapy and radiation when the extent of the primary disease would require a total laryngectomy. An EORTC[54] study consisted of patients with locally advanced hypopharyngeal carcinoma limited to the pyriform sinus or hypopharyngeal aspect of the aryepiglottic fold. They were randomized to either receive standard surgery (total laryngectomy, partial pharyngectomy, neck dissection) and postoperative radiation therapy (5,000 to 7,000 cGy at 200 cGy/fraction) versus induction chemotherapy with

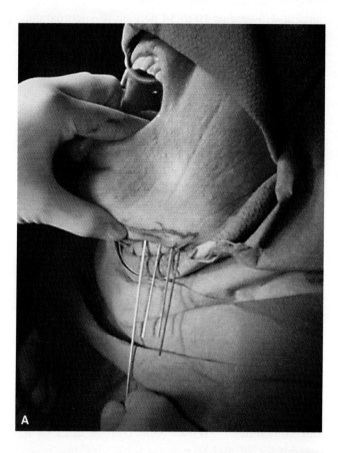

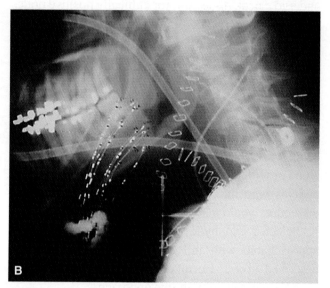

Figure 21–6. Patient with a T2N2cM0 squamous cell carcinoma of the base of tongue. He was treated with external beam radiation therapy to the primary area and regional lymph nodes to a dosage of 5,400 cGy, and 5,000 cGy to the low anterior neck nodes. Subsequently a bilateral neck dissection was performed showing no pathologic evidence of metastatic disease. At the same surgery, he underwent a temporary afterloaded interstitial implant (A). Lateral film after the procedure shows the orientation of the catheters with the implants in place (B).

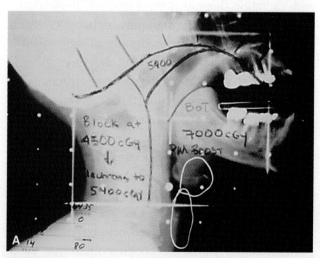

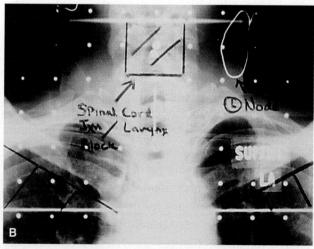

Figure 21–7. A and B, Patient with a T3N2CM0 squamous cell carcinoma of the base of the tongue. He was treated with cisplatin chemotherapy on day 1 and 22 concurrent with accelerated fractionation radiotherapy with a delayed concomitant boost to the sites of tumor to a dosage of 7000 cGy.

cisplatin + 5FU for up to 3 cycles and radiation therapy (7,000 cGy at 200 cGy/fraction) for those who achieve a complete clinical response at the primary site. Those with less than a complete response at the primary site underwent standard surgery and postoperative radiation therapy. Results revealed a 3-year survival of 57 percent with chemotherapy-radiation therapy versus 43 percent with the surgery-radiation therapy arm; however the survival advantage was not maintained at 5 years. The 3-year disease-free survival with a functional larynx was 64 percent in those patients with a complete response to induction chemotherapy. Zelefsky and colleagues[55] reported on the Memorial Sloan-Kettering Cancer Center experience and found that the survival was comparable between patients treated with chemotherapy-radiation therapy and those who underwent standard surgery with postoperative radiation therapy for advanced hypopharyngeal cancers.

At Memorial Sloan-Kettering Cancer Center, we would administer cisplatin on days 1 and 22, concurrent with radiation therapy using accelerated fractionation with a concomitant boost to the primary lesion and lymphadenopathy to a dosage of 7,000 cGy. 5,000 to 5,400 cGy would be administered for elective nodal irradiation. Surgery is saved for salvage.

Posterior Pharyngeal Wall

This region is adjacent to the retropharyngeal space and is contiguous with the pharyngeal wall of the oropharynx with superior extension to the base of skull and inferiorly to the cervical esophagus. Primary tumors in this region are usually large and infiltrate deeply along the retropharyngeal space with lymph node metastasis in the retropharyngeal and cervical nodes.

Because of the extent of most of these tumors at presentation, surgical resection is usually not possible. Radiation therapy is the main therapeutic modality. Consideration of altered fractionation approaches would be reasonable. At Memorial Sloan-Kettering Cancer Center, we would treat the unresectable lesions with cisplatin chemotherapy delayed concurrent with radiation therapy using accelerated fractionation with a concurrent boost to

7,000 cGy to the primary tumor and lymphadenopathy; 5,000 to 5,400 would be administered for elective nodal irradiation.

Larynx

Supraglottic Larynx

T1 lesions are limited to one subsite with a normal vocal cord mobility. T2 lesions invade the mucosa of more than one adjacent subsite of the supraglottis or the glottis, vallecula, mucosa of the base of tongue, or the medial wall of the pyriform sinus, but do not have fixation of the larynx. The incidence of lymph node metastasis is high at 25 to 50 percent. The risk for bilateral nodal involvement is substantial as well. These early stage lesions are highly curable by either surgery or radiation therapy in general.

Small, superficial, exophytic lesions with no palpable neck nodes or a solitary node ≤ 2cm can be treated with radiation therapy alone. Thin, nonbulky lesions are more likely to be controlled with radiation. However, ulcerative lesions, those located in the petiole and thick, bulky lesions may be more difficult to control by radiation therapy.

Primary radiation therapy for a T1 lesion would involve a treatment field encompassing the supraglottis, glottis, subglottis, and regional lymph nodes. The field arrangements would be via right/left lateral portals opposed and the low anterior neck nodes via a direct AP portal. For small, non-bulky lesions, conventional fractionation can be considered to a total dosage of 7,000 cGy to the primary lesion and 5,000 to 5,400 cGy for elective nodal irradiation. For larger, more extensive lesions, accelerated fractionation with a delayed concomitant boost to a dosage of 7,000 cGy would be favored. Local control rates of radiation therapy have been reported at 73 percent, 90 percent and 100 percent.[56–58]

Radiation therapy for T2 lesions would be similarly treated using accelerated fractionation with a delayed concomitant boost. Local control rates with hyperfractionation have been reported at 90 percent and with conventional fractionation it is 80 percent.[58] With surgical salvage, the latter rates increase to 88 percent.

Surgery involves a supraglottic laryngectomy with removal of the epiglottis, aryepiglottic fold, false cords and upper half of the adjacent thyroid cartilage. The hyoid bone may or may not be removed. Bilateral staging neck dissections are indicated as the risk for lymph node metastasis bilaterally is high. It is vital that patients undergo rigorous preoperative medical evaluation as this procedure is not well tolerated in patients with chronic obstructive pulmonary disease due to subsequent swallowing difficulties and possible aspiration. Som reported an overall 68 percent 5-year survival.[59] Ogura and Biller noted an 85 percent 3-year survival with epiglottic lesions; however, when there was extension to the false cord, this dropped to 71 percent.[60]

If the pathology specimen shows close or positive margins or nodal metastasis, postoperative radiation therapy may be indicated. However, there is a risk for development of severe laryngeal edema with a 20 percent incidence of a prolonged tracheostomy and a 4 percent risk for a completion laryngectomy. We would treat the primary area and regional lymph node at 180 cGy per fraction, 1 fraction per day, 5 days a week to a total dosage of 6,300 cGy.[23]

T3 lesions involve vocal cord fixation and/or invasion of the postcricoid area or preepiglottic tissues. Selected lesions with preepiglottic extension without vocal cord involvement can be treated with a supraglottic laryngectomy for preservation of the voice. Results show a 75 percent 3-year survival with a 10 percent local recurrence rate.[61]

All other T3 and T4 lesions will require a total laryngectomy. In these cases, we would initially employ a laryngeal preservation approach with chemotherapy and radiation therapy while reserving total laryngectomy for salvage. At Memorial Sloan-Kettering Cancer Center, we would use cisplatin chemotherapy on days 1 and 22 concurrent with radiation therapy with an accelerated fractionation and a delayed concomitant boost to a total dosage of 7,000 cGy to the primary lesion and lymphadenopathy.[61a] 5,000 to 5,400 cGy is administered for elective nodal irradiation. Results for primary conventional radiation therapy alone for T3 or T4 lesions are poor.

Glottic Larynx

Squamous cell carcinoma in situ of the true vocal cords is initially treated surgically, and usually with micro-excision. However, if there is evidence of microinvasive squamous cell carcinoma in the specimen or if there are rapid or multiple recurrences, radiation therapy can be administered with an approach identical to that for T1 invasive lesions. Wang[24] reported a 92 percent 5-year local control and a 98 percent 5-year disease-free survival. The results in voice quality are good.

T1 invasive vocal cord lesions are limited to the cord with a normal mobility and are treated with surgery or radiation therapy with equally high effectiveness. Generally, the treatment of choice is radiation therapy while surgery is reserved for salvage of radiation failures. Bulky lesions in general and especially those located in the anterior commissure as well as extension of glottic lesions to the far anterior and posterior aspects of the larynx can decrease local control rates with radiation therapy. Radiation and surgery both result in an equivalent high local control rate but irradiated patients have superior voice quality.[62] The treatment field has a superior margin below the hyoid bone, an inferior margin at the bottom of the cricoid cartilage and an anterior margin with a 2 cm flash. The posterior margin is at the anterior 25 to 30 percent of the vertebral body for cobalt 60 teletherapy units; for 4 MV linear accelerators, anterior vocal cord lesions have a posterior portal margin at the anterior border of the vertebral body while posterior lesions have a portal margin similar to that noted for cobalt 60 teletherapy units. Because of the sparse lymphatics in the true vocal cords, the risk for nodal metastasis is quite low at 5 percent for T1 lesions[63] and thus the regional lymph nodes are not included in the treatment field. The field arrangements are via the right/left lateral opposed portals. Treatment should be administered on a cobalt 60 teletherapy unit (Figure 21–8) with 1.25 MV gamma rays or a linear accelerator with 4 MV x-rays, since higher energy units (Figure 21–9) may create a dosimetry problem, particularly for anterior commissure lesions with an underdosage to this region because of the greater maximum depth dose in this anatomically narrowed area.[64] If a linear accelerator with 6 MV x-rays is used, a bolus of appropriate thickness will be needed to compensate for this dosimetry concern; however, this will be associated with an increased acute skin reaction. A

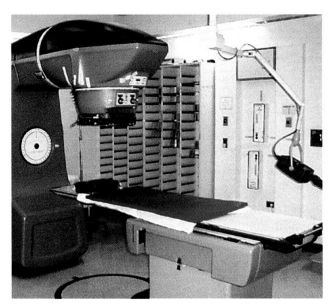

Figure 21–8. Cobalt 60 teletherapy unit administers 1.25 MV gamma rays.

larynx compensator would be used to improve the dose homogeneity. The dose per fraction would be 200 cGy or higher as lower fraction sizes have been associated with higher local recurrence rates.[65,66] The total dosage would be 6,600 cGy. Radiation therapy local control rates for T1 lesions have been reported at 93 percent, 91 percent and 93 percent (Figure 21–10A to C).[24,67,68]

Surgery for T1 lesions is with a vertical hemi-laryngectomy with the removal of the involved vocal cord, the ipsilateral false cord and the adjacent thyroid cartilage. Local control rates have been reported at 78 percent[69] and 87 percent.[70] This procedure is most frequently used for salvage of radiation therapy failures.

T2 glottic lesions involve the transglottic extension of tumor to the supraglottis and/or subglottis with or without impaired vocal cord mobility. In general, the risk of lymph node metastasis is rather low at 8 percent.[63] This is a heterogeneous group. C.C. Wang has advocated dividing this stage into a T2a with normal vocal cord mobility and T2b with impaired mobility. Primary radiation therapy results are quite good with T2a but suboptimal for T2b lesions which appear to behave more like T3 lesions.

For T2a lesions, radiation therapy is generally the treatment of choice. With disease that is primarily on the vocal cord with low volume extension onto the

adjacent supraglottis or subglottis, one would consider designing a generous treatment volume similar to a T1 glottis that would encompass 2 cm around all of the tumor. Generally, we would not include the regional lymph nodes in the treatment volume; however, with extensive moderate to high volume involvement of the adjacent supraglottis or sublottis, we would consider treatment of adjacent lymph nodes based on the extent of the disease. One should note that if there is such an extensive amount of bulk and volume in the adjacent supraglottic or subglottic subsites with respect to the true vocal cord involvement, one may need to reconsider whether this lesion may indeed be a primary site in these other structures rather than the true vocal cord, and thus be treated as such. This would include regional nodal irradiation. Field arrangements are via right/left lateral opposed portals. Substantial lesions involving these adjacent subsites that are rich in lymphatics will require that the regional lymph nodes be treated as well. For small volume, less bulky lesions, conventional fractionation radiation therapy can be considered at 200 cGy per fraction to a total dosage of

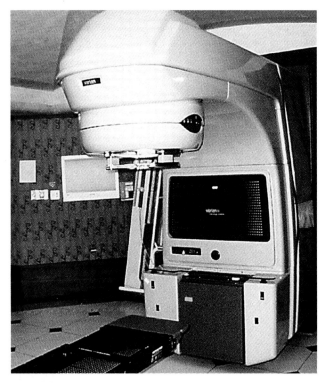

Figure 21–9. Linear accelerator with dual energy x-rays and multiple electron energy capabilities. Dynamic multi-leaf collimation allows for its use in IMRT cases.

7,000 cGy. However, for more extensive lesions, we would use accelerated fractionation with a delayed concomitant boost to a dosage of 7,000 cGy. Local control rates with radiation therapy have been reported at 86 percent.[71] Primary surgery is usually a vertical hemilaryngectomy and has 3-year survival rates in the low 80 percent range.[70] In men, surgery can be considered for lesions that involve one entire vocal cord and up to one-third of the opposite cord; however for women, one vocal cord and only a few millimeters of the opposite cord may be resected without causing airway compromise. For subglottic extension, the maximum extent allowable for a ver-

tical hemilaryngectomy is 9 mm anteriorly and 5 mm posteriorly in order to preserve the functional integrity of the cricoid cartilage. The postoperative voice quality is inferior to that of post-radiation therapy and the patient will have a persistent hoarseness. Therefore, surgery is usually reserved for salvage of radiation failures. However, if the lesion extends to involve the epiglottis, false cord, or both arytenoids, a total laryngectomy is needed if surgery is used. In such cases, we would consider initially treating the patient with a larynx preservation approach using chemotherapy and radiation therapy and saving surgery for salvage.

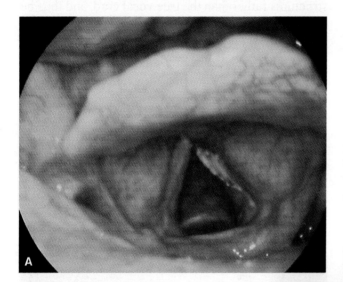

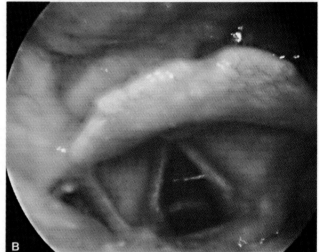

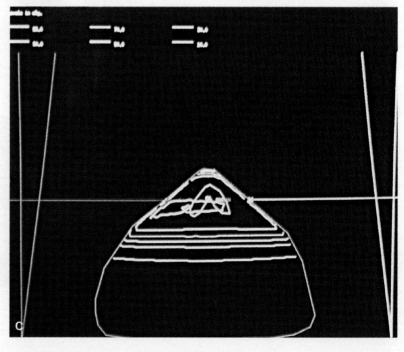

Figure 21–10.   Patient with a T1aN0 squamous cell carcinoma of the right true vocal cord before (*A*) and several months after (*B*) full course external beam radiation therapy showing a complete clinical response. Treatment plan with the use of wedges to create a more homogenous dose distribution (*C*).

For T2b lesions, primary radiation therapy can be considered particularly for small, non-bulky lesions. Local control rates of radiation alone are in the range of 60 to 70 percent. Wang reported a local control rate of 63 percent.[71] Large, bulky masses may be approached with surgery if a vertical hemi-laryngectomy can be performed. However, if a total laryngectomy is required, it would be reasonable to consider the laryngeal preservation approach with chemotherapy and radiation therapy, reserving surgery for salvage.

T3 lesions have a fixed vocal cord while T4 lesions involve extension into the thyroid cartilage, thyroid gland, and soft tissues of the neck and esophagus. The risk of lymph node metastasis is 15 percent for T3 lesions and 20 to 30 percent for T4 lesions.[63] The initial therapeutic approach should be with larynx preservation as surgical therapy would require a total laryngectomy and this can be reserved for salvage. Data from the Veterans Affairs Laryngeal Cancer Study Group[72] evaluating stage III and IV larynx cancers in 1991 is based on using neoadjuvant cisplatin and 5-FU chemotherapy for 2 to 3 cycles and then conventional fractionation radiation therapy to a total dosage of 7,000 cGy for partial or complete responders. They reported a 68 percent 2-year survival rate which was equivalent to that of the total laryngectomy-postoperative radiation therapy arm. However, there was a 64 percent larynx preservation in the chemotherapy-radiation therapy arm. At Memorial Sloan-Kettering Cancer Center, we have usually employed cisplatin chemotherapy on days 1 and 22 concurrent with radiation therapy using accelerated fractionation with a delayed concomitant boost to a total dosage of 7,000 cGy to the primary site and lymphadenopathy.[61a] When elective lymph node irradiation is administered, we would deliver 5,000 to 5,400 cGy.

Subglottic Larynx

Primary subglottic larynx cancers account for only 4 to 6 percent of all larynx cancers. Most lesions involving the subglottic region represent transglottic extension of glottic malignancies.

It is uncommon for primary subglottic cancers to present at an early stage as they are asymptomatic until quite advanced. The risk of lymph node metastasis is 20 to 30 percent with bilateral involvement being common.

T1 lesions are those that are confined to the subglottis and T2 lesions involve the vocal cord with normal or impaired mobility. In view of the low incidence of such early lesions, there is not much meaningful therapeutic data available. It would be reasonable to consider low volume, low bulk disease for treatment with radiation therapy alone, saving surgery for salvage. Conventional fractionation radiation therapy 5-year survival results have been reported to be 36 to 40 percent.[26,69]

T3 lesions involve vocal cord fixation, and T4 lesions invade the thyroid/cricoid cartilages, the thyroid gland, soft tissue of the neck, the trachea, or the esophagus. These advanced stages are associated with symptoms such as hoarseness and dyspnea. Surgical therapy would require a total laryngectomy and paratracheal lymph node dissection. Shaha and Shah[73] reported a 70 percent 5-year control rate while Vermund noted only a 42 percent rate.[74] Postoperative radiation therapy would be administered. Consideration of the laryngeal preservation approach with chemotherapy and radiation therapy is reasonable. However, it is important to note that the Veteran Affairs Laryngeal Study Group data did not have any primary subglottic lesions.

At Memorial Sloan-Kettering Cancer Center, we would consider using cisplatin chemotherapy on days 1 and 22 concurrent with radiation therapy using accelerated fractionation with a delayed concomitant boost to a total dosage of 7,000 cGy to the primary site and lymphadenopathy, using three-dimensional conformal or intensity-modulated radiation therapy treatment planning techniques;[61a] 5,000 to 5,400 cGy would be administered for elective nodal irradiation.

Nasal Area

Nasal Vestibule

This rare tumor has a distinct clinical behavior that is different from the nasal cavity. The area is lined by skin and malignancies of the region are squamous cell carcinoma or basal cell carcinoma. The incidence of lymph node metastasis is low at < 10 percent. However, nodal metastasis is a poor prognostic sign.

T1 and T2 lesions can be effectively treated with either surgery or radiation therapy with local control rates of over 90 percent.[75] If surgery is used, a relatively large amount of the external nose is resected with a resultant significant cosmetic defect. Therefore, primary treatment with radiation therapy is preferred. Radiation therapy can be administered with external beam radiation (6,000 to 7,000 cGy/30/35 fractions), brachytherapy alone (low dose rate IR 192 6,500 to 7,500 cGy in 6 to 7 days), or a combination of these two modalities (external beam radiation therapy 5,000 cGy/5 weeks and Ir 192 2,000 cGy). Some data suggest that brachytherapy alone provides superior results compared with external beam radiation therapy alone but is equivalent to the results obtained with surgery.[76]

T3 and T4 lesions may involve the cartilage of bone and there is controversy regarding its treatment. Some have reported good control with radiation therapy alone that is comparable to surgery. McCollough and colleagues[75] reported local control rates of 60 to 70 percent using external beam radiation therapy and brachytherapy. However, others lean toward surgery and postoperative radiation therapy when there is bone invasion. McCollough and colleagues[75] have reported that local control correlated better with tumor volume than with whether or not there was bone or cartilage involvement.

Nasal Cavity

The nasal cavity is composed anatomically of an antrum and the olfactory region which is associated with the cribriform plate of the ethmoid bone. This region has sparse lymphatics and therefore lymph node metastasis is uncommon. Tumors are primarily squamous cell carcinomas but also can be minor salivary gland malignancies or esthesioneuroblastomas among other less frequent histopathologies. The extent of the disease needs to be accurately determined and thus requires a thorough radiographic evaluation with a CT and/or MRI scan. In some cases, a lateral rhinotomy may be required to determine the extent of the disease. Lesions in the superior portion are more biologi-

cally aggressive than those located in the anterior and inferior areas.

Early lesions in the anterior-inferior aspect of the nasal cavity can be treated either with surgery or radiation therapy with equally excellent cure rates. However, even small lesions of the anterior nasal septum and turbinates may have early invasion of the adjacent bone and cartilage, which will significantly impact the therapeutic decision. Selected small, early lesions may be treated with primary radiation therapy consisting of external beam radiation therapy alone, brachytherapy alone, or a combination of these two modalities.[77] Logue and colleagues.[78] report local control rates of 93 percent for T1 and 83 percent for T2 lesions treated with radiation therapy alone. Ang and colleagues.[77] reviewed control rates for stage I and II lesions treated with radiation therapy alone at M.D. Anderson Cancer Center and noted a 94 percent control with external beam radiation and 100 percent with brachytherapy alone. Because it may be difficult to accurately ascertain the extent of disease unless a lateral rhinotomy is performed, there is often a preference to approach these lesions with surgery and, if indicated, postoperative radiation therapy. Negative surgical margins noted on the pathology report do not assure success. Spiro and colleagues[79] reviewed the records of 27 patients at Memorial Sloan-Kettering Cancer Center with squamous cell carcinoma of the nasal cavity who were treated solely with surgery. They noted only a 43 percent 5-year determinant cure rate. The most common site of failure was in the nasal cavity—despite negative margins.

Early lesions located in the posterosuperior region of the nasal cavity tend to be high-grade malignancies. These biologically more aggressive lesions are generally treated with surgical resection. Despite pathology reports showing negative margins, these lesions have a high risk for local recurrence and thus postoperative radiation therapy is generally employed. Local failure rates following radical surgery alone have ranged from 10 to 40 percent despite negative margins.

Advanced disease is approached with surgery and postoperative external beam radiation therapy within 6 weeks from the procedure. Conventional fractionation is used to deliver up to 6,300 cGy for high-risk cases if at all possible. Lesions that are marginally resectable or are unresectable can be considered for neoadjuvant radiation therapy to a dosage of 4,500 to 5,400 cGy with or without chemotherapy to try and shrink the tumor and make it more operable. We would approach clearly unresectable lesions with cisplatin chemotherapy on days 1 and 22 concurrent with radiation therapy using accelerated fractionation and a delayed concomitant boost to a dosage 7,000 cGy to the primary site using three-dimensional treatment planning.

Paranasal Sinuses

Maxillary Antrum

Radical en bloc resection of the tumor is the initial treatment of choice if possible. Contraindications include extension of disease to the nasopharynx, base of skull, pterygoid fossa and distant metastases.

T1 lesions are limited to the antral mucosa with no erosion or destruction of bone. A partial maxillectomy, usually through a lateral rhinotomy, is performed, removing the tumor in an en bloc fashion. Postoperative radiation therapy is indicated except for early, locally confined, well-differentiated squamous cell carcinomas where surgery alone is sufficient.

T2 lesions involve bone erosion or destruction, except for the posterior antral wall, and include extension into the hard palate and/or the middle nasal meatus. These are treated with a total maxillectomy and en bloc resection of tumor usually through a Weber-Ferguson approach. Surgery alone is sufficient for early, locally confined well-differentiated squamous cell carcinomas. Otherwise, postoperative radiation therapy is indicated, as the ability to achieve good clear surgical margins is most difficult. Treatment would be administered within 6 weeks after the procedure using conventional fractionation to a total dosage of 6,300 cGy using three-dimensional conformal treatment planning.

T3 lesions are extensive and involve the bone of the posterior wall of the maxillary sinus, subcutaneous tissues, skin of the cheek, floor or medial wall of the orbit, the infratemporal fossa, the pterygoid plates and the ethmoid sinuses. If these can be approached surgically, a total maxillectomy with an en bloc resection of all involved structures is performed. Postoperative radiation therapy is adminis-

tered in a fashion similar to that described above. A combined modality approach would provide better local control than either treatment alone.

T4 lesions represent massive disease and involve invasion of the orbital contents beyond the floor or medial wall, including the orbital apex, cribriform plate, base of skull, nasopharynx, sphenoid and frontal sinuses. Occasionally these may be resectable through the use of a craniofacial approach. Postoperative radiation therapy would be indicated in the fashion described above.

For resectable lesions, the indications for postoperative radiation therapy include: (1) T3 and T4 disease, (2) positive or close margins, (3) perineural/vascular invasion and (4) the surgeon's concerns regarding adequacy of resection (eg, tumor spillage, piecemeal resection, margins status irrespective of the pathology report).

There are no prospective trials comparing preoperative versus postoperative radiation therapy for paranasal sinus tumors. Retrospective studies show no clear advantage of one approach over the other.

5-year survival rates are in the 25 to 30 percent range with single treatment modalities.[80] A combined modality approach using surgery and postoperative radiation therapy produces somewhat improved results with local control rates of 50 to 60 percent and 5-year survival rates of 40 to 50 percent.[81]

At Memorial Sloan-Kettering Cancer Center, we prefer postoperative radiation therapy using three-dimensional conformal treatment planning based on a heavily weighted AP portal and right/left lateral opposed portals (Figure 21–11). We are investigating the use of intensity modulated radiation therapy in selected cases. The treatment volume would include the total nasal cavity, complete ethmoid sinuses, partial or subtotal frontal sinuses, sphenoid sinus, nasopharynx, hard palate, the ipsilateral maxillary antrum and the medial aspect of the contralateral maxillary antrum. The incidence of lymph node metastasis is relatively low at 15 to 20 percent and therefore elective nodal irradiation is not performed. Postoperatively, conventional fractionation is used delivering 180 cGy per fraction to a total dosage of 6,300 cGy if possible. Because of the close proximity of vital structures such as the brain stem, orbits, optic nerves, optic chiasm and spinal cord, special

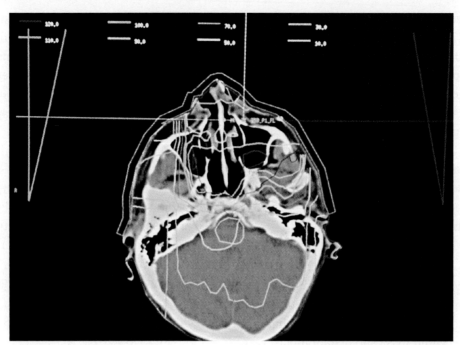

Figure 21–11. Computer-generated three-dimensional conformal treatment plan for a maxillary antrum tumor using two lateral portals with wedges and an anterior portal.

attention must be paid to evaluating the dose given to these areas and this may modify the total dosage administered.

In selective cases, neoadjuvant radiation therapy with or without chemotherapy can be considered for initially unresectable or only marginally resectable lesions. Conventional fractionation at 180 cGy per fraction to a total dosage of 4,500 to 5,400 cGy is administered to try and cause tumor shrinkage and thus possibly improve resectability.

Advanced unresectable disease can be considered for treatment with chemotherapy and radiation therapy. Complex three-dimensional conformal treatment planning is used to produce fields described above. At Memorial Sloan-Kettering Cancer Center, we would administer cisplatin chemotherapy on days 1 and 22 concurrent with radiation therapy using accelerated fractionation with a delayed concomitant boost to a dosage of 7,000 cGy. The use of neutrons has been reported with 30 percent 3-year survival rates.[82]

Ethmoid Sinus

Lesions of the ethmoid sinuses tend to be of high grade and are associated with a significant risk for local recurrences despite negative margins. The generally preferred approach is with surgery and postoperative radiation therapy. Early lesions in the anterior ethmoid sinus can often be excised surgically. For involvement of the middle and/or posterior ethmoid sinuses and for extensive disease, craniofacial resection and sometimes orbital exenteration may be necessary. Postoperative radiation therapy with three-dimensional conformal or even intensity modulated treatment planning should be considered, in that clear margins may be difficult to achieve in this region and the surgical technique may be suboptimal, thus placing the patient at high risk for local recurrence. Radiation therapy would be initiated within 6 weeks following surgery using conventional fractionation to doses upward of 6,300 cGy. The dose to the adjacent vital structures would need to be carefully evaluated and this may modulate the total dosage possible.

Advanced lesions that are unresectable would be considered for treatment with cisplatin chemotherapy on days 1 and 22 concurrent with radiation therapy using accelerated fractionation with a delayed concomitant boost to a dosage of 7,000 cGy using three-dimensional conformal or even intensity modulated treatment planning. The dosage to the orbits, optic nerves, optic chiasms and brain will need to be evaluated closely. Because of the anatomic location of the visual structures, blindness may be a necessary complication if tumoricidal doses of radiation are to be administered. This will need to be discussed at length with the patient before proceeding.

Sphenoid Sinus

Early lesions with disease confined to the sphenoid sinus can be approached surgically through either a sub-labial or lateral rhinotomy approach. A cutting burr is then used to achieve a good exposure, which will allow dissection of the tumor. Disease extending into the surrounding anatomy sometimes can be resected using an infratemporal approach and a craniotomy. In both circumstances, postoperative radiation therapy within 6 weeks following the procedure will be necessary.

Primary radiation therapy with three-dimensional conformal or even intensity modulated treatment planning is a major treatment modality in these regions. Small to moderate volume lesions can be effectively irradiated. Large lesions, particularly those that are unresectable, may be approached with chemotherapy and altered fractionation. However, great care must be taken when deciding on the dose to be administered to the surrounding vital structures; this may modulate the total dosage possible.

Salivary Gland

Parotid Gland

Surgery is the treatment of choice for both primary and locally recurrent salivary gland tumors. Lumpectomy, enucleation or an excisional biopsy should not be performed because the recurrence rate is high even for benign lesions. The size and location of the mass would determine the extent of surgical resection with the goal of an adequate en bloc procedure.[83]

T1 and T2 lesions with a low-grade malignancy are approached with a superficial parotidectomy if the anatomic location and extent of tumor will permit. Otherwise, a total parotidectomy with preservation of the facial nerve is performed. For high-grade lesions, a total parotidectomy with preservation of the facial nerve, unless it is involved and a neck dissection for a clinically involved neck, is performed.

T3 lesions all undergo total parotidectomy and a neck dissection for a clinically involved neck.

T4 lesions are extensive and require a total parotidectomy with resection of adjacent soft tissue and/or bone as necessary in order to achieve free surgical margins.

For unresectable primary or recurrent lesions, the use of neutrons is indicated. Results from the randomized multi-institutional study conducted by the RTOG (United States) and the MRC (England) revealed a 10-year local control rate of 56 percent with neutrons compared to only 17 percent with photons.[84]

Postoperative radiation therapy is an important part of treatment and is indicated as follows:[85,86] (1) resectable primary T4 and recurrent tumors, (2) high grade lesions, (3) positive or close margins, (4) perineural/vascular invasion, (5) concern of the surgeon over the margins irrespective of the pathology report and (6) locoregional lymph node metastasis.

Postoperative radiation therapy improves locoregional control substantially. Spiro and colleagues[87] reported on 264 patients with parotid malignancies who were treated primarily with surgery (only 12 received postoperative radiation therapy). The recurrence rates were: stage I, 7 percent; stage II, 21 percent; stage III, 58 percent. Harrison and colleagues[86] reported on patients with postoperative radiation therapy for major salivary gland malignancies with 5-year actuarial local control rates as follows: T1, 100 percent; T2, 83 percent; T3, 80 percent; T4, 43 percent. If the patient had no neck node involvement, there was an 83 percent local control versus those with nodal metastasis who had a 58 percent control rate. Fu and colleagues.[88] reviewed 35 patients with minor and major salivary gland carcinomas with known microscopic disease at or close to the surgical margins following curative surgery at the University of California, San Francisco. Those who did not undergo postoperative radiation therapy had a 54 percent (7/13) recurrence rate while the irradiated patients only had a 14 percent (3/22) rate.

At Memorial Sloan-Kettering Cancer Center, we would use CT simulation and three-dimensional conformal treatment planning. The primary area usually is approached using a lateral oblique wedge pair. If the lymph nodes are to be treated, ipsilateral AP/PA opposed portals off the spinal cord are employed. 6 MV x-rays are administered, and if the treatment is postoperative, 180 cGy per fraction is given to a total dosage at 6,300 cGy to the primary area and high-risk lymph node levels. 5,000 to 5,400 cGy is administered for elective nodal irradiation when indicated. If the treatment is for unresectable primary or recurrent lesions that are not being treated with neutrons, we would administer concurrent cisplatin chemotherapy with radiation therapy using accelerated fractionation with a delayed concomitant boost to a total dosage of 7,000 cGy.

If the histopathology is adenoid cystic carcinoma, the radiation portal will include the cranial nerve pathways to the base of skull, as tumors of this type have a high incidence of neurotropism and thus the potential for tracking of disease intracranially must be addressed.

Thyroid

Differentiated Thyroid Cancers

The two primary types of differentiated thyroid cancers are papillary and follicular. Several variants exist and include a follicular variant of papillary carcinoma, a tall cell variant of papillary carcinoma and a Hürthle cell carcinoma which is a variant of follicular carcinoma. The latter two subtypes are more ominous lesions.

Primary surgery is the initial treatment approach. The surgical therapeutic decisions are based on prognostic variables. At Memorial Sloan-Kettering Cancer Center, those patients who are felt to be at high risk are assessed based on "GAMES," for example: (1) Grade: high, (2) Age: > 45 years, (3) Metastasis: positive, (4) Extracapsular extension: positive, (5) Size > 4 cm.[89] The patients at low risk do well irrespective of the extent of surgery. The surgical goal is to remove all gross disease that is clinically detectable. The different operations represent the variations in the volume of the thyroid gland that is resected and include partial thyroidectomy and total thyroidectomy. Partial thyroidectomy encompasses the following procedures: (1) lumpectomy, (2) lobectomy, (3) isthmectomy, (4) lobectomy and isthmectomy, and (5) near-

total thyroidectomy. Shah and colleagues.[90] reviewed the Memorial Sloan-Kettering Cancer Center experience of 931 previously untreated patients in a matched pair analysis to evaluate the extent of surgical resection necessary for differentiated thyroid cancer clinically confined to one lobe. They noted that a large (> 4 cm) primary tumor size and presence of extra-thyroidal extension were associated with a poor prognosis. However, multifocal lesions were not associated with an adverse prognosis. The presence of microscopic disease in the contralateral thyroid lobe was found to have very few clinical consequences with respect to overall survival. In this review, 73 patients ≥ 45 years of age who had undergone a lobectomy for a thyroid cancer confined to one lobe were stratified for significant prognostic factors and matched with 73 other similar patients who had undergone a total thyroidectomy. The 20-year survival rate was roughly equivalent at around 80 percent for both arms. It was concluded that patients at low risk[89] undergoing lobectomy were likely to do as well as those who underwent a total thyroidectomy. A lobectomy with isthmectomy is felt to be the minimal surgical procedure that could be considered in a patient with a solitary thyroid nodule. However, if a patient is felt to need postoperative RAI, then a total thyroidectomy should be performed.

The issue of regional lymph nodes needs to be addressed surgically as well. Papillary thyroid cancers are at high risk for cervical node metastasis while follicular thyroid cancers are at a relatively low risk for this process. The surgical approach is one of conservatism. For papillary carcinomas with an N0 neck, one can consider a central compartment clean-out versus monitoring the patient. If the primary lesion is greater than 2 cm and/or there is extra-thyroidal extension, one can consider a central compartment resection—removing the highest risk lymph nodes. For follicular carcinomas with an N0 neck, monitoring the patient can be justified. However if the patient has palpable neck nodes, central compartment and neck dissections involving levels II through V are warranted. If gross lymphadenopathy is present in the superior mediastinal lymph nodes, dissection at that level is necessary as well.

Postoperative radioactive iodine (I–131) should be considered but is not required for all cases. To be therapeutic, the I–131 must be well concentrated in any residual normal or malignant thyroid cell. Uptake varies by histology: papillary and follicular: 60 to 90 percent; Hürthle cell: 36 percent. Also, locally-invasive thyroid cancer in contrast to lymph node recurrence many times will not concentrate RAI.[91] This emits a beta particle with a 2 mm zone of effective irradiation. Its use is to: (1) ablate residual normal thyroid tissue, and (2) treat the residual cancer.

I–131 indications include: (1) high postoperative risk for microscopic disease in the thyroid bed and regional lymph nodes (eg, extensive extracapsular extension in the adjacent tissues), (2) postoperative macroscopic residual disease (thyroid bed and lymph nodes), (3) gross disease: recurrent primary or nodal disease or unresectable primary or nodal disease (4) persistently elevated thyroglobulin without clinical evidence of disease, and (5) metastatic disease: lung, bone (iodine uptake is only approximately 50 percent overall and is rather low for bone metastasis).

Contraindications for I–131 include: (1) low-risk papillary carcinoma: age < 40 to 45 years, size < 1.0 to 1.5 cm, no clinical evidence for nodal metastasis, and (2) low-risk follicular carcinoma: age < 40 to 45 years, size < 2.5 cm, no clinical evidence for nodal metastasis, minimal invasiveness.

The use of postoperative external beam radiation therapy is controversial but there is data to support its use.[92,93] However, there are no phase III, controlled randomized studies available. Thyroid carcinomas are not any more or less curable than squamous cell carcinomas of equivalent volume when treated by external beam radiation.[9] With adequate doses (5,000 to 5,400 cGy for elective nodal irradiation/ 6,300 cGy or more for high-risk disease) and contemporary complex treatment planning using CT-PET fusion (Figures 21–12A and B) and intensity-modulated radiation therapy (IMRT), the efficacy of external beam radiation therapy may become more substantiated.

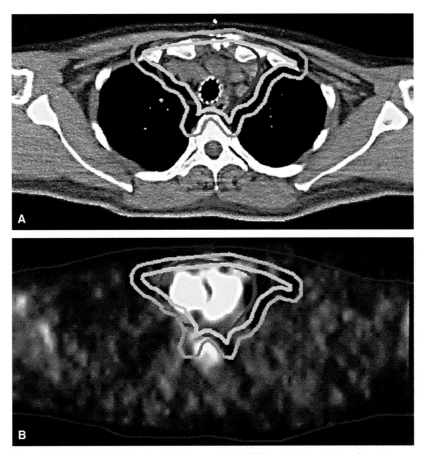

Figure 21–12. CT-PET fusion technique using IMRT treatment planning for a locoregionally recurrent differentiated thyroid cancer. (*A, B*).

Possible indications for external beam radiation therapy[92,93] include: (1) postoperative high risk for microscopic disease in the thyroid bed and regional lymph nodes (eg, locally-advanced disease with extracapsular tumor extension),[91,94–97] (2) postoperative macroscopic residual disease (thyroid bed and nodes,[91,94,96,97] (3) gross disease: recurrent primary or nodal disease or unresectable primary or nodal disease,[96–98] (4) poor uptake of RAI with above high-risk features,[96] (5) persistent/recurrent disease after RAI therapy,[99] (6) persistently elevated thyroglobulin with no evidence of disease, and (7) metastatic disease: brain metastasis, painful bone metastasis.[98]

At Memorial Sloan-Kettering Cancer Center, our initial treatment volume includes the thyroid bed, cervical-retropharyngeal nodes (up to the mastoid tip-mandibular rim level), supraclavical nodes and superior mediastinal nodes (down to around the level just above the carina or at the angle of Louis. IMRT is employed as a recent evaluation of our experience comparing two-dimensional, three-dimensional and IMRT plans (Figures 21–13A to D) revealed a more homogenous dose distribution and improved sparing of adjacent vital organs, particularly the spinal cord, with IMRT.[100] Elective nodal irradiation is taken to a dosage of 5,000 to 5,400 cGy. High-risk primary and nodal sites are administered 6,300 cGy and may go up to 7,000 cGy for gross disease as a cone down which is based on our current research using PET scan fusion with the CT simulation scans for treatment planning. Often we consider planned postoperative I–131 and then external beam radiation therapy 6 weeks later for selected high-risk patients.

Medullary Thyroid Carcinoma

The initial treatment of choice is surgery. Because of the high incidence of multicentric disease, a total thyroidectomy is performed.

Postoperative RAI is not administered since medullary carcinoma does not take up iodine.

Postoperative considerations for external beam radiation therapy are the same as noted above for the differentiated thyroid carcinomas. In particular, this would include persistently elevated calcitonin with no clinical evidence of disease.[96]

Anaplastic Thyroid Carcinoma

This aggressive thyroid cancer is generally quite large and is associated with extra-thyroidal extension and is usually not respectable. For the occasional case where the lesion is small and intra-thyroidal, resection may be considered. Early development of distant metastasis and an aggressive course make this a most deadly disease.

Iodine is not concentrated by these malignant cells and thus I–131 is not used for treatment. Altered fractionation external beam radiation therapy usually is administered for primary therapy along with consideration of concurrent radiosensitizing chemotherapy such as low-dose Adriamycin.[101–103] Kim and Leeper[102] from Memorial Sloan-Kettering Cancer Center administered 160 cGy bid, 3 consecutive days per week, to a total dosage of 5,760 cGy in 40 days with concurrent pretreatment low-dose Adriamycin (10 mg/m^2) given once weekly 1.5 hours prior to irradiation. They achieved a 68 percent 2-year local control rate. The best subgroup was in those patients who were able to undergo some surgery that involved more than just biopsy.

CLINCIAL ANALYSIS OF THE HEAD AND NECK CANCER PATIENT

Primary Tumor

Site

There exist significant differences in radio-responsiveness for some head and neck cancer subsites. Adjacent anatomic regions separated by 1 to 2 centimeters may show markedly contrasting responses to treatment. There is no known scientific or clinical explanation for this observation.

Squamous cell carcinoma of the oral tongue is much less frequently controlled by external beam radiation therapy than are comparable lesions in the base of tongue. Similarly, squamous cell carcinoma of the tonsillar pillar has a much poorer control rate with external beam radiation therapy than do lesions in the tonsillar fossa.

Size

The probability of control of a primary head and neck tumor by radiation therapy depends in part on the

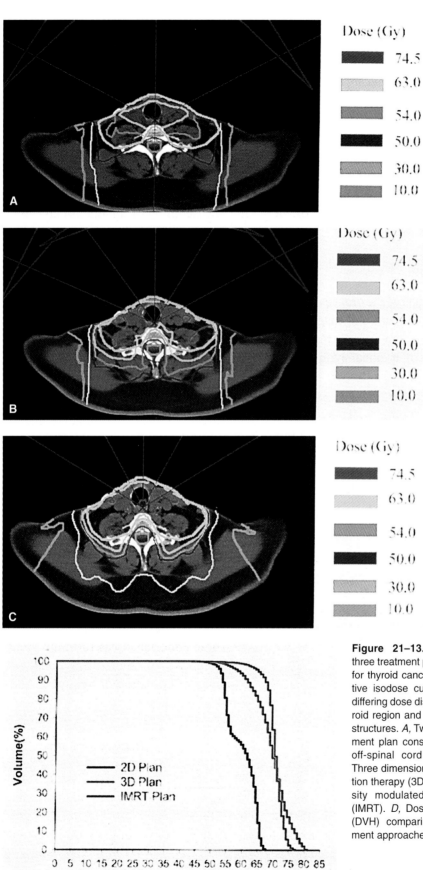

Figure 21–13. Comparisons of three treatment planning approaches for thyroid cancer. Note the respective isodose curves that show the differing dose distributions to the thyroid region and to the adjacent vital structures. *A,* Two dimensional treatment plan consisting of AP/PA and off-spinal cord oblique fields. *B,* Three dimensional conformed radiation therapy (3DCRT) plan. *C,* Intensity modulated radiation therapy (IMRT). *D,* Dose-volume histogram (DVH) comparing the three treatment approaches.

number of tumor clonogens present which is related to the volume of the mass. Since radiation cell kill is exponential, each fraction of radiation administered results in a set proportion of cells that are killed which is in contradistinction to an absolute number of cells killed. The larger the tumor mass, the greater the total cumulative dosage of radiation that is required to achieve control. The total dosage administered is based on the initial tumor volume and should not be decreased based on the rate of regression of the lesion, as this can result in an under-dosage of the tumor with an increased risk of recurrence.

Depth

For squamous cell carcinomas of the oral cavity, particularly in the floor of mouth and oral tongue subsites, the depth of invasion of the primary tumor has been correlated with risk of regional lymph node metastasis.[104] A general primary tumor invasion depth versus lymph node correlation risk is as follows: (1) mucosa (< 2 mm depth): < 10 percent risk; (2) mucosa and superficial submucosal (2 to 8 mm depth): > 25 percent risk; and (3) deep submucosa (> 8 mm depth): > 40 percent risk.

Topography

The initial clinical appearance of the primary head and neck tumor can be described as exophytic or endophytic-infiltrative. This characterization has very important therapeutic implications. Exophytic tumors are associated with a decreased rate of lymph node metastasis and respond better to surgical and radiation therapy intervention. Conversely, the infiltrative lesions which are often poorly differentiated have an increased rate of lymph node metastasis and do not respond as well to radiation therapy.

Histopathology

There is no major difference in the potential radiocurability rates among the varying epithelial malignancies of comparable size of the head and neck. Thus similarly staged T1 and T2 lesions of squamous cell carcinomas, basal cell carcinomas, mucoepidermoid carcinomas, and adenocarcinomas have an equal potential for cure by radiation.[105] The only exception would be lymphoepitheliomas, which have a better locoregional control and survival when treated with radiation therapy as compared to classic squamous cell carcinomas.

The differentiation of the tumor does not affect the radiocurability rate, however, it may affect its clinical response with well-differentiated lesions regressing more slowly than their poorly-differentiated counterparts. Less-differentiated tumors do have an increased risk for regional nodal and distant metastasis. Among the diverse group of squamous cell carcinomas of the head and neck, there exists a significant variation between them in radiosensitivity.

Fractionation

The conventional fractionation schedule using 180 to 200 cGy per fraction, one fraction per day, 5 days per week for $6^1/_2$ to $7^1/_2$ weeks to a total dosage of 6,500 to 7,000 cGy has been the standard regimen of curative head and neck radiation therapy for many years. Significant clinical data on acute and late treatment effects and complications and tumor control rates have been based on this approach. However, it should be acknowledged that this standard evolved empirically and while its familiarity and known relative efficacy can provide a modicum of comfort to the clinician, its wholesale use for all primary head and neck cancers must come under critical scrutiny. Based on both laboratory and clinical research, it is now apparent that the conventional fractionation scheme may not be the best approach for all tumors, particularly those in the head neck region.

Three important areas form the foundation of the evolving use of altered fractionation: (1) tissue response, (2) duration of treatment, and (3) fraction size and number.

Tissue Response

There are two categories of tissue responses to radiation: early or acutely responding tissues (including most tumors), and late responding tissues.

Acutely responding tissues are rather active in ongoing cellular proliferation. Since most tumors (except perhaps prostate cancer and melanoma) share this characteristic, they are felt to respond similarly to radiation. Normal tissues that are considered to be acutely responding include skin, mucous membranes and gastrointestinal epithelium. These highly proliferative tissues have a high α/β ratio that is estimated to be in the range of 800 to 2,000 cGy. Their cell survival curve characteristics are different from late responding tissues. These tissues are most affected by the overall treatment duration rather than by the size or number of fractions used. Thus, by decreasing the treatment duration and keeping the total dose constant, there is a greater risk for increasing the severity of the acute side effects from radiation such as mucositis, dysphagia and odynophagia.

Late responding tissues have a low proliferative rate. These include the spinal cord, brain, bone and cartilage. Their α/β ratio is low and is estimated to be in the range of 200 to 500 cGy. The corresponding cell survival curves are distinctly different from those representing acutely reacting tissues. These tissues are most affected by the size and number of fractions rather than by treatment duration. Thus by decreasing the dose per fraction, there would be a sparing of these late responding tissues and vice versa. Because there is minimal or no regeneration of these cells during therapy, a reduction in overall treatment time should not increase the severity of late effects, provided there is sufficient inter-fraction time to complete repair of sublethal damage.

The fundamental difference between acutely responding tissues and late responding tissues is due to differences in the repair capabilities. Early responding tissues have a larger shoulder in the cell survival curve corresponding to an increased repair ability, versus the situation for late responding tissues, which is just the opposite.

Duration of Treatment

Local tumor control, as well as acutely responding normal tissue reactions, is strongly dependent on the overall treatment duration rather than on the size or number of fractions.

Human cancers have a relatively slow growth rate with tumor doubling times of around 2 months. However, when squamous carcinoma of the head and neck is exposed to radiation therapy, the tumor clonogens within the lesion develop an accelerated repopulation approximately 3 to 5 weeks after commencement of treatment.[5] It has been estimated that the tumor clonogen doubling time (T_{pot}) is about 4 days.[106] This burst of tumor cell proliferation can overwhelm the ongoing treatment effects of radiation and ultimately lead to local failure. Of further clinical importance is the fact that this accelerated growth of tumor clonogens during treatment is not detectable on examination. Thus even with significant progressive regression of the primary tumor mass, local failure could still ultimately result. Therefore, with this accelerated regrowth of tumor clonogens occurring about 4 weeks into a course of curative well-fractionated radiation therapy, it is essential to complete treatment in as short a time as possible consistent with an acceptable level of acute toxicity. By shortening the treatment duration, the period of time over which this accelerated growth could occur is minimized as are the effects of such proliferation, which may result in an increased chance for local control.

Fraction Size and Number

Late responding normal tissues are most sensitive to fractionation issues rather than the overall treatment duration, which is in contradistinction to acutely responding tissues and tumors. By decreasing the size of the dose per fraction, the result is the sparing of the late responding tissues. Likewise, if the dose per fraction is significantly increased, the total dosage will need to be correspondingly reduced to maintain similar late effects in the late responding tissues. However, while there may possibly be some effect on the acutely responding tissues and tumors, it would not have nearly the magnitude of reaction as it would have on late responding tissues.

Altered Fractionation

The evolution of altered fractionation schemes came in response to the realization of the points presented above. The goal has been to improve the therapeutic ratio by maximizing the tumor-killing effect and minimizing acute and late toxicities while using readily available low LET radiation. The mechanism has involved alterations in the overall treatment duration and/or fractionation. The differential points between the various altered fractionation schemes have revolved around a delicate balance between local tumor control and acute and late effects through modification of the fractionation scheme and/or treatment duration.

There are two major categories of altered fractionation schemes: hyperfractionation and accelerated fractionation. They share basic radiobiologic principles yet have their own particular features. It should be noted that there are many hybrid schemes that have developed which combine features of these two categories. It is felt that for the very rapidly proliferating tumors, accelerated fractionation is the strategy of choice; with more slowly proliferating tumors, hyperfractionation may yield better results.[106] However a recent randomized RTOG study 90–03[107] has provided important information in the use of low LET radiation alone for squamous cell carcinoma of the head and neck (sites: oral cavity, oropharynx, hypopharynx, supraglottic larynx; stage: III or IV/stage II for base of tongue and hypopharynx/no distant metastasis) using altered fractionation. This study compared treatment using conventional fractionation (arm 1), hyperfractionation (arm 2), accelerated hyperfractionation with split (arm 3), and accelerated fractionation with concomitant boost (arm 4). The preliminary results show a significantly better 2-year locoregional control (p = 0.035) and disease-free survival rates (p = 0.042) with accelerated fractionation with a concomitant boost compared with those treated with standard fractionation. Patients treated with hyperfractionation also had a trend toward better 2-year locoregional control (p = 0.07) and disease-free survival (p = 0.07) rates versus those treated with standard fractionation. Patients treated with accelerated fractionation with a split had an outcome similar to patients treated with standard fractionation. Based on these results, accelerated fractionation with a concomitant boost will serve as the control arm for future RTOG phase III trials evaluating locally-advanced head and neck cancer treatments.

Hyperfractionation

An improvement in the therapeutic ratio is obtained primarily through redistribution of tumor cells into more radiosensitive phases due to multiple fractions, and differential sparing of late responding normal tissues due to a decrease in size of the dose per fraction. It is theorized that this fraction scheme may be best for more slowly proliferating tumor cells.[106] This is characterized by: (1) decreased size of the dose per fraction (115 to 120 cGy) compared with conventional fractionation (180 to 200 cGy), (2) bid to tid fractionation, (3) increased total dosage (7,440 to 8,160 cGy) over conventional fractionation (7,000 cGy), and (4) similar overall treatment duration to conventional fractionation.

An EORTC randomized trial (22791) evaluated patients with oropharyngeal cancer (stage T2 to T3 N0 to N1 with node size < 3 cm) who were treated with either conventional fractionation or hyperfractionation for head and neck cancer. There was a 19 percent improvement in 5-year local control with hyperfractionation and a borderline significant advantage in 5-year survival.

Accelerated Fractionation

The major therapeutic gain is based on the concept that tumor clonogens undergo an accelerated rate of proliferation 3 to 5 weeks after initiation of conventional fractionation radiotherapy. By shortening the overall treatment duration, the opportunity for accelerated repopulation would be reduced.[106,108] It is felt that this treatment scheme would be best for very rapidly growing tumors. This is characterized by: (1) dose per fraction size similar to conventional fractionation, (2) bid-tid fractionation, (3) similar total dosage to conventional fractionation, and (4) shortened overall treatment duration compared to conventional fractionation.

Fractionation Equivalence

Cell survival curves which plot radiation dose against cellular survival can be described mathematically by the linear-quadratic equation:

$$\mathrm{Log_e}S = \alpha\,D + \beta\,D^2$$

S represents cell survival and D is dose; α is the linear (first order dose-dependent) component of cell killing that is caused by nonreparable radiation damage; β is the quadratic (second order dose dependent) component of cell killing that is associated with an accumulation of reparable radiation damage.

The ratio α/β represents the dosage at which the two components of cell killing are equal. For acutely responding tissues and radio-responsive tumors (eg, lymphomas), this ratio is estimated to be between 800 to 2,000 cGy. For late responding tissues and poorly responsive tumors (eg, melanoma), this ratio is estimated to be between 200 to 500 cGy. Clinically the α/β ratio gives the fractionation sensitivity of tissues.

Based on the linear-quadratic equation, a formula has been developed that allows for the calculation of a biologically equivalent dose:

$$BED = D_x = D_r \frac{\alpha/\beta + dr}{\alpha/\beta + dx}$$

D_x is the new total dosage (with different fractionation schedule); D_r is the known reference total dosage; dr is the known reference fraction size; Dx is the new fractionation dose.

SPECIAL THERAPEUTIC CONSIDERATIONS

Squamous Cell Carcinoma Metastatic to Cervical Nodes from an Unknown Head and Neck Primary

Patients with a primary squamous cell carcinoma of the upper aerodigestive tract frequently will present with cervical lymphadenopathy generally in the mid- to upper neck levels. After thorough evaluation, approximately 90 percent of these cases will have the primary site detected. The remaining 10 percent of patients are presumed to have a primary malignancy of the upper aerodigestive region; however, the actual site cannot be diagnosed despite thorough clinical examination, radiographic studies and examination under anesthesia, including directed biopsies of suspicious areas. Currently, the utility of PET scans in identifying occult primary sites is being investigated in such patients.[114,115]

The majority of these patients will have involvement of the mid- to upper jugular nodes, which is associated with five possible mucosal sites which may harbor the primary tumor source: (1) nasopharynx, (2) tonsillar region, (3) base of tongue, (4) pyriform sinus, and (5) supraglottic larynx. Shah[116] reviewed the Memorial Sloan-Kettering Cancer Center experience with 1,081 previously untreated patients with squamous cell carcinomas of the upper aerodigestive tract who underwent an initial elective or therapeutic classic neck dissection. He correlated the primary sites with their propensity to metastasize to particular lymph node levels: (1) oral cavity: levels I to III, (2) oropharynx: levels II to IV, (3) hypopharynx: levels II to IV, and (4) larynx: levels II to IV.

Two special circumstances merit notation:

1. Submandibular lymphadenopathy (level I): involvement of the submandibular nodes suggests a probable primary oral cavity lesion. While head and neck nodal metastases generally occur in an orderly, predictable pattern, Byers and colleagues[28] found that 15 percent of patients with a primary oral tongue cancer exhibited skip metastasis. The first echelon of nodes (levels I/II) were bypassed in favor of more inferior regions such as level IV. Spiro and colleagues. from Memorial Sloan-Kettering Cancer Center reported an overall incidence of 5 percent of such skip metastases in oral cavity cancers.[27]

2. Level II and upper level V lymphadenopathy (particularly bulky): involvement of these regions is particularly suggestive of a primary nasopharyngeal carcinoma. The suspicion is further increased under the following situations: (a) the histopathology is a lymphoepithelioma or a very poorly-differentiated carcinoma, (b) the patient is of Chinese ethnicity, (c) the nasopharyngeal carcinoma serology is positive (Epstein-Barr virus titre), (d) there is retropharyngeal node involvement. Davidson and colleagues[117] analyzed 1,123 previously untreated Memorial Sloan-Kettering Cancer Center patients with squamous cell carcinoma of the upper aerodigestive tract who underwent 1,277 classic radical neck dissections. Only 3 percent were found to have involvement of posterior triangle (level V) nodes. The sub-sites with the highest percentage of level V adenopathy were the oropharynx (6%) and the hypopharynx (7%).

The therapeutic approach to this group of patients is based on the nodal stage and the high-risk mucosal sites. Patients who clinically present with a mid- to high neck node that is felt to be ≤ 3 cm in diameter can undergo a fine-needle aspiration biopsy to establish the diagnosis of cancer, rather than an excisional or incisional biopsy which may contaminate the wound. If the search for a primary is negative, then the patient can undergo a neck dissection. Should the pathologic diagnosis show a clear, uncomplicated N1 node, then the patient may be considered only for monitoring as the risk of regional neck recurrence for this select group is roughly 10 percent with primary surgery or radiation therapy. Combined therapy is not necessary.[18] The risk of subsequently developing a primary site manifestation ranges from 6 to 50 percent in the world's literature.[118–122] In a review from M.D. Anderson Hospital Cancer Center, 20 percent of the patients who were managed initially with surgery alone for the cervical lymphadenopathy subsequently developed a primary lesion.[121] However, if the pathology evaluation reveals stages N2a, N2b or N2c or extracapsular extension, then the patient should undergo postoperative radiotherapy. Also, if the patient had undergone an incisional or excisional biopsy of the node prior to the cervical through supraclavicular dissection, postoperative radiotherapy is also recommended. Radiation for these high-risk groups would be administered to the neck nodes as well as to the suspected possible primary mucosal sites. To only irradiate the high-risk neck would compromise the ability to subsequently irradiate the mucosal primary site should the disease subsequently become clinically apparent. Our practice at Memorial Sloan-Kettering Cancer Center is to include the nasopharynx in the treatment volume only if enough risk factors merit its treatment.

The nodal areas would be treated with conventional fractionation to 5,400 cGy at 180 cGy per fraction with a subsequent boost to high-risk nodal regions to a total dosage of 6,300 cGy. The possible primary mucosal sites would be similarly irradiated to a total dosage of 5,400 cGy. The low neck nodes would be taken to 5,000 cGy to maximum dose point (Dmax) at 200 cGy per fraction. It is an important clinical point that these patients must be closely evaluated for the development of tumoritis, a mucosal inflammation that may occur around 2,000 cGy and which may indicate the location of the primary lesion.[24]

Numerous retrospective studies suggest that elective mucosal irradiation is effective in decreasing the risk of subsequent local failure.[121] However, there have been no randomized trials to confirm this observation.

Primary Cervical Nodal Metastasis Treated with Radiation Therapy Alone

Primary radiation therapy can be considered for definitive treatment of cervical nodal metastasis in highly selected patients: (1) node size: ≤ 2 cm (solitary metastatic node < 3cm has been associated with a 92 percent control with radiation therapy alone),[18] (2) primary site: nasopharynx, oropharynx and larynx (these primary sites are associated with excellent nodal control with radiation therapy; in particular, even multiple large and bulky nodal metastases from nasopharyngeal carcinoma often can be controlled with radiation therapy alone), (3) mobility: movable or tethered lymph nodes have an 84 percent control rate with radiation therapy (fixed lymph nodes have a poor control rate of 55 percent with radiation alone),[123] (4) number of lymph nodes involved: solitary (multiple nodes that are < 3cm had only a 65 to 75 percent control rate with radiation therapy).[18]

The dosage required for sterilization is dependent on the lymph node size: (1) ≤ 1 cm: 6,500 cGy, (2) ≥ 1 cm to 2 cm: 7,000 cGy, (3) > 2 cm to 3 cm: 7,500 cGy.

At Memorial Sloan-Kettering Cancer Center, we generally would consider a solitary, mobile, ≤ 2 cm lymph node for treatment with radiation therapy alone if the primary lesion is to be treated with full course radiation therapy. The entire cervical and supraclavicular nodes would be treated electively to 5,000 to 5,400 cGy followed by a boost to the area of the palpable adenopathy to a total cumulative dosage as noted above depending on the size of the lymph node. Following treatment, if there is no palpable or radiographic evidence of residual disease, the patient can be considered for close follow-up rather than undergo a neck dissection.

Elective Nodal Irradiation

A clinically negative neck on examination may still contain micro-metastatic deposits in the lymph nodes—so-called occult metastasis. The risk for this depends on several factors:

1. the anatomic site of the primary head and neck lesion will influence the risk for occult nodal metastasis. Lesions in the nasopharynx, base of tongue, supraglottic larynx and pyriform sinus are at particularly high risk (≥ 30%) for subclinical nodal disease irrespective of the T stage.[124]
2. advanced T3 and T4 head and neck primary lesions carry a high risk for subclinical neck disease.

The use of elective nodal irradiation to eradicate occult disease is very effective.[124] The doses administered are in the range of 5,000 to 5,400 cGy using conventional fractionation. Initial therapy of the clinically negative neck will decrease the incidence of relapse in the neck and may ultimately decrease the risk of distant metastasis.[125]

The treatment volume would include the entire cervical and supraclavicular nodes.

Locoregional Recurrence After Primary Radiation Therapy

Patients who suffer a local and/or regional recurrence after having undergone a full course of radiation therapy with curative doses present a therapeutic challenge. These patients must be carefully evaluated to determine the extent of the locoregional disease as well as whether distant metastasis has also developed. It is important to analyze whether the lesion is truly a recurrence versus a persistence of the initial disease at the primary site or a complication from radiation therapy. Head and neck cancer patients must be followed closely after treatment as this may allow the detection of locoregional recurrences perhaps at an early, localized state. Limited disease would be more amenable for consideration of possible aggressive therapeutic intervention. The vast majority of recurrences occur within the first 2 to 3 years following completion of treatment.

Generally, surgery would be the treatment of choice for locoregional recurrences after radiation therapy. However, the lesion would need to be surgically resectable and the patient able to tolerate the procedure, undergo the necessary postoperative rehabilitation and tolerate any functional deficit.

Additional radiation therapy can sometimes be considered for this group of patients who are not surgical candidates. However, it is important that any potential patient be chosen carefully and judiciously. Carte blanche use of re-irradiation is associated with a high major complication risk (eg, necrosis) and poor therapeutic results. The recurrent malignant cells very likely would be in a rather hypoxic environment due to the effects of the initial radiation therapy (such as scarring) and this could decrease the efficacy of treatment. These patients would need to be evaluated with respect to the following criteria: (1) general condition of the patient, (2) time interval since completion of initial radiation therapy, (3) radiation dosage initially administered to the tumor and adjacent vital organs, (4) tolerance of radiation therapy and development of any complications, (5) anatomic location, extent of recurrence and adjacent vital organs, (6) condition of previously irradiated tissues, (7) symptoms related to recurrence, and (8) life expectancy.

Contraindications to re-irradiation include: (1) poor general condition, (2) recurrence less than 6 months from initial radiation therapy, (3) prior ultra-high radiation doses, (4) massive tumor recurrence equivalent to advanced T3 and T4 lesions, and (5) location of recurrence in or around the central nervous system.

If re-irradiation is recommended, high doses in the range of 6,000 to 6,500 cGy will need to be administered.[126–128] Both conventional fractionation and hyperfractionation have been reported in the literature. Moderate doses of 4,500 cGy or less will mostly likely not be effective and may not even provide substantive palliation. The use of concurrent chemotherapy, external beam radiation therapy alone, external beam radiation therapy with brachytherapy, or brachytherapy alone will need to be assessed based on the characteristics of the recurrence. Due caution must be exercised when re-irradiating the alveolar ridge and floor of mouth regions as these two anatomic areas have a relatively low radiation tolerance and would be at high risk for development of soft-tissue necrosis and/or osteoradionecrosis. Good treatment planning and careful radiation technique is required. At Memorial Sloan-Kettering Cancer Center we have been using IMRT for these cases. The margins around the tumor sites should be relatively tight at 1.5 to no more than 2 cm. The brain and spinal cord must not be re-irradiated.

Re-irradiation has been used primarily for localized recurrent nasopharyngeal carcinomas with a stage equivalence of a T1 and T2 lesion.[129,130] Limited volume external beam radiation therapy and a fractionated intracavitary boost with brachytherapy can potentially provide good local control. Re-irradiation also has been used on a limited basis for recurrences of squamous cell carcinoma in the glottic larynx.[131] While surgery is the preferred treatment, there are some patients who have refused surgery and were treated with re-irradiation with good results. More recently, clinical research in re-irradiation has expanded to include tumors in other head and neck sites with promising preliminary results. These studies have shown a good palliation of symptoms and even some long-term survivors with a 20 percent 2-year survival and 15 to 17 percent 5-year survival rate.[126,127] The results appear better than with the use of chemotherapy alone.

The incidence of late toxicity is greater than that usually experienced after a first course of radiation therapy; however, several studies have suggested that the adverse events are still acceptable.[17,132] In the well-selected patient, re-irradiation may be feasible and efficacious. However, the patient must be aware of the high risks involved and be willing to accept the possibility of complications.

Chemoradiotherapy

The use of primary chemotherapy with radiation therapy in the treatment of selected head and neck cancers is an exciting and rapidly evolving area of oncologic research with substantial information available from preliminary clinical results. The goals of combining these two treatment modalities are: (1) increase locoregional control (chemotherapy acts as a radiosensitizer and has direct cytotoxic effects on the tumor in addition to the effect of the radiation), (2) decreases distant metastasis (chemotherapeutic eradication of systemic microscopic disease), and (3) improves survival (increased locoregional control and decreased metastases).

There are 4 categories of sequencing chemotherapy and radiation therapy: (1) induction (neoadjuvant) chemotherapy, (2) concurrent chemotherapy and radiation therapy, (3) alternating chemotherapy and radiation therapy, and (4) adjuvant chemotherapy.

In induction (neoadjuvant) chemotherapy, several cycles of drugs are given prior to initiation of radiation therapy. The chemotherapy frequently results in high response rates. However, there is no significant improvement in survival or in locoregional control.[133] It has been suggested that induction chemotherapy may cause a tumor to initially regress but also may result in the surviving tumor clonogens undergoing accelerated growth just as the radiation phase begins. This would result in a much more difficult group of tumor cells with which the radiation therapy must deal.

An important area of research in this category with significant clinical impact is the use of chemotherapy with radiation for organ preservation. The Department of Veterans Affairs Laryngeal Cancer Study Group[72] data and the EORTC[54] study of locally-advanced hypopharyngeal cancer are two major controlled, randomized studies supporting the use of neoadjuvant chemotherapy and radiation therapy as primary treatment for larynx preservation with total laryngectomy reserved for salvage.

Patients who have a complete response to induction chemotherapy have a better prognosis than those who have no response.[134] Those who responded well to chemotherapy also tended to respond to radiation therapy. While severe and sometimes fatal toxicities occurred with chemotherapy, the morbidity of subsequent radiotherapy was not increased.[135]

Concurrent chemotherapy and radiation therapy requires that the drugs be given on days 1 and 22 with the radiation therapy. This approach has resulted in increased locoregional control, relapse-free survival and overall survival rates. There is a significantly increased acute radiation reaction, however. When more than one chemotherapeutic agent is used, the acute side effects are even worse. It is theorized that cells which have acquired resistance to radiation may be sensitive to it in the presence of chemotherapeutic drugs.[136]

Forastiere and colleagues[61a] reported on Intergroup Trial R91-11—a randomized study that evaluated larynx preservation in the treatment of 510 patients with stage III and IV squamous cell carcinoma of the larynx. The 3 arms in this study included sequential cisplatin + 5FU and radiation therapy (control arm), concomitant cisplatin chemotherapy administered on day 1, 22, and 43 with radiation therapy, and radiation therapy alone to a dosage of 7000cGy (200cGy/fraction). 12% of patients in the concomitant arm versus 26% of patients in the sequential chemotherapy-radiation arm (control) and 31% of patients in the radiation treatment alone arm required a laryngectomy at 2 years. The time to laryngectomy was significantly improved with concomitant chemotherapy-radiation therapy. It was concluded that the standard for laynx preservation should be concomitant cisplatin chemotherapy and radiation therapy.

Alternating chemotherapy and radiotherapy sequences the drugs during the break in a split-course radiation therapy schedule. The data suggests that prolongation of the radiation therapy duration to twice the normal time of conventional fractionation does not adversely affect local control rates when aggressive cell cycle-specific drugs are given during the break intervals. Results show an improved complete response and median overall survival comparable to radiation therapy alone.[136]

Adjuvant chemotherapy regimens schedule the initiation of drugs after completion of the radiation therapy phase. This has shown no improvement in survival but there has been a decreased incidence in distant metastasis.

Overall, various studies suggest that the concomitant chemo-radiotherapy approach very well may result in superior locoregional control rates compared with the other sequencing schemes.[61a] Preliminary data also suggests that it may convey a survival advantage. However, the final answer is still forthcoming. The use of altered rather than conventional fractionation schemes in conjunction with chemotherapy also may enhance results and this approach is currently under active investigation. At this time, our practice at Memorial Sloan-Kettering Cancer Center is to use chemotherapy for larynx preservation in advanced T3 and T4 head and neck cancers where surgery would require a total laryngectomy. For patients with advanced nasopharyn-

geal carcinoma, cisplatin (administered on days 1 and 22) concurrent with accelerated fractionation with a concomitant boost to 7,000 cGy using intensity-modulated radiation therapy, and subsequent adjuvant cisplatin + 5-FU for 3 cycles is our standard approach. Patients with unresectable paranasal sinus tumors also are treated similarly. Active clinical investigation continues with the use of concurrent chemotherapy and radiation therapy for advanced unresectable lesions or in cases where the massive lesion may be technically resectable but associated with major functional sequelae.

TREATMENT PLANNING

Simulation

The first step in setting-up the radiation fields involves simulation. This can be accomplished using either a fluoroscopically (two-dimensional treatment planning) or a CT (three-dimensional treatment planning) assisted approach. The tumor site, lymph nodes and adjacent tissues at risk are determined by the radiation oncologist at consultation.

The patient will initially have any visible, palpable and technically reachable lesion in the oral cavity or oropharynx marked by the implantation of gold seeds at strategic points along its perimeter for later radiographic visualization on the simulation films. Topical anesthetic is sprayed over the tumor region and a seed injector is employed to interstitially implant one or several gold seeds to an approximate depth of 1 cm. Direct pressure using sponges is applied to any areas of bleeding until controlled.

The patient is then placed in a supine position on the simulation table and properly adjusted using an appropriate head holder to position the head at the desired angle. A shoulder pull board is used to maximally bring the shoulders into a caudad position with the patient gripping straps that wrap around the soles of the feet. All incisional scars, strategic anatomic locations and masses are marked or outlined with appropriate material for later radiographic visualization.

A bite-block made of thermoplastic material with a lead wire placed in the longitudinal direction for later radiographic visualization is designed for those patients in whom it is desired to separate the hard palate region from the mandible to spare it from radiation. If dental guards are necessary, they should be placed into position. A thermoplastic face mask is then fabricated to firmly hold the head in proper position (Figure 21–14A).

If the patient will require conventional simulation with two-dimensional treatment planning (Figure 21–14B), then the process can begin using fluoroscopy to determine the portal margins under the direction of the radiation oncologist. Simulation films are special radiographs with cross-hair wires marking the isocenter, delineator wires at the perimeter noting the portal margins, and graticule marks 2 cm apart creating a grid of dots approximately 3 mm in diameter which serve as reference markers. The films are evaluated and any changes are then made and repeat simulation films obtained until the setup has been approved by the radiation oncologist. Block positions are drawn on the films with a wax pencil and they will subsequently be fabricated into cerrobend blocks which will be mounted on the treatment unit head during therapy. Every effort is made to avoid irradiation of the larynx for oral cavity and oropharyngeal cancers by placing the inferior margin of the lateral portals above the thyroid notch. Therefore the larynx will be placed in the treatment volume of the adjacent low anterior neck portal and is completely blocked. This will also serve a dual role as a spinal cord junction block. However, if the larynx is in the treatment volume as is the case for lesions in the hypopharynx or larynx, a larynx compensator is created to make the dose more homogenous at that level, resulting in a decrease in the excessive dose to the true vocal cords. At the completion of the conventional simulation, Polaroid pictures are taken to show the patient setup. Tattoos are then strategically and discretely placed on the patient to delineate the setup reference points. The patient will then be scheduled to undergo beam films and initiation of treatment in the near future.

Patients with lesions in the nasopharynx, paranasal sinus, parotid gland and thyroid gland will require CT simulation in preparation for either three-dimensional conformal treatment planning or intensity-modulated radiation therapy treatment planning (Figure 21–15). After the initial preparation has been performed as previously presented, the patient will be moved to the CT simulation suite and repositioned. If IV contrast is required, then this will be administered using an apparatus that delivers the contrast slowly and continuously. CT cuts of 3 mm are obtained of the head and neck regions. Upon completion of the procedure, the radiation oncolo-

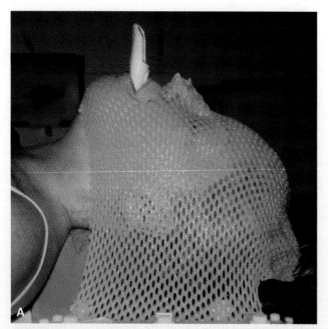 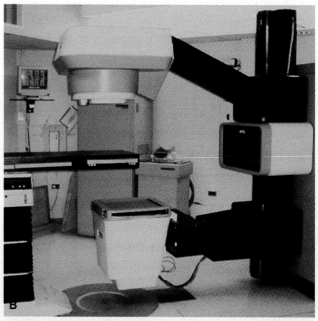

Figure 21–14. *A,* Patient undergoing a fluoroscopically-assisted simulation with a customized face mask and bite block in place. *B,* Fluoroscopically-assisted simulator which is used in conventional two-dimensional treatment planning techniques.

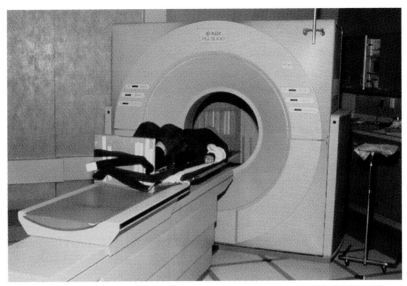

Figure 21–15. Computed tomography simulator which is used in 3DCRT and IMRT treatment planning.

gist determines the superior and inferior margins of the field on the CT images, which allows for the determination of the isocenter which is transferred to the patient by the use of tattoos for future setup reference points. The computerized data is then transferred to a treatment planning computer in the Division of Radiation Oncology Physics where contours of vital organs (eg, spinal cord, brain stem, optic nerves, optic chiasm, orbits) and the tumor region are digitized on the CT slices. At this time, the complex process of three-dimensional computerized treatment planning will begin.

Three-dimensional Conformal Treatment Planning

Using CT simulation computer data, beam placement in 3 dimensions using non-coplanar beam arrangements that conform to the target are developed. This approach replaces the conventional simulation and two dimensional treatment planning with a computer-based "virtual simulation." A beam's eye view (BEV) perspective is created and linked to the treatment unit via digitally reconstructed radiographs (DRR) that will correspond to the port films taken to verify the patient treatment position. Complicated three-dimensional dose calculations allow for accurate administration of radiation to the target regions based on the computer-generated isodose curves. Dose-volume histograms

(DVH) are available for analysis by the radiation oncologist to determine the three-dimensional dose distribution to both the tumor and vital structures.

Intensity-modulated Radiation Therapy

Intensity-modulated radiation therapy (IMRT) is an advanced form of three-dimensional conformal treatment planning which involves the use of the most sophisticated computer-generated treatment planning and clinical linear accelerators available. It is indicated in the treatment of lesions with complex anatomy that are adjacent to vital structures such as the spinal cord or brain stem. IMRT improves the therapeutic ratio by optimizing the dose to the tumor target and by decreasing both the dose given to and the volume of the surrounding normal tissues. This approach creates multiple nonuniform, non-coplanar beam profiles by means of wedges and physical compensators to modulate the intensity of the beam for each unique port. Many small beams with different intensities are thus created, resulting in a beam intensity that will vary across the treatment field. Conceptually, this involves using the inverse planning technique whereby the target and adjacent vital organ doses are first determined. Then, the process works backward to generate the appropriate delivery parameters that would result in the preset, ideal dose distributions.

Our preliminary research has indicated that in cases of nasopharyngeal carcinoma, there is improved target coverage and lower normal tissue dosage with IMRT compared to two- and three-dimensional treatment plans.[31] Similar results have been found for the use of IMRT in thyroid carcinoma.

Thus far, current usage of IMRT provides an improvement in the therapeutic ratio with respect to the dosage administered to adjacent vital organs which will decrease acute and late effects. Current research involves dose escalation studies.

The clinical application of IMRT requires a sophisticated linear accelerator with a computer-driven dynamic multi-leaf collimator capability. These treatment plans typically involve multiple portals and can run as high as 7 to 14 fields that would otherwise take a prohibitive amount of time to employ with the conventional cut block as well as the static multi-leaf collimator units.

Radiation Oncology Dose Nomenclature

Radiation dose exposure in air is measured in roentgens (R). However, it is the direct measurement of the absorbed radiation dose in tissue that is of importance in radiation oncology. To actually perform this measurement is difficult and impractical. Instead, the amount of ionization in air (roentgens) is measured and this value in conjunction with information on the energy used, the type of radiation, and the absorption coefficient of the absorbing material can be employed to compute the radiation absorbed dose (rad). One roentgen of exposure in air is approximately equal to 0.95 cGy absorbed dose in tissue.

In contemporary clinical radiation oncology, dose is expressed as the amount of energy absorbed per unit mass of absorbing material. In the past, this was termed the "rad (r)" which stood for radiation absorbed dose. One rad is equal to 100 ergs absorbed per gram. Over the past decade and a half, the rad has been replaced by the gray (Gy) or centigray (cGy): 100 rad = 100 cGy = 1.00 Gy.

Clinical Course of Radiation Therapy

The patient undergoing radiation therapy will need to be seen for routine status evaluation at least once a week. At that time, a pertinent interval history is obtained with special attention paid to the development of a sore mouth or throat, dysphagia, hoarseness, taste problems, xerostomia, skin symptomology, and even ear symtoms when the portal includes the external auditory canal and/or eustachian tube. A directed examination will evaluate the tumor status with measurements and an estimation of the mobility and texture when appropriate. Failure of head and neck cancers to achieve a complete response at or shortly after completion of radiation is associated with an increased risk of local failure. Therefore close monitoring and weekly documentation of the tumor is necessary. The patient should be checked for mucositis, oral *Candida* and dermal reactions. The general condition, weight status and complete blood count will need to be monitored.

An occasional patient will develop acute parotitis which can occur within the first 12 hours after initiation of irradiation to portals including the parotid gland. This is due to an acute inflammatory reaction within the parotid gland due to radiation. These patients will complain of parotid area swelling, localized pain and perhaps even a low-grade temperature. This is a self-limited problem that will usually resolve spontaneously after several hours. However, we generally prescribe a nonsteroidal anti-inflammatory drug and reassure the patient.

During the second week of treatment at around the 2,000 cGy dosage, the patient should be checked for development of tumoritis, a mucosal inflammation which indicates the true extent of tumor and thus may necessitate a modification of the portal.[24] If tumors do not show reasonable regression or if they actually progress during radiation therapy, immediate reevaluation by all of the physicians on the case is mandatory, as this may be an indication that surgery is necessary. However, we have seen an occasional patient in whom their lymphadenopathy had actually increased in size during treatment and while preparing to undergo surgery, it had regressed to its baseline dimensions. We elected to complete the initially planned radiation therapy and had very good results. These unusual situations may be related to a transitory inflammatory response in the lymph nodes from an undetermined cause.

Patients can develop progressive weight loss and dehydration by the fourth to fifth week of treatment.

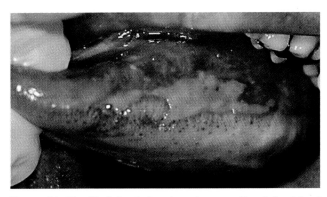

Figure 21–16. Radiation-induced acute mucositis of the lateral aspect of the oral tongue. Note the erythema and the more pale area of fibrinous exudate.

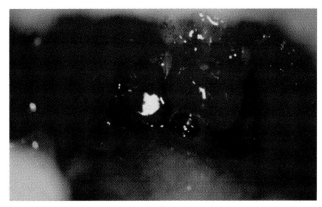

Figure 21–17. Radiation-induced acute brisk mucositis of the oropharynx.

This is particularly prominent in patients undergoing concurrent chemotherapy and radiation therapy. They initially may require intravenous hydration as outpatients but often will ultimately need to have a percutaneous endoscopic gastrostomy tube placed for more intensive daily hydration and caloric administration.

Patients will develop mucositis (Figures 21–16 and 17) which can become quite severe by the fourth to fifth week of treatment, particularly in patients who are receiving concurrent chemotherapy and radiation therapy. Acetaminophen with codeine either in tablet or liquid form can be palliative initially. However, not infrequently, we have needed to advance the medication to a long-acting morphine sulfate or fentanyl patch with immediate-release morphine sulfate for rescue.

A fair number of patients will develop an oral *Candida* infection (Figure 21–18). Some may be asymptomatic at presentation while others may complain of an acute development or exacerbation of their sore mouth or throat. Immediate initiation of antifungal medication will usually resolve the problem in short order.

Post-treatment Follow-up

The highest risk for locoregional recurrence after definitive treatment for head and neck cancer patients is generally within the first 2 to 3 years after therapy. It is therefore imperative that they be followed closely, routinely and diligently.

Immediately after radiation therapy, we may follow those patients with particularly severe mucositis and weight loss on a weekly basis until sufficient recovery has occurred—which may take 3 to 4 weeks. Otherwise, they are seen monthly, usually for 2 months, at which point most patients have had sufficient recovery from the significant acute radiation reaction. We then follow them every 1 to 2 months, often alternating with the other physicians on the case unless we are monitoring the response of a mass. If indicated, a baseline CT or MRI study of the head and neck can be obtained 2 to 3 months after radiation therapy and then routinely in perhaps 4 months. CT scans are particularly helpful in evaluating for nodal involvement and bone invasion while MRI scans are useful for soft-tissue and intracranial extension. Current research is investigating the use of PET scans for the post-therapy follow-up of head and neck cancers. It has been reported that this study is more accurate for detecting recurrence than MRI scans.[137]

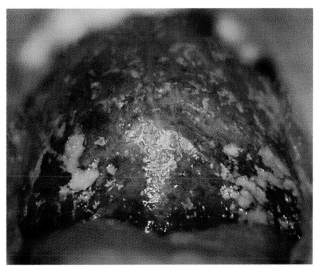

Figure 21–18. Oral candidiasis.

Long-term follow-up for endocrine complications requires appropriate laboratory monitoring as abnormalities can occur late.

Thyroid function tests including TSH are obtained every 6 months post-treatment for up to 5 years for all patients who received radiation to the thyroid gland area. Clinical hypothyroidism develops in approximately 5 percent of adults and a bit higher in children irradiated to the thyroid region. There is a 20 to 25 percent incidence of chemical hypothyroidism which increases to 66 percent in patients who have also undergone a hemithyroidectomy. If the TSH rises above a normal range, the patients are started on thyroid hormone replacement therapy irrespective of the T3 and T4 values, which very well may be within normal limits. The thyroid gland is a very radiosensitive organ and should be routinely monitored after radiation therapy. If the hypothalamic-pituitary axis has been irradiated as well, then a complete endocrine screening should also be similarly obtained.

Patients who receive radiation to the oral cavity or oropharyngeal areas should be seen routinely by the dental service for an indefinite time. The fluoride prophylaxis routine which was initiated prior to treatment should be continued. No gingival surgery or tooth extraction should occur without the dentist knowing the history of the prior radiation therapy volume and dosage as well as the potential risks for osteoradionecrosis subsequent to the planned dental surgery. During the follow-up evaluation, the radiation oncologist will need to pay special attention to eliciting history of mandibular or tooth pain. An examination should be carried out to look for any exposed bone in the oral cavity. These findings may suggest the development of osteoradionecrosis and necessitate a thorough work-up including detailed radiologic evaluation.

Some patients who received radiation to the cervical spine may develop Lhermitte's syndrome, a benign, transient myelopathy thought to be due to demyelination, that can appear from 1 to 3 months after radiation therapy and can last for up to 9 months or more with an average of 3 to 4 months. The syndrome is characterized by the development of a symmetrical instantaneous, shooting, electrical sensation radiating down the spine and extremities with neck flexion. There are no other associated neurologic problems. This is self-limited and requires no therapy. However, if these symptoms should develop for the first time 9 to 12 months after radiation therapy, one must be very concerned that this may be a harbinger for the development of radiation myelitis.

The patient should be evaluated for trismus, which may be due to either post-radiation fibrosis versus recurrence or progression of tumor. Routine daily range of motion exercises must be encouraged for the jaw, tongue, neck, and shoulders to minimize post-treatment functional deficits from fibrosis and scarring.

Occasionally, a patient who received high-dose radiation therapy to the head and neck, particularly with chemotherapy, may develop chronic dysphagia secondary to fibrosis. This will require an esophagoscopy to rule out tumor. If benign stricture is noted within the cervical or upper thoracic esophagus, then occasional dilatation procedures are indicated and can be most helpful.

Special Radiation Oncology Therapeutic Modalities

Brachytherapy

Brachytherapy (from the Greek term "brachio" which means short) is the subspecialty of radiation oncology which uses selected radioisotopes and specialized instruments to directly administer radiation to a tumor mass or bed. The radiation source is placed either adjacent to the surface of a tumor mass or bed or inside the mass itself. Depending on the technique employed, the treatment may involve a permanent implantation of a radioactive source (eg, permanent I^{125} seeds injected into a recurrent nasopharyngeal mass) or may involve temporary exposure after which it is removed (eg, intracavitary insertion of I^{125} seeds for a localized recurrent nasopharyngeal carcinoma, temporary interstitial catheter implantation for afterloading with Ir192 sources for a neck mass or tumor bed).

Brachytherapy radiation travels only a short distance to the desired target region. Its dose intensity has a rapid falloff with distance according to the

Table 21–4. TYPES OF HEAD AND NECK BRACHYTHERAPY	
Permanent	**Temporary**
LDR I125 implanted into a mass by free hand technique using an applicator (eg, recurrent nasopharyngeal lesion)	Interstitial implantation of catheters to the tumor bed or mass afterloading with Ir192 (eg, squamous cell carcinoma of the lip or base of tongue)
LDR I125 Vicryl™ suture placed into tumor bed (eg, resected neck mass with close or positive margins)	Intracavitary insertion of brachytherapy instruments afterloading with high activity I125/LDR or HDR Ir192 (eg, recurrent nasopharyngeal cancer)
	Intraoperative radiation therapy (IORT) using HAM applicator applied to the tumor bed using HDR Ir192

LDR = low dose rate; HDR = high dose rate; HAM = Harrison-Anderson-Mick applicator.

inverse square law ($I \propto 1/D^2$) which allows for a sharp decrease in the dosage in the surrounding normal tissue. The dose rate can be low and continuous (low dose rate = LDR with a rate of 40 to 200 cGy/hour) or high and administered in a hyperfractionated fashion (high dose rate = HDR with dose rate > 1,200 cGy/hour). The radiation dose is delivered to a relatively small, well-defined volume.

Radiobiologically, low dose rate brachytherapy treatment is a continuous low dose rate of radiation and is likened to fractionated radiation with an infinite number of small individual doses. This allows redistribution of the tumor cell within the cell cycle, resulting in a greater percentage of malignant cells in the more radiosensitive phases. However, this probably has little clinical consequence. This approach also allows time for reoxygenation of hypoxic cells during the treatment and thus results in an increase in their radiosensitivity. This effect varies tremendously between different tumor types. Repair is the major radiobiological factor in low dose rate brachytherapy. This favors late responding normal tissues relative to tumors. Repopulation occurs but unfortunately benefits tumors.

High dose rate treatments need to be well-fractionated (hypofractionation with only 1 to 3 fractions per week) as this approach is at a greater risk for complications with late responding tissues, particularly since the dose per fraction is usually rather high.

Brachytherapy may be used as the primary treatment or more commonly as a local boost in conjunction with external beam radiation therapy and perhaps surgery. It is usually employed with a curative intent but can be used for highly selected patients needing palliative care. The isotopes most commonly used in head and neck cancer treatments

are I125 and Ir192 (Tables 21–4 and 5). The implants can be planar (single plane) or volumetric (more than one parallel plane separated by 1 to 1.5 cm). Pretreatment planning with respect to any surgical or anatomic considerations as well as dosimetric concerns is critical.

Head and neck tumor sites commonly considered for possible brachytherapy include the lip, floor of mouth, oral tongue, base of tongue (Figure 21–19), buccal mucosa, tonsillar region, nasopharynx, skull base and neck nodes (Figure 21–20) (Table 21–6). The size and volume of the primary lesion, anatomic extent, topography, adjacent vital organs, any prior therapy, and the medical and psychologic condition of the patient must be critically evaluated when considering a case for possible brachytherapy intervention. In the oral tongue and floor of mouth regions, while T1 and T2 lesions can be treated with brachytherapy alone or with external beam radiation therapy with good therapeutic results, the risk of possible complications from treatment such as soft-tissue or bone necrosis must be weighed against consideration of a primary surgical approach with its low complication rate. In the case where the radioactive sources are in close proximity to the mandibular mucosa and bone, the risk of complications greatly increases and thus this would be a contraindication to brachytherapy. If an implant cannot adequately encompass the tumor region with margin or if the

TABLE 21–5. HEAD AND NECK BRACHYTHERAPY ISOTOPES			
Isotope	**Type of Radiation**	**KeV Energy**	**Half Life**
I125	X-rays	27–32	60 days
Ir192	Gamma rays	340	74 days

TABLE 21–6. COMMON HEAD AND NECK BRACHYTHERAPY PROCEDURES

Site	Stage	Procedures
Lip	T1, T2 (small)	Interstitial implant alone, EBRT + interstitial implant
Oral tongue	T1 (small)	Interstitial implant alone
	T1, T2, T3	EBRT + implant
Base of tongue	T1, T2, T3, T4	EBRT + implant
Floor of mouth	T1 (small)	Interstitial implant alone
	T1, T2	EBRT + interstitial implant
Buccal mucosa	T1, T2 (early)	Implant alone
	T2, T3	EBRT + interstitial implant
Base of tongue	T1, T2,	EBRT + interstitial implant
Nasopharynx	Recurrent T1, T2	EBRT + intracavitary insertion
Neck nodes	Adherent to carotid artery	Surgery with intraoperative planar implant of I125 Vicryl™ suture permanent seed implant or placement of afterloading catheters or IORT with HDR Ir192 (add EBRT with all of the above if never irradiated)

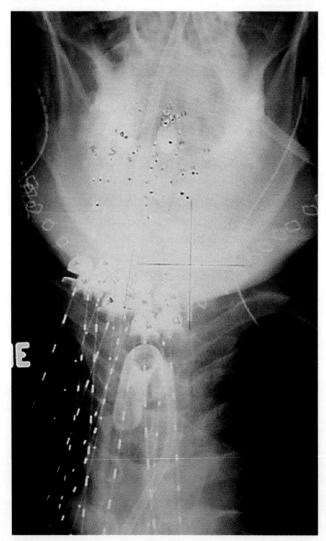

Figure 21–19.   Base of tongue implant.

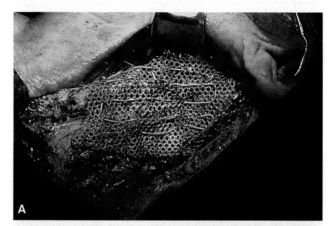

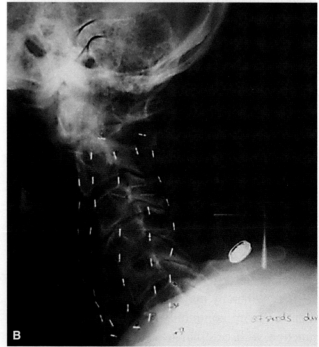

Figure 21–20.   Locally recurrent squamous cell carcinoma in the neck following prior external beam radiation therapy. The mass was resected but was fixed to underlying tissues. *A*, A permanent low dose rate I125 seed implant was performed. *B*, A lateral film shows the seed implant.

region is not technically approachable, then brachytherapy should not be performed.

Neutron Therapy

This densely ionizing high linear energy transfer particulate radiation has a limited but important role in clinical radiation oncology. Fast neutrons can be contrasted to photons in th following ways:

1. the biologic effectiveness is much less influenced by hypoxic environments.
2. lethal effects are less dependent on the cell cycle phase.
3. the ability of malignant cells to rcpair sublethal damage matters less.
4. is biologically more effective with a relative biologic effectiveness (RBE) of 2.6 or greater.

Clinically, fast neutrons lack skin sparing and therefore can cause more acute dermal reactions compared to photons. The overall severe late complication rate has been reported at 19 percent which is related to its increased RBE. Several major randomized studies evaluating the efficacy of fast neutrons versus photons in the treatment of head and neck cancer have shown similar local tumor control and overall survival rates.[139] However, there was a higher control of lymph node metastasis[138] and a poor survival rate with laryngeal carcinoma treated with neutrons.[138,140]

The specific indication for neutron therapy in clinical practice is with unresectable primary and recurrent salivary gland tumors. A major randomized multi-institutional study under the auspices of RTOG (United States) and the MRC (England) has shown a 10-year local control rate of 56 percent with neutrons and 17 percent with photons.[84]

REFERENCES

1. Selman J. The basic physics of radiation therapy. 2nd ed. Springfield (IL): Charles C. Thomas; 1976.
2. Fuks Z, Haimovitz-Friedman A, Kolesnick RN. The role of the sphingomyelin pathway and protein kinase C in radiation-induced cell kill. IMP Adv Oncol 1995;19–31.
3. Ang KK, Peters LJ, Weber RS, et al. Concomitant boost radiotherapy schedules in the treatment of carcinoma of the oropharynx and nasopharynx. Int J Radiat Oncol Biol Phys 1990;19:1339–45.
4. Phillips TL. Treatment: radiation therapy. In: Silverman S Jr, editor. Oral Cancer. 4th ed. Hamilton: BC Decker Inc. 1998:80–5.
5. Withers HR, Taylor JMG, Maciejewski B. The hazard of accelerated tumor clonogen repopulation during radiotherapy. Acta Oncologica 1988;27:131–46.
6. Bush RS. The significance of anemia in clinical therapy. Int J Radiat Oncol Biol Phys 1986;12:2047–50.
7. Bush RS, Jenkin RDT, Allt WEC, et al. Definitive evidence for hypoxic cells influencing cure in cancer therapy. Br J Cancer 1978;37(Suppl 3):302–306.
8. Strong EW. Preoperative radiation and neck dissection. Surg Clin North Am 1969;49:271.
9. Million RR, Cassisi NJ. Management of head and neck cancer: a multidisciplinary approach. 2nd ed. Philadelphia (PA): J. B. Lippincott; 1984.
10. Vikram B, Strong EW, Shah JP, Spiro RH. Failure at the primary site following multimodality treatment in advanced head and neck cancer. Head Neck Surg 1984;6:720–3.
11. Looser KG, Shah JP, Strong EW. The significance of "positive" margins in surgically resected epidermoid carcinomas. Head Neck Surg 1978;1:107–11.
12. Scholl P, Byers RM, Batsakis JG, et al. Microscopic cut through of cancer in the surgical treatment of squamous cell carcinoma of the tongue: prognostic and therapeutic implications. Am J Surg 1987;152:354–60.
13. Byrne M, Koppang HS, Lillieng R, et al. Malignancy grading of the deep invasive margins of oral squamous cell carcinomas has high prognostic value. J Pathol 1992;166:375–81.
14. Kramer S, Gelber RB, Snow JB, et al. Combined radiation therapy and surgery in the management of advanced head and neck cancer: Final report of study 73-03 of the Radiation Therapy Oncology Group. Head Neck Surg 1997;10:19.
15. Carter RL, Bliss JM, Soo K, O'Brien CJ. Radical neck dissection for squamous carcinomas: Particular findings and their clinical implications with particular reference to transcapsular spread. Int J Radiat Oncol Biol Phys 1987;13:825.
16. Olsen KD, Caruso M, Foote RL, et al. Primary head and neck cancer. Histopathologic predictors of recurrence after neck resection in patients with lymph node involvement. Arch Otolarngol Head Neck Surg 1994;120:1370–4.
17. Barkley HT Jr, Fletcher GH, Jesse RH, Lindberg RD. Management of cervical lymph node metastases in squamous cell carcinoma of the tonsillar fossa, base of tongue, supraglottic larynx and hypopharynx. Am J Surg 1972;124:462.
18. Mendenhall WM, Million RR, Cassisi NJ. Squamous cell carcinoma of the head and neck treated with radiation therapy: the role of neck dissection for clinically positive neck nodes. Int J Radiat Oncol Biol Phys 1986;12:733–40.
19. Zelefsky MJ, Raben A, Strong EW, et al. Long term results of postoperative radiotherapy for squamous cell cancers of the head and neck [abstract]. Proc Int Conf Head Neck Cancer 1996;289:131.
20. Vikram B. Importance of the time interval between surgery and postoperative radiation therapy in the combined man-

agement of head and neck cancer. Int J Radiat Oncol Biol Phys 1979;5:1837–40.

21. Schiff PB, Harrison LB, Strong EW, et al. Impact of the time interval between surgery and the postoperative radiation therapy on local regional control in advanced head and neck cancer. J Surg Oncol 1990;160:415–9.

22. Vikram B, Strong EW, Shah JP, Spiro RH. Failure in the neck following multimodality treatment for advanced head and neck cancer. Head Neck Surg 1984;6:724–9.

23. Peters LJ, Goepfert H, Ang KK, et al. Evaluation of the dose for postoperative radiation therapy of head and neck cancer: First report of the prospective randomized trial. Int J Radiat Oncol Biol Phys 1993;26:3.

24. Wang CC. Radiation therapy for head and neck neoplasms. 3rd ed. New York: Wiley-Liss; 1997.

25. Jorgensen K, Elbron O, Anderson AP. Carcinoma of the lip; a series of 869 cases. Acta Radiol 1973;12:177–90.

26. Lederman M. Cancer of the larynx. I. Natural history in relation to treatment. Br J Radiol 1971;44:569–78.

27. Spiro JD, Spiro RH, Shah JP, et al. Critical assessment of supraomohyoid neck dissection. Amer J Surg 1988;156:286–9.

28. Byers RM, Weber RS, Andrews T, et al. Frequency and therapeutic implications of "skip metastases" in the neck from squamous carcinoma of the oral tongue. Head Neck 1997;19:14–9.

29. Mazeron J, Grimard L, Raynal M, et al. Ir-192 curietherapy for T1 and T2 epidermoid carcinomas of the floor of mouth. Int J Radiat Oncol Biol Phys 1990;18:1299.

30. Fein DA, Mendenhall WM, Parson JT, et al. Carcinoma of the oral tongue: a comparison of results and complications of treatment with radiotherapy and/or surgery. Head Neck 1994;16:358–65.

31. Hunt M, Zelefsky M, Losso T, et al. Treatment planning and delivery of intensity modulated radiation therapy for primary nasopharynx cancer. ASTRO Abstract 1999.

31a. Wolden SL, Zelefsky MJ, Hunt MA, et al. Failure of a 3D conformal boost to improve radiotherapy for nasopharyngeal carcinoma. Int J Radiat Oncol Biol Phys 2001;49:1229–34.

32. Bedwinek JM, Perez CA, Keys DJ. Analysis of failures after definition irradiation for epidermoid carcinoma of the nasopharynx. Cancer 1980;45:2725–9.

33. Hoppe RT, Goffinet DR, Bagshaw MA. Carcinoma of the nasopharynx: eighteen years' experience with megavoltage radiation therapy. Cancer 1976;37:2605–12.

34. Mesic JB, Fletcher GM, Goepfert H. Megavoltage irradiation of epithelial tumors of the nasopharynx. Int J Radiat Oncol Biol Phys 1981;7(4):447–53.

35. Walsh CS, McIntyre JF, Okunieff P, Wang CC. Control of cervical lymph node disease in carcinoma of the Waldeyers ring: results and complications following twice a day radiotherapy [abstract]. Int J Radiat Biol Phys 1988;15 (Suppl 1).

36. Al-Sarraf M, Le Blanc M, Giri S. Chemoradiotherapy versus radiotherapy in patients with advanced nasopharyngeal cancer: Phase III randomized Intergroup Study 0099. J Clin Oncol 1998;16:1310–7.

36a. Wolden SL, Zelefsky MJ, Kraus DH, et al. Accelerated concomitant boost radiotherapy and chemotherapy for advanced nasopharyngeal carcinoma. J Clin Oncol 2001;19:1105–10.

37. Nell HB. Nasopharyngeal carcinoma: diagnosis, staging and management. Oncology 1992;692:87–95.

38. Mazeron JJ, Marinello G, Crook J, et al. Definitive radiation treatment for early stage carcinoma of the soft palate and uvula: the indications for iridium 192 implantation. Int J Radiat Oncol Biol Phys 1987;13;1829–37.

39. Esche BA, Haie CM, Gerbaulet AP, et al. Interstitial and external radiotherapy in carcinoma of the soft palate and uvula. Int J Radiat Oncol Biol Phys 1988;15:619–25.

40. Amdur RJ, Mendenhall WM, Parson JT, et al. Carcinoma of the soft palate treated with irradiation: analysis of results and complication. Radiother Oncol 1987;9:185–94.

41. Million RR. Squamous cell carcinoma of the head and neck: combined therapy surgery and post-operative irradiation. Int J Radiat Biol Phys 1979;5:2161–2.

42. Remmler D, Medina JE, Byers RM, et al. Treatment of choice for squamous carcinoma of the tonsillar fossa. Head Neck Surg 1985;7:206–11.

43. Hinerman RW, Parsons JT, Mendenhall WM, et al. External beam irradiation alone or combined with neck dissection for base of tongue carcinoma: an alternative to primary surgery. Laryngoscope 1994;104:1466–70.

44. Foote RL, Olsen KD, David DL, et al. Base of tongue carcinoma: patterns of failure and predictions of recurrence after surgery alone. Head Neck 1993;15:300–7.

45. Weber RS, Gidley P, Morrison WM, et al. Treatment selection for carcinoma of the base of tongue. Am J Surg 1990;160:415–9.

46. Harrison LB, Kraus DM, Zelefsky MJ, et al. Long term results of primary radiation therapy for squamous cell cancer of the base of tongue [abstract]. Proc Int Mtg Head Neck Cancer 1996;71.

47. Harrison LB, Lee M, Kraus DM, et al. Long term results of primary radiation therapy for squamous cancer of the base of tongue [abstract]. Radiother Oncol 1996;39:56.

48. Harrison LB, Sessions RB, Strong EW, et al. Brachytherapy as part of the definitive management of squamous cancer of the base of tongue. Int J Radiat Oncol Biol Phys 1989;17:1309–12.

49. Harrison LB, Zelefsky MJ, Sessions RB, et al. Base of tongue cancer treated with external beam irradiation plus brachytherapy: Oncologic and functional outcome. Radiology 1992;184:267–70.

50. Dupont JB, Guillamondegui OM, Jesse RM. Surgical treatment of advanced carcinoma of the base of tongue. Am J Surg 1978;136:501–3.

51. Mendenhall WM, Parsons JT, Devine JW, et al. Squamous cell carcinoma of the pyriform sinus treated with surgery and/or radiotherapy. Head Neck Surg 1987;10:88.

52. Mendenhall WM, Parsons JT, Stringer SP, et al. Radiotherapy alone or combined with neck dissection for T1-2 carcinoma of the pyriform sinus: an alternative to conservation surgery. Int J Radiat Oncol Biol Phys 1993;27:1017.

53. Laccourreye O, Merite-Dranc A, Brasnu D, et al. Supracricoid hemilaryngopharyngectomy in selected pyriform sinus carcinoma staged as T2. Laryngoscope 1993;103:1373.

54. Lefèbvre J-L, Chevalier D, Luboinski B, et al. Larynx preser-

vation in pyriform sinus cancer: preliminary results of a European Organization for Research and Treatment of Cancer phase III trial. J Natl Cancer Inst 1996;88:890.

55. Zelefsky MJ, Kraus DM, Pfister DG, et al. Combined chemotherapy and radiotherapy versus surgery and postoperative radiotherapy for advanced hypopharyngeal cancer. Head Neck 1996;18:405.

55a. Hunt MA, Zelefsky MJ, Wolden S, et al. Treatment planning and delivery of intensity modulated radiation therapy for primary nasopharynx cancer. Int J Radiat Oncol Biol Phys 2001;49:623–32.

56. Wang CC, Schulz M, Miller D. Combined radiotherapy and surgery for carcinoma of the supraglottis and pyriform sinus. Am J Surg 1972;124:551.

57. Fletcher G, Lindberg R, Hamburger H, et al. Reasons for irradiation failure in squamous cell carcinoma of the larynx. Laryngoscope 1975;85:987.

58. Mendenhall W, Parsons JT, Stringer S. Carcinoma of the supraglottic larynx: a basis for comparing the results of radiotherapy and surgery. Head Neck 1990;12:204.

59. Som M. Conservation surgery for carcinoma of the superglottis. J Laryngol Otol. 1970;84:655.

60. Ogura J, Biller M. Conservative surgery in cancer of the head and neck. Otolaryngol Clin North Am 1969;2:641.

61. Soo KC, Shah JP, Gopinath KS, et al. Analysis of prognostic variables and results after supraglottic partial laryngectomy. Am J Surg 1988;156:301.

61a. Forastiere AA, Berkey B, Maor M, et al. Phase III trial to preserve the larynx: induction chemotherapy and radiation therapy versus concomitant chemoradiotherapy versus radiotherapy alone, Intergroup Trial R91-11. Proceedings of ASCO 2001. 2001;20:2a.

62. Harrison L, Solomon B, Miller S, et al. Prospective computer assisted voice analysis for patients with early stage glottic cancer: a preliminary report of the functional result of laryngeal irradiation. Int J Radiat Oncol Phys 1990; 19:123.

63. Daly CJ, Strong EW. Carcinoma of the glottic larynx. Am J Surg 1975;130:489–92.

64. Sombeck MD, Kalbough KJ, Mendenhall WM, et al. Radiotherapy for early vocal cord cancer: dosimetric analysis of co^{60} versus 6 mv photons. Head Neck 1996;18:167–72.

65. Kim RY, Marks ME, Salter MM. Early stage glottic cancer: importance of dose fractionation in radiation therapy. Radiology 1990;182:273–5.

66. Schwaibold F, Scariato A, Nunno M, et al. The effect of fraction size on control of early glottic cancer. Int J Radiat Oncol Biol Phys 1988;14:451–4.

67. Harwood A. Cancer of the larynx—the Toronto experience. J Otolaryngol 1982;11:1.

68. Pellitteri P, Kennedy T, Vrabec D, et al. Radiotherapy, the mainstay in the treatment of early glottic carcinoma. Arch Otolaryngol Head Neck Surg 1991;117:297.

69. Kirchner JA, Owen JR. Five-hundred cancers of the larynx and pyriform sinus. Results of treatment of radiation and surgery. Laryngoscope 1977;87:1288–303.

70. Ogura J, Sessions D, Spector G. Analysis of surgical therapy for epidermoid carcinoma of the laryngeal glottis. Laryngoscope 1975;85:1522.

71. Wang CC. Treatment of glottic carcinoma by megavoltage radiation therapy and results. Am J Roentgenol Radium Ther Nucl Med 1974;120:157.

72. Department of Veterans Affairs Laryngeal Cancer Study Group. Induction chemotherapy plus radiation compared with surgery plus irradiation in patients with advanced laryngeal cancer. N Engl J Med 1991;324:1685–90.

73. American Joint Committee on Cancer. Manual for staging cancer. 5th ed. Philadelphia: Lippincott-Raven; 1998.

74. Vermund H. Role of radiotherapy in cancer of the larynx as related to the TNM system of staging. Cancer 1970; 25:485.

75. McCollough WM, Mendenhall NP, Parsons JT, et al. Radiotherapy alone for squamous cell carcinoma of the nasal vestibule: management of the primary site and regional lymphatics. Int J Radiat Oncol Biol Phys 1993;26:73–9.

76. Poulsen M, Turner S. Radiation therapy for squamous cell carcinoma of the nasal vestibule. Int J Radiat Oncol Biol Phys 1992;7:267.

77. Ang KK, Jiang GL, Frankenthaler RA, et al. Carcinomas of the nasal cavity. Radiother Oncol 1992;24:163.

78. Logue JP, Slewin NJ. Carcinoma of the nasal cavity and paranasal sinuses: an analysis of radical radiotherapy. Clin Oncol 1991;3:84–9.

79. Spiro JD, Soo K, Spiro RH. Squamous carcinoma of the nasal cavity and paranasal sinus. Am J Surg 1991;158:328–32.

80. St. Pierre S, Baker SR. Squamous cell carcinoma of the maxillary sinus: analysis of 77 cases. Head Neck Surg 1983; 5:508–13.

81. Isaacs J, Mooney S, Mendenhall W, et al. Cancer of the maxillary antrum treated with surgery and/or radiation therapy. Am J Surg 1990;56:327–30.

82. Griffin TW, Pajak TF, Maor MH, et al. Mixed neutron/photon irradiation of unresectable squamous cell carcinomas of the head and neck: the full report of a randomized cooperation trial. Int J Radiat Oncol Biol Phys 1989;17:959.

83. Spiro RH. Management of malignant tumors of the salivary glands. Oncology 1998;12:671–83.

84. Griffin TW, Pajak TF, Laramore GE, et al. Neutron versus photon irradiation of inoperable salivary gland tumors: Results of an RTOG-MRC cooperative randomized study. Int J Radiat Onco Biol Phys 1988;15:1085–90.

85. Armstrong JG, Harrison LB, Spiro RH, et al. Malignant tumors of major salivary gland origin. Arch Otolaryngol Head Neck Surg 1990;116:290–3.

86. Harrison LB, Armstrong JG, Spiro RH, et al. Postoperative radiation therapy for major salivary gland malignancies. J Surg Oncol 1990;45:52–5.

87. Spiro RH, Huros AG, Strong EW. Cancer of the parotid gland: a clinicopathologic study of 288 primary cases. Am J Surg 1975;130:457.

88. Fu KK, Leibel SA, Levine ML, et al. Carcinoma of the major and minor salivary glands. Cancer 1977; 40:2882–90.

89. Shah JP, Loree TR, Dharker D, Strong EW, et al. Prognostic factors in differentiated carcinoma of the thyroid gland. Am J Surg 1992;164:658–61.

90. Shah JP, Loree TR, Dharker D, Strong EW. Lobectomy versus total thyroidectomy for differentiated carcinoma of the thyroid; a matched-pair analysis. Am J Surg 1993;166.

91. Tsang RW, Brierley JD, Simpson WJ, et al. The effects of surgery, radioiodine, and external radiation therapy on the

clinical outcome of patients with differentiated thyroid carcinoma. Cancer 1998;82:375–88.

92. Tubiana M, Haddead E, Schlumberger M, et al. External radiotherapy in thyroid cancers. Cancer 1985;55:2062.

93. O'Connell ME, A'Hern RP, Harmer CL. Results of external beam radiotherapy in differentiated thyroid carcinoma: a retrospective study from the Royal Marsden Hospital. Eur J Cancer 1994;6:733.

94. Philips P, Hanzen C, Andry G, et al. Postoperative irradiation for thyroid cancer. Eur J Surg Oncol 1993;19(5):399–404.

95. Sheline GE, Galante M, Lindsay S. Radiation therapy in the control of persistent thyroid cancer. Am J Roentgenol Radium Ther Nucl Med Rad 1966;97:923–30.

96. Simpson WJ. Radioiodine and radiotherapy in the management of thyroid cancers. Otolaryngol Clin North Am 1990;23(3):509–21.

97. Simpson WJ, Carruthers JS. The role of external radiation in the management of papillary and follicular thyroid cancer. Am J Surg 1978;136(4):457–60.

98. Brierley JD, Sang Tsang RW. External-beam radiation therapy in the treatment of differentiated thyroid cancer. Semin Surg Oncol 1999;16(1):42–9.

99. Haugen BR. Management of the patient with progressive radio iodine non-responsive disease. Semin Surg Oncol 1999;16(1):34–41.

100. Happersett L, Hunt M, Chong L, et al. Intensity modulated radiation therapy for the treatment of thyroid cancer. ASTRO Poster Presentation; Boston (MA): 2000.

101. Ain KB. Anaplastic thyroid carcinoma: a therapeutic challenge. Semin Surg Oncol 1999;16(1):64–9.

102. Kim J, Leeper R. Treatment of locally advanced thyroid cancer with combination of doxorubicin and radiation therapy. Cancer 1987;60:10.

103. Levendag PC, De Porre PM, Van Putten WL. Anaplastic carcinoma of the thyroid gland treated by radiation therapy. Int J Radiat Oncol Biol Phys 1993;26(1):125–8.

104. Spiro RH, Huvos AG, Wong GY, Spiro JD. Predictive value of tumor thickness in squamous cell carcinoma confined to the tongue and floor of the mouth. Am J Surg 1986;152:354–50.

105. Fletcher GH. Basic principles of the combination of irradiation and surgery. Int J Radiat Oncol Biol Phys 1979;5:2091–6.

106. Thames HD, Peters LJ, Withers HR, Fletcher JH. Accelerated fractionation versus hyperfractionation: Rationale for several treatments per day. Int J Radiat Oncol Biol Phys 1983;9:127–38.

107. Fu KK, Pajak TF, Trotti A, et al. A radiation therapy oncology group (RTOG) phase III randomized study to compare hyperfractionation and two variants of accelerated fractionation to standard fractionation radiotherapy for head and neck squamous cell carcinomas: first report of RTOG 9003. Int J Radiat Biol Phys 2000;48:7–16.

108. Peters LJ, Ang KK, Thames HD Jr. Accelerated fractionation in the radiation therapy of head and neck cancer. A critical comparison of different strategies. Acta Oncol 1988;27:185–94.

109. Ang KK, Peters LJ. Concomitant boost radiotherapy in the treatment of head and neck cancers. Sem Radiat Oncol 1992;2:31–3.

110. Dische S, Saunders MI. The rationale for continuous, hyperfractionated, accelerated radiotherapy (CHART). Int J Radiat Oncol Biol Phys 1990;19:1317–20.

111. Saunders MI, Dische S. Continuous hyperfractionated accelerated radiotherapy (CHART). Sem Radiat Oncol 1992;2:31–44.

112. Saunders MI, Dische, S, Hong A, et al. Continuous hyperfractionated accelerated radiotherapy in locally advanced carcinoma of the head and neck lesion. Int J Radiat Oncol Biol Phys 1989;17:1287–93.

113. McGinn CJ, Harari PM, Fowler JF, et al. Dose intensification in curative head and neck cancer radiotherapy-linear quadratic analysis and preliminary assessment of clinical results. Int J Radiat Oncol Biol Phys 1993;27:363–9.

114. Bonner JA. Use of monoclonal antibodies as radiosensitizers. American Society of Clinical Oncology 1999 Educational Book. Baltimore (MD): Lippincott Williams & Wilkins; 1999.

115. Safa AA, Tran LM, Rege S, et al. The role of positron emission tomography in occult primary head and neck cancers. Cancer Journal 1999;5:214–8.

116. Shah JP. Patterns of cervical lymph node metastasis from squamous carcinomas of the upper aerodigestive tract. Am J Surg 1990;160:405–9.

117. Davidson BJ, Kulkarny V, Delacure MD, Shah JP. Posterior triangle metastases of squamous cell carcinoma of the upper aerodigestive tract. Am J Surg 1993;166:395–8.

118. Coker DD, Casterline PF, Chambers RG, Jaques DA. Metastases to lymph nodes of the head and neck from an unknown primary site. Am J Surg 1977;134:517–22.

119. Fitzpatrick PJ, Kotalik JF. Cervical metastases from an unknown primary tumor. Radiology 1974;110:659–63.

120. Jesse RH, Neff LE. Metastatic carcinoma in cervical nodes with an unknown primary. Am J Surg 1966;112:547–50.

121. Jesse RH, Perez CA, Fletcher GH. Cervical lymph node metastasis of unknown primary cancer. Cancer 1973;31:854–9.

122. Johnson JT, Newman RK. The anatomic location of neck metastasis for occult squamous cell carcinoma. Otolaryngol Head Neck Surg 1981;89:54–8.

123. Mendenhall WM, Million RR, Cassisi NJ. Elective neck irradiation in squamous cell carcinoma of the head and neck. Head Neck Surg 1980;3:15.

124. Fletcher G. Elective irradiation of subclinical disease in cancers of the head and neck. Cancer 1972;29:1450.

125. Jesse RH, Barkley HT Jr, Lindberg RD, Fletcher GH. Cancer of the oral cavity: Is elective neck dissection beneficial? Am J Surg 1970;120:505.

126. De Crevoisier R, Bourhis J, Bomenge C, et al. Full-dose reirradiation for unresectable head and neck carcinoma: Experience at the Gustave-Roussy Institute in a series of 169 patients. J. Clin Oncol 1998;16:3556–62.

127. Stevens KR Jr, Britsch A, Moss WT. High-dose reirradiation of head and neck cancer with a curative intent. Int J Radiat Oncol Biol Phys 1994;29:687–98.

128. Wang CC. To reirradiate or not to reirradiate. Int J Radiat Oncol Biol Phys 1994;20:913.

129. Teo TML, Kwan WH, Chan et al. How successful is high dose (≥ 60 Gy) reirradiation using mainly external beams in salvaging local failures of nasopharyngeal carcinoma? Int J Radiat Oncol Biol Phys 1998;40:897–913.

130. Wang CC. Decision making for re-irradiation of nasopharyngeal carcinoma. Int J Radiat Oncol Biol Phys 1993; 26:903.

131. Wang CC, McIntyre J. Re-irradiation of laryngeal carcinoma-techniques and results. Int J Radiat Oncol Biol Phy 1993;26:783–5.

132. Lampe I. The place of radiation therapy in the treatment of carcinoma of the lower lip. Plast Reconstr Surg 1959; 24:34.

133. Fu K. Combined-modality therapy for head and neck cancer. Oncology 1997;11:1781–800.

134. Vokes EE, Weichselbaum RR, Lippman SM, Hong WK. Head and neck cancer. N Engl J Med 1993;328:184–94.

135. Pfister DG, Harrison LB, Strong EW, Bosl GJ. Current status of larynx preservation with multimodality therapy. Oncology 1992;6(3):33–43.

136. Merlano M, Benasso M, Corro R, et al. Five year update of a randomized trial of alternating radiotherapy and chemotherapy compared with radiotherapy alone in treatment of unresectable squamous cell carcinoma of the head and neck. J Natl Cancer Inst 1996;88:583.

137. Anzai Y, Carroll WR, Quint DJ, et al. Recurrence of head and neck cancer after surgery or irradiation: prospective comparison of 2-deoxy-2- [F-18] fluoro-D-glucose-PET and MR imaging diagnoses. Radiology 1996;200:135–41.

138. Cohen L. The absence of a demonstrable gain factor for neutron beam therapy of epidermoid carcinoma of the head and neck. Int J Radiat Oncol Biol Phys 1982;8:2173–6.

139. Maor MH, Hussey DH, Barkley HT, Peters, LJ. Neutron therapy for head and neck cancer. II. Further follow-up on the MD Anderson TAMVEC randomized clinical trial. Int J Radiat Oncol Biol Phys 1983;9:1261–5.

140. Catterall M, Sutherland I, Bewley DK. First results of a randomized clinical trial of fast neutrons compared with x or gamma rays in treatment of advanced tumors of the head and neck. Br Med J 1975;2:653–6.

22

Chemotherapy and Chemoprevention in Head and Neck Cancer

FERNANDO C. MALUF, MD
ERIC SHERMAN, MD
DAVID G. PFISTER, MD

For most epithelial tumors of the head and neck, surgery and/or radiation therapy have historically been the principal treatment modalities. Systemic drug therapy alone in most instances does not have curative potential, and previously had been reserved for the palliative treatment of recurrent and/or distant metastatic disease. Over the last decade, this has changed dramatically, especially for squamous cell carcinomas of the upper aerodigestive tract, the most common type of invasive malignancy to occur in this body region if skin cancers are excluded. Randomized trials have demonstrated that integrated chemotherapy/radiation programs improve disease control rates relative to those obtained with radiation therapy alone in patients with unresectable squamous cell carcinomas of the head and neck,[1–4] as well as in those with advanced nasopharyngeal[5] and oropharyngeal[6] cancers. Combined modality programs including chemotherapy and radiation, with surgery to the primary site reserved for salvage, facilitate larynx preservation in patients with advanced cancers of the larynx or hypopharynx.[7,8] More recently, drug therapy is being explored to decrease the significant incidence of second primary cancers, widely recognized as frequent sources of morbidity and mortality in these patients,[9–12] and to decrease the side effects of therapy.[13,14]

The primary goal of this chapter is to describe and discuss the evolving role of chemotherapy for squamous cell cancers of the upper aerodigestive tract. When available, the results of randomized trials will be emphasized. Due to important differences in etiology and biologic behavior, the treatment of nasopharyngeal carcinoma will be discussed in a separate section. The chemotherapy for salivary gland and thyroid cancers also will be briefly reviewed, since these tumors are unique to this body region.

Background Considerations

Interpreting the available literature on the use of chemotherapy in patients with squamous cell head and neck cancer poses many challenges. To facilitate accrual, primary sites with potentially different natural histories, prognoses, responsiveness to systemic therapies, and presenting different management issues are frequently combined. Many randomized trials have sample sizes too small to rule out false-negative results, a problem exacerbated by the risk of mortality due to second primary cancers and medical co-morbidities in these patients,[15,16] as well as suboptimal compliance with therapy, which is especially prominent in the context of adjuvant chemotherapy.[17] Trials evaluating new combined modality therapies often change more than one variable at a time (eg, type of chemotherapy, dosing, integration with radiation, radiotherapy schedule), making the assessment of the incremental impact of any one treatment variable difficult to delineate. In studies of patients with locoregionally advanced, M0 disease, distinctions between resectable, unresectable, and medically inoperable are often not clearly stated.[18]

A number of drugs have activity against squamous cell head and neck cancer. Many also have the ability to enhance radiation when given concurrently with this modality.[19] Methotrexate, cisplatin/carboplatin, 5-fluorouracil, and more recently, paclitaxel, docetaxel, and ifosfamide are among the most widely used.[20–31] This list, however, is far from complete—some drugs have proven activity (eg, bleomycin), but offer no advantage in terms of activity, may be cumbersome to use and have been displaced from common clinical practice; others are undergoing clinical evaluation to define their role in the disease (eg, gemcitabine).[32] Most of the data regarding chemotherapy is derived from patients with advanced disease, since outcomes with standard therapy are disappointing for them. Much less data is available regarding the use of chemotherapy in patients with early stage disease, for whom single modality surgery or radiation therapy frequently yields excellent survival and functional results. Among these patients with more favorable prognoses, chemopreventive agents intended to decrease the rate of second primary cancers are the drug intervention receiving the greatest attention.[9–12,33]

The expected response rates depend on the clinical circumstances in which the chemotherapy is administered, and whether the particular drug is given alone, in combination with other drugs, or with radiation. For example, the use of single-agent therapy in patients with recurrent disease refractory to surgery and radiotherapy leads to a major response rate of 10 to 20 percent (based on randomized trials—response rates of up to 40 percent are noted in selected phase II studies,[20,21]) and rare complete regressions; the durability of these responses is disappointing, generally lasting weeks to less than 6 months.[24] Better activity is seen in patients with locoregionally advanced, previously untreated, M0 disease, in whom treatment with a widely used combination chemotherapy such as cisplatin (100 mg/m^2 IV day 1) and 5-fluorouracil (1000 mg/m^2 continuous infusion days 1 to 5) will yield a major response in 60 to 90 percent of patients, with complete shrinkages in 20 to 50 percent, many of whom will show no tumor on biopsy.[21,34–36] It should be emphasized, however, that even among complete responders to chemotherapy alone, progression will gener-

ally occur unless some type of definitive treatment modality addresses the site of bulk disease. Newer combination chemotherapy regimens are being developed and evaluated in hopes of improving both the frequency and durability of complete responses (Table 22–1). One of the attractive features of the concomitant integration of chemotherapy with radiation is the durability of the observed responses, even in the previously treated setting.[43,44]

Chemotherapy can be associated with a variety of side effects, such as nausea/vomiting, blood count suppression with an increased risk of infection, anemia and bleeding, renal dysfunction, hearing loss, and neuropathy, which are not unique to patients with head and neck cancer. Since many of these patients have medical co-morbidities and/or are treated with function preservation intent, a careful consideration of potential drug options and their side effects is an important part of the treatment planning process. The integration of chemotherapy with radiotherapy can lead to enhanced locoregional toxicity within the radiation field, and a spectrum of side effects more unique to this patient population. This is especially true when newer altered fractionation schedules and concomitant chemotherapy are utilized.[45–47] Mucositis, dysphagia, and xerostomia are common sequelae. There has been increasing interest in developing strategies to ameliorate these toxicities, both to improve patient tolerance of therapy and to facilitate dose intensity. Randomized studies have demonstrated the efficacy of selected drugs to ameliorate some of these toxicities.[13,14] These agents, while not chemotherapy agents in the usual sense, are nonetheless important, and are discussed in a separate section in this chapter.

CHEMOTHERAPY IN THE TREATMENT OF ADVANCED LOCOREGIONAL DISEASE

Sequential Chemotherapy

The sequential integration of chemotherapy with locoregional treatment can be done in three main ways: as induction or neoadjuvant chemotherapy prior to surgery and/or radiation, as an adjuvant after locoregional treatment, or as a combination of these approaches. Given the impressive response rates

Table 22–1. PHASE I/II TRIALS EVALUATING NEW CHEMOTHERAPEUTIC COMBINATION REGIMENS' ACTIVITY IN PREVIOUSLY UNTREATED PATIENTS WITH LOCALLY ADVANCED HEAD AND NECK CANCER

Author	No. of Patients	Chemotherapy Regimen	Overall/Complete Response Rates (%)	Commentary
Dunphy[37]	26	PCLT/CBDCA	54/27	Patient with advanced, stage III or IV head and neck tumors; induction chemotherapy followed by radiation therapy or surgery; paclitaxel 3-hour infusion
Hitt[38]	27	PCLT/CDDP	77/40	Patients with locally advanced head and neck tumors; no previous chemotherapy or radiation therapy; paclitaxel 3-hour infusion; G-CSF support
Colevas[36]	23	DCT/CDDP/5-FU/L	100/61	Patients with locally advanced head and neck tumors; no previous chemotherapy
Wang[39]	113	T/L/CDDP	62/26	Patients with advanced head and neck tumors; chemotherapy followed by locoregional treatment
Gebbia[40]	60	VNRB/CDDP/5-FU	88/23	Patients with locally advanced head and neck tumors; locoregional treatment included surgery or radiotherapy
Rivera[41]	37	VNRB/UFT/CDDP	91/50	Patients with locally advanced and resectable head and neck tumors; total of 4 cycles; radiation therapy with larynx preservation or surgery decided according to the response to the induction chemotherapy
Pai[42]	21	GCT/CDDP/IFM	71/07	Patients with locally advanced and resectable head and neck tumors; chemotherapy followed by surgery or radiotherapy

CBDCA = carboplatin; CDDP = cisplatin; DCT = docetaxel; 5-FU = 5-fluorouracil; GCT = gemcitabine; IFM = ifosfamide; L = leucovorin; PCLT = paclitaxel; T = tegafur; UFT = oral uracil and ftorafur; VNRB = vinorelbine.

observed in untreated patients with the cisplatin-based combination chemotherapy discussed previously, there initially was great enthusiasm from phase II studies that sequential strategies would improve survival in these patients.[48] As summarized below, randomized trials failed to demonstrate a significant survival benefit, although in selected studies the pattern of failure was altered compatible with a biologic effect of the chemotherapy, with a decrease in the rate of distant metastases among patients treated with chemotherapy.[17,35,49,50]

Selected, larger (> 100 patients per arm) randomized trials evaluating the use of neoadjuvant/induction or adjuvant chemotherapy integrated with locoregional treatment are summarized in Tables 22–2 and 22–3. Interpreting some of the neoadjuvant studies is complicated by the inclusion of both resectable and unresectable patients, as was the case in the study reported by Paccagnella and colleagues.[35] In this latter trial, if there was any benefit with the addition of chemotherapy, it was seen on subset analysis in the unresectable group only (3-year

Table 22–2. SELECTED RANDOMIZED TRIALS COMPARING NEOADJUVANT CHEMOTHERAPY FOLLOWED BY LOCOREGIONAL TREATMENT VERSUS LOCOREGIONAL TREATMENT ONLY IN PATIENTS WITH ADVANCED HEAD AND NECK CANCER

Author or Group	Total No. of patients	Chemotherapy Regimen	Resectability Status	LCT	Overall Survival Benefit (p < 0.05)
[†]Head and Neck Contracts Program[17]	443	CDDP/BLM	Resectable	S+RT	No
Richard[51]	222	BLM/VCR (IA)	Resectable	S ± RT	*No
Depondt[52]	324	CBDCA/5-FU	Resectable	S and/or RT	No
Paccagnella[35]	237	CDDP/5-FU	Resectable Unresectable	S → RT RT	**No
Dalley[53]	280	CDDP/5-FU	N/S	N/S	No

* Overall survival benefit limited to patients with floor of the mouth tumors.
** Overall survival benefit limited to patients with unresectable tumors (p = 0.04).
† Also included neoadjuvant/adjuvant arm—please see text.
BLM = bleomycin; CBDCA = carboplatin; CDDP = cisplatin; 5-FU = 5-fluorouracil; IA = intra-arterial; LCT = locoregional treatment; N/S = not specified; RT = radiotherapy; S = surgery; VCR = vincristine.

Table 22–3. SELECTED RANDOMIZED TRIALS COMPARING LOCOREGIONAL TREATMENT WITH OR WITHOUT ADJUVANT CHEMOTHERAPY IN RESECTABLE HEAD AND NECK CANCER

Author	Total No. of Patients	Postoperative Radiation Therapy	Chemotherapy Regimen	Decreased Distant Metastases	Overall Survival Benefit (p < 0.05)
Intergroup Study 0034[50]	448	Yes	CDDP/5-FU q3w x 3 cycles (before RT)	Yes	No
Domenge[54]	287	Yes	CDDP/BLM/MTX	*No	*No
Horiuchi[55]	424	No	UFT (orally) for 1 year	Yes	No

* Adjuvant chemotherapy arm had higher incidence of distant metastases and inferior overall survival compared to the standard arm.
BLM = bleomycin; CDDP = cisplatin; 5-FU = 5-fluorouracil; MTX = methotrexate; UFT = tegafur and uracil: RT = radiotherapy.

overall survival rate 24% vs. 10%, p = 0.04). Only one other study, the one reported by Richard and colleagues, which utilized an intra-arterial approach with vincristine and bleomycin, demonstrated improvement in survival outcome in selected subset of patients with the use of chemotherapy.[51] The study reported by Di Blasio and colleagues (69 patients entered, not listed in Table 22–2) favored the standard treatment arm.[56] Comparing these neoadjuvant studies can be difficult since a variety of chemotherapy regimens were used. However, when only studies using standard cisplatin and infusional 5-fluorouracil published in the 1990s were reviewed by Adelstein and colleagues (5 studies, over 800 patients), there was no convincing improvement in outcome.[48]

Fewer adjuvant studies have been published. These trials were limited to patients with resectable disease, although neither the eligibility criteria nor the integration of chemotherapy were identical in all the studies. For example, in the Intergroup Study 0034, patients, after the completion of the resection, were stratified as good-risk or poor-risk;[50] in the French study,[54] only patients with extracapsular nodal spread were eligible. Furthermore, chemotherapy was sandwiched between the surgery and radiation in the Intergroup trial,[50] rather than after all treatment.[54,55] As with the neoadjuvant chemotherapy approach, no convincing evidence of survival benefit was demonstrated. In fact, the trial reported by Domenge and colleagues favored the standard treatment arm.[54] Compliance with adjuvant therapy after locoregional treatment can be a challenge. In the Intergroup study, even though the adjuvant chemotherapy was given before radiation, only 62 percent of patients received chemotherapy per protocol or with a minor variation.[50] In the arm of the Head and Neck Contracts program that received adju-

vant chemotherapy (discussed below), only 9 percent of patients received the planned six cycles of adjuvant single-agent cisplatin.[17]

Randomized studies evaluating the incorporation of both neoadjuvant and adjuvant therapy at the same time with locoregional treatment are the least common. Perhaps the best example is the Head and Neck Contracts program, the first large-scale study evaluating the role of sequential chemotherapy in the management of advanced squamous cell head and neck cancer.[17] The study included 443 evaluable patients with resectable disease randomized to three arms: standard treatment—surgery followed by postoperative radiotherapy; neoadjuvant arm— neoadjuvant chemotherapy consisting of a single course of cisplatin and bleomycin by infusion, followed by surgery and radiotherapy; and neoadjuvant/adjuvant arm—the same induction chemotherapy followed by surgery, postoperative radiotherapy and six cycles of single-agent cisplatin. Radiation therapy was administered as a once daily dose in all three arms. The 5-year disease-free and overall survival times among the three arms of the study were comparable. Also, no significant difference in terms of locoregional control was observed among the arms. The neoadjuvant/adjuvant chemotherapy arm, however, was associated with an improved distant disease control (distant recurrences at first relapse 19%, 19%, and 9%, for standard arm [p = 0.025], neoadjuvant arm [p = 0.021], and neoadjuvant/adjuvant arm, respectively; time to distant failure was also improved). Poor compliance with adjuvant chemotherapy possibly contributed to the lack of observed survival benefit. As noted, only 9 percent received all six cycles of cisplatin, and 27 percent received at least three cycles.[17] On a subsequent multivariate analysis, patients with N2 disease appeared to derive the largest benefit from the addition of adjuvant chemotherapy.[57]

Another noteworthy study evaluating a neoadjuvant/adjuvant strategy was reported by Ervin and colleagues. In this trial, 114 patients with advanced disease received induction chemotherapy with cisplatin/bleomycin/methotrexate/leucovorin, then underwent locoregional treatment; responders to induction therapy were randomized either to observation or three cycles of the same adjuvant chemotherapy. Patients allocated to receive adjuvant chemotherapy had superior 3-year failure-free survival (88% vs. 57%, p = 0.03). Of interest, the patients who were partial responders to induction chemotherapy derived the greatest benefit from adjuvant therapy.[58]

In summary, these studies failed to demonstrate a consistent improvement in overall survival among these advanced disease patients with the incorporation of sequential chemotherapy. Subsequent meta-analyses also failed to convincingly detect a significant improvement in survival.[46,59–62] Selected studies demonstrated a change in the pattern of failure with less distant metastases[17,35,50] compatible with a biologic effect of the chemotherapy, but neither this nor the impact on other sources of failure was sufficiently large to improve survival outcome. Due to this lack of survival benefit, such strategies, especially in patients with advanced resectable squamous cell carcinoma of the head and neck in the setting of a planned resection, are not recommended outside of an investigational protocol.

Concomitant Chemotherapy

The concomitant integration of chemotherapy and radiation therapy for the treatment of advanced disease has been one of the areas of greatest interest in head and neck oncology during the last decade. Potential radiation enhancement, the simultaneous treatment of both locoregional and distant disease in a dose-intense manner, and shorter treatment times make the approach particularly appealing. Interestingly, the approach is much older than the relatively recent surge in interest would suggest. Randomized studies suggesting a benefit with the concomitant integration of chemotherapy with radiation therapy

date back over 2 decades.[1–6,63–68] Interest in strategies incorporating sequential chemotherapy was of greater interest during the 1980s, at the expense of the development of concomitant ones. Given the prospect for improved local control, unresectable disease has been the focus more often than not in studies to date. Encouraging results as summarized below, however, are prompting evaluation in the resectable disease setting, either as part of organ preservation strategies or as adjuvant therapy after surgery in high-risk patients.

There are an enormous number of concomitant treatment schedules. They can generally be classified into three main types: concomitant chemotherapy—typically a single agent, with continuous-course radiation therapy; concomitant chemotherapy—more frequently a combination regimen with split-course radiation; and an alternating integration of chemotherapy with radiotherapy (rather than a strict sequential integration of the modalities). Obviously, within each of these categories there is considerable variation. The commonly altered treatment variables include the chemotherapy drug(s), doses, timing, as well as radiation dose, fraction size, and fractionation schedule. Most randomized trials to date compare radiotherapy alone to chemotherapy/radiotherapy, not one chemotherapy/radiotherapy schedule versus another. Accordingly, the relative effectiveness of different combined modality programs is difficult to assess at this time.

Tables 22–4 and 22–5 review representative randomized trials comparing concomitant chemotherapy (single agent and combination chemotherapy, respectively) with radiation therapy versus radiation therapy alone. Unlike the sequential integration data, a number of these studies demonstrate improved outcomes, including an improvement in overall survival as an endpoint. Two recent meta-analyses have similarly confirmed the potential benefit of a concomitant approach.[46,62] For example, El-Sayed and Nelson found that concurrent treatment reduced the mortality by 22 percent (95% confidence interval, 8 to 33%) compared to radiation alone, albeit at the expense of greater toxicity.[46] Munro reported a 12.1 percent increase in survival (95% confidence interval, 5 to 19%) with the use of single-agent chemotherapy with radiotherapy compared to radiotherapy alone.[62] A few

Table 22–4. SELECTED RANDOMIZED TRIALS COMPARING CONCURRENT SINGLE-AGENT CHEMOTHERAPY WITH RADIATION THERAPY IN PATIENTS WITH ADVANCED HEAD AND NECK CANCER

Author	Total No. of Patients	Drug	RT Fractionation	Overall Survival Benefit (p < 0.05)
Arcangeli[69]	142	MTX (IA)	Standard	Yes
Shanta and Krishnamurthi[63]	157	BLM	Standard	Yes
Fu[70]	104	BLM	Standard	†No
Eschwege[71]	199	BLM	Standard	No
Vermund[72]	222	BLM	Standard	No
Gabriele[73]	130	CBDCA	Standard	Yes
Haselow[74]	319	CDDP	Standard	No
Bachaud[75]	83	CDDP	Standard	§Yes
Sanchiz[64]	600	5-FU	Standard	#Yes
Lo[68]	136	5-FU	Standard	**No
Browman[65]	175	5-FU	Standard	‡No
Gupta[66]	313	MTX	Standard	‡No
*Weissberg[67]	117	MMC	Standard	‖No
Dobrowsky[76]	188	MMC	Hyperfractionated	††Yes

* Resectable patients were also included. A subgroup received the chemotherapy/radiotherapy as an adjuvant.
† Relapse-free survival (p = 0.04) and locoregional control (p = 0.001) benefit.
‡ Trend in survival benefit (p = 0.07—Gupta study and p = 0.08—Browman study).
§ Adjuvant chemotherapy and radiation administered after complete resection.
‖ Local recurrence-free survival benefit (p < 0.02).
Three-arm trial: survival benefit compared to the conventional radiotherapy alone arm (p < 0.001); no survival benefit compared to the hyperfractionated radiation arm.
** Patients with oral cavity, base of the tongue, and oropharynx tumors entered the trial. Survival benefit restricted to patients with oral cavity tumors.
†† Survival benefit compared to the two other arms: conventional and hyperfractionated radiation alone (p < 0.05).
BLM: bleomycin; CBDCA = carboplatin; CDDP = cisplatin; 5-FU = 5-fluorouracil; IA = intra-arterial; MTX = methotrexate; MMC = mitomycin C; RT = radiotherapy.

selected studies warrant further discussion, and are reviewed in more detail below.

One of the critiques commonly encountered when discussing randomized trials of concomitant chemotherapy/radiotherapy is that the radiation-alone control arm did not use the most effective radiation dosing strategy. The trial reported by Brizel and colleagues is relevant in this regard. The radiation-alone control arm in this study utilized hyperfractionated radiation therapy (1.25 Gy twice a day to a total dose of 75 Gy). The chemotherapy/radiation arm utilized split-course radiotherapy to a lower total dose (1.25 Gy twice a day to 70 Gy) with concurrent cisplatin and infusional 5-fluorouracil. Of 121 randomized patients with T3 to T4 squamous cell head and neck cancer stratified by resectability and hemoglobin level, 116 were analyzed. Locoregional control (44% vs. 70%, p = 0.01), 3-year relapse-free survival (41% vs. 61%, p = 0.08), and 3-year overall survival (34% vs. 55%, p = 0.07) all favored the

Table 22–5. SELECTED RANDOMIZED TRIALS COMPARING COMBINATION CHEMOTHERAPY AND RADIATION THERAPY WITH RADIATION THERAPY ALONE IN PATIENTS WITH LOCALLY ADVANCED HEAD AND NECK CANCER

Author	Total No. of patients	CT/RT Schedule	CT Regimen	RT Fraction*	Overall Survival Benefit (p < 0.05)
GORTEC[6]	226	Concurrent	CBDCA/5-FU	Standard	Yes
Adelstein[77,78]	100	Concurrent	CDDP/5-FU	Standard	†No
Wendt[3]	270	Concurrent	CDDP/5-FU	Hyperfractionated	Yes
Keane[79]	212	Concurrent	MMC/5-FU	Standard	No
Brizel[2]	122	Concurrent	CDDP/5-FU	Hyperfractionated	‡No
Merlano[4]	157	Alternating	CDDP/5-FU	Standard	Yes

*All studies except the GORTEC study required a planned split in the radiation when combined with chemotherapy.
†Relapse-free survival benefit (p = 0.03).
‡Trend in survival benefit (p = 0.07).
BLM = bleomycin; CBDCA = carboplatin; CDDP = cisplatin; CT = chemotherapy; 5-FU = 5-fluorouracil; MMC = mitomycin C; RT = radiotherapy.

combined modality arm. When a multivariate adjustment was made for the randomization of less advanced nodal disease to favor the chemotherapy/radiotherapy arm, the corrected p values were 0.01, 0.12, and 0.11, respectively. Of note, the placement of feeding tubes (29% vs. 44%) was more common, and the resolution of mucositis slower (4 vs. 6 weeks) on the combined modality arm.[2]

The GORTEC ("Groupe d'Oncologie Radiotherapie Tête et Cou") study is important in that it represents one of the few site-specific, randomized studies evaluating a concomitant approach. Patients with stage III or IV squamous cell oropharynx cancer were randomized to radiotherapy alone (70 Gy, 2 Gy per fraction, 5 fractions per week), or the same radiation schedule with three cycles of concomitant carboplatin (70 mg/m^2) and 5-fluorouracil (600 mg/m^2 continuous infusion), days 1 to 4, 22 to 25, and 43 to 46 with the same schedule of radiotherapy. Locoregional control (42% vs. 66%, p = 0.03), 3-year disease-free survival (20% vs. 42%, p = 0.04), and 3-year overall survival (31% vs. 51%, p = 0.02) all favored the combined modality arm. Grades 3 and 4 mucositis (39% vs. 71%) were more common with combined modality treatment, as was the need for a feeding tube.[6]

The Cleveland Clinic experience reported by Adelstein and Lavertu[77,78,80] is relevant for two main reasons. First, the study was limited to patients with resectable disease, so the fact that the organ preservation rate with their program of concomitant cisplatin/5-fluorouracil and radiation therapy was superior to that obtained with radiation alone (5-year survival with primary site preservation, 34% vs. 42%, p = 0.02) has implications with regard to potential organ preservation strategies. The second is that one of the concerns surrounding the use of aggressive combined chemotherapy/radiotherapy programs in the organ preservation setting is that the morbidity of salvage surgery, if necessary, may be increased. When analyzing their data, however, they did not find that the incidence of major or minor complications was higher among patients previously treated with concomitant chemotherapy and radiation compared to radiation therapy alone.[80] The specific complications, however, may have been more serious in the former group, as more resources (eg, duration of surgery, length of stay) were necessary to address them.

There are more limited data available regarding the use of concomitant chemotherapy/radiotherapy as an adjuvant after resection. Bachaud and colleagues evaluated in a phase III trial the combination of single-agent cisplatin at the dose of 50 mg (total dose) weekly for 7 to 9 cycles given concurrently with postoperative, conventionally-fractionated radiation. The control arm received radiation alone. A total of 83 patients were included. The chemoradiation arm was associated with better locoregional control (p = 0.08), and higher disease-free (p < 0.02) and overall survival rates (p < 0.01). There was no increased toxicity observed in the combined modality treatment arm.[75] The results of a major intergroup randomized trial comparing radiation therapy alone versus concomitant cisplatin (100 mg/m^2 IV days 1, 22, and 43) with radiation in resected, poor-risk patients is currently pending.

When chemotherapy is given concomitantly with radiation, often both chemotherapy and radiation dosing is affected. The net effect is that each modality by itself is arguably given in a less optimal way. For example, chemotherapy doses may be reduced, or a single agent will be used instead of combination therapy. The radiation dose may be reduced, or the course may be split instead of being continuous. Accordingly, the relative effectiveness of sequential versus concomitant chemotherapy with radiation therapy is of great interest. As noted in the next section, it also has major implications with regard to organ preservation strategies in patients with resectable disease.

Four randomized trials have compared treatment arms where the same drugs were integrated with radiotherapy either sequentially or concomitantly.[81–84] These trials are summarized in Table 22–6. Only one study revealed a significant difference between the arms in overall survival as endpoint.[83] In certain studies, the risk of a false-negative result was significant given the sizes of the samples randomized. When other disease endpoints were considered, however, the results favored the concomitant arms, although toxicity was higher. Of note, the previously discussed meta-analyses by El-Sayed and Nelson[46] and Munro,[62] also demonstrated an apparent advantage for concomitant therapy over a sequential approach. Current randomized studies

Table 22–6. RANDOMIZED TRIALS CONCURRENT VERSUS SEQUENTIAL CHEMOTHERAPY WITH RADIATION THERAPY IN LOCALLY ADVANCED HEAD AND NECK CANCER

Author or Group	Total No. of Patients	CT Regimen	Resectability Status	Overall Survival Benefit-Arm (p < 0.05)
SECOG[81]	267	BLM/MTX/VCR ± 5-FU	N/S	‡No
Adelstein[82]	54	CDDP/5-FU	Unresectable	†No
Merlano[83]	116	BLM/MTX/L/VBL	Unresectable	Yes
Taylor[84]	214	CDDP/5-FU	Unresectable	‡No

†Relapse-free survival benefit for patients receiving the concurrent arm (p = 0.03).
‡Disease-free survival benefit for patients receiving the concurrent arm (p = 0.04—SECOG study; p = 0.01—Taylor study).
BLM = bleomycin; CDDP = cisplatin; CT = chemotherapy; 5-FU = 5-fluorouracil; L = leucovorin; MTX = methotrexate; N/S = not specified; SECOG = South-East Cooperative Oncology Group; VBL = vinblastine; VCR = vincristine.

in the organ preservation setting should provide further insights in this regard.

Combining sequential and concomitant strategies offers the advantage of optimizing distant and locoregional control. Compliance as described previously can be suboptimal for adjuvant chemotherapy after locoregional therapy.[17] Accordingly, there has been increased interest in the delivery of neoadjuvant chemotherapy followed by concomitant chemoradiation. For example, Kies and colleagues evaluated (in 93 patients with stage III or IV disease) the induction regimen of cisplatin, infusional 5-fluorouracil, *l*-leucovorin, and interferon-α for a total of three cycles, followed by concurrent chemoradiotherapy with hydroxyurea and infusional 5-fluorouracil. The results were encouraging with 5-year progression-free and overall survival of 68 percent and 62 percent, respectively. Locoregional and distant failure rates at 5 years were 25 percent and 10 percent, respectively. However, the toxicity was appreciable, and there were 6 treatment-related deaths.[85] Investigators at Memorial Sloan-Kettering Cancer Center compared the results of two consecutive larynx-preservation protocols. From 1988 to 1990, 70 patients were treated with the combination of cisplatin and infusional 5-fluorouracil for a total of three cycles followed by conventional, definitive-dose radiation therapy. A latter group of 103 patients were treated from 1991 to 1995, with similar neoadjuvant chemotherapy followed by the concurrent administration of single-agent cisplatin 100 mg/m² on days 1 and 22 during definitive radiation therapy with a concomitant boost. In the multivariate analysis controlling for a wide range of potential confounders, the latter protocol was associated with significant

improvement in the locoregional control rates without total laryngectomy, or the need for tracheostomy or gastrostomy. Since more than one treatment variable was changed between these studies, the relative benefits can not be delineated, especially given the non-randomized design.[86] Whether strategies like these offer a significant advantage over other chemoradiation approaches awaits further evaluation and randomized comparison to other regimens.

The Role of Chemotherapy in Larynx/Organ Preservation

The trials evaluating induction chemotherapy, while disappointing with regard to improving survival as an endpoint, did provide the backdrop for current organ preservation strategies. Investigators observed that some patients refused surgery after initial chemotherapy and proceeded with radiation alone.[87] Some of these patients were controlled over the long term without surgery, and there appeared to be a positive correlation between initial response at the primary site to induction chemotherapy and the likelihood of disease control with radiation alone. Pilot organ preservation studies demonstrated that induction chemotherapy followed by definitive dose radiation, with surgery to the primary site reserved for non-response or relapse, was a feasible approach.[88,89] Reported survival results in selected patients were comparable to those anticipated with standard surgery and radiotherapy, but surgery to the primary site was avoided in a significant proportion of patients (Figure 22–1). Avoiding total laryngectomy was the focus of many of these studies, as the procedure is widely acknowledged to be among those most feared by

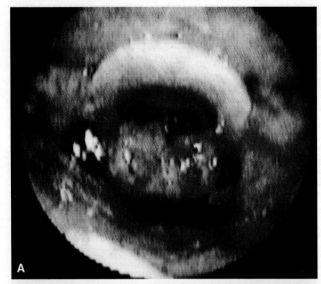

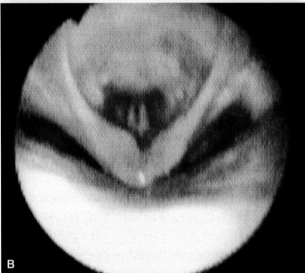

Figure 22–1. Photographs of a larynx cancer treated with chemotherapy/radiotherapy with larynx preservation intent. *A*, Pre-treatment; *B*, Post-treatment.

patients. The potential negative impact on the quality of life of patients who undergo it are well described in the literature,[90,91] and include loss of functional voice, impairment of deglutition, permanent tracheotomy, and adverse effect on cosmetic appearance. Larynx preservation studies serve as a paradigm for the application of organ preservation to other primary sites and will be discussed in more detail.

In patients with locally advanced but resectable tumors of the larynx and surrounding structures, standard surgical management will jeopardize the larynx in the majority of patients. Unfortunately, an organ-preserving surgical procedure will be applica-

ble to only selected patients with locally advanced disease. Radiation alone may cure some patients, but anticipated local control rates when radiation alone is used as a single modality are disappointing.[92,93] Accordingly, combined modality treatment strategies that decrease surgical morbidity without compromising locoregional control rates and overall survival have generated considerable interest. The best studied approach to date uses induction chemotherapy followed by definitive-dose radiation therapy, with surgery reserved for non-response to chemotherapy, persistent disease after radiation, or relapse. Three randomized studies have compared variations on this approach to standard surgical treatment (Table 22–7).

The Veterans Affairs Laryngeal Cancer Study Group (VALCSG) evaluated 332 patients with resectable stage III or IV laryngeal cancer. The chemotherapy regimen included standard cisplatin and infusional 5-fluorouracil given for three cycles. The radiation treatment after the chemotherapy for responding patients included daily fractions of 180 to 200 cGy to a total dose of 6,600 to 7,600 cGy. If necessary, neck dissection was done after radiation therapy. Patients who presented with progression of disease during any chemotherapy cycle, or a lack of major objective response at the primary site after the second chemotherapy cycle, underwent salvage surgery. Larynx preservation was achieved in 31 percent of patients randomized to the induction chemotherapy arm (62% of survivors).[7] With a median follow-up of 98 months, the overall and median survival rates were comparable between both arms. Patients who received salvage laryngectomy after initial chemotherapy had similar survival outcome, compared with patients randomized directly to surgical treatment, suggesting that the delay in the surgery caused by the administration of chemotherapy did not adversely affect survival.[7,95] Follow-up data suggests that quality of life outcomes were superior on the chemotherapy/radiotherapy arm.[96]

The European Organization for Research and Treatment of Cancer (EORTC) study, reported by Lefebvre and colleagues, included 202 patients with squamous cell carcinoma of the pyriform sinus or of the hypopharyngeal aspect of the aryepiglottic fold. Patients with stage T2 to T4 disease were eligible.

Table 22–7. RESULTS OF RANDOMIZED LARYNX PRESERVATION TRIALS							
Group	**No of Patients**	**Tumor Site**	**Regimen**	**Schedule**	**Control Arm**	**Organ Preservation**	**Survival Comparison**
VALCSG[7]	332	Larynx	CDDP + 5-FU up to 3 cycles	Sequential	S → RT	31% at 3 years	Comparable to surgery plus RT
EORTC[8]	202	Hypopharynx	CDDP + 5-FU up to 3 cycles	Sequential	S → RT	42% at 3 years	Comparable to surgery plus RT
GETTEC[94]	68	Larynx	CDDP + 5-FU up to 3 cycles	Sequential	S → RT	20% at 3 years	Inferior to surgery plus RT

CDDP = cisplatin; EORTC = European Organization for Research and Treatment of Cancer; GETTEC = Groupe d'Etudes des Tumeurs de la Tête et du Cou; 5-FU = 5-fluorouracil; RT = radiotherapy; S = surgery; VALCSG = Veterans Affairs Laryngeal Cancer Study Group.

As with the VALCSG study, the chemotherapy regimen also consisted of standard cisplatin and infusional 5-fluorouracil administered for three cycles followed by radiotherapy. The surgical procedure performed in the standard arm was total laryngectomy with partial pharyngectomy and neck dissection followed by postoperative radiation therapy. Patients in the chemotherapy arm had to achieve a complete response, including normalization of vocal cord mobility to proceed to definitive radiation therapy. The time of neck dissection was left to the discretion of the involved surgeon. With a median follow-up of 51 months, there was no statistical difference in terms of 5-year overall and disease-free survival between the arms. Disease control rates at 3 and 5 years without total laryngectomy, need for tracheostomy or gastrostomy, and with the larynx preserved were 42 percent and 35 percent, respectively.[8] As with the VALCSG study, delay in local therapy caused by non-response to induction chemotherapy did not appear to adversely affect survival outcome.[7]

The third study was performed by the Groupe d'Études des Tumeurs de la Tête et du Cou (GETTEC) trial, and 68 patients (total planned: 300 patients) with locally advanced and resectable larynx cancer were accrued. More than 90 percent of the patients presented with stage III disease, and glottic tumors predominated. Salvage surgery was performed for those who failed to achieve at least a partial response. The locoregional control rates, as well as 3-year disease-free and overall survival rates, were significantly better on the surgery/radiation arm.[94] Limitations of this trial include the poor patient accrual, imbalance between arms (more patients with stage IV disease in the chemother-

apy/radiation arm), and lack of uniformity in the radiographic tests required for disease staging.[94]

A meta-analysis including the above described three studies showed a 5-year overall survival of 39 percent and 45 percent for patients randomized to chemotherapy/radiotherapy and surgery/radiotherapy, respectively (95% confidence interval = 0.97 to 1.47, $p = 0.1$). The 5-year disease-free survival was 34 percent and 40 percent, respectively (95% confidence interval = 0.97 to 1.44, $p = 0.1$). The locoregional failure rates were greater in the chemotherapy/radiotherapy arm (35% vs. 20%), although the incidence of distant metastasis was higher in the surgery/radiotherapy arm.[97] When taken collectively, these data suggest that sequential chemotherapy and radiation, with surgery reserved for salvage, yield survival rates comparable to, but certainly no better than, that observed with "up-front" total laryngectomy and postoperative radiotherapy. Such an approach is appropriately offered to patients with advanced squamous cell carcinomas of the larynx or hypopharynx seeking to avoid the morbidities of total laryngectomy. Close interdisciplinary communication and cooperation is fundamental to the success of such an approach.

Randomized trials in progress are currently addressing important questions. The United States Intergroup Trial 91–11 will include 546 patients with resectable stage III or IV laryngeal cancer (excluding T1 and unfavorable T4 lesions) for a comparison in a three-arm trial of the following treatment strategies: sequential chemotherapy (cisplatin/5-fluorouracil) followed by radiotherapy, versus concurrent chemotherapy (cisplatin) and radiotherapy, versus radiotherapy alone, with all arms including surgery for salvage. This study addresses one of the criticisms of the VALCSG study—the lack of a radiation-alone control arm. The EORTC Trial 24954 is planning accrual of 564 patients with stages T3/T4, N0 to N2 larynx cancer and stages T2 to T4, N0 to N2 hypopharynx cancer for a two-arm randomized trial comparing sequential (like the VALCSG and EORTC studies) versus an alternating chemotherapy and radiation therapy program. Both of these trials should provide insights regarding the optimal chemotherapy/radiotherapy schedule in the larynx preservation setting.

Toxicity Amelioration

One of the greatest concerns for patients with head and neck cancer is the adverse effects secondary to chemotherapy and/or radiotherapy exposure. Improvements in local control and survival with newer combined modality approaches often come at the expense of more side effects, especially xerostomia and mucositis. Xerostomia contributes to a higher incidence of abnormalities of speech, oral cavity infections, and dental caries.[45] Complications secondary to the mucositis include local pain, malnutrition, gastrostomy tube placement, and a higher incidence of aerodigestive tract infections. Therefore, potential approaches to prevent these treatment-related toxicities are of great interest.

Amifostine (Ethyol-WR-2721) is a thiol that has been studied as a chemo- and radiotherapy-protectant agent. Briefly, this agent acts selectively as a scavenger of oxygen-derived free radicals in normal cells. The selective targeting effect of amifostine is at least in part related to the property of higher thiol uptake, due to vascularization and pH, demonstrated in normal cells rather than tumor cells. Although of theoretical concern, reports to date have not documented evidence of "tumor protection".[98] The potential role of amifostine was outlined in a randomized trial including 315 patients with advanced head and neck cancer treated with conventional radiotherapy with or without daily amifostine. The incidence of grade ≥ 2 acute and late xerostomia (assessed by saliva production measurement, questionnaire, and the Radiation Therapy Oncology Group [RTOG] clas-

sification) were significantly lower in the amifostine arm. The incidence of grade ≥ 3 mucositis was comparable between the two arms.[13] The protective effect of amifostine was also observed in patients who received concurrent chemotherapy with single-agent carboplatin and radiotherapy,[99] as well as in patients receiving radioiodine.[100] Amifostine-related toxicity includes nausea, vomiting, hypotension, and less frequently, allergic reactions and hypocalcemia.[98] Evidence-based guidelines for the use of amifostine were recently published by the American Society of Clinical Oncology.[98] The results of clinical trials to date indicate that the use of amifostine may be considered in patients with locally advanced head and neck cancer who are undergoing radiation therapy (particularly radiation that is accelerated/hyperfractionated, or with large fields with or without chemotherapy), in order to decrease the incidence of acute and late xerostomia. Other toxicities, such as nephrotoxicity and neutropenia, may also be reduced with amifostine. The potential benefit of amifostine in reducing the incidence of severe mucositis warrants further study.

Pilocarpine, a cholinomimetic natural alkaloid with muscarinic action, has been shown to be, in two prospective double-blind, placebo-controlled, multicenter phase III trials, associated with increasing saliva production, as measured by sialometry and symptom improvement (intraoral dryness, ability to speak, mouth comfort) as assessed by questionnaires. In both trials, patients received radiation therapy alone at doses ≥ 4000 cGy and received pilocarpine after the radiation treatment.[14] There is also evidence, according to an open-label randomized trial, that a maintenance dose of oral pilocarpine for 36 months following radiation treatment improves oral function. Mild-to-moderate sweating is the most common side effect, and urinary frequency, lacrimation and rhinitis may occur less frequently.[101]

Keranocyte growth factor, recognized as a potent mitogen of normal epithelial cells from the skin, oral mucosa and gastrointestinal tract, is being evaluated as a mucosal protectant agent.[102] Other options to prevent oral toxicity are also being explored.[103] One would anticipate that this area will remain one of great investigational interest.

CHEMOTHERAPY IN THE TREATMENT OF RECURRENT AND/OR METASTATIC DISEASE

Patients with recurrent and/or metastatic squamous cell carcinoma of the head and neck that is not amenable to surgery or radiation have a poor prognosis. Cure in these cases is rare; palliation of symptoms and, if possible, prolongation of survival become the major goals. The minority of patients will typically have a major response. The median survival for these patients ranges from 5 to 8 months, with no significant survival advantage offered by combination drug therapy.[104–106] Three recent, representative phase III trials in patients with recurrent and/or metastatic head and neck cancers comparing single agents versus combination chemotherapy regimens are summarized in Table 22–8.

Browman and Cronin analyzed in a meta-analysis the results of studies that evaluated single-agent therapy versus combination treatment with standard cisplatin/5-fluorouracil. Their analysis showed that combination chemotherapy regimens are associated with higher response rates but also greater toxicity than single-agent chemotherapy, with no significant difference in the median survival.[60] Accordingly, these data failed to support the routine use of combination chemotherapy in those patients. Some would argue that the higher response rates of combination therapy translate into better symptom palliation. The severity of symptoms requiring palliation, a patient's performance status and preferences, and the related toxicity of therapy all need to be considered when making the treatment decision.

In past years, there was great concern regarding re-irradiation, let alone the addition of chemotherapy to it. There is a growing appreciation, especially with the use of newer conformal techniques, that such an approach is feasible and deserves consideration in certain settings. For example, De Crevoisier and colleagues reported their experience at the Institute Gustave-Roussy with full-dose re-irradiation plus or minus chemotherapy in 169 patients. This approach led to complete remissions ranging from 12 to 111 months in 13 patients. Late toxicity was increased compared with their historical experience with single courses of radiation, but was within an acceptable range.[44]

For these patients, investigational protocols, including phase I trials, deserve consideration. A summary of potentially promising investigational options is beyond the scope of this chapter. Initiatives involving injectable gene therapy[107] and the use of receptor-specific antibodies[108] are among the most exciting strategies.

Nasopharyngeal Cancer

The biologic behavior of nasopharyngeal carcinoma, especially among the undifferentiated histologic subtype, is characterized by high proliferation rates and the development of metastases early in the course of the disease. Lymph node involvement in the neck is common. The incidence of distant metas-

Author	Total No. of Patients	Chemotherapeutic Regimen	Response Rates (%)	Median Survival (months)
Forastiere[104]	88	MTX	10	5.6
	86	CBDCA/5-FU	21*	5.0
	87	CDDP/5-FU	32**	6.6
Jacobs[105]	83	CDDP	17	5.0
	83	5-FU	13	6.1
	79	CDDP/5-FU	32***	5.5
Clavel[106]	113	CDDP	15	5.3
	116	CDDP/5-FU	31****	6.2
	127	CDDP/MTX/BLM/VCR	34*****	8.2

TABLE 22–8. RANDOMIZED STUDIES IN PATIENTS WITH RECURRENT AND/OR METASTATIC HEAD AND NECK TUMORS COMPARING SINGLE-AGENTS VERSUS COMBINATION CHEMOTHERAPY REGIMENS

BLM = bleomycin; CBDCA = carboplatin; CDDP = cisplatin; 5-FU = 5-fluorouracil; MTX = methotrexate; VCR = vincristine
* $P = 0.5$ vs. MTX; ** $P = 0.01$ vs. MTX; ***$P = 0.035$ vs. CDDP and $P = 0.005$ vs. 5-FU; **** $P = 0.003$ vs. CDDP; ***** $P < 0.001$ vs. CDDP.

tasis is higher compared with more typical squamous cell carcinomas of the head and neck. Approximately 5 to 11 percent of patients will present with clinical evidence of metastatic disease initially, although studies that included extensive staging evaluation, including radiographic studies and bone marrow assessment, have shown distant metastasis in approximately 40 percent of cases.[109]

Radiation alone is the cornerstone of treatment. Nasopharyngeal carcinoma can be quite responsive to chemotherapy, and given the propensity for distant metastasis in many patients, there has been interest in the potential ability of chemotherapy when combined with radiation to improve on results. Relevant studies are summarized in Table 22–9.

The three studies evaluating the addition of sequential chemotherapy failed to demonstrate an impact on overall survival.[110–112] The largest of these trials was performed under the direction of the Institute Gustave-Roussy and included 339 patients with advanced nasopharyngeal carcinoma. The treatment arms compared neoadjuvant chemotherapy with bleomycin, epirubicin, and cisplatin followed by radiation therapy versus the same dose of radiotherapy alone. The median follow-up was 49 months. The complete response rate in the chemotherapy/ radiotherapy arm was significantly higher compared with the radiotherapy alone arm. Also a lower number of failures were reported in the chemotherapy arm (32.7% vs. 54.7%, $p < 0.01$), as well a superior disease-free survival ($p < 0.01$). However, there was no statistical difference in the overall survival between the two arms, and the treatment-related mortality was higher in the chemotherapy/radiotherapy arm as well (8% vs. 1%).[110]

The other two sequential chemotherapy studies not only failed to show any significant advantage in overall survival with the addition of chemotherapy, but also disease-free survival seemed unaffected.[111,112] The negative results of the National Milan Institute study cannot be explained by poor patient compliance, as only 9 percent of the entire patient population randomized to the chemotherapy arm refused to undergo chemotherapy. However, two major criticisms of this trial are that the chemotherapy regimen utilized (vincristine, oral cyclophosphamide, and doxorubicin) did not include the most active chemotherapeutic agents for this disease, and patients who achieved a major response, but still had residual disease, were randomized.[111] The randomized study performed at the Prince of Wales Hospital included only 82 patients with nasopharyngeal carcinoma (nodal stage N3 or with lymph node ≥ 4 cm). Besides the risk of a false-negative result, another limitation was that the cisplatin/5-fluorouracil was administered using a nonstandard dosing schedule.[112]

The Intergroup 0099 trial used a fundamentally different treatment design. This study evaluated the role of chemotherapy (cisplatin 100 mg/m^2 IV on days 1, 22, and 43) administered concurrently with radiation therapy followed by three cycles of cisplatin and infusional 5-fluorouracil versus the same radiotherapy dosing alone (70 Gy in 35 fractions over 7 weeks) in patients with locally advanced stage III or IV nasopharyngeal carcinoma. Toxicity was greater in the chemotherapy/radiotherapy arm as only 63 percent and 55 percent of patients were able to complete the concurrent and adjuvant chemotherapies, respectively. The chemoradiation arm was associated with higher 3-year progression-

Table 22–9. RANDOMIZED TRIALS OF COMBINED MODALITY THERAPY VERSUS RADIATION THERAPY ALONE IN THE TREATMENT OF ADVANCED NASOPHARYNGEAL CARCINOMA						
Author or Group	Total No. of Patients	CT/RT Schedule	CT Regimen	Control Arm— Fractionation	Overall Survival Benefit (p < 0.05)
Gustave Roussy Institute[111]	339	Neoadjuvant	CDDP/BLM/EPI	RT—standard	*No
National Milan Institute[112]	229	Adjuvant	VCR/CTX/ DOXO	RT—standard	No
Prince of Wales Hospital[113]	82	Neoadjuvant + adjuvant	CDDP/5-FU	RT—standard	No
Intergroup 0099[5]	193	Concurrent + adjuvant	CDDP-concurrent CDDP/5-FU-adjuvant	RT—standard	Yes

* Superior disease-free survival at 49 months follow-up for the induction chemotherapy arm (p < 0.01).
BLM = bleomycin; CDDP = cisplatin; CT = chemotherapy; CTX = cyclophosphamide; DOXO = doxorubicin; 5-FU = 5-fluorouracil; EPI = epirubicin; RT = radiotherapy; VCR = vincristine

free (69% vs. 24%, p < 0.001) and overall survival (78% vs. 47%, p=0.005).[5] The compelling results of this study have had a dramatic impact on the management of nasopharynx cancer. This program is now widely applied as the standard approach to patients with advanced locoregional disease.

In the recurrent/metastatic disease setting, nasopharynx cancer may be somewhat more responsive than more typical squamous cell carcinomas of the head and neck. Although such disease is incurable in most cases, durable complete responses have been reported in selected patients.[113,114] Drugs are chosen based on activity demonstrated in other epithelial cancers of the upper aerodigestive tract. There are, however, a limited number of site-specific nasopharynx cancer studies. 4'-epidoxorubicin and mitoxantrone, both as single agents, are associated with response rates of approximately 20 percent.[115,116] Paclitaxel is an active drug in the treatment of recurrent/metastatic nasopharynx carcinoma as demonstrated by Au and colleagues.[117] Paclitaxel was administered at a dose of 175 mg/m^2 by a 3-hour infusion in 23 patients, and a major response rate of 26 percent was reported. All patients included had prior exposure to radiation therapy but none of them had had previous chemotherapy as a part of their initial treatment.

With regard to the activity of combination regimens in this recurrent/metastatic disease population, Mahjoubi and colleagues evaluated the combination of bleomycin, epirubicin and cisplatin, and reported overall and complete response rates of 45 percent and 20 percent, respectively. Approximately 10 percent of the patients were still in complete remission with a follow-up ranging from 30 to 46+ months.[116] Taamma and colleagues investigated the combination of cisplatin, 5-fluorouracil, bleomycin and epirubicin, and reported an overall response rate of 75 percent, with two patients having complete responses. Of note, all the patients had received prior radiation treatment and half of them had previously been treated with chemotherapy. The median duration of response was 10 months.[118] The major toxicities in both trials were myelosuppression and mucositis.[114,118]

CHEMOPREVENTION

Slaughter and colleagues popularized the concept of "field cancerization" over 40 years ago.[119] Advances in our understanding of the molecular biology of head and neck cancer and integration of this information with clinicopathologic observations have subsequently supported the concept of a multi-step process for head and neck carcinogenesis.[120,121] Unfortunately, even among individuals with a history of head and neck cancer that cease tobacco and/or alcohol consumption, the risk of second primary cancers persists at a rate of 3 to 7 percent/year.[16,122]

The goal of chemoprevention is to intervene with natural or synthetic compounds during the earlier stages of carcinogenesis in hopes of suppressing, or even reversing, the cascade of events leading to invasive cancer. The promise of chemoprevention is not limited to head and neck cancers.[33] An enormous number and spectrum of drugs are under evaluation, the rationale for certain classes of agents often derived from supporting epidemiologic data. Chemoprevention has generated special interest in head and neck cancers, given concerns regarding field cancerization; the high incidence of oral premalignant lesions with significant rates of progression to cancer and concurrent/metachronous cancers; the multifocality of these lesions that are often not amenable to surgical resection; and feasible response monitoring. Reversal of an evaluable premalignant lesion as a measure of a particular agent's activity is one mechanism used to identify compounds that offer potential promise as adjuvant therapies (Figure 22–2).

Vitamin A and its analogues, especially the retinoids, form the class of drugs most studied in chemoprevention.[33] Retinoids may be either natural (eg, all-*trans*-retinoic acid, retinyl-palmitate) or synthesized (eg, 13-*cis*-retinoic acid, fenretiditine). They are capable of modifying and modulating cell growth, differentiation, proliferation and apoptosis of normal, dysplatic and malignant tissue through a variety of mechanisms.[123] These activities are mediated by their binding to the retinoid acid receptors (RARs/RXRs and subtypes), and ligand-activated DNA proteins, with further modulation of gene transcription.[124] They have differences regarding mechanisms of action and function (RARs appear to affect cell differentiation and RXRs affect apoptosis) and ligands.[125]

Hong and colleagues demonstrated the ability of isotretinoin (13-*cis*-retinoic acid) to reverse leuko-

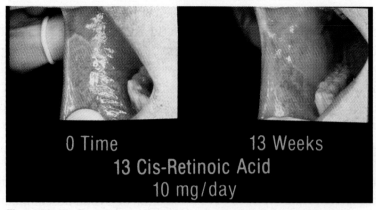

0 Time   13 Weeks
13 Cis-Retinoic Acid
10 mg/day

Figure 22–2.   Regression of leukoplakia after treatment with isotretinoin.

plakia in a trial that included 44 patients randomized to receive high-dose isotretinoin at the dose of 1 to 2 mg/kg/day or placebo for 3 months. The patients were followed for 6 months. Partial and complete remissions were more often seen in the retinoid arm (67% vs. 10%, p = 0.0002). The reversal of dysplasia was reported in 54 percent of patients in the treatment arm versus 10 percent of those in the placebo arm (p = 0.01). However, nine of the 16 patients of the isotretinoin arm relapsed 2 to 3 months after therapy discontinuation, suggesting the need for maintenance therapy. Common toxicities included skin dryness and/or peeling, cheilitis, hypertriglyceridemia and conjunctivitis, but these were reversible after treatment.[9] Vitamin A has also been demonstrated, according to randomized trials, to cause regression of leukoplakia.[126]

The concern regarding the high relapse rates after treatment discontinuation, as well as associated treatment-related toxicity with higher-dose isotretinoin, led the investigators at the M.D. Anderson Cancer Center to design a randomized trial that included maintenance therapy with low-dose isotretinoin administered after the induction part of the treatment. After induction therapy with 1.5 mg/kg/day for 3 months, patients with responding or stable premalignant lesions were randomized for 9 months to low-dose isotretinoin at the daily dose of 0.5 mg/kg/day or to beta carotene 30 mg/day. The 1-year premalignant lesion progression rates were lower in the retinoid arm (8% vs. 55%, p < 0.001),[10] although with a longer follow-up (66 months) there was no significant difference between the two arms regarding the inci-

dence of in situ or invasive carcinoma, as well as overall time to cancer development.[127] The short-term duration of the maintenance therapy and the limited number of patients included might have contributed to the lack of observed difference between arms in these endpoints. Fenretidine was evaluated as maintenance therapy for 12 months after resection of premalignant lesions, and decreased the rate of relapse compared to no therapy.[128]

Randomized trials assessing application of chemopreventive agents as an adjuvant strategy in head and neck cancer are less common. Hong and colleagues randomized 103 patients with head and neck carcinomas, stages I to IV, who had prior surgery, radiation therapy or both, to receive high-dose isotretinoin or placebo for 12 months. The initial dose of isotretinoin was 100 mg/m^2, but was subsequently reduced to 50 mg/m^2 because of the high toxicity rate. The rates of local, regional, and distant disease progression were similar between the two arms, as was the median survival. With a median follow-up of 55 months, however, the rate of second primaries was higher in the placebo arm (31% versus 14%, p = 0.004), as was the incidence of tobacco-related second primary cancer (p = 0.008). The incidence of skin dryness, cheilitis, and hypertriglyceridemia (p = 0.019) were higher in the isotretinoin arm. The treatment was not completed in 33 percent of patients in the retinoid arm because of toxicity.[11,129] Based on what was learned from this study, the current Intergroup chemoprevention study is evaluating a lower-dose, presumably less toxic isotretinoin dosing schedule, and only patients with a history of stage I and II cancer, who are less likely to die from their index disease, are eligible.

Bolla and colleagues evaluated the second generation retinoid, etretinate, as an adjuvant strategy in 324 patients with oral or oropharynx carcinoma staged T1 or T2, N0 or N1 ≤ 3 cm, and M0 status post locoregional treatment. Patients were randomized to etretinate or placebo for 24 months. Unlike the M.D. Anderson Cancer Center trial, this study did not show an effect on the incidence of second primary tumors. The survival between the arms was also not significantly different. There was a higher incidence of labial, cutaneous, and ocular toxicity, and onycholysis, seen on the etretinate arm.[12] In this study, the proportion of patients who stopped smoking after the definitive locoregional treatment was not recorded, nor was patient compliance recorded, which may influence the results. Also, the second primary tumor incidence in this trial was higher overall compared to other trials that evaluated the efficacy of retinoic acid intervention.

Other studies are evaluating the combination of vitamin A, *N*-acetylcysteine, and beta carotene as adjuvants.[130,131] One study of note is the so-called Euroscan being done in patients with early stage head and neck cancer (60.2%) and lung cancer (39.8%). A total of 2,592 patients from 15 countries are included. Patients were randomized to receive retinyl-palmitate 300,000 IU daily for the first year, and half of the dose for the second year, or *N*-acetylcysteine 600 mg daily for 2 years, or the combination of both, or observation. The patients in the retinyl-palmitate arm presented with higher incidence of overall and severe toxicity. The final results are pending.[130]

Clinical trials to date have yielded provocative information regarding the use and potential impact of chemopreventive agents. Until more information is available, however, these data fail to support the routine use of these drugs as part of standard treatment. It should be emphasized that in certain trials addressing lung cancer prevention, the chemopreventive agent may have adversely affected outcome.[132,133] Ongoing and planned randomized trials should provide important insights. The identification of reliable intermediate markers of risk may facilitate such studies, as they currently require very large numbers of patients and a long follow-up period.

Chemotherapy for Salivary Gland Cancers

Major and minor salivary gland cancers represent approximately 5 to 10 percent of head and neck malignancies.[134,135] In general, surgery and/or radiation have been the principle treatment modalities, with chemotherapy primarily used in the recurrent/metastatic disease setting. As a single modality, chemotherapy is not curative.

Because of the relative rarity and heterogeneity of these tumors, the available data on the efficacy of systemic therapy is often of poor quality. Many series are small, are developed in a retrospective manner, and combine different salivary gland cancer subtypes even though drug activity may vary among them.[136] Single-agent activity has been shown for doxorubicin, cisplatin, 5-fluorouracil, and selected other drugs.[137–142] The minority of patients will have a major response. In general, the response rates associated with combination therapy are higher than those with a single agent. Selected combination regimens are summarized in Table 22–10. The combination of cyclophosphamide, doxorubicin and cisplatin is probably the most widely used. The clinical benefit of combination versus single-agent therapy, however, has not been well studied. Considering investigational, even phase I, studies from the outset for such patients is quite reasonable. There is currently no demonstrated role for induction or adjuvant chemotherapy. As with squamous cell head and neck cancers, concurrent chemotherapy/radiation is often considered for unresectable tumors, although the practice guidelines for one major organization specify radiation alone (neutrons or photons) as the recommended therapy for these patients.[147]

Often initial close observation is the best treatment option for certain patients. Many of these tumors may behave in an indolent manner. A good example is adenoid cystic carcinoma, a subtype that, even while associated with frequent distant metastases, can relapse late and grow slowly for years, especially when the metastases are limited to the lung (Figure 22–3).

Chemotherapy for Thyroid Cancer

As with salivary gland tumors, thyroid cancer constitutes a spectrum of histologic subtypes and clinical

Table 22–10. COMBINATION CHEMOTHERAPY IN SALIVARY GLAND CANCER				
Author	No. of Patients	CT Regimen	Subtype	Overall Response Rates (%)
Triozzi[143]	8	5-FU/CTX/VCR	Adenoid cystic	25
Posner[144]	3	CDDP/BLM/MTX	Mucoepidermoid	33
Airoldi[141]	3	CDDP/5-FU	Mucoepidermoid	33
Venook[145]	17	CDDP/DOXO/5-FU	*Variable	35
Airoldi[141]	9	CDDP/EPI/5-FU or CTX	*Variable	45
Posner[144]	11	CTX/DOXO	*Variable	45
Dimery[146]	16	CTX/DOXO/CDDP	*Variable	50

* Variable: includes adenoid cystic carcinoma and mucoepidermoid carcinoma as the most common histologies.
BLM = bleomycin; CDDP = cisplatin; CT = chemotherapy; CTX = cyclophosphamide; DOXO = doxorubicin; 5-FU = 5-fluorouracil; EPI = epirubicin; MTX = methotrexate; VCR = vincristine.

behaviors that should be considered when making decisions regarding the role of systemic therapy. Chemotherapy is most commonly considered after surgery and/or radiation therapy (external beam, and if applicable, radioactive iodine [RAI]) have failed, as induction/adjuvant chemotherapy is of unproven benefit. Chemotherapy by itself is not a curative modality. The available data to aid clinical decision-making is limited in both quantity and quality. Investigational studies from the start are appropriate to consider.

For differentiated histologies (eg, papillary or follicular), radioactive iodine (RAI) is the initial systemic therapy of choice. Before considering chemotherapy, evaluating the adequacy and quality of prior therapy with RAI should be the first step. For example, recent intravenous iodinated contrast, consumption of an iodine-rich diet, inadequate levels of thyroid stimulating hormone (TSH), or persistence of a significant amount of native thyroid cancer may all affect the efficacy of RAI treatment for the tumor. For RAI-refractory disease, initial observation is appropriate for selected patients, as the tumor may grow slowly. If chemotherapy is indicated, doxorubicin is the most studied and widely used drug, with response rates in the 30 to 40 percent range.[148,149] Cisplatin, carboplatin, methotrexate, and etoposide also have activity.[150] Combination chemotherapy may improve response rate but has unproven benefit in terms of palliation and survival. Chemotherapy and radiation have been combined for the treatment of compelling local disease with good local effect in most patients.[151,152] The possible use of agents intended to

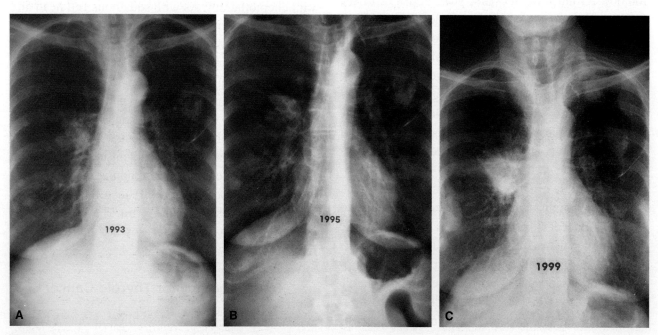

Figure 22–3.   Chest-radiographs, years apart, in a patient with adenoid cystic cancer with no treatment.

differentiate the tumor (eg, retinoids) and help it regain RAI avidity is an area of active interest.[153]

Anaplastic thyroid cancer is an aggressive subtype with a poor prognosis even with the best available therapy. Generally these tumors are unresectable at presentation and are not RAI avid. Combined modality chemotherapy/radiation programs [151,152] are commonly employed initially in the management of these cancers with reported improvement compared to historical results with radiation alone. There are, however, no randomized data, and survival statistics remain disappointing. When chemotherapy is employed alone, one randomized trial reported a higher complete response when doxorubicin and cisplatin were combined compared to doxorubicin alone.[154] Of note, a large cell lymphoma of the thyroid can present in a manner similar to anaplastic thyroid cancer, but the former will have a better prognosis and chemotherapy for the disease is much more effective. Accordingly, the initial pathology review is extremely important.

Medullary carcinoma is another cancer that can behave in an indolent manner, where initial observation in order to get a sense of disease trajectory is often a good option for the patient. Streptozocin, cyclophosphamide, dacarbazine, and 5-fluorouracil appear to have some activity, alone or in combination, but only a minority of patients will have a major response.[155,156] Many of these patients will suffer from troublesome diarrhea for which debulking of gross tumor or a trial of octreotide or interferon-α may be helpful.[157,158] Occasionally these patients will present to the medical oncologist without appropriate screening studies having been done to rule out a familial syndrome. If so, an appropriate screening evaluation should be initiated.

REFERENCES

1. Weissler MC, Melin S, Sailer SL, et al. Simultaneous chemoradiation in the treatment of advanced head and neck cancer. Arch Otolaryngol Head Neck Surg 1992; 118:806–10.
2. Brizel DM, Albers ME, Fisher SR, et al. Hyperfractionated irradiation with or without chemotherapy for locally advanced head and neck cancer. N Engl J Med 1997;338:1798–804.
3. Wendt TG, Grabenbauer GG, Rödel CM, et al. Simultaneous radiochemotherapy versus radiotherapy alone in advanced head and neck cancer: a randomized study. J Clin Oncol 1998;16:1318–24.
4. Merlano M, Benasso M, Corvo R, et al. Five-year update of a randomized trial of alternating radiotherapy and chemotherapy compared with radiotherapy alone in treatment of unresectable squamous cell carcinoma of the head and neck. J Natl Cancer Inst 1996;88:583–9.
5. Al-Sarraf M, LeBlanc M, Giri PGS, et al. Chemoradiotherapy versus radiotherapy in patients with advanced nasopharyngeal cancer: phase III randomized Intergroup Study 0099. J Clin Oncol 1998;16:1310–7.
6. Calais G, Alfonsi M, Bardet E, et al. Randomized trial of radiation therapy versus concomitant chemotherapy and radiation therapy for advanced-stage oropharynx carcinoma. J Natl Cancer Inst 1999;91:2081–86.
7. The Department of Veterans Affairs Laryngeal Cancer Study Group. Induction chemotherapy plus radiation compared with surgery plus radiation in patients with advanced laryngeal cancer. N Engl J Med 1991;324:1685–90.
8. Lefebvre JL, Chevalier D, Luboinski B, et al. Larynx preservation in pyriform sinus cancer: preliminary results from a European Organization for Research and Treatment of Cancer phase III trial. EORTC Head and Neck Cancer Cooperative Group. J Natl Cancer Inst 1996;88:890–9.
9. Hong WK, Endicott J, Itri LM, et al. 13-*cis*-retinoic acid in the treatment of oral leukoplakia. N Engl J Med 1986; 315:1501–5.
10. Lippman SM, Batsakis JG, Toth BB, et al. Comparison of low-dose isotretinoin with beta carotene to prevent oral carcinogenesis. N Engl J Med 1993;328:15–20.
11. Hong WK, Lippman SM, Itri LM, et al. Prevention of second primary tumors with isotretinoin in squamous-cell carcinoma of the head and neck. N Engl J Med 1990;323: 795–801.
12. Bolla M, Lefur R, Ton Van J, et al. Prevention of second primary tumors with etretinate in squamous cell carcinoma of the oral cavity and oropharynx. Results of a multicentric double-blind randomised study. Eur J Cancer 1994; 30A:767–72.
13. Sauer R, Wannenmacher M, Wasserman T, et al. Randomized phase III trial of radiation with or without amifostine in patients with head and neck cancer. Proc Am Soc Clin Oncol 1999;18:392.
14. Rieke JW, Hafermann MD, Johnson JT, et al. Oral pilocarpine for radiation-induced xerostomia: integrated efficacy and safety results from two prospective randomized clinical trials. Int J Radiat Oncol Biol Phys 1995;31:661–9.
15. Piccirillo JF. Inclusion comorbidity in a staging system for head and neck cancer. Oncology 1995;9:831–6.
16. Shaha AR, Hoover EL, Mitrani M, et al. Synchronicity, multicentricity and metachronicity of the head and neck cancer. Head Neck 1988;10:225–8.
17. Head and Neck Contracts Program. Adjuvant chemotherapy for advanced head and neck squamous carcinoma: final report of the Head and Neck Contracts Program. Cancer 1987;60:301–11.
18. Beziak A, Grilli R, Browman G. Non-resectability in radiotherapy trials in squamous cell carcinoma of the head and neck—implications for generalizability of trials results. Proc Am Soc Clin Oncol 1995;14:296.

19. Vokes EE, Weichselbaum RR. Concomitant chemoradiotherapy: rationale and clinical experience in patients with solid tumors. J Clin Oncol 1990;8:911–34.

20. Schantz SP, Harrison LB, Forastiere AA. Tumors of nasal cavity and paranasal sinuses, nasopharynx, oral cavity, and oropharynx. In: De Vita V Jr, Hellman S, Rosenberg SA, editors. Principles of Practice and Oncology. 5th ed. Philadelphia: Lippincott-Raven Publishers; 1997. p. 741–801.

21. Smith RE, Thornton DE, Allen J. A phase II trial of paclitaxel in squamous cell carcinoma of the head and neck with correlative laboratories studies. Semin Oncol 1995;22 (3 Suppl 6):41–46.

22. Gebbia V, Testa G, Cannata G, et al. Single agent paclitaxel in advanced squamous cell head and neck carcinoma. Eur J Cancer 1996;32A:901–2.

23. Forastiere AA, Shank D, Neuberg D, et al. Final report of a phase II evaluation of paclitaxel with advanced squamous cell carcinoma of the head and neck. Cancer 1998;82:2270–4.

24. Vermorken JB, Catimel G, de Mulder P, et al. Randomized phase II trial of weekly methotrexate (MTX) versus two schedules or triweekly paclitaxel (Taxol®) in patients with metastatic or recurrent squamous cell carcinoma of the head and neck (SCCHN). Proc Am Soc Clin Oncol 1999;18:395.

25. Catimel G, Verwij J, Hanauske A. Docetaxel (taxotere): an active drug for the treatment of patients with advanced squamous cell carcinoma of the head and neck. Ann Oncol 1994;5:533–7.

26. Dreyfuss AI, Clark J, Norris C, et al. Docetaxel: an active drug for squamous cell carcinoma of the head and neck. J Clin Oncol 1996;14:1672–8.

27. Colevas D, Posner MR. Docetaxel in head and neck cancer. Am J Clin Oncol 1998;21:482–6.

28. Huber MH, Lippman SM, Benner SE, et al. A phase II study of ifosfamide in recurrent squamous cell carcinoma of the head and neck. Am J Clin Oncol 1996;19:379–83.

29. Buesa JM, Fernandez R, Esteban E, et al. Phase II trial of ifosfamide in recurrent and metastatic head and neck cancer. Ann Oncol 1991;2:151–2.

30. Martin M, Diaz-Rubio E, Gonzales-Larriba JL, et al. Ifosfamide in advanced epidermoid head and neck cancer. Cancer Chemother Pharmacol 1993;31:340–2.

31. Cervellino JC, Araujo CE, Pirisi C, et al. Ifosfamide and mesna for the treatment of advanced squamous cell head and neck cancer. Oncology 1991;48:89–92.

32. Catimel G, Vermorken JB, Clavel M, et al. A phase II study of gemcitabine (LY 188011) in patients with advanced squamous cell carcinoma of the head and neck. Ann Oncol 1994;5:543–7.

33. Lippman SM, Bronner SE, Hong WK. Cancer chemoprevention. J Clin Oncol 1994;12:851–73.

34. Kish J, Drelichman A, Jacobs J, et al. Clinical trial of cisplatin and 5-FU infusion as initial treatment for advanced squamous cell carcinoma of the head and neck. Cancer Treat Rep 1982;66:471–4.

35. Paccagnella A, Orlando A, Marchiori C, et al. Phase III trial of initial chemotherapy in stage III and IV head and neck cancers: a study by the Gruppo di Studio sui Tumori della Testa e del Collo. J Natl Cancer Inst 1994;86:265–72.

36. Colevas AD, Busse PM, Norris CM, et al. Induction chemotherapy with docetaxel, cisplatin, 5-fluorouracil, leucovorin (TPFL5) for squamous cell carcinoma of the head and neck: a phase I/II trial. J Clin Oncol 1998;16:1331–9.

37. Dunphy F, Boyd J, Dunleavy T. Paclitaxel and carboplatin in head and neck cancer. Semin Oncol 1997;24(6 Suppl 19):25–27.

38. Hitt R, Hornedo J, Colomer R, et al. Study of escalating doses of paclitaxel and cisplatin in patients with inoperable head and neck cancer. Semin Oncol 1997;24(1 Suppl 2):58–64.

39. Wang H-M, Wang C-H, Chen J-S, Lin Y-C. Cisplatin (C), tegafur (T), leucovorin (L): an effective, less toxic, and outpatient neoadjuvant chemotherapy (CT) for squamous cell carcinoma of the head and neck (SCCHN). Proc Am Soc Clin Oncol 1999;18:400.

40. Gebbia V, Mantovani G, Farris A, et al. Vinorelbine, cisplatin, and 5-fluorouracil as initial treatment for previously untreated, unresectable squamous cell carcinoma of the head and neck: results of a phase II study. Cancer 1997;79:1394–400.

41. Rivera F, López-Brea M, Pascual C, et al. Interim analysis of a phase III study of cisplatin and 5-FU continuous infusion (PF) vs. cisplatin, UFT and vinorelbine (UFTVP) as induction chemotherapy (IC) in locally advanced squamous cell head and neck cancer (SCHNC). Proc Am Soc Clin Oncol 1999;18:399.

42. Pai VR, Mazumdar AT, Parikh DM, et al. Gemcitabine with ifosfamide, cisplatin combination chemotherapy in advanced head and neck cancer. Proc Am Soc Clin Oncol 1999;18:408.

43. Hartsell WF, Thomas CR, Murthy AK, et al. Pilot study for the evaluation of simultaneous cisplatin/5-fluorouracil infusion and limited radiation therapy in regionally recurrent head and neck cancer. Am J Clin Oncol 1998;17:338–43.

44. De Crevoisier R, Bouhris J, Domenge C, et al. Full-dose reirradiation for unresectable head and neck carcinoma: experience at the Gustave-Roussy Institute in a series of 169 patients. J Clin Oncol 1998;16:3556–62.

45. Mossman KL. Frequent short-term oral complications of head and neck radiotherapy. Ear Nose Throat J 1994;73:316–20.

46. El-Sayed S, Nelson N. Adjuvant and adjunctive chemotherapy in the management of squamous cell carcinoma of the head and neck region: a meta-analysis of prospective randomized trials. J Clin Oncol 1996;14:838–47.

47. Fu KK, Pajak TF, Trotti A, et al. A Radiation Therapy Oncology Group (RTOG) phase III randomized study to compare hyperfractionation and two variants of accelerated fractionation to standard fractionation radiotherapy for head and neck squamous cell carcinomas: preliminary results ot RTOG 9003. Int J Radiat Oncol Biol Phys 1999;45:145.

48. Adelstein DJ. Induction chemotherapy in head and neck cancer. Hematol Oncol Clin North Am 1999;13:689–98.

49. Schuller DE, Metch B, Mattox D, et al. Preoperative chemotherapy in advanced resectable head and neck cancer: final report of the Southwest Oncology Group. Laryngoscope 1988;98:1205–11.

50. Laramore GE, Scott CB, Al-Sarraf M, et al, Adjuvant chemotherapy for resectable squamous cell carcinomas of the head and neck: report on Intergroup study 0034.Int J Radiat Oncol Biol Phys 1992;23:705–13.

51. Richard JM, Kramar A, Molinari R, et al. Randomised EORTC head and neck cooperative group trial of preoperative intra-arterial chemotherapy in oral cavity and oropharynx carcinoma. Eur J Cancer 1991;27:821–7.

52. Depondt J, Gehanno P, Martin M, et al. Neoadjuvant chemotherapy with carboplatin/5-fluorouracil in head and neck cancer. Oncology 1993;50(Suppl 2):23-7.

53. Dalley D, Beller E, Aroney R, et al. The value of chemotherapy (CT) prior to definitive local therapy (DLT) in patients with locally advanced squamous cell carcinoma (SCC) of the head and neck (HN). Proc Am Soc Clin Oncol 1995;14:297.

54. Domenge C, Marandas P, Vignoud J, et al. Post-surgical adjuvant chemotherapy in extra-capsular spread invaded node (N + R +) of epidermoid carcinoma of the head and neck. A randomized multicentric trial. Second International Conference in Head and Neck, Boston, 1988. Am Soc Head Neck Surg 1988;74.

55. Horiuchi M, Inuyama Y, Miyake H, and the Head and Neck UFT Study Group. Efficacy of surgical adjuvant with tegafur and uracil (UFT) in resectable head and neck cancer: a prospective randomized study. Proc Am Soc Clin Oncol 1994;13:284.

56. Di Blasio B, Barbieri W, Bozzetti A, et al. A prospective randomized trial in resectable head and neck carcinoma: loco-regional treatment with and without neoadjuvant chemotherapy. Proc Am Soc Clin Oncol 1994;13:279.

57. Jacobs C, Makuch R. Efficacy of adjuvant chemotherapy for patients with resectable head and neck cancer: a subset analysis of the head and neck contracts program. J Clin Oncol 1990;8:838–47.

58. Ervin TJ, Clark JR, Weichselbaum RR, et al. An analysis of induction and adjuvant chemotherapy in the multidisciplinary treatment of squamous-cell carcinoma of the head and neck. J Clin Oncol 1987;5:10–20.

59. Stell PM. Adjuvant chemotherapy in head and neck cancer. Semin Radiat Oncol 1992;2:195–205.

60. Browman GP, Cronin L. Standard chemotherapy in squamous cell head and neck cancer: what we have learned from randomized trials. Semin Oncol 1994;21:311–9.

61. Bourhis J, Pignon JP, Designé L, et al. Meta-analysis of chemotherapy in head and neck (MACH-NC): (1) Loco-regional treatment vs same treatment + chemotherapy (CT). Proc Am Soc Clin Oncol 1998;17:386.

62. Munro AJ. An overview of randomised controlled trials of adjuvant chemotherapy in head and neck cancer. Br J Cancer 1995;71:83–91.

63. Shanta V, Krishnamurthi S. Combined bleomycin and radiotherapy in oral cancer. Clin Radiol 1980;31:617–20.

64. Sanchíz F, Milla A, Torner J, et al. Single-fraction per day versus two fractions per day versus radiochemotherapy in the treatment of head and neck cancer. Int J Radiat Oncol Biol Phys 1990;19:1347–50.

65. Browman GP, Cripps C, Hodson DI, et al. Placebo-controlled randomized trial of infusional fluorouracil during standard radiotherapy in locally advanced head and neck cancer. J Clin Oncol 1994;12:2648–53.

66. Gupta NK, Pointon RCS, Wilkinson PM. A randomized clinical trial to contrast radiotherapy with radiotherapy and methotrexate given synchronously in head and neck cancer. Clin Radiol 1987;38:575–81.

67. Weissberg JB, Son YH, Papac RJ, et al. Randomized clinical trial of mitomycin C as an adjunct to radiotherapy in head and neck cancer. Int J Radiat Oncol Biol Phys 1989;17:3–9.

68. Lo TC, Wiley AL Jr, Ansfield FJ, et al. Combined radiation therapy and 5-fluorouracil for advanced squamous cell carcinoma of the oral cavity and oropharynx: a randomized study. Am J Roentgenol 1976;126:229–35.

69. Arcangeli G, Nervi C, Righini R, et al. Combined radiation and drugs: the effect of intra-arterial chemotherapy followed by radiotherapy in head and neck cancer. Radiother Oncol 1983;1:101–7.

70. Fu KK, Phillips TL, Silverberg IJ, et al. Combined radiotherapy and chemotherapy with bleomycin and methotrexate for advanced inoperable head and neck cancer: update of a Northern California Oncology Group randomized trial. J Clin Oncol 1987;5:1410–8.

71. Eschwege F, Sancho-Garnier H, Gerard JP, et al. Ten-year results of randomized trial comparing radiotherapy and concomitant bleomycin to radiotherapy alone in epidermoid carcinomas of the oropharynx: experience of the European Organization for Research and Treatment of Cancer. NCI Monogr 1988;6:275–8.

72. Vermund H, Kaalhus O, Winther F, et al. Bleomycin and radiation therapy in squamous cell carcinoma of the upper aero-digestive tract: a phase III clinical trial. Int J Radiat Oncol Biol Phys 1985;11:1877–86.

73. Gabriele P, Tessa M, Ragona R, et al. An interim analysis of phase III study on radiotherapy (RT) versus RT plus carboplatin (CBDCA) in inoperable stage III-IV head and neck (H&N) carcinoma. Proceedings of the 4th International Conference on Head and Neck Cancer 1996; Toronto, Canada.

74. Haselow RE, Warshaw MG, Oken MM, et al. Radiation alone versus radiation with weekly low-dose cisplatinum in unresectable cancer of the head and neck. In: Fee WE Jr, Goepfert H, Johns ME, et al., editors. Head and Neck, vol. II. Philadelphia: JB Lippincott; 1990. p. 279–81.

75. Bachaud JM, Cohen-Jonathan E, Alzieu C, David JM, et al. Combined postoperative radiotherapy and weekly cisplatin infusion for locally advanced head and neck carcinoma: final report of a randomized trial. Int J Radiat Oncol Biol Phys 1996;36:999–1004.

76. Dobrowsky W, Naude J, Widder J, et al. Continuous hyperfractionated radiotherapy with/without mitomycin C in head and neck cancer. Int J Radiat Oncol Biol Phys 1998;42:803–6.

77. Aldelstein DJ, Saxton JP, Lavertu P, et al. A phase III trial comparing concurrent chemotherapy and radiotherapy with radiotherapy alone in resectable stage III and IV squamous cell head and neck cancer: preliminary results. Head Neck 1997;19:567–75.

78. Adelstein DJ, Lavertu P, Saxton JP, et al. Long-term results of a phase III randomized trial comparing concurrent chemoradiotherapy and radiation therapy (RT) alone in squamous cell head and neck cancer (SCHNC). Proc Am Soc Clin Oncol 1999;18:394.

79. Keane TJ, Cummings BJ, O'Sullivan B, et al. A randomized trial of radiation therapy compared to split course radiation therapy combined with mitomycin C and 5-fluorouracil as initial treatment for advanced laryngeal and hypopharyngeal squamous carcinoma. Int J Radiat Oncol Biol Phys 1993;25:613–8.

80. Lavertu P, Bonafede JP, Aldestein DJ, et al. Comparison of surgical complications after organ-preservation therapy in patients with stage III or IV squamous cell head and neck cancer. Arch Otolaryngol Head Neck Surg 1998;124:401–6.

81. A randomized trial of combined multidrug chemotherapy and radiotherapy in advanced squamous cell carcinoma of the head and neck. An interim report from the SECOG participants. South-East Co-operative Oncology Group. Eur J Surg Oncol 1986;12:289–95.

82. Adelstein DJ, Sharan VM, Earle AS, et al. Simultaneous versus sequential combined technique therapy for squamous cell head and neck cancer. Cancer 1990;65:1685–91.

83. Merlano M, Rosso R, Sertoli MR, et al. Randomized comparison of two chemotherapy, radiotherapy schemes for stage III and IV unresectable squamous cell carcinoma of the head and neck. Laryngoscope 1990;100:531–5.

84. Taylor IVSG, Murthy AK, Vannetzel JM, et al. Randomized comparison of neoadjuvant cisplatin and fluorouracil infusion followed by radiation versus concomitant treatment in advanced head and neck cancer. J Clin Oncol 1994;12:385–95.

85. Kies MS, Haraf DJ, Athanasiadis I, et al. Induction chemotherapy followed by concurrent chemoradiation for advanced head and neck cancer: improved disease control and survival. J Clin Oncol 1998;16:2715–21.

86. Sherman E, Pfister DG, Harrison L, et al. A comparison of concomitant cisplatin with accelerated radiation therapy versus conventional RT as part of larynx preservation strategy: results of multivariate analysis. Proc Am Soc Clin Oncol 1998.

87. Pfister DG, Harrison LB, Strong EW, Bosl GJ. Current status of larynx preservation with multimodality therapy. Oncol 1994;6:33–43.

88. Pfister DG, Strong E, Harrison L, et al. Larynx preservation with combined chemotherapy and radiation therapy in advanced but resectable head and neck cancer. J Clin Oncol 1991;9:850–9.

89. Karp DD, Vaughan CW, Carter R, et al. Larynx preservation using induction chemotherapy plus radiation therapy as an alternative to laryngectomy in advanced head and neck cancer. A long-term follow-up report. Am J Clin Oncol 1991;14:273–9.

90. McNeil BJ, Weichselbaum R, Pauker SG. Speech and survival: trade-offs between quality of life in laryngeal cancer. N Engl J Med 1981;305:982–7.

91. Harwood AR, Rawlinson E. The quality of life of patients following treatment for advanced laryngeal cancer. Int J Radiat Oncol Biol Phys 1983;9:335–8.

92. De Santo LW. T3 glottic cancer: options and consequences of the options. Laryngoscope 1984;94:1311–5.

93. Kazem I, van den Broek P, Huygen PL. Planned preoperative radiation therapy vs. definitive radiotherapy for advanced laryngeal carcinoma. Laryngoscope 1984;94:1355–8.

94. Richard JM, Sancho-Garnier H, Pessey JJ, et al. Randomized trial of induction chemotherapy in larynx carcinoma. Oral Oncol 1998;34:224–8.

95. Wolf GT, Hong WK, Fisher SG. Neoadjuvant chemotherapy for organ preservation: current status. Proceedings of the 4th International Conference in Head and Neck Cancer 1996;4:89–97.

96. Terrel JE, Fisher SG, Wolf GT. Long-term quality of life after the treatment of laryngeal cancer. Arch Otolaryngol Head Neck Surg 1998;124:964–71.

97. Lefebvre JL, Wolf G, Luboinski B, et al. Meta-analysis of chemotherapy in head and neck cancer (MACH-NC): (2) Larynx preservation using neoadjuvant chemotherapy (CT) in laryngeal and hypopharyngeal carcinoma. Proc Am Soc Clin Oncol 1998;17:382.

98. Hensley ML, Schuchter LM, Lindley C, et al. American Society of Clinical Oncology clinical practice guidelines for the use of chemotherapy and radiotherapy protectants. J Clin Oncol 1999;17:3333–55.

99. Buntzel J, Kuttner K, Frohlich, Glatzel M. Selective cytoprotection with amifostine in concurrent radiochemotherapy for head and neck cancer. Ann Oncol 1998;9:505–9.

100. Bohuslavizki KH, Klutmann S, Brenner W, et al. Salivary gland protection by amifostine in high-dose radioiodine treatment: results of a double-blind placebo-controlled study. J Clin Oncol 1998;16:3542–9.

101. Jacobs CD, van der Pas M. A multicenter maintenance study of oral pilocarpine tablets for radiation-induced xerostomia. Oncology (Huntingt) 1996;10 (3 Suppl):16–20.

102. Ning S, Shuii C, Khan WB, et al. Effects of keranocyte growth factor on the proliferation and radiation survival of human squamous cell carcinoma in vitro and in vivo. Int J Radiat Oncol Biol Phys 1997;40:177–87.

103. Plevová P. Prevention and treatment of chemotherapy—and radiotherapy—induced oral mucositis: a review. Oral Oncol 1999;35:453–70.

104. Forastiere AA, Metch B, Schuller DE, et al. Randomized comparison of cisplatin plus fluorouracil and carboplatin plus fluorouracil versus methotrexate in advanced squamous-cell carcinoma of the head and neck: a Southwest Oncology Group study. J Clin Oncol 1992;10:1245–51.

105. Jacobs C, Lyman G, Velez-Garcia E, et al. A phase III randomized study comparing cisplatin and fluorouracil as single agents and in combination for advanced squamous cell carcinoma of the head and neck. J Clin Oncol 1992;10:257–63.

106. Clavel M, Vermoken JB, Cognetti F, et al. A randomized comparison of cisplatin, methotrexate, bleomycin and vincristine (CABO) versus cisplatin and 5-fluorouracil (CF) versus cisplatin in recurrent or metastatic squamous cell carcinoma of the head and neck. Ann Oncol 1994;5:521–6.

107. Clayman GL, el-Naggar AK, Lipmann SM, et al. Adenovirus-mediated p53 transfer in patients with advanced recurrent head and neck squamous cell carcinoma. J Clin Oncol 1998;16:2221–32.

108. Brown D, Wang R, Russel P. Antiepidermal growth factor receptor antibodies augment cytotoxicity of chemotherapeutic agents on squamous cell carcinoma cell lines. Otolaryngol Head Neck Surg 2000;122:75–83.

109. Micheau C, Boussen H, Klijanienko J, et al. Bone marrow

biopsies in patients with undifferentiated carcinoma of nasopharyngeal type. Cancer 1987;60:2459–64.

110. International Nasopharynx Cancer Study Group: VUMCA I trial. Preliminary results of a randomized trial comparing neoadjuvant chemotherapy (cisplatin, epirubicin, bleomycin) plus radiotherapy vs. radiotherapy alone in stage IV (≥ N2, M0) undifferentiated nasopharyngeal carcinoma: a positive effect on progression-free survival. Int J Radiat Oncol Biol Phys 1996;35:463–9.

111. Rossi A, Molinari R, Boracchi M, et al. Adjuvant chemotherapy with vincristine, cyclophosphamide, and adriamycin after radiotherapy in loco-regional nasopharyngeal cancer: result of a 4-year multicenter randomized study. J Clin Oncol 1988;6:1401–10.

112. Chan ATC, Teo PML, Leung WT, et al. A prospective randomized study of chemotherapy adjunctive to definitive radiotherapy in advanced nasopharyngeal carcinoma. Int J Radiat Biol Phys 1995;33:569–77.

113. Fandi A, Altun M, Azli M, et al. Nasopharyngeal cancer: epidemiology, staging, and treatment. Semin Oncol 1994; 21:382–97.

114. Mahjoubi R, Azli N, Bachouchi M, et al. Metastatic (MTS) undifferentiated carcinoma of nasopharyngeal type (UCNT) treated with bleomycin (B), epirubucin (E) and cisplatin (P) (BEC). Final report. Proc Am Soc Clin Oncol 1992;11:772.

115. Shiu WCT, Tsao SY. Efficacy of 4'-epidoxorubicin (pharmorubicin) in advanced nasopharyngeal carcinoma. Clinical Trials Journal 1989;26:419.

116. Dugan M, Choy D, Ngai A, et al. Multicenter phase II trial of mitoxantrone in patients with advanced nasopharyngeal carcinoma in Southeast Asia: an Asian-Oceanic Clinical Oncology Association Group study. J Clin Oncol 1993; 11:70–6.

117. Au E, Ang PT, Chua EJ. Paclitaxel in metastatic nasopharyngeal cancer. Proc Am Soc Clin Oncol 1996;15:919.

118. Taamma A, Fandi A, Azli N, et al. 5 fluorouracil (FU), bleomycin (BLM), epirubicin (E), cisplatin (P) in locally advanced (LA), recurrent and/or metastatic (REC/MTS) undifferentiated carcinoma nasopharyngeal type. (UCNT) preliminary activity/toxicity report. Proc Am Soc Clin Oncol 1996;15:909.

119. Slaughter DP, Southwick HW, Smejkal W. "Field cancerization" in oral stratified squamous epithelium: clinical implications of multicentric origin. Cancer 1953;6:963–8.

120. Shin DM, Kim J, Ro JY, et al. Activation of p53 gene expression in premalignant lesions during head and neck tumorigenesis. Cancer Res 1994;54:321–6.

121. Renan MJ. How many mutations are required for tumorigenesis? Implications from human cancer data. Mol Carcinog 1993;7:139–46.

122. Vokes EE, Weichselbaum RR, Lipman S, Hong WK. Head and neck cancer. N Engl J Med 1993;328:184–94.

123. Lotan R. Retinoids in cancer chemoprevention. FASEB J 1996;10:1031–9.

124. Mangelsdorf DJ, Umesono K, Evans RM. The retinoid receptors. In:Sporn MB, Roberts AB, Goodman DS, editors. The retinoids. New York: Raven Press; 1994. p. 319–49.

125. Nagy L, Thomazy VA, Shipley GL, et al. Activation of retinoid X receptors induces apoptosis in HL-60 cell lines. Mol Cell Biol 1995;15:3540–51.

126. Stich HF, Hornby AP, Mathew B, et al. Response of oral leukoplakias to the administration of vitamin A. Cancer Lett 1988;40:93–101.

127. Papadimitrakopoulou VA, Hong WK, Lee JS, et al. Low-dose isotretinoin versus β-carotene to prevent oral carcinogenesis: long-term follow-up. J Natl Cancer Inst 1997;89:257–8.

128. Chiesa F, Tradati N, Marazza M, et al. Fenretidine (4-HPR) in chemoprevention of oral leukoplakia. J Cell Biochem Suppl 1993;17:255–61.

129. Benner SE, Pajak TF, Lippman SM, et al. Prevention of second primary tumors with isotretinoin in squamous cell carcinoma of the head and neck: long-term follow-up. J Natl Cancer Inst 1994;86:140–1.

130. Van Zandwijk N, Pastorino U, De Vries N, et al. Randomized trial of chemoprevention with vitamin A and N-acetylcysteine in patients with cancer of the upper and lower airways: the Euroscan study. Proc Am Soc Clin Oncol 1999; 18:464.

131. Papadimitrakopoulou VA, Shin DM, Hong WK. Chemoprevention of head and neck cancer. In: Harrison LB, Sessions RB, Hong WK, editors. Head and neck cancer: a multidisciplinary approach. Philadelphia: Lippincott-Raven Publishers; 1999. p. 49–75.

132. Omenn GS, Goodman GE, Thornquist MD, et al. Risk factors for lung cancer and for intervention effects in CARET, the beta-carotene and retinol efficacy trial. J Natl Cancer Inst 1996;88:1550–9.

133. Albanes D, Heinonen OP, Taylor PR, et al. α-Tocopherol and β-carotene supplements and lung cancer incidence in the Alpha-Tocopherol, Beta-Carotene Cancer Prevention study: effects of base-line characteristics and study compliance. J Natl Cancer Inst 1996;88:1560–70.

134. Spiro RH, Koss LG, Hajdu SI, et al. Tumors of minor salivary gland origin: a clinicopathologic study of 492 cases. Cancer 1973;31:117–30.

135. Spiro R, Spiro J. Cancer of the salivary glands. In: Meyers E, Suen J, editors. Cancer of the head and neck. 2nd ed. New York: Churchill Livingstone; 1984. p. 644–99.

136. Suen J, Johns M. Chemotherapy for salivary gland cancer. Laryngoscope 1982;92:235–9.

137. Tannock IF, Sutherland DJ. Chemotherapy for adenocystic carcinoma. Cancer 1980;46:452–4.

138. Schramm V Jr, Srodes C, Myers C. Cisplatin therapy for adenoid cystic carcinoma. Arch Otolaryngol 1981;107:739–41.

139. Licitra L, Marchini S, Spinazze S, et al. Cisplatin in advanced salivary gland carcinoma. A phase II study of 25 patients. Cancer 1991;68:1874–7.

140. Jones AS, Phillips DE, Cook JA, Helliwell TR. A randomized phase II trial of epirubicin and 5-fluorouracil versus cisplatinum in the palliation of advanced and recurrent malignant tumour of the salivary glands. Br J Cancer 1993;37:112–4.

141. Airoldi M, Brando V, Giordano C, et al. Chemotherapy for recurrent salivary gland malignancies: experience of the ENT Department of Turin University. ORL J Otorhinolaryngol Relat Spec 1994;56:105–11.

142. Rentscheler R, Burgess MA, Byers R. Chemotherapy for malignant salivary gland neoplasms: a 25-year review of M.D. Anderson Hospital experience. Cancer 1977;40:619–24.

143. Triozzi PL, Brantley A, Fisher S, et al. 5-fluourouracil, cyclophosphamide, and vincristine for adenoid cystic carcinoma of the head and neck. Cancer 1987;59:887–90.

144. Posner MR, Ervin TJ, Weichselbaum RR, Fabian RL. Chemotherapy of advanced salivary gland neoplasms. Cancer 1982;50:2261–4.

145. Venook AP, Tseng A, Meyers FJ, Silverberg I. Cisplatin, doxorubicin, and 5-fluorouracil chemotherapy for salivary gland malignancies: a pilot study of the Northern California Oncology Group. J Clin Oncol 1987;5:951–5.

146. Dimery IW, Legha SS, Shirinian M, Hong WK. Fluorouracil, doxorubicin, cyclophosphamide, and cisplatin combination chemotherapy in advanced or recurrent salivary gland carcinoma. J Clin Oncol 1990;8:1056–62.

147. National Comprehensive Cancer Network guidelines. Oncology. In press. 2000.

148. Gottlieb JA, Hill CS Jr. Chemotherapy of thyroid cancer with adriamycin. Experience with 30 patients. N Engl J Med 1974;290:193–7.

149. Haugen BR. Management of the patient with progressive radioiodine non-responsive disease. Semin Surg Oncol 1999;16:34–41.

150. Hoskin PJ, Harmer C. Chemotherapy for thyroid cancer. Radiother Oncol 1987;10:187–94.

151. Kim JH, Leeper RD. Treatment of locally advanced thyroid carcinoma with combination doxorubicin and radiation therapy. Cancer 1987;60:2372–5.

152. Tennwall J, Lundell G, Hallquist A, Wahlberg P. Combined doxorubicin, hyperfractionated radiotherapy, surgery in anaplastic thyroid carcinoma: report on two protocols. Cancer 1994;74:1348–54.

153. Börner AR, Simon D, Müller-Gärtner HW. Isotretinoin in metastatic thyroid cancer. Ann Int Med 1997;127:246.

154. Shimaoka K, Schoenfeld DA, DeWys WD, Creech RH. Randomized trial of doxorubicin versus doxorubicin plus cisplatin with advanced thyroid carcinoma. Cancer 1985; 56:2155–60.

155. Schlumberger M, Abdelmoumene N, Deslisle NJ, the Groupe d'Études des Tumeurs a Calcitonine (GETC). Treatment for advanced medullary thyroid cancer with an alternating combination of 5-FU-streptozocin and 5 FU-dacarbazine. Brit J Cancer 1995;71:363–5.

156. Wu LT, Averbuch SD, Ball DW, et al. Treatment of advanced medullary thyroid carcinoma with a combination of cyclophosphamide, vincristine, and dacarbazine. Cancer 1994;73:432–6.

157. Vitale G, Tagliaferri P, Caraglia M, et al. Slow release lanreotide in combination with interferon-alpha2b in the treatment of symptomatic advanced thyroid carcinoma. J Clin Endocrinol Metab 2000;85:983–8.

158. Lupoli G, Cascone E, Arlotta F, et al. Treatment of advanced medullary thyroid carcinoma with a combination of recombinant interferon alpha-2b and octreotide. Cancer 1995;78:1114–8.

23

Rehabilitation and Quality of Life Assessment in Head and Neck Cancer

BHUVANESH SINGH, MD

In 1947, the World Health Organization (WHO) expanded its definition of health beyond the "absence of disease and infirmity," to include the "state of physical, mental, and social being." This milestone change in connotation elevated the study of health-related quality of life to an accepted endpoint for clinical studies and promulgated investigator interest.[1,2] Reflecting its increased use in medical studies, quality of life was introduced as a category in the Index Medicus in 1966.[1] Since then, the number of health-related quality of life publications had grown exponentially in the medical literature (Figure 23–1).

Of all disease states, the role of quality of life (QOL) assessment is most persuasively essential in patients with cancer. Stressing this importance, the National Institutes of Health and the Food and Drug Administration implemented several initiatives to encourage the more routine inclusion of the QOL assessment in oncology trials. As a result, the number of quality of life related studies in oncology burgeoned in the medical literature (see Figure 23–1). In sequence, QOL also became important in the management of head and neck cancer (HNC), particularly given the multitude of QOL-associated problems and the absence of survival differences between therapeutic modalities used in the treatment of these patients.[3–5] The comment made by Hays Martin in the 1940s remains valid today: "In deciding a method of treatment we should not, in our eagerness to achieve cure, lightly disregard the crippling that may result from our surgical endeavors."[3–5]

In conformity with this statement, studies have shown that patients are willing to sacrifice survival in favor of QOL issues.[6] List and colleagues have shown that in order of preference, patients with head and neck cancer rank being cured first, followed by living as long as possible, having no pain, being able to swallow, and having a normal amount of energy at the top end of their desired outcomes from cancer treatment.[7] This chapter presents an overview of QOL assessment in patients with HNC and reviews its impact on treatment, rehabilitation, and support policies in head and neck cancer management.

Definition of Quality of Life

Since its inception, assessment of QOL has remained controversial, mainly due to the ambiguity in its definition and the difficulties with the objective assessment of a subjective phenomenon. The variability in the concept of QOL can be seen by several different definitions published in the literature. Calman defined quality of life as the gap between the patient's expectations and achievements.[8] Spitzer, on the other hand, suggested that the measurement of quality of life should be restricted to the assessment of a series of characteristics among individuals that are sick.[2] Schipper and colleagues reported that quality of life represented the functional effect of an illness and its therapy on a patient, as perceived by that individual. Ware concluded that quality of life should measure both health and the full spectrum of health

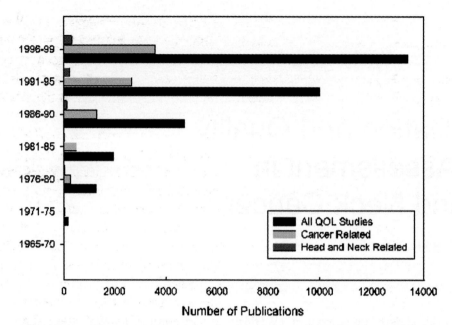

Figure 23–1.   Quality of life publications by year. Searches performed using the following terms: "quality of life" (MeSH term or Text word) and crossed with year of publication and "cancer OR neoplasms" (MeSH term or Text word) or "head and neck neoplasms" (MeSH term or Text word).

states ranging from disease to well-being.[9b] Torrance suggested that quality of life is measured at each point in time between birth and death, suggesting that this is an all-inclusive concept that incorporates all factors that affect the individual.[10] Kaplan and colleagues limit their assessment of health-related quality of life to three functions, namely: mobility, physical activity, and social activity.[11] This wide variation in definitions is reflected in the diversity of assessments provided by available quality of life instruments. Clearly, given the differences in the evaluation target, the choice of QOL instruments depends on the desired assessments.

Quality of Life Instruments

As the science of QOL assessment has matured, standardized testing has been implemented to validate QOL instruments, centered on establishing reliability, validity, and normative data.[1] Reliability can best be defined as the usability of a particular instrument, which can be divided into four concepts: namely test-retest reliability, alternate-form reliability, internal consistency, and interobserver reliability. Test-retest reliability measures the stability of the test over time. Typically, the same test is given to

a group of individuals twice, with an intervening period of time. In order for the quality of life measures to meet the requirements for test-retest reliability, there should be minimal change in the score obtained between the two measurements in a stable population. Alternate-form reliability is the comparison of the test instrument with an established quality of life measure. Internal consistency is a concept applied to quality of life instruments that are aiming to measure the same characteristics. This is a test of correlation among individual items contained in the instrument to determine the extent to which each instrument correlates with the total score. The last form of reliability, interobserver reliability, is based on the correlation of the use of an instrument by two different observers of the same individual.

Validity is a measure of the instrument's stability to assess the characteristics it aims to assess. Although reliability is necessary to determine its validity of a QOL measure, it is inadequate for establishing validity independently. Validity can be assessed in several ways. Face-validity is not truly a technical form of validity assessment, and refers to the integrity of the instrument as judged by the experimenter. Social validity is the assessment of whether the information measured by an instrument is what the researcher intends. Content validity is a measure of the completeness of the instrument in assessing its desired endpoints. Criteria grid validity is associated with the empirical relationship between a measure and the reliable criteria for comparison. Construct-validity refers to the inclusion of a group of related behaviors to assess a single psychosocial construct. Finally, sensitivity to change refers to the ability of a measure to identify changes occurring in the given population.

Instrument norms are a standard for comparison for QOL instruments. When good normative data is established, instruments can be used to compare individuals to a reference group. Norms should be based on a representative population of sufficient sample size. The normative data should be broken down into subcategories, such as age and gender. Finally, normative data should be available in the form of percentiles and standard scores.

Even with the significant advances and statistical scrutiny applied to QOL assessment, the complexity of studying QOL still results in inconsistencies in reporting. Gill and Feinstein confirmed this in a study of representative QOL publications in the medical literature. Their analysis found several flaws, including that investigators conceptually defined quality of life in only 11 of the 75 articles reviewed (15%), identified the target domain in only 47 percent, gave reasons for selecting the chosen quality of life instrument in only 35 percent, and aggregated their results into a composite QOL score

in only 38 percent of the eligible articles. These authors concluded that since QOL is a unique personal perception, most measurements in the medical literature seem to aim at the wrong target; thus they made several specific recommendations to improve QOL assessment. In addition to the issue identified by Gil and Feinstien, HNC-QOL studies have also been plagued by other recurrent problems, including cross-sectional analyses, limited sample size, inclusion of a diversity of tumor types, and a lack of uniformity in reporting.[12] However, as experience with QOL measures increases, newer studies on HNC promise to deliver significant and usable information, allowing their direct clinical application.

Quality of life measures can be grouped into three different categories, namely general measures, disease-specific measures, and the use of a battery of integrated instruments. The general measures of QOL are designed for employment independent of the type of disease, treatment, or treatment interventions that are provided. The use of general instruments allows a QOL ranking that is comparable across disease states. Disease-specific measures focus their attention on the assessment of responsiveness to a particular treatment or course of a specific disease process. Table 23–1 reviews some of the most commonly used general measures for the assessment of quality of life, and Table 23–2 shows the available measures for the assessment of head and neck cancer-specific quality of life.

Table 23–1. SELECTED GENERAL QUALITY OF LIFE INSTRUMENTS			
Measure	No. of Items	Reliability/ Validity	Comments
Medical Outcomes Study Short Form 36 (MOS-SF-36)	36	Yes	A self-administered assessment that requires 10 minutes to complete. This is not a cancer-specific measure
Sickness Impact Profile	136	Yes	Designed for use as a self-administered or interviewer-administered assessment that requires 30 minutes to complete. This is not a cancer-specific measure
Nottingham Health Profile (NHP)	45	Yes	A general QOL tool that is well validated but is not a cancer-specific measure. It requires 10 minutes to complete
Functional Living Index-Cancer (FLIC)	22	Yes	A general measure for patients with cancer that has sub-scales, and requires 10 minutes to complete
European Organization for Research and Treatment of Cancer Quality of Life Questionnaire (EORTC-QLQ-C30)	30	Yes	A well validated general instrument for use in cancer populations. Has a sub-scale for head and neck cancer. Requires 30 minutes to complete
Functional Assessment of Cancer Therapy (FACT)	28	Yes	Well validated measure with a sub-scale for head and neck cancer. Requires 10 minutes to complete

Table 23–2. HEAD AND NECK-SPECIFIC QUALITY OF LIFE INSTRUMENTS—HEAD AND NECK			
Measure	**No. of Items**	**Reliability/ Validity**	**Comments**
University of Washington Quality of Life Head and Neck (UW-QOL)	9	Yes	Easy to use, completed in less than 5 minutes, with excellent sensitivity in patients with head and neck cancer. A revised version has been published recently
Head and Neck Performance Status Scale	3 sub-scales	Yes	Designed as a clinician-rated survey, but has been used as a self-administered questionnaire
Head and Neck Survey	11	Yes	Formulated by an expert panel with the goal of assessing unique dimensions of head and neck-specific health
EORTC-QLQ-C30—Head and Neck Module	21	Yes	Initially developed on radiation-treated patients. Designed for use in combination with the well-validated EORTC-QLQ-C30
Functional Assessment of Cancer Therapy (FACT)—Head and Neck Module	11	No	Usually in combination with the FACT-G measure (28 items), which is well validated
Functional Status in Head and Neck Cancer—Self Report (FSH&N-SR)	15	Yes	Assesses symptomatic and functional outcome in patients treated for head and neck cancer
Head and Neck Quality of Life Questionnaire	20	Yes	Includes components of 2 previously validated measures within a new instrument
McMaster University Head and Neck Radiotherapy Questionnaire	22	Yes	Designed for assessment of acute radiation toxicity
Quality of Life—Radiation Therapy Instrument—Head and Neck Module	14	Yes	Designed for use in patients undergoing radiation treatment for head and neck neoplasms. Validated in a single small-scale study
Mayo Clinic Post-laryngectomy Questionnaire	48	No	Only used in a single study of surgical patients at the Mayo Clinic. Multiple items may make it comprehensive but cumbersome to use
Linear Analog Self-Assessment Scale for Voice Quality (LASA)	16	No	Designed for voice assessment after treatment for larynx cancer

General measures are well validated for use in the assessment of quality of life by their widespread use. In contrast, the head and neck cancer-specific measures are relatively new and therefore have not been thoroughly investigated. However, given that studies have shown a better correlation with head and neck-related domains when compared to general measures, it is evident that HNC-specific instruments do have some advantages over general measures.[13] The last approach for QOL analysis surmounts the dilemma over selection of QOL measures, by the use of a battery of instruments. This allows a broad-based assessment of QOL, which can include both general and disease-specific measures. Nonetheless, there are associated shortcomings in the required time, resources, and patient compliance with the use of this approach, resulting from the increased number of items.

Given the diversity and divergent information potentially yielded, the selection of QOL instruments is of paramount importance in QOL analysis.

There is no single ideal QOL instrument, but rather instruments that function better in specific scenarios. Selection of a non-validated instrument, without good normalized data, will yield information of limited value. Conversely, the selection of an established instrument that is too cumbersome for routine use also limits the acquired data quality. The main factors impacting on the selection of a QOL instrument include: the intended analytic endpoints, the method of administration, feasibility of completing the analysis, and the usability of the data obtained. In addition, many instruments are now available for QOL assessment in patients with head and neck cancer (see Table 23–1). With respect to HNC-specific measures, most instruments are designed for global use in all HNC patients, while others are designed for treatment-specific analyses. Algorithms and checklists for the selection of an appropriate QOL instrument for an intended study are available, and are based on the evaluation of a study's needs and the availability of resources.[1]

QUALITY OF LIFE ASSESSMENT IN HEAD AND NECK CANCER

The limitations in QOL assessment in HNC, detailed previously, confound the usefulness of the derived information. Nonetheless, several themes are recurrent in QOL studies and have resulted in changes in therapeutic and rehabilitative interventions.[4,5,13–18] Perhaps the most significant contribution of these studies has been a change in the dictum of "cure at all costs," to incorporate the impact of treatment interventions on patient functioning. In this regard, it is important to understand that the physician's perception of QOL is often quite different from that of the patient, as confirmed in analytic studies. In one study assessing QOL concerns in 20 laryngectomy patients and 20 health care professionals, the patients' main concerns were with the physical consequences of surgery and interference with social activities, while physicians primarily focused on communication, and self-image and self-esteem problems.[19] Accordingly, QOL assessment must be patient-based to more accurately direct methods for outcome quantification and improvement.

Given the limitations in QOL assessment in the literature, the following section includes selected representative data—extracted from HNC-QOL, functional, and rehabilitative studies—presented to provide perspective and highlight important aspects of the impact of QOL analysis on the management of HNC.

Global Quality of Life Assessment

Global quality of life assessments form a basis for QOL comparisons between disease states and to normative data. These studies have shown that the relative impact of HNC and its treatment on QOL is more significant than other cancers. Terrell and colleagues looked at 397 patients with HNC using the SF-36 in combination with disease-specific measures.[18,20] They found that the QOL of patients with HNC was significantly poorer than the Medical Outcomes Study Group's results for similar age patients. A study by Gritz and colleagues prospectively assessed QOL in 105 previously untreated patients using PSS-HNC, Profile of Mood States, and Cancer Rehabilitation Evaluation System-Short Form.[21] They noted that the QOL of patients treated for HNC was poorer than for lung or colon cancer. The QOL for patients with active head and neck cancer is poorer than normative data from male cancer patients, male non-prostate cancer patients and female breast cancer patients.[21]

Global assessments show that the perception of overall quality of life in patients with HNC is affected by several factors, including the mode and duration of treatment. Continuous surveillance of patient QOL is therefore required. Gritz noted that QOL-HNC changed significantly in the first 12 months after treatment of head and neck cancer.[21] Although most domains improved with time, domains of marital and sexual functioning showed progressive declines. These authors also showed that patients treated with primary radiation therapy had declines in QOL with time.[21] A study by Rogers and colleagues showed similar results, with return to pretreatment QOL scores occurring by 12 months using the UW-QOL questionnaire.[22] Huguenin and colleagues, using the EORTC QLQ-C30 and the Head and Neck module, showed that QOL in patients receiving radiation treatment was influenced by the location of the lesion, with nasopharyngeal cancer patients having the worst outcome due to increased target volume.[23]

Speech and Swallowing

The impact of surgery on speech and swallowing functions are logical, however, these disabilities also extend to patients receiving radiation treatment, with or without chemotherapy. Studies have shown that resections within the oral cavity are mainly associated with problems in bolus preparation and oral transit; oropharyngeal resections, on the other hand, result in impairment of the pharyngeal phase of swallowing in addition to the oral phase. Partial resection of the larynx, especially the supraglottis, disrupts the pharyngeal phase and also increases the risk of aspiration.[24,25] Many swallowing maneuvers have been developed to augment swallowing function in these patients.[24,26–28] In addition, changes in surgical practice to include free tissue transfer and sensory innervation show promise for improving outcome. In a study by Wilson and colleagues, patients reconstructed with rigid fixation after hemimandibulectomy had better scores in eating ability and overall quality of life, in addition to physical appearance.[29]

Functional assessment has confirmed the deleterious impact of radiation on speech and swallowing, showing reduction in oral and pharyngeal efficiency and motility.[30] In Epstein's study utilizing EORTC-QLQ-C30 with an oral symptom and function scale for the assessment of 100 patients treated with radiation therapy for HNC, 63 percent of patients had complaints of dysphagia and 51 percent had difficulties relating to speech.[31]

The presence of functional disorders in speech and swallowing has a profound impact on QOL. A study by List and colleagues showed that only 33 percent of patients achieved a perfect score for normalcy of diet and 60 percent for eating in public in a cross-sectional study of 181 patients undergoing treatment for head and neck cancer.[32] These authors also reported that only 55 percent of patients have a perfect score for comprehensibility of speech. In another study, List and colleagues longitudinally assessed QOL in 64 patients undergoing concomitant chemoradiation treatment for HNC using FACT-HN, PSS-HN, and the McMaster University Head and Neck Radiotherapy Questionnaire.[33] They found significant alterations in speech and swallowing function that showed some patients improved over 12 months, but residual deficits remained in a significant number of cases. However, they did not find a direct relationship between function and QOL outcome.[34]

Perhaps speech and swallowing issues are most pertinent in patients with laryngeal cancer. In the absence of outcome differences, studies showing improved speech outcome in patients with early (T1/T2) larynx cancers have shifted the treatment paradigm in favor of radiation therapy. Interestingly, in a review of five studies directed at the assessment of voice quality in radiation versus surgical treatment, three showed no clear advantage in voice quality. This reflects the deleterious impact of radiation treatment on voice quality. Stoicheff and colleagues showed, in 223 patients treated with radiation, that 83 percent were judged to be normal subjectively, yet 80 percent of patients self-reported voice difficulties, ranging from voice fatigue and reduced volume to lack of clarity.[35] Functionally, the negative effect of radiation on voice can be correlated to decreased phonatory time and frequency range, increased jitter and shimmer, and diminished or absent mucosal waves in patients undergoing radiation treatment for T1/T2 glottic cancer.[36]

In patients with advanced HNC, especially larynx and hypopharynx cancers, organ preservation strategies are as effective as laryngectomy-based treatment with respect to survival.[37] However, larynx preservation is achieved in up to 64 percent of cases in the organ preservation arm. This information has led to increased use of chemoradiation treatment in patients with advanced cancers. Interesting accumulating studies have shown a lack of correlation between speech preservation and overall QOL. A study by De Santo and colleagues on 111 patients with total laryngectomy, 38 with near-total laryngectomy, and 23 with partial laryngectomy, using the Psychological Adjustment to Illness Scale (PAIS) and the Mayo Clinic Post-laryngectomy Questionnaire, showed that QOL and speech function are independent, and that satisfactory QOL can be achieved independent of altered speech.[38] In another study, looking at 46 of 65 survivors from the Veterans Affairs (VA) Laryngeal Cancer Study Group No. 268, Terrell and colleagues showed that QOL was superior in patients in the organ preservation arm, mainly due to improved freedom from pain, greater emotional well-being, and lower levels of depression, rather than improved speech outcomes.[39] This is reflective of the lack of significant differences in technician-assessed speech intelligibility scores in 24-month survivors. This was judged to be acceptable in 96 percent of the organ preservation group, 91 percent of the chemoradiation group, and 85 percent for the total laryngectomy group from the VA study population.[40] Similarly, a report by Deleyiannis and colleagues failed to correlate functional disability with QOL scores in patients undergoing laryngectomy.[41] Finizia and colleagues, in a case-matched study, showed that although patients treated with radiation for larynx cancer fared better functionally, QOL in this group was not dissimilar from laryngectomized patients.[42] These studies indirectly reflect the negative impact of chemoradiation treatment on speech function, the positive effects of speech rehabilitation in patients with total laryngectomy, and a limited impact of functional outcome on QOL.

Recovery and rehabilitation of post-treatment speech and swallowing is dependent on several factors, including the stage of disease, the extent of surgery, the technique and dose of radiation, and use of rehabilitative measures.[31,43] Several techniques are available for swallowing rehabilitation, of which time post-treatment and adaptation often are the most valuable. In contrast, direct intervention with early speech therapy interaction, electro-larynx utilization, training in esophageal speech, and most importantly tracheoesophageal prosthesis placement has had significant impact on communication capability of patients with head and neck cancer. Urken and colleagues showed that the use of free tissue transfer in oromandibular reconstruction yielded superior functional outcome compared with similar patients who did not have bony mandibular reconstruction.[44] The use of an oral prosthesis improves both speech and swallowing in the patient completing treatment for HNC. Placement of these prostheses correlates with improved eating, esthetic satisfaction, reduced pain, and improved physical and mental well-being.[45] The role of the prosthodontist in improvement of swallowing function is multifold, and can help compensate for deficits in the hard and soft palate, tongue, and tongue base.[46]

Olfaction and Gustation

Nasal airflow and intact sensory innervation are essential for normal olfaction and gustation. All of the modalities used in the treatment of patients with HNC have a potential to adversely impact olfaction and gustation. Surgery has direct effects in terms of sacrifice of sensory nerves for olfaction (craniofacial resection) and taste (lingual nerve resection), resection of taste organs and occlusion of nasal airway. It can also have indirect effects, as in laryngectomy patients who no longer have air passing through the nasal cavity. Van Dam and colleagues showed the presence of olfactory dysfunction in two-thirds of 65 patients undergoing laryngectomy.[47] They noted that patients who were able to smell actively employed several different methods, most notably the use of facial muscles. Moreover, gustatory dysfunction in these patients was directly correlated to olfactory function.

A study by Epstein and colleagues, using the European Organization for Research and Treatment of Cancer (EORTC) Quality of Life (QLQ)–C30 index with an added oral symptom and function scale, identified complaints of changes in taste in 75 percent of 65 patients treated with radiation therapy for oropharyngeal cancer.[31] Several agents, such as amifostine and pilocarpine, have been employed in attempts to limit radiation therapy-induced xerostomia and gustatory dysfunction. A study by Buntzel and colleagues showed a 38 percent reduction in severe xerostomia (grade 2) and a 64 percent reduction in loss of taste with the addition of amifostine.[48] Another study by Zimmerman and colleagues reported similar results with the use of pilocarpine.[49] Johnson and colleagues showed that the addition of pilocarpine was beneficial in improving post-radiation oral dryness in 44 percent of cases, oral discomfort in 31 percent, and speaking ability in 33 percent.[50] In a study assessing taste, Ripamonti and colleagues showed the presence of gustatory dysfunction in 100 percent of patients receiving radiation, the severity and recovery of which was improved by the use of zinc sulfate during treatment.[51]

Pain

Pain is a common complaint among patients with cancer, especially patients with head and neck cancer. Pain can be acute, as a consequence of surgery, or chronic, as in shoulder disability secondary to accessory nerve sacrifice (Figure 23–2).[52,53] Pfister and colleagues found a 31 percent prevalence of frequent or persistent pain in a cross-sectional analysis of 194 treated patients, 67 percent of which was moderate or great in intensity. Pain scores tend to improve with time in this population, but a small but significant percentage have persistent, often disabling pain. A study by Chaplin and Morton showed that the presence of pain diminished from 48 percent at diagnosis to 26 percent after treatment. Interestingly the prevalence of shoulder pain increased with time.[54]

The precise cause of pain and its perception cannot be identified in all cases. A study by Chua and colleagues showed that pain in HNC patients is related to cancer recurrence (35%), treatment sequelae (30%), multiple etiologies (25%), and unrelated causes (10%).[55] The most common pain type is mixed nociceptive and neuropathic (37.5%), but nociceptive pain alone (32.5%), myofacial (13%), neuropathic (7.5%) and other mixed types of pain (7.5%) also occur. The character and severity of pain is influenced by the location of the cancer, type of treatment and time after treatment.[56]

Studies have shown a direct correlation between the presence of pain and lower quality of life in patients with head and neck cancer, with the most significant impact on general well-being and psychosocial distress.[54] Accordingly, QOL improvements can be impacted by the use of effective pain control schema. Cancer pain management paradigms have been established to allow a directed approach to pain control. The use of the WHO analgesic ladder is highly successful in controlling HNC-associated pain, with all but two patients experiencing relief in a study of 62 consecutive terminal HNC patients.[57] Finally, integral to pharmacologic interventions is the use of adjunctive measures, such as intervention for depression, and physical therapy in patients with shoulder disability.

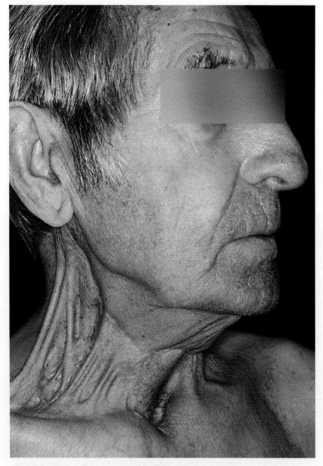

Figure 23–2. The deformity following radical neck dissection.

Psychosocial Impact

The psychosocial impact of a cancer diagnosis and its treatment often supersede the physical consequences of treatment. Psychosocial issues can be addressed via several different domains including emotional well-being, role functioning, social relations, sexuality and assessment of anxiety or stress. Affected patients have increased psychosocial stressors with resultant increases in depression and suicides.[58] One study found that cancer patients accounted for one-quarter of all hospital-based suicides, of which 19 percent had head and neck cancers.[59]

Coping methods are important in overcoming the psychologic impact of cancer. In addition, evidence from prospective studies suggests that coping methods have a significant impact on cancer outcome. A classic article, prospectively examining the outcome of patients with early-stage breast cancer, showed that patients with a "fighting spirit" or denial type of coping approach had better survival outcomes than those exhibiting stoicism or helplessness. These results have been echoed in studies of melanoma patients as well. A recent study of patients with HNC showed that patients with significant psychosocial complaints prior to treatment did better than stoic patients who did not express their negative feelings.[60] Often coping can be enhanced by the presence of strong social support groups, as well as through health care worker involvement. De Boer and colleagues showed a positive correlation between rehabilitation outcomes and open discussion of illness in the family, social support from others, and adequate information from specialists.[60,61] Hammerlid and colleagues confirmed the usefulness of support groups and short-term psycho-educational programs for improving psychosocial outcome and QOL in HNC patients.[62]

Taken as a whole, assaults on psychosocial functioning in patients with HNC are multifactorial, but can be grouped into immediate and delayed concerns. In the immediate period, the overriding issues in these patients are fear of the unknown and the apprehension of the physical, social, and functional effects of cancer treatment. Many of these concerns can be addressed by detailed explanation of the anticipated course of events, reassurance, and establishment of a support network. In the long-term, work situation, functional status, communication concerns, issues of intimacy, sexuality, self-image and identity become more relevant. One study showed that over 45 percent of patients report self-image problems after treatment for HNC.[63] Often patients concerned about image and appearance isolate themselves from family, friends and support groups.[60,61] In addition, a decrease in or lack of sexual contact are reported by 8 to 48 percent of patients treated for HNC.[61,64]

Several methods can be employed to improve psychosocial outcomes; it is paramount that these issues be addressed with the patient and their importance reinforced. The use of educational programs, exposure to cancer survivors, discussions with appropriate health care professionals such as speech therapists prior to initiating treatment, and the establishment of clear lines of communication are basic to the management of all cancer patients. Studies have confirmed that patients who are informed about their condition and its treatment have better adjustment in interpersonal relationships and intimacy with family.[60,61] Consultation and treatment with an appropriate psychiatric professional is indicated in many situations. Often the alleviation of treatment sequelae has a significant impact on psychosocial outcomes. Studies from the Netherlands Cancer Institute show that when physical symptoms of treatment are ameliorated, such as correction of excess sputum production, coughing, and the need for frequent forced expectoration in laryngectomy patients, psychological stress is reduced, social contacts are increased, and overall QOL is improved. Similarly, better psychosocial outcome can be achieved by addressing cosmetic concerns. For example, even though there is no functional benefit, better psychosocial results are reported for patients undergoing mandible resection if mandibular reconstruction with free tissue transfer is performed.

CONCLUSION

Although still in its infancy, quality of life assessment has already impacted on our approach to the management of patients with head and neck cancer. With improved methodology, validation of head and neck cancer-specific instruments, and the completion of phase III trials where it is a primary endpoint, the impact of QOL assessment on the management of head and neck cancer will likely expand. At present, lessons learned from available QOL data support the use of specific treatments, patient education programs, rehabilitative efforts, and indicate a need for diligence in identifying and addressing QOL issues.

REFERENCES

1. McSweeny AJ, Creer TL. Health-related quality-of-life assessment in medical care. Dis Mon 1995;41(1):1–71.
2. Spitzer WO. State of science 1986: quality of life and functional status as target variables for research. J Chronic Dis 1987;40(6):465–71.
3. Moore GJ. Quality of life after radiation therapy for base of tongue cancer. Oncology (Huntingt) 1996;10(11):1643–8.
4. Morton RP. Evolution of quality of life assessment in head and neck cancer. J Laryngol Otol 1995;109(11):1029–35.
5. Morton RP, Witterick IJ. Rationale and development of a quality-of-life instrument for head-and-neck cancer patients. Am J Otolaryngol 1995;16(5):284–93.
6. McNeil BJ, Weichselbaum R, Pauker SG. Speech and survival: tradeoffs between quality and quantity of life in laryngeal cancer. N Engl J Med 1981;305(17):982–7.
7. List MA, Stracks J, Colangelo L, et al. How do head and neck cancer patients prioritize treatment outcomes before initiating treatment? J Clin Oncol 2000;18(4):877–84.
8. Calman KC. Quality of life in cancer patients—an hypothesis. J Med Ethics 1984;10(3):124–7.
9a. Schipper H, Clinch J, Powell V. Definitions and conceptual issues. In: Spilker B, ed. Quality of life assessments in clinical trials. New York: Raven, 1990:11–24.
9b. Ware JE Jr. Standards for validating health measures: definition and content. J Chronic Dis 1987;40(6):473–80.
10. Torrance GW. Utility approach to measuring health-related quality of life. J Chronic Dis 1987;40(6):593–603.
11. Kaplan RM, Anderson JP, Wu AW, et al. The Quality of Well-being Scale. Applications in AIDS, cystic fibrosis, and arthritis. Med Care 1989;27(3 Suppl):27–43.
12. Gill TM, Feinstein AR. A critical appraisal of the quality of quality-of-life measurements. JAMA 1994;272(8):619–26.
13. Gliklich RE, Goldsmith TA, Funk GF. Are head and neck specific quality of life measures necessary? Head Neck 1997;19(6):474–80.
14. Allison PJ, Locker D, Wood-Dauphinee S, et al. Correlates of health-related quality of life in upper aerodigestive tract cancer patients. Qual Life Res 1998;7(8):713–22.
15. List MA, Ritter-Sterr CA, Baker TM, et al. Longitudinal assessment of quality of life in laryngeal cancer patients. Head Neck 1996;18(1):1–10.
16. Moore C. Quality of life. Laryngoscope 1978;88(1 Pt 2 Suppl 8):87–8.
17. Morton RP. Life-satisfaction in patients with head and neck cancer. Clin Otolaryngol 1995;20(6):499–503.
18. Terrell JE. Quality of life assessment in head and neck cancer patients. Hematol Oncol Clin North Am 1999;13(4):849–65.

19. Mohide EA, Archibald SD, Tew M, et al. Postlaryngectomy quality-of-life dimensions identified by patients and health care professionals. Am J Surg 1992;164(6): 619–22.

20. Terrell JE, Nanavati KA, Esclamado RM, et al. Head and neck cancer-specific quality of life: instrument validation. Arch Otolaryngol Head Neck Surg 1997;123(10):1125–32.

21. Gritz ER, Carmack CL, de Moor C, et al. First year after head and neck cancer: quality of life. J Clin Oncol 1999;17 (1):352–60.

22. Rogers SN, Lowe D, Brown JS, Vaughan ED. The University of Washington head and neck cancer measure as a predictor of outcome following primary surgery for oral cancer. Head Neck 1999;21(5):394–401.

23. Huguenin PU, Taussky D, Moe K, et al. Quality of life in patients cured from a carcinoma of the head and neck by radiotherapy: the importance of the target volume. Int J Radiat Oncol Biol Phys 1999;45(1):47–52.

24. Logemann JA. The role of the speech language pathologist in the management of dysphagia. Otolaryngol Clin North Am 1988;21(4):783–8.

25. Logemann JA, Bytell DE. Swallowing disorders in three types of head and neck surgical patients. Cancer 1979; 44(3):1095–105.

26. Rademaker AW, Logemann JA, Pauloski BR, et al. Recovery of postoperative swallowing in patients undergoing partial laryngectomy. Head Neck 1993;15(4):325–34.

27. Lazarus CL, Logemann JA, Rademaker AW, et al. Effects of bolus volume, viscosity, and repeated swallows in non-stroke subjects and stroke patients. Arch Phys Med Rehabil 1993;74(10):1066–70.

28. Pauloski BR, Logemann JA, Rademaker AW, et al. Speech and swallowing function after anterior tongue and floor of mouth resection with distal flap reconstruction. J Speech Lang Hear Res 1993;36(2):267–76.

29. Wilson KM, Rizk NM, Armstrong SL, Gluckman JL. Effects of hemimandibulectomy on quality of life. Laryngoscope 1998;108(10):1574–7.

30. Lazarus CL, Logemann JA, Pauloski BR, et al. Swallowing disorders in head and neck cancer patients treated with radiotherapy and adjuvant chemotherapy. Laryngoscope 1996;106(9 Pt 1):1157–66.

31. Epstein JB, Emerton S, Kolbinson DA, et al. Quality of life and oral function following radiotherapy for head and neck cancer. Head Neck 1999;21(1):1–11.

32. List MA, D'Antonio LL, Cella DF, et al. The Performance Status Scale for Head and Neck Cancer Patients and the Functional Assessment of Cancer Therapy-Head and Neck Scale. A study of utility and validity. Cancer 1996; 77(11):2294–301.

33. List MA, Mumby P, Haraf D, et al. Performance and quality of life outcome in patients completing concomitant chemoradiotherapy protocols for head and neck cancer. Qual Life Res 1997;6(3):274–84.

34. List MA, Siston A, Haraf D, et al. Quality of life and performance in advanced head and neck cancer patients on concomitant chemoradiotherapy: a prospective examination. J Clin Oncol 1999;17(3):1020–8.

35. Stoicheff ML. Voice following radiotherapy. Laryngoscope 1975;85(4):608–18.

36. Lehman JJ, Bless DM, Brandenburg JH. An objective assessment of voice production after radiation therapy for stage I squamous cell carcinoma of the glottis. Otolaryngol Head Neck Surg 1988;98(2):121–9.

37. Induction chemotherapy plus radiation compared with surgery plus radiation in patients with advanced laryngeal cancer. The Department of Veterans Affairs Laryngeal Cancer Study Group. N Engl J Med 1991;324(24):1685–90.

38. DeSanto LW, Olsen KD, Perry WC, et al. Quality of life after surgical treatment of cancer of the larynx. Ann Otol Rhinol Laryngol 1995;104(10 Pt 1):763–9.

39. Terrell JE, Fisher SG, Wolf GT. Long-term quality of life after treatment of laryngeal cancer. The Veterans Affairs Laryngeal Cancer Study Group. Arch Otolaryngol Head Neck Surg 1998;124(9):964–71.

40. Hillman RE, Walsh MJ, Wolf GT, et al. Functional outcomes following treatment for advanced laryngeal cancer. Part I—Voice preservation in advanced laryngeal cancer. Part II—Laryngectomy rehabilitation: the state of the art in the VA System. Research Speech-Language Pathologists. Department of Veterans Affairs Laryngeal Cancer Study Group. Ann Otol Rhinol Laryngol Suppl 1998;172:1–27.

41. Deleyiannis FW, Weymuller EA Jr, Coltrera MD, Futran N. Quality of life after laryngectomy: are functional disabilities important? Head Neck 1999;21(4):319–24.

42. Finizia C, Hammerlid E, Westin T, Lindstrom J. Quality of life and voice in patients with laryngeal carcinoma: a post-treatment comparison of laryngectomy (salvage surgery) versus radiotherapy. Laryngoscope 1998;108(10):1566–73.

43. De Graeff A, de Leeuw RJ, Ros WJ, et al. A prospective study on quality of life of laryngeal cancer patients treated with radiotherapy. Head Neck 1999;21(4):291–6.

44. Urken ML, Buchbinder D, Weinberg H, et al. Functional evaluation following microvascular oromandibular reconstruction of the oral cancer patient: a comparative study of reconstructed and nonreconstructed patients. Laryngoscope 1991;101(9):935–50.

45. Moroi HH, Okimoto K, Terada Y. The effect of an oral prosthesis on the quality of life for head and neck cancer patients. J Oral Rehabil 1999;26(4):265–73.

46. Hurst PS. The role of the prosthodontist in the correction of swallowing disorders. Otolaryngol Clin North Am 1988;21(4):771–81.

47. Van Dam FS, Hilgers FJ, Emsbroek G, et al. Deterioration of olfaction and gustation as a consequence of total laryngectomy. Laryngoscope 1999;109(7 Pt 1):1150–5.

48. Buntzel J, Kuttner K, Frohlich D, Glatzel M. Selective cytoprotection with amifostine in concurrent radiochemotherapy for head and neck cancer. Ann Oncol 1998;9(5):505–9.

49. Zimmerman RP, Mark RJ, Tran LM, Juillard GF. Concomitant pilocarpine during head and neck irradiation is associated with decreased post-treatment xerostomia. Int J Radiat Oncol Biol Phys 1997;37(3):571–5.

50. Johnson JT, Ferretti GA, Nethery WJ, et al. Oral pilocarpine for post-irradiation xerostomia in patients with head and neck cancer. N Engl J Med 1993;329(6):390–5.

51. Ripamonti C, Zecca E, Brunelli C, et al. A randomized, controlled clinical trial to evaluate the effects of zinc sulfate on cancer patients with taste alterations caused by head and neck irradiation. Cancer 1998;82(10):1938–45.

52. Remmler D, Byers R, Scheetz J, et al. A prospective study of shoulder disability resulting from radical and modified neck dissections. Head Neck Surg 1986;8(4):280–6.

53. Ewing M, Martin H. Disability following radical neck dissection. Cancer 1952;5:873–9.

54. Chaplin JM, Morton RP. A prospective, longitudinal study of pain in head and neck cancer patients. Head Neck 1999; 21(6):531–7.

55. Chua KS, Reddy SK, Lee MC, Patt RB. Pain and loss of function in head and neck cancer survivors. J Pain Symptom Manage 1999;18(3):193–202.

56. Keefe FJ, Manuel G, Brantley A, Crisson J. Pain in the head and neck cancer patient: changes over treatment. Head Neck Surg 1986;8(3):169–76.

57. Talmi YP, Waller A, Bercovici M, et al. Pain experienced by patients with terminal head and neck carcinoma. Cancer 1997;80(6):1117–23.

58. Davies AD, Davies C, Delpo MC. Depression and anxiety in patients undergoing diagnostic investigations for head and neck cancers. Br J Psychiatry 1986;149:491–3.

59. Ferrence RG, Johnson FG. Factors affecting reported rates of self-injury. Life Threat Behav 1974;4(1):54–66.

60. De Boer MF, Van den Borne B, Pruyn JF, et al. Psychosocial and physical correlates of survival and recurrence in patients with head and neck carcinoma: results of a 6-year longitudinal study. Cancer 1998;83(12):2567–79.

61. De Boer MF, McCormick LK, Pruyn JF, et al. Physical and psychosocial correlates of head and neck cancer: a review of the literature. Otolaryngol Head Neck Surg 1999;120 (3):427–36.

62. Hammerlid E, Persson LO, Sullivan M, Westin T. Quality-of-life effects of psychosocial intervention in patients with head and neck cancer. Otolaryngol Head Neck Surg 1999; 120(4):507–16.

63. Gamba A, Romano M, Grosso IM, et al. Psychosocial adjustment of patients surgically treated for head and neck cancer. Head Neck 1992;14(3):218–23.

64. Monga U, Tan G, Ostermann HJ, Monga TN. Sexuality in head and neck cancer patients. Arch Phys Med Rehabil 1997;78(3):298–304.

Index